S0-AHC-217

Dentistry,
Dental Practice,
and the
Community

The Resource Center

Property of
High-Tech Institute of Sacramento, CA
Library/Resource Center

Dentistry, Dental Practice, and the Community

5th Edition

Brian A. Burt, BDS, MPH, PhD

Program in Dental Public Health
School of Public Health
The University of Michigan
Ann Arbor, Michigan

Stephen A. Eklund, DDS, MHSA, DrPH

Program in Dental Public Health
School of Public Health
The University of Michigan
Ann Arbor, Michigan

with a chapter contributed by
Amid I. Ismail

W.B. SAUNDERS COMPANY
A Division of Harcourt Brace and Company
Philadelphia London Toronto Montreal Sydney Tokyo

W.B. SAUNDERS COMPANY
A Division of Harcourt Brace & Company

The Curtis Center
Independence Square West
Philadelphia, Pennsylvania 19106

Library of Congress Cataloging-in-Publication Data

Dentistry, dental practice, and the community / Brian A. Burt, Stephen A. Eklund; with a chapter contributed by Amid I. Ismail.—5th ed.

p.   cm.

Includes bibliographical references and index.

ISBN 0-7216-7309-0

1. Dental public health.   2. Dentistry—Practice.   I. Eklund, Stephen A.
II. Ismail, Amid I.   III. Title.   [DNLM: 1. Public Health Dentistry.
2. Preventive Dentistry.   WU 113B973d 1999]

RK52.B87 1999   617.6—dc21

DNLM/DLC   98–28551

Property of
High-Tech Institute of Sacramento, CA
Library/Resource Center

DENTISTRY, DENTAL PRACTICE, AND THE COMMUNITY   ISBN 0–7216–7309–0

Copyright © 1999, 1992, 1983, 1969, 1964 by W.B. Saunders Company.

All rights reserved. No part of this publication may be reproduced or transmitted in any form or by any means, electronic or mechanical, including photocopy, recording, or any information storage and retrieval system, without permission in writing from the publisher.

Printed in the United States of America.

Last digit is the print number: 9   8   7   6   5   4   3   2

To Lizzie and Sue

NOTICE

Dentistry is an ever-changing field. Standard safety precautions must be followed, but as new research and clinical experience broaden our knowledge, changes in treatment and drug therapy become necessary or appropriate. Readers are advised to check the product information currently provided by the manufacturer of each drug to be administered to verify the recommended dose, the method and duration of administration, and the contraindications. It is the responsibility of the treating physician, relying on experience and knowledge of the patient, to determine dosages and the best treatment for the patient. Neither the publisher nor the editor assumes any responsibility for any injury and/or damage to persons or property.

THE PUBLISHER

Preface to the Fifth Edition

The preface to the fourth edition of this book began with this statement: "Death and taxes notwithstanding, it has been said that change is the only constant in life." That is still true. Since the last edition of this book in 1992 the economy of the United States has rebounded in a way that few predicted at that time. As the 20th century draws to a close we have high employment, a buoyant stock market, and our leaders promising us a balanced national budget. This could be the introduction to a new era, or the chill winds from the collapsed Asian economies could still blow us away in this age of the interdependent global economy.

The purpose of this book is to present dentistry and dental practice against the backdrop of social events: economic, technological, and demographic trends, as well as the distribution of the oral diseases that dental professionals treat and prevent. The pace of change in these areas can be bewildering, and substantial rewriting of many parts of this book has thus been required. Since the 1992 edition came out we have seen an attempt to introduce a national health system under the name of "health care reform" get soundly rejected because of suspicions about "big government" and "socialized medicine." So, instead of having the United States' first comprehensive national health system, we have been engulfed by something called managed care, under which we have delegated important decisions on our health care to bottom-line money managers instead of government panels. Not everyone is convinced that we have got this one right, and further change is inevitable. It may manifest as constant tinkering with the system, or it could be a revolution in health care.

Our guiding principle in this fifth edition is that on all matters discussed we should lay out the facts and interpret them as we see them. We express our opinions, and leave the reader to develop his or her own views. We see health as a major factor in a higher quality of life rather than an end in itself. We have no doubt that good oral health significantly improves the quality of life, and that the constant improvement of the public's oral health is a worthy goal.

The lineage of this book can be traced from the landmark work of Pelton and Wisan's *Dentistry in Public Health*, first published in 1949, up to our fourth edition in 1992. We have now substantially revised and reorganized the material for this fifth edition. There are more chapters than before; some of the longer chapters in the fourth edition burst their boundaries and regrouped into several new ones. So we now have 29 chapters collated into five sections. Section I looks at the professions and the public they serve and deals with ethics, the public–private partnership, and health promotion. Section II deals with the structure and financing of dental practice, types of personnel, infection control and mercury safety, and an expanded section on keeping up with the dental literature. The chapter on Dental Care in Canada is contributed by Dr. Amid Ismail, formerly of Dalhousie University in Halifax and now at the University of Michigan. This chapter is not just for Canadian readers, for it illustrates many aspects of providing dental care. Section III is the nitty-gritty of oral epidemiology, from research designs and survey methods through to the various indexes used to measure oral disease, and Section IV looks at the distribution of these diseases in the population and the various risk factors associated with them. In conclusion, Section V deals with the prevention of oral diseases and conditions.

In matters of style, we favor liberal referencing. This gives readers a chance to pursue further the issues that interest them, and the references give the basis for our interpretation of the more contentious issues. Although most references reflect current work, we have retained a lot of older ones to illustrate how issues have developed over

time and to show the richness of the dental
literature. Landmark reports and our
historical development should never be
forgotten. We have continued our method of
dealing with the gender-specific personal
pronoun by making it feminine in the odd-
numbered chapters, masculine in the even-
numbered. The "her" of Chapter 1 thus
becomes the "his" of Chapter 2. In our
frequent use of the term *dental professionals*,
we include both dental hygienists and
dentists as colleagues working together.

Since our previous edition, there has
been a major revolution in how we find
information, for the Worldwide Web—just a
curiosity to most of us in 1992—has now
become a standard source of information.
There is a great deal of information in this
book that has come from various websites.
The depth and breadth of information to be
found in the websites of the Health Care
Financing Administration, Centers for
Disease Control and Prevention,
Occupational Safety and Health
Administration, and the American Dental
Association, to name just a few, is truly
breathtaking. Given that the Web is in a state
of rapid evolution, and because Web
addresses can change frequently, we have
not given specific Web addresses for our
data sources on the grounds that they could
be totally different by the time someone
reads this book. In fact, by the first decade
of the new millennium the whole concept of
the Worldwide Web could be fundamentally
changed. It's an exciting time for
developments in the world of information,
and no one can predict what even the near
future will hold.

Contrasts have to be made at times
between how things are done in the richer
parts of the world compared to the poorer.

We use the term *developed countries*, or
sometimes *industrialized* countries, to refer to
those nations such as the United States,
Canada, most European countries, Australia,
New Zealand, and Japan, which have
industrial and service-based economies, high
levels of literacy, a large middle class,
sophisticated transport systems, and mass
distribution of goods far from their points of
origin. The developing nations, by contrast,
are those in which those factors are just
beginning to be seen, or in which they do
not exist at all. In addition, there are many
nations which don't clearly fit either
category but lie somewhere between the
two. Without going into details of world
economics, we frequently use those
oversimplified categories of "developed"
and "developing" to illustate broad
differences.

We owe a debt of gratitude to those
who have helped us get this book out. In no
particular order, we want to thank our in-
house helpers Keith Heller, Monica Fisher,
and Woosung Sohn for data analysis and
general production assistance. Discussions
with Jim Beck helped clarify the concept of
risk, and Ralph Katz always has stimulating
thoughts on root caries. Joan McGowan and
Scott Tomar were very helpful in locating
material on tobacco issues. All these people
made our task a little easier, though we
emphasize that responsibility for every word
in this book lies with us, and with us alone.

So who knows what lies ahead in the
new millennium? We certainly don't pretend
to, other than to state the obvious: it will be
challenging and exciting times for dentistry.
To thrive and progress, dental professionals
require a mindset which permits them to
adapt to changing circumstances. We hope
that this book will help readers to develop
that mindset.

Brian A. Burt
Stephen A. Eklund

Contents

SECTION I
Dentistry and the Community

chapter 1
The Professions of Dentistry and Dental Hygiene 3

chapter 2
The Public Served by Dentistry 13

chapter 3
Ethics and Responsibility in Dental Care 27

chapter 4
The Practice of Dental Public Health 34

chapter 5
Promotion of Oral Health 43

SECTION II
Dental Practice

chapter 6
The Healthy Dental Practice: Infection Control and Mercury Safety 57

chapter 7
The Structure of Dental Practice 71

chapter 8
Financing Dental Care 89

chapter 9
Dental Personnel 115

chapter 10
Dental Care in Canada 134
   Amid I. Ismail

chapter 11
Reading the Dental Literature 150

SECTION III
The Methods of Oral Epidemiology

chapter 12
Research Designs in Epidemiology 159

chapter 13
The Measurement of Oral Disease 168

chapter 14
Measuring Dental Caries 178

chapter 15
Measuring Periodontal Diseases 185

chapter 16
Measuring Dental Fluorosis 191

chapter 17
Measuring Other Conditions in Oral Epidemiology 197

SECTION IV
The Distribution of Oral Diseases and Conditions

chapter 18
Tooth Loss 203

chapter 19
Dental Caries 212

chapter 20
Periodontal Diseases 237

chapter 21
Dental Fluorosis 259

chapter 22
Oral Cancer and Other Oral Conditions 267

SECTION V
Prevention of Oral Diseases in Public Health

chapter 23
Fluoride: Human Health and Caries Prevention 279

chapter 24
Fluoridation of Drinking Water 297

chapter 25
Other Uses of Fluoride in Caries Prevention 315

chapter 26
Fissure Sealants 334

chapter 27
Diet and Plaque Control 347

chapter 28
Prevention of Periodontal Diseases 358

chapter 29
Smokeless Tobacco, Oral Cancer, and Antitobacco Initiatives 371

Index 377

section I

Dentistry and the Community

1

The Professions of Dentistry and Dental Hygiene

What is a Profession? ◆ Historical Development ◆
The Professions of Dentistry and Dental Hygiene ◆
Dental Organizations in the United States: ADA, NDA,
HDA, FDI, ADHA ◆ Careers in Dentistry and Dental
Hygiene: Private Practice, Salaried Practice,
Academic Careers

Dental practice has existed in some form since the dawn of time, but it is only in comparatively recent years that its practitioners in the economically-developed nations have achieved the status of a profession. In most of the developing world, dental practice is still more of a craft. In countries with a moderate level of economic development, dentistry exhibits some aspects of a profession, but not all.

Webster's dictionary defines a *profession* as "a calling requiring specialized knowledge and often long and intensive academic preparation" and "the whole body of persons engaged in a calling." The definition of *professionalism* is "the conduct, aims, or qualities that characterize or mark a profession or professional person." These terse dictionary definitions, however, do not capture the essence of a profession or of professionalism: commitment to patient welfare, ethics, and other professional ideals are not included. The word *professional* can have subtleties of meaning: it can be the opposite of *amateur,* sometimes in a derogatory sense, or it can be the converse of *voluntary.* Nor are all aspects of professionalism necessarily high-minded or noble; admission to some professional groups can be based on self-perpetuation rather than public good, and aspects of "closed shop" practices have not been uncommon.[20]

Three models of professionalism have been described,[17] none of which by itself fully describes dentistry although collectively they may do so. The first is the *commercial model,* in which dental care is viewed as a commodity sold by the practitioner. The services are thus not based primarily on the client's needs, but rather on what the client is able or willing to buy. This rather crass view is distasteful to many, although there are aspects of it in dental practice. The second is the *guild model,* in which dental care is a privilege with the professional dominant in practitioner-patient relations. In the guild model, the professional is the repository of all knowledge and wisdom, the patient is a passive recipient, and the practitioner has an ethical trust to provide the best quality care. This model has probably been dominant in the United States, although it may be slowly merging with the third model, the *interactive model,* in which dental care is a partnership of equals. In this model, practitioner and patient jointly determine care provided through a combination of professional expertise and patient values.

What are the criteria that characterize a profession, and how can a profession be distinguished from, for example, a trade union? The first is the criterion given in the dictionary definition, a substantial body of knowledge, a corollory of which is the obligation to keep that knowledge up to date through continuing education. The second is self-regulation, a tradition whereby society delegates to professional groups the legal responsibility for determining who shall join them in serving the public, and for disciplining those members who do not meet the profession's requirements. A third, and perhaps the main distinguishing criterion of a profession, is a code of ethics, guidelines for professional conduct that are rooted in a moral imperative rather than in law or regulation (Chapter 3). A profession sets its own code of ethics and its own procedures for dealing with infringements.

A profession can then be defined as a calling with a body of specialized knowledge requiring intensive academic preparation to qualify for admission, the members of which act as a cohesive group in matters affecting their relationship to the public they serve. Taking the various criteria mentioned, a profession is distinguished by the following features:

- An existing body of knowledge that is constantly being expanded, updated, and archived in a literature record. The purpose is constant improvement of the quality of the profession's service to individuals and to the public.
- Academic preparation carried out in specialized institutions.
- The profession and its members accept a lifelong commitment to continuing education.
- Society awards it the privilege of self-regulation, which means determining the requirements for entering and remaining in the profession, and dealing with those members who do not meet the requirements.
- Its members subscribe to a code of ethics drawn up by the profession itself.
- The members form organized societies to enhance the development of the group and its societal mission, and to serve its individual members.

We can define a *health profession* by paraphrasing Webster's definition above: a calling in the health sciences requiring specialized knowledge, and one which meets the other criteria listed. Dentistry meets all the requirements of a profession. Dental hygiene is usually considered a profession within dentistry, although for the most part it is not self-regulating. Exceptions within the United States are found in Connecticut, where dental hygiene is regulated through the state's public health agency, and in New Mexico and Wash-

ington, where quasi-independent committees of the dental boards are the regulatory agencies.

DEVELOPMENT OF THE DENTAL PROFESSIONS

Dentistry

Dental diseases have afflicted the human race since the dawn of recorded history.[15, 19] Dentistry, however, has existed as a vocation only in recent years; it was not until modern times that the care of oral diseases developed any sort of scientific basis. One landmark event was the 1728 publication of Pierre Fauchard: *Le Chirurgien Dentiste, ou Traite des Dents*, a two-volume book of more than 800 pages. Fauchard, a Frenchman, is a seminal figure in the evolution of the dental profession. His work was the first complete treatise on dentistry published in the western world, and it remained an authoritative document for more than 100 years. Fauchard, despite the lack of formal training, was clearly a first-class empiricist with keen powers of observation.

Aspiring dentists of the time served as apprentices. It is worth noting that even the formal education of G. V. Black, one of the profession's most notable 19th century pioneers, did not exceed 20 months. His introduction to dentistry consisted of "a few weeks" with a Dr. Speers, who was not considered a particularly good dentist and whose dental library consisted of one book.[4] Fortunately, Dr. Black was a true professional and followed the old precept that "a professional person has no choice other than to be a continuous student."

The first dental school was the Baltimore College of Dental Surgery, later part of the University of Maryland, established in 1840. The course was 16 weeks long after a year or more of apprenticeship; the initial enrollment was 5, of whom 2 graduated. At about the same time, the first national professional dental journal appeared, *The American Journal of Dental Science*, and the first national professional dental organization, the American Society of Dental Surgeons, was established. The genesis of the dental profession in the United States can thus be dated fairly precisely to the 1840s. The path of professional progress, however, was not entirely smooth, for the emergence of dentistry as a fledgling profession was followed by an undignified scramble to open proprietary dental schools. In the best

American traditions of free enterprise and entrepreneurship, most of these places were run strictly for profit. In the years before public and professional regulation, the proprietary schools turned out thousands of graduates whose professional abilities covered the full range from respectable to dreadful.

The anarchic events of the time, however, led to dentistry's development in the United States as a profession separate from medicine, a position that has been maintained to the present day. This separate development actually occurred more by chance than by deliberate policy, for it was intended that the Baltimore dental school would be established within the medical school. It was not, but only because of lack of space and internal friction among medical school faculty. The separation of dentistry from medicine is characteristic of the English-speaking world, Scandinavia, and some other European countries; but in central and southern Europe, there was a division between stomatologists, physicians with specialty training in clinical dentistry, and dentists, who in this context were a second-level provider. This division of labor is thought to have not benefitted oral health in most of these countries[7] and has been abandoned in some of them as the European Community moves toward standardization of professional training.

Dentistry in the 20th Century

The era of modern dentistry dates from the closing of the last proprietary school in 1929, which came shortly after the landmark Gies report on dental education.[13] Gies collected a mass of information from the dental schools of the time and concluded that the dental profession would progress only when dental education became university-based and subject to the maintenance of high standards through accreditation. Despite the adoption of Gies' recommendations, however, dental practice during the economic depression of the 1930s was largely a matter of survival, with few patients able to afford dental care. World War II followed, during which dentists were drafted along with other health professionals into the armed forces. As part of the national mobilization for the war effort, American dental schools compressed the curriculum of 4 academic years into 3 calendar years. This expedient was dropped when the war ended in 1945, although it was flirted with again for a short time in the 1970s.

The 1930s and 1940s were a hard time for dental education. The teaching of basic science was often perfunctory, and the emphasis in the clinical sciences was almost entirely on restorative dentistry and prosthetics. Subjects such as radiology, oral diagnosis, endodontics, periodontics, and pediatric dentistry were neglected in many dental schools; and full-time faculty were the exception rather than the rule. There were few educational programs for the preparation of specialists, and the few that did exist varied in quality and length.[13] One of the few bright spots during this difficult period was the beginning of the first controlled water fluoridation projects in 1945 (Chapter 24).

With a rapidly expanding postwar economy and population, added to accelerating technologic growth and a spirit of optimism, dentistry entered what many see as a "golden age" during the 1950s. New dental materials expanded treatment horizons, and the arrival of the high-speed air-turbine engine in 1957 revolutionized dental practice. Dental research, stimulated by the establishment of the National Institute of Dental Research* in 1948, grew rapidly, and the publication of *The Survey of Dentistry* in 1961[11] led to improvements in education and practice. Semi-stagnant dental schools were revitalized with the passage of the Health Professions Educational Assistance Act in 1963. This act authorized federal funds for construction and student aid; later renewals in 1971 and 1976 included per capita funding to support the basic instructional program. In the 15 years from 1963 to 1978, the addition of federal money to state, local, and private sources spurred the reconstruction of the entire physical plant of dental education.[9] New schools were built; the 39 dental schools in 1930 had increased to 59 by 1980.[1]

The 1960s and 1970s saw increasing interest in comprehensive care rather than tooth-oriented treatment, growth in use of auxiliaries, the beginnings of prepaid dental insurance, and the development of a community outlook in dentistry. Growth in the number of dentists and in dental business was robust, in retrospect perhaps too robust. The economic downturn after the Vietnam War (1964–1975), plus the decline in dental caries among children (Chapter 19), added to a growing perception of an oversupply of dentists, despite increasing public utilization of

---

*Now the National Institute of Dental and Craniofacial Research (NIDCR)

services (Chapter 2) and continued growth of dental insurance (Chapter 8). During the 1980s, enrollment in dental schools dropped substantially from its peak during the 1977–1979 period and rose only a little from these levels through the mid-1990s (Chapter 9). Five dental schools announced their closing during the 1980s (Emory, Fairleigh Dickinson, Georgetown, Oral Roberts, Washington University), and Loyola of Chicago followed a few years later. The biggest jolt came with the closing of the dental school at Northwestern University, the home of G. V. Black, in late 1997. On the other side of the ledger, a private university in Florida (Nova Southeastern University) opened a new dental school in 1997.

At the turn of the 21st century, dentistry is on the brink of new types of practice, as the major diseases are now better controlled than ever. Research in molecular biology is promising new understanding of many diseases, including oral diseases that currently are poorly understood and that to date have not been treated in dental practice. Other features that will shape dental practice in the 21st century are the development of new restorative materials, the changing demographic profile (Chapter 2), and disease patterns (Chapters 18–22). Infection control procedures and their associated regulations had become a standard part of dental practice by the 1990s (Chapter 6).

Dental Hygiene

Dr. Alfred Fones, an 1890 graduate of the New York College of Dentistry, developed a technique of scaling and polishing teeth and also taught his patients to carry out home care procedures. By 1906, acting under the preventive dictum that "a clean tooth never decays," Dr. Fones was sure that the oral health of his patients was improved through his oral prophylactic practices. He trained his assistant to practice dental hygiene, and in 1907 he was instrumental in having dental hygiene legally recognized in Connecticut as an adjunct to dental practice. Fones went on to establish the first school of dental hygiene in 1913. Accepting only "young ladies of good character," the school was located in a carriage house on the grounds of the Fones residence.[16] Connecticut passed legislation specifically describing the practice of dental hygiene in 1916. Ten states had similar legislation in place by 1920, and the total rose to 34 in 1935. Not until 1951, however, did the

practice acts of all states, the District of Columbia, and the Commonwealth of Puerto Rico include provisions for the practice of dental hygiene.[8]

This leisurely development of dental hygiene was largely tied to the development of dental schools. In 1945, of the 16 dental hygiene programs then in existence, 13 were associated with schools of dentistry. By 1974, however, only 37 of 158 were so affiliated. The explosive growth after 1960 mostly took place in junior and community colleges,[8] stimulated by federal funds for vocational-technical education in health occupation training centers. By 1980, the number of programs was 204. With subsequent cuts in federal funding, the number had diminished to 190 by the end of the 1980s, but was back to about 215 again by the mid-1990s (Chapter 9).

During the first 30 years of dental hygiene education, there was no uniformity in either prerequisites or curriculum. These variations were due to differences in state licensing acts, problems of integrating a 2-year clinical program into a 4-year baccalaureate degree curriculum, and the lack of nationally approved standards. The latter problem was remedied in 1947, when the Council on Dental Education of the American Dental Association (ADA) adopted the first accreditation requirements for dental hygiene schools. In 1952, the council began an active program in accreditation of dental hygiene schools; the requirements developed then still essentially stand today.

For training as a dental hygienist, a 2-year curriculum must meet the standards of the ADA's Commission on Accreditation. The candidate, after passing an examination for licensure, may use the initials RDH (Registered Dental Hygienist) following the name. In all states except Alabama, which recognizes preceptorship, the completion of an accredited 2-year curriculum is the minimum requirement for admittance to licensure examination by a state dental board. An individual enrolled in a 4-year baccalaureate degree program must also meet university standards for that degree. Some dental hygienists earn advanced degrees (MS, MPH, PhD, DrPH), for which the requirements of the university's graduate school also must be met.

ORGANIZATION OF THE DENTAL PROFESSIONS IN THE UNITED STATES

The legal basis for dental practice in the United States is the Dental Practice Act in each state. It is not a federal matter. The effect of these acts on dental practice is discussed more fully in Chapter 9. Here we look at the professional organizations in dentistry.

The American Dental Association

The precursor organization of the ADA, as already noted, first appeared as a tiny organization in 1840; today it represents 73% of the nation's 160,000 active dentists. It is the largest and most influential dental organization in the country. The ADA operates on a tripartite basis, that is, members must join the local society (a component), the state society (a constituent), and the national ADA; they cannot be members of just 1 or 2 (with the exception of students and dentists in the federal services, who may join the national ADA directly). There are 54 constituent societies and 529 components.

The tripartite system has been in place since 1913, when it was modelled on the structure of the American Medical Association. The purpose of adopting the tripartite structure was to unify a profession, which at the time was highly fragmented, and to improve efficiency through avoiding duplication of effort. The tripartite structure was challenged by 4 Arizona dentists in 1972, who argued that by requiring membership at all levels the ADA had instituted an illegal arrangement. The District Court ruled against the dentists in 1980, stating that the membership requirement did not suppress competition between dentists, and it also disagreed with the charge that the associations or their members held a monopoly on the practice of dentistry in Arizona. The decision was upheld in the Court of Appeals in 1982, so the legal basis for the ADA's tripartite structure seems secure.[14]

Dentists apply for membership in a component society, which represents a county, a group of counties, or a large city. If accepted at this local level, the dentist automatically becomes a member of the state dental society and of the ADA. Traditionally, membership standards have included graduation from an accredited dental school, a license to practice in the jurisdiction, and "good moral standing," a vague term that has been interpreted in various ways.

ADA membership provides access to a number of fringe benefits that are important to a self-employed practitioner, such as group insurance plans and the availability of expert consultative services. The ADA also serves its members, and indirectly the public, primarily in 3 other areas:

- Holding scientific meetings at the local, state, and national level. These meetings are an important mechanism for the exchange of scientific information within the profession. This exchange is enhanced by the publication of a variety of scientific journals.
- Establishing standards, such as accreditation of professional schools for dentists, dental hygienists, dental assistants, and dental laboratory technicians. The ADA also sets the standards for specialty training. Standards are also established for materials, drugs, and devices used by dentists in practice and for some products offered for sale to the public. These standards are established by having experts in specialized fields serve as members of reviewing councils and committees.
- Obtaining a consensus among the profession on major issues and transmitting this consensus to government agencies and others concerned with establishing policies for public health.

The ADA is a cohesive and well-organized body. Although its membership of 73% of American dentists is lower than it was some years ago, it is still higher than the 44% representation in the American Medical Association and the 50% of lawyers who belong to the American Bar Association.[14] Its ultimate governing body is the House of Delegates.[2] This 423-member body is composed of elected representatives from the 50 states, the District of Columbia, the Commonwealth of Puerto Rico, the Panama Canal, and the Virgin Islands. Like the U.S. House of Representatives, state delegations are proportional to state dental populations; they range from 1 delegate (the Virgin Islands and Panama Canal) to California's 46. The House of Delegates includes 1 representative of each federal administrative unit, including the Air Force, Army, Navy, U.S. Public Health Service, and the Department of Veterans Affairs. It also includes a representative of the American Student Dental Association.

The Board of Trustees, charged with day-to-day responsibility for the ADA's operations, is made up of a trustee from each of 16 geographic districts of roughly equal numbers of dentists, plus the president, president-elect, and first and second vice-presidents. The Board reports on its activities to the

House of Delegates. It also reviews most resolutions on their way to the House and recommends action to be taken on them.

The House of Delegates conducts business once a year for 5 days during the annual session. Resolutions may be introduced by the Board of Trustees, the ADA's commissions and councils, the trustee districts, constituent and component societies, or directly by delegates. Resolutions, along with supporting documentation, are referred for hearing to one of 7 reference committees: Budget and Business Matters; Communications and Membership Services; Dental Benefits, Practice, and Health; Dental Education and Related Matters; Legal and Legislative Matters; President's Address and Administrative Matters; and Scientific Matters. Depending on the issues in any given year, special (generally single-issue) committees and variations of the committees listed are established. The hearings of the reference committees are open to all members of the association. At these meetings members are encouraged to speak their minds and advise the House of Delegates of their positions on specific issues or on the status of the association as a whole. The reference committees prepare reports that are transmitted to the House of Delegates. As the House considers the issues, it usually has the original resolution and background report, the comments and recommendations of the Board of Trustees, and the report and recommendations of the reference committee. On the basis of this information, the House acts to adopt, defeat, amend, substitute, or refer.

The ADA has long been keenly aware of the public image of dentistry and has conducted many campaigns to promote it. Children's Dental Health Month, which grew from an original 1-week campaign and is held in February each year, is the ADA's oldest annual public relations exercise. Others have come and gone, such as Senior Smile Week and Smile America![3] The impact of these campaigns is discussed in Chapter 5.

Dentistry might be a bit preoccupied with its image, for many public opinion polls show that the public consistently ranks dentists high in terms of professional trust.[5] The sometimes prickly sensitivity of dentistry to its image is seen in the chorus of complaints when dentists are portrayed in movies or TV as bumbling, obsessive, or sadistic, or when newscasters refer to "doctors and dentists." (One that gets under our skin is reference to "medical treatment" and "dental work").

These things can grate at times, but they seem to be part of the territory. When viewed in the perspective of how all professions are treated in the media, it is doubtful if any real harm is done by media imagery.

The National Dental Association (NDA)

Reflecting the rigid racial attitudes of former years, most component dental societies used not to accept dentists of African-American origin. This led to the creation of the National Dental Association (NDA) to meet the needs of African-American dentists. Those days are now happily gone; both the ADA and the NDA have stated that their objective is complete integration of the dental profession. White dentists now belong to the NDA and African-American dentists belong to the ADA, and there is a good cooperative relationship between the two organizations. They continue to exist separately, however, for traditional reasons. The National Dental Hygienists' Association was officially recognized as an affiliate of the NDA in 1963.

Hispanic Dental Association (HDA)

Established in 1990, the Hispanic Dental Association (HDA) is a national dental organization whose focus is the interests of both Hispanic professionals and patients. This active organization already has several hundred members and a number of affiliate groups throughout the country. The HDA mission is to improve the oral health of the Hispanic community, and to that end it sponsors continuing education and oral health promotional activities directed at the Hispanic population. The HDA has further information on its mission and its activities available from its website.

Other Groups in Dentistry

Beyond the major national organizations and their constituent and component societies, each specialty group has its own organization: the American Academy of Periodontics, the American Association of Oral and Maxillofacial Surgeons, the American Association of Public Health Dentistry, and others. These specialty organizations are sponsors of the specialty certifying bodies, whose role is discussed in Chapter 9. At another level still, myriad study clubs and groups of dentists are brought together by common specific interests.

World Dental Federation (FDI)

Practically every country with a recognizable dental profession has a working national organization, an equivalent of the ADA, although no other national dental association has resources as extensive as those of the ADA. On the international scene, the World Dental Federation (formerly the Fédération Dentaire Internationale, hence the initials FDI) is an organization of national dental associations. Formed in the early 20th century as a loose grouping of several European national associations, the FDI now represents more than 100 national dental organizations. Headquartered in London, the FDI has a full-time executive-secretary, a large staff, and a structure that resembles that of the United Nations. Its work is both scientific and political. Its technical committees bring international experts together to develop state-of-the-art reports and recommendations for further action. Politically, the FDI has been helpful in the development of the dental professions and dental care services in many countries where the local profession has little political clout. It publishes the *International Dental Journal,* a respected journal in the dental literature.

The American Dental Hygienists' Association (ADHA)

In 1923, 46 dental hygienists from 11 states met in Cleveland, Ohio, to organize the ADHA. They received strong support from the dental profession. Although early growth was not spectacular, between 1925 and 1945, active membership increased from several hundred to about 2000. In the next 10 years (1945 to 1955) membership more than doubled to nearly 4400, and by the end of the 1980s it was approximately 25,000.

The organization of the ADHA closely parallels that of the ADA. There are 7 classifications of membership (including student membership for a modest fee), but the basic category of "active" membership must be held through constituent and component associations if such exist. There are 51 constituent associations. The House of Delegates meets once a year and is the supreme authoritative body of the association, having all legislative and policy-making powers. The Board of Trustees is composed of the elective officers (except the Speaker of the House), 12 trustees, and the immediate past president, and has responsibility for supervising the day-to-day operations. It reviews reports and makes recommendations and relates all of its activities to the House. The *Journal of the American Dental Hygienists' Association* was established in 1927. In 1972 the name was changed to *Dental Hygiene,* and in 1988 it became the *Journal of Dental Hygiene.*

CAREERS IN DENTISTRY AND DENTAL HYGIENE

Private Practice

Private practice, in which the dentist invests capital into land, buildings, equipment, and furnishings, and in turn seeks to attract patients who will pay for dental services, is the primary career choice for most dentists in the United States. Private practice is a small business and, from the career perspective, has all the advantages and disadvantages of small business operation.

The advantages are considerable. A dentist has an almost unlimited choice of where to locate her practice (provided of course that a license to practice in the chosen state can be secured). Other advantages are usually a good income, high status in the community, and the freedom that comes from being one's own boss. There is also the satisfaction of knowing that the profession is generally held in high esteem by the public,[10] although studies in the 1990s indicated that dentists themselves were less positive about the future of the profession than they used to be.[10, 18] Disadvantages of private practice also relate to the small business aspects: overhead costs for utilities, insurance, staff benefits, equipment maintenance; the necessity to plan for retirement; and income maintenance in the event of disability. The need to adhere to various government regulations also requires some effort. Dental practice is highly physical in nature, and conditions that are only an inconvenience in many occupations, such as mild arthritis, a bad back, or failing eyesight, can be career-threatening for a private practitioner.

The choice of practice location is naturally based on personal preference: going back to a hometown or moving to somewhere new, the prospects for a spouse's career, the quality of the schools, access to cultural facilities and recreational interests, the climate, all the things that anyone factors into an idea of good quality life. Rather than just pick one's dream town, the new graduate is well advised to investigate those matters that will directly affect professional life.[6] The presence of established practices, the socioeconomic status of the community, and the extent of dental insurance among the potential patients all have a direct bearing on practice prospects. The ADA has an extensive set of materials to help the new graduate select a practice location.

An associate in an established practice is usually paid by salary, or salary plus percentage of gross. These arrangements allow practice patterns to be sharpened before establishing one's own practice and can lead to buying into an established practice. Partnership, too, can ease the financial burden of starting practice, as can entering a group practice. Partnerships can provide more flexibility in practicing pattern than solo practice, but partners setting out together should be as sure as they can be that they are of the right personality to make joint decisions, and that they are mutually compatible. An unhappy business partnership can be as emotionally traumatic and financially devastating as a broken marriage.

Dental specialists generally earn higher incomes than generalists. Achievement of specialty status requires at least an extra 2 years of education beyond dental school, followed by specialty board examinations (Chapter 9). For specialists, the process of choosing a practice location parallels that for general practitioners, with two important exceptions. First, the choice usually is limited to the larger population centers; second, the referral potential of the practitioners in the area, as well as the number of specialists already located there, must be assessed. In at least the early years of a specialty practice, the supply of patients depends primarily on referrals from the general practitioners. Where the general practitioners all have busy, established practices, they will usually refer patients more readily than will younger generalists attempting to establish their own practices. In the latter instance, referrals may be few and limited to the most extreme problems. The choices for the 2 types of specialists who usually work only in salaried positions, oral pathologists and public health dentists, are limited by positions available.

Colorado is the only state that permits independent practice of dental hygiene, although few hygienists established their own practices there after the 1986 law that permitted independent practice. Most hygienists, in Colorado as elsewhere, begin their careers treating patients in the offices of private dental practitioners. They are reimbursed on either a straight salaried basis or a combination of a salary and commission.

Salaried Practice

The advantages and disadvantages of salaried practice, like those of private practice, are most related to whether the dentist is temperamentally comfortable in an organization as opposed to being a private entrepreneur. Even if a new graduate does not wish to stay in salaried service permanently, it is often a good place to start. Advantages include the opportunity to reduce dental school debts before incurring more, an immediate specified income, a chance to improve clinical experience, and a time to think about careers before deciding to establish a practice or go back to graduate school.

For some dentists, however, salaried practice appeals as a life career, especially as a new private practice cannot assume the certainty of success that it could a generation or two ago. A reasonably good salary (although not as high as peak earnings in private practice), fringe benefits such as health and disability insurance, liability coverage, a retirement plan, paid vacation time, and freedom from the overhead costs and day-to-day worries of private practice can combine to make the long-term financial prospects of salaried employment attractive. Many organizations provide opportunities for continuing education or even advanced graduate degrees.

For the new dentist interested in general practice, a general practice residency offers a form of short-term salaried practice that combines advanced educational opportunities with the ability to earn. More than 1200 training positions in general practice residencies and advanced general dentistry programs are accredited by the ADA; all are 12 or 24 months long and offer stipends. They generally include rotations through such areas as medicine, emergency care, anesthesia, and various special areas of clinical dentistry. This excellent clinical experience would be broadened even further if general practice residencies included some public health perspectives (Chapter 4).

Dentists in the U.S. Public Health Service (USPHS), a component of the Department of

Health and Human Services, serve as commissioned officers of the federal government and enjoy essentially the same pay, rank, and privileges as their counterparts in the Army, Navy, and Air Force. The USPHS's broad mission relates to the health of the entire nation, in recognition of which its chief officer is commissioned as Surgeon-General of the United States. The USPHS carries out major responsibilities in health research (principally through the National Institutes of Health) and in the promotion of health through public health efforts. Clinical care is provided primarily to merchant seamen, the Coast Guard, American Indians and Alaska Natives, residents of federal prisons, and certain other special populations. USPHS dental officers serve in a wide variety of assignments in all states. The clinics of the Indian Health Service, for example, range from Point Barrow, Alaska (the farthest northern point of the United States above the Arctic Circle), to Arizona, just north of the Mexican border. Although the USPHS is the oldest health service of the federal government, beginning as the Marine Hospital Service in 1798 and with its Commissioned Corps dating from 1873, it remained relatively unknown to the public before Surgeon-General Koop gave it high visibility during his campaigns against smoking and in favor of AIDS education during the 1980s.[12]

Other major federal dental services are the dental corps of the Army, Navy (which also serves the Marine Corps), and Air Force. Availability of positions varies with the degree of military activity, although some openings are virtually always present. The dentist in the armed services receives all the advantages of a service career, meaning a reasonably good income, generous fringe benefits, usually excellent clinical facilities, and rewarding professional opportunities such as graduate education. Dentists serve on military bases in the United States and overseas. In the Navy, duty is also available on ships.

Another major federal dental service, the Department of Veterans Affairs (previously the Veterans Administration, and hence still referred to as the VA), was established in 1920 to improve services to veterans of American wars. It is a major participant in postdoctoral dental education and it offers, in addition to specialty programs, more than half of the general practice residencies available in the federal services. Many VA institutions are affiliated with dental schools. Care is provided in VA hospitals and outpatient clinics; occasionally it is purchased from private practitioners. Like all federal dental programs, the VA offers equal employment opportunities for male and female dentists. Under some circumstances, the VA has been able to accommodate married couples where both are health professionals.

Dental hygienists are employed by the USPHS, both through Civil Service and the Commissioned Corps. Expanded opportunities in the federal service are available for dental hygienists with a degree of Master of Public Health (MPH); a number of hygienists with this degree have advanced into leadership positions. Civilian hygienists are employed in the Army, Navy, and Air Force, although a major share of clinical procedures ordinarily performed by hygienists are carried out by specially trained enlisted personnel.

Outside of the federal dental services, there are other opportunities for salaried employment. Most states have a position of state dental director in the state's health department, usually filled by a dentist or hygienist with advanced training in public health, most commonly the MPH degree. Dentists and dental hygienists are also employed by state and local health departments, group dental practices, prepaid dental programs, industry-sponsored clinics, and institutions such as hospitals, prisons, schools for the mentally retarded, and homes for the mentally ill. These positions may involve public health and administrative activities, clinical practice, or a combination of both.

Academia: Dental Education and Research

Dental schools, as seen earlier in this chapter, used to be staffed largely by part-time faculty whose primary task was to grade students' clinical treatment. Academic careers have evolved, however, and the emphasis now is on full-time teachers and researchers; most schools have drastically reduced their part-time faculty. The ability to conduct independent research has become a major criterion for an academic career as research grant funds increasingly form an important part of a school's budget.

An advanced degree is virtually mandatory for the new dentist or hygienist who is thinking of an academic career. The most common is the MS (Master of Science), the usual 2-year degree taken to fulfill specialty training requirements, which mixes advanced clinical training with some research training. Those who want to make their careers in research need doctoral-level training in the philosophy and methods of research through the degrees of PhD (Doctor of Philosophy), DrPH (Doctor of Public Health), or DSc (Doctor of Science). The National Institute of Dental Research in Bethesda, Maryland, has information on research training programs that it supports.

Academic positions for dental professionals with advanced degrees have attractive salaries and fringe benefits. They can be intellectually demanding, and university politics can be just as vigorous as politics anywhere else. The future of dentistry rests with its dental education institutions and research institutes. Those employed in these institutions have the rewards and challenges of being on the cutting edge of new developments, of interacting with talented fellow faculty members, and of relating to students who represent the future.

REFERENCES

1. American Dental Association. Summary of the 1979-1980 annual report on dental education. J Am Dent Assoc 1980;100:926–30.
2. American Dental Association, House of Delegates. Structure and function of the ADA's policy-making body. J Am Dent Assoc 1976;93:708–12.
3. Berry JH. Dentistry's public image: Does it need a boost? J Am Dent Assoc 1989;118:687–92.
4. Bremner MDK. The story of dentistry; from the dawn of civilization to the present. 3rd ed. Brooklyn NY: Dental Items of Interest, 1954.
5. DiMatteo MR, McBride CA, Shugars DA, O'Neill EH. Public attitudes towards dentists: A U.S. household survey. J Am Dent Assoc 1995;126:1563–70.
6. Dunlap JE. The beginning dental practice: The first year. Tulsa: Dental Economic/PPC Books, 1978.
7. Ennis J. The story of the Fédération Dentaire Internationale. London: FDI, 1967.
8. Fales MJH. History of dental hygiene education in the United States, 1913 to 1975 [dissertation]. Ann Arbor MI: University of Michigan, 1975.
9. Galagan DJ. Back from the brink: how and why U.S. dental schools were rebuilt. Dent Survey 1978;54:14–8.
10. Gerbert B, Bernzweig J, Bleecker T, Bader J, Miyasaki C. How dentists see themselves, their profession, the public. J Am Dent Assoc 1992;123:72–8.
11. Hollinshead BS, director. The survey of dentistry: The final report. Washington DC: American Council on Education, 1961.
12. Koop CE, Ginzburg HM. The revitalization of the Public Health Service Commissioned Corps. Public Health Rep 1989;104:105–10.
13. Mann WR. Dental education. In: Hollinshead BS. The survey of dentistry: The final report. Washington DC: American Council on Education, 1961;239–422.
14. McCann D. Tripartite system: Working together for a common goal. J Am Dent Assoc 1989;119:241–7.
15. Moore WJ, Corbett ME. The distribution of dental caries in ancient British populations. II. Iron Age, Romano-British and Mediæval periods. Caries Res 1973;7:139–53.
16. Motley WE. Ethics, jurisprudence, and history for the dental hygienist. 3rd ed. Philadelphia: Lea and Febiger, 1976.
17. Ozar DT. Three models of professionalism and professional obligation in dentistry. J Am Dent Assoc 1985;110:173–7.
18. Romberg E, Cohen L. Dentists' outlook toward their profession. J Dent Pract Admin 1990;7:39–43.
19. Weinberger BH. An introduction to the history of dentistry, with medical and dental chronology and bibliographic data. St. Louis: Mosby, 1948.
20. Wolfenden. What makes a profession? Br Dent J 1975;139:61–5.

2

The Public
Served by Dentistry

Population Trends in the United States ◆ Population Size
and Growth ◆ Age Distribution ◆
Geographic Distribution ◆ Racial and Ethnic
Composition ◆ Economic Distribution ◆ Utilization of
Dental Services ◆ Annual Dental Attendance ◆
Factors Associated with the Use of Dental Services:
Gender, Age, Socioeconomic Status, Race and
Ethnicity, Geographic Location, General Health,
Dental Insurance ◆ Future Use of Dental Services

Dentistry exists to serve the public. Many aspects of that broad statement will be examined throughout this book, and in this chapter we start by looking at the structure of the US population. The age distribution of the population, its ethnic makeup, and its geographic distribution within the country all profoundly affect the practice of dentistry. We then look at the public's use of dental services and the factors that affect that use.

POPULATION TRENDS IN THE UNITED STATES

Population Size and Growth

The Census Bureau listed the population of the United States in 1994 as 260.7 million, about 5% of the world's population. Life expectancy in 1993 reached 72.1 years for males (whites 73.0 and African-Americans 67.4 years) and 78.9 years for females (whites 79.5 and African-Americans 75.5 years).[7] Life expectancy is expected to increase into the 21st century,[10] although the disparities between males and females and between whites and African-Americans are likely to persist.

Figure 2–1 is a population pyramid, a graphic method of showing age distribution, for the United States in 1994. The bulge of the "baby-boomer" generation, the large number

of children born between 1946 and 1964 in the aftermath of World War II, is clearly evident between 30 and 49 years. The lower rates of growth subsequent to this generation are seen in the shorter bars under the "boomers."

The Census Bureau estimates that the total population of the United States in the year 2010 will be 300.4 million, and in 2025 it will be 338.3 million.[12] The annual rate of population increase during the 1980–1995 period was generally around 0.9%, which does not seem large but is still more than 2 million people per year. By contrast with the low growth rates of modern times, the annual average growth rate was 2.0% at the beginning of the 20th century, 1.7% in the 1950s, and 1.2% in the 1960s.[8] For a global perspective, the contrast between current and projected population growth rates in some economically developed countries and those in some developing nations of Latin America and Africa is shown in Figure 2–2. The highest rates of population growth are clearly coming from the developing world. In the year 2000, the population in the economically developed countries will be only about one fifth of the world's total.

Age Distribution

Low fertility rates since the late 1960s have combined with increasing life expec-

13

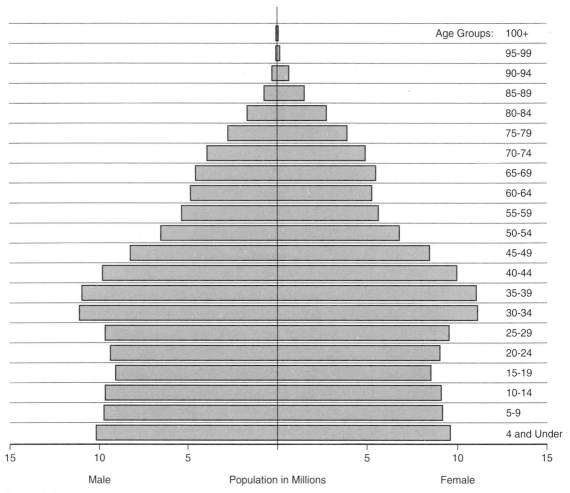

Figure 2–1. Population pyramid for the United States, 1994. (From US Department of Commerce, Bureau of the Census. Statistical abstract of the United States: 1995, 115th ed. Washington DC: Government Printing Office, 1995.)

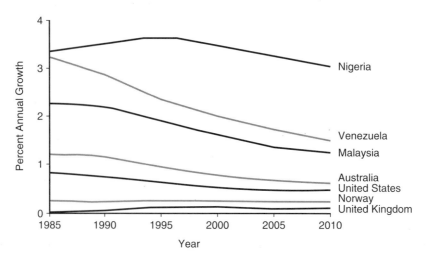

Figure 2–2. Estimated rates of population growth in seven countries from 1985 to 2010. (From Vu MT: World population projections 1984. Washington DC: World Bank, 1984.)

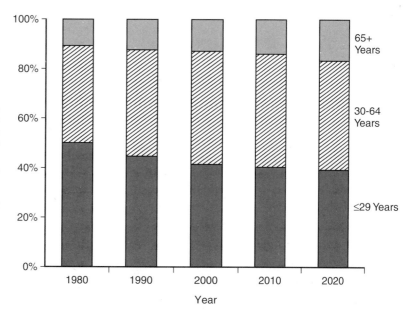

Figure 2–3. Projected population distribution by age-group for the United States from 1980 to 2020. (From US Department of Commerce, Bureau of the Census: US population estimates by age, sex, race, and Hispanic origin: 1993 to 2050. Series P-25 No 1104. Washington DC: Government Printing Office, 1994.)

tancy to lead to the "graying of America," the name often given to the nation's constantly increasing average age. Those aged 65 and over were 11.2% of the population in 1979,[9] 12.8% in 1994,[12] estimated to be 13.4% by 2010, and 18.4% in 2025 as the last of the "baby boomers" approaches 65.[12] Figure 2–3 shows the change in age distribution of the United States population between 1980 and 1990, with Census Bureau projections to the year 2020. The main points to note are the continuing diminution of the 29-and-under group as a proportion of the total, and the continuing growth in the 65-and-older group. As noted, these trends will become even more pronounced in the years to come.

The elderly population is not spread evenly around the country. Although the proportion of persons aged 65 or older in the United States was 12.8% in 1994, it ranged from 18.4% in Florida to 4.6% in Alaska. This aging trend, already well recognized in dentistry by the growing emphasis on education in geriatric dentistry, will clearly affect the types and distribution of dental services in future years. For example, from population trends alone there is likely to be a greater need for periodontic and prosthetic care, at the expense of treatment for children, even apart from trends in the oral diseases (Chapters 18–22).

Geographic Distribution

Extensive migration of people from one region to another has long been a characteristic of the United States. It still is, with 18% of the population moving each year.[13] A major trend since 1970 has been the shift from the northeastern, north central, and midwest regions to the South and West; the rate of population growth in the 1990s has been most pronounced in the mountain states. Figure 2–4 shows the percentage of population by region for 1994; Figure 2–5 shows the projected degree of population growth in each region between 1995 and 2010. Since interregional migrants tend to be younger people, the median age in the South, mountain regions, and the West is already less than it is in the northeast regions, and the interregional differences are expected to increase into the 21st century.[10]

Reasons for the "Sunbelt migration" since 1970 are primarily economic. The nation's industrial base, once concentrated in the Northeast and Midwest, has become more spread out, and businesses in the computer age have greater flexibility in choice of location than they used to. The growing importance of the Pacific Rim nations in the American economy ensures that the West Coast will remain a leading business area, as well as a stopping place for immigrants from Asia. However, there are some potential constraints to this pattern of growth. The main one concerns water supplies, for much of the "Sunbelt" could become the "Thirstbelt" in the future. If the rapidly growing cities in the region also develop the social problems of the older northern cities, they may become less attractive places to live.

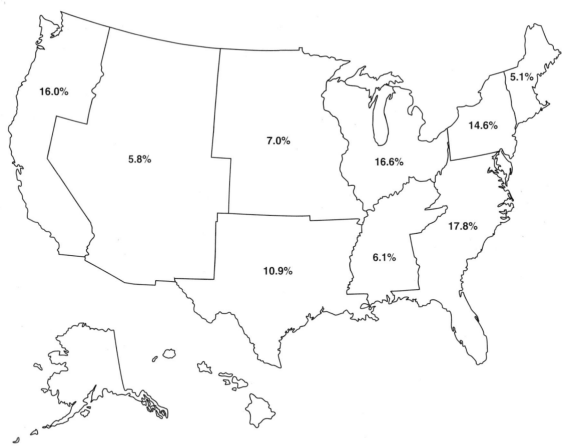

Figure 2–4. Population distribution by geographic regions in the United States in 1994. (From US Department of Commerce, Bureau of the Census. Statistical abstract of the United States: 1995, 115th ed. Washington DC: Government Printing Office, 1995.)

At a different level, big cities continue to lose population to suburbs and small towns and are financially troubled as job opportunities move out. The provision of dental services in these inner city areas is one of many functions that are adversely affected by these population movements.

Racial and Ethnic Composition

The 1994 population of the United States included 32.7 million African-Americans, or 12.5% of the total. Persons of Hispanic descent numbered 26.1 million, 10% of the total.[11, 12] Because the racial/ethnic groups now considered "minorities" are growing rapidly, the term *minority groups* will lose much of its current meaning in the 21st century. Figure 2–6 shows the percentages of racial and ethnic groups in the United States in 1995, compared with the projected distribu-

tion in the year 2020. The main features of Figure 2–6 are the doubling of the Asian-Pacific Islander population from 3% to 6%, the growth of Hispanics from 10% to 16%, and the decrease in the proportion of non-Hispanic whites from 74% to 64% of all Americans.

The main feature of population growth among the various ethnic groups in the United States at the end of the 20th century is the emergence of the Hispanic population as the main minority group. The term *Hispanic* is a generic term for Spanish-speaking persons and covers a variety of cultures and even races. Two thirds of the Hispanic population is of Mexican heritage living in the Southwest. A large New York Hispanic population is predominantly Puerto Rican, and the Cuban population is centered in Miami.[2]

A striking reminder of the growing ethnic diversity of the United States is the fact that minority populations grew 14% in the

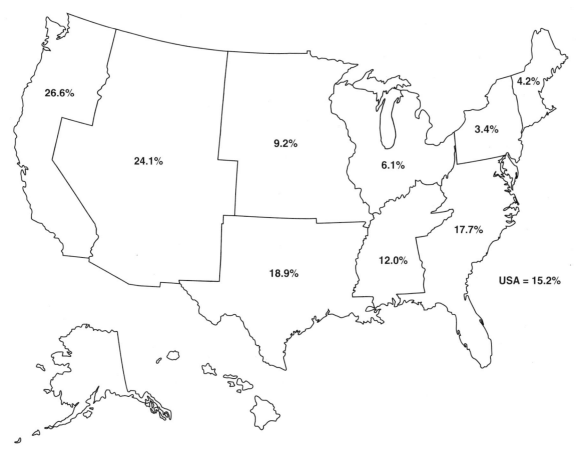

Figure 2-5. Projected population growth for geographic regions of the United States, 1995–2010. (From: US Department of Commerce, Bureau of the Census: Projections of the population of states by age, sex, and race: 1988 to 2010. Series P-25 No 1017. Washington DC: Government Printing Office, 1989.)

first half of the 1990s, whereas the non-Hispanic white population grew only 3%.[2]

Economic Distribution

A disturbing trend that became evident during the 1980s was the increase in the proportion of Americans living in poverty. (The federal definition of poverty changes with inflation and in 1993 was set as an annual income of $14,763 for a nonfarm family of four). The proportion of Americans in poverty through the 1980s was 13% to 15%.[14] It was not decreasing in the 1990s, and rose to 15.1% in 1993. Poverty was more common in minority groups, for that 1993 national figure of 15.1% comprised 12.2% of the white population, 33.1% of African-Americans, and 30.6% of Hispanics. Median annual income in 1993 was $39,300 for white families, $21,542 for African-Americans, and $23,654 for Hispanics. Although the national median income was still rising in the 1990s, the rate of in-

crease had slowed down from that seen during the 1970s and 1980s.

A further breakdown of these figures shows that the problem of poverty is even more pronounced among America's children. The proportion of the nation's children living in poverty reached 22.0% in 1993, the highest ever recorded, and it has been climbing steadily since reaching 19% in 1988.[14] This figure comprises 17.0% of white children, 45.9% of African-Americans, and 39.9% of Hispanics.

This increase in the proportion of children and families who are poor has implications for the provision of dental care, for the problem of untreated oral disease is considerably greater among people of low income and education. (This issue will be illustrated frequently throughout the book).

Summary

The American population is aging, and the so-called minority groups are comprising

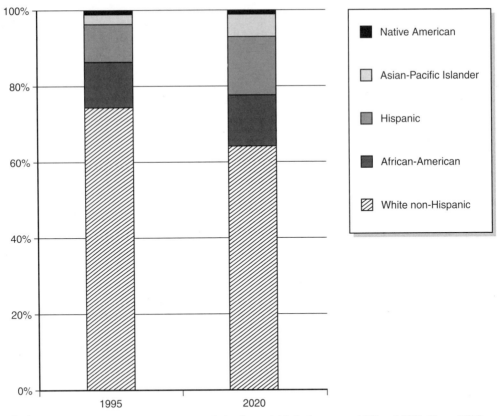

Figure 2–6. Distribution of the United States population by racial/ethnic groups, 1995 and 2020. (From US Department of Commerce, Bureau of the Census: US population estimates by age, sex, race, and Hispanic origin: 1980 to 1991. Series P-25 No 1095. Washington DC: Government Printing Office, 1993.)

an ever-growing proportion of it. The polarization between richer and poorer segments grew more pronounced during the 1990s, and population continued to shift south and west. Some dental implications are that patients in their 80s and 90s, possibly even some over 100, will become more common, and all dental personnel will need training in the special needs of the older patient. The dental professions will need to face the problems of providing care for the increasing proportion of people in poverty, for the lack of access to dental care among these groups is already a major public health problem and is likely to grow in the absence of programmatic action. Adequate provision of dental care for the growing minority populations may require more dentists from those groups, as well as a better understanding of the various ethnic cultures, if dental care is to achieve the status in their lives that it has in the lives of the majority.

UTILIZATION OF DENTAL SERVICES

Need for dental care can be defined as that quantity of dental treatment that expert opinion judges ought to be consumed over a certain period for people to achieve the status of being dentally healthy.[5] This professionally-determined dental need is sometimes referred to in the literature as *normative need.* Need for an individual or population can be expressed as (1) individual items of care required, such as those entered on a patient's chart; (2) total professional time needed for treatment; (3) the numbers of professionals needed for a particular time; or (4) the total cost of such care. *Perceived need,* also referred to as subjective need or felt need, is need for dental care as determined by a patient or the public. Perceived need can often differ considerably from normative need. For example, a dentist judges that the patient needs a root canal treatment followed by a crown when the patient wants the tooth extracted.

Demand for dental care is the expression by a patient or the public of a desire to receive dental care to attend to their perceived needs.[4] Related terms are *potential demand,* or *latent demand,* meaning a desire for care that is not being met for some reason, usually a problem with access. *Utilization* is the actual attendance by members of the public at dental treatment facilities to receive dental care. Utilization is expressed as the proportion of a population who attended a dentist within a given time, usually a year, or as the average number of visits per person made during a year. The latter measure usually uses the whole population as denominator, so it is weighted by people who did not visit the dentist at all over the time in question. In much of the dental literature, the terms *demand* and *utilization* are used almost synonomously. Economists almost invariably use the term *demand* (meaning utilization) in their studies of the dental care market.

Annual Dental Attendance

Information on the use of dental services, in addition to a lot of other health-related information, comes from the continuing series of household interviews conducted by the National Center for Health Statistics, an agency within the US Department of Health and Human Services. In 1989, 57.2% of people in the United States reported that they had visited a dentist within the last year, the highest proportion ever to do so.[20] By way of contrast with utilization some 30 years before, only 37.0% reported visiting a dentist within the last year in 1957–1958.[17] The average number of dental visits per person in 1989 was 2.1, again the highest ever recorded.

Utilization of dental services in the United States, as measured by those making at least one dental visit over the last year, rose modestly during the 1960s, plateaued at about 50% during the 1970s, then rose noticeably during the 1980s. At all times, more women than men visited the dentist, both in terms of annual proportion and number of visits per year. The trend of increasing annual utilization over recent years, for both men and women, is shown in Figure 2–7.

FACTORS ASSOCIATED WITH THE USE OF DENTAL SERVICES

The use of dental services is not spread evenly over the population. The profile of the most frequent user of dental services is a white, female, college-educated suburbanite in a higher income bracket, who enjoys good

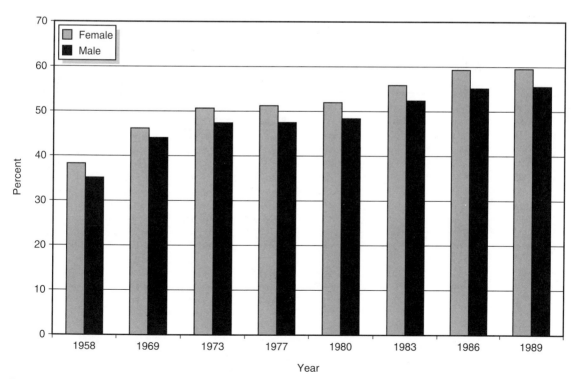

Figure 2–7. Proportion of the population who reported having visited a dentist within the previous year, for males and females. United States, 1958–1989. (Data from references 17–20.)

general health and has dental insurance. The variations in dental service utilization by demographic and other variables provide some basis for predicting how dental services may be used in the future.

Gender

As mentioned earlier, and as seen in Figure 2–7, women report using dental services more than men do. This finding is so consistent over time, and so constant in all countries that have studied the issue,[1] that it seems virtually universal—one of the few issues of which we can say it "always" happens.

It is not easy to say why women use dental services more; numerous attempts to explore the issue have not come up with convincing explanations. In the past, vanity has been suggested as a reason, but are women really more vain than men? Vague "cultural factors" is another, but the trend is seen across a wide variety of cultures. It has also been hypothesized that a largely male dental profession is part of the answer, but that breaks down with evidence from countries such as Finland, where the dental profession

is predominantly female.[6] Women also make more physician contacts than do men,[16] so perhaps the reason is related to the way that women view life.

Age

The peak ages for dental visits have traditionally been the late teenage years and early adulthood, with a gradual tailing-off with increasing age. Service use has always been relatively low in preschool years. The distribution of dental service use is also the antithesis of how physician services are used, for use of physician services is highest among the youngest and the oldest, giving rise to the U-shaped utilization curve shown in Figure 2–8. The contrast between use of medical and dental services is particularly important for administration of managed care plans (Chapter 8).

The traditional tailing-off of dental service use with increasing age, however, is changing quite rapidly as tooth retention among older adults increases. Figure 2–9 shows utilization by age in 1969 compared with that in 1989; the marked increase in the

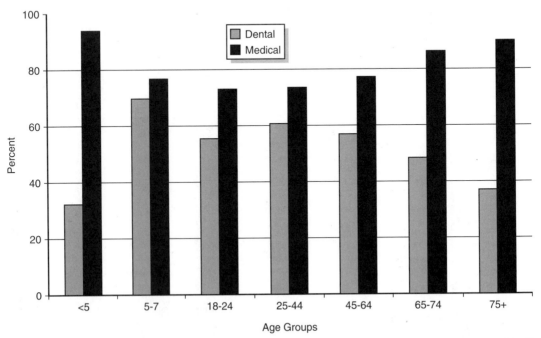

Figure 2–8. Contrasting patterns of the utilization of medical and dental services, by age. United States, 1989. (Data from US Public Health Service, National Center for Health Statistics. Current estimates from the National Health Interview Survey, 1989. DHHS Publication No. [PHS] 90-1504, Series 10 No 176. Washington DC: Government Printing Office 1990; US Public Health Service, National Center for Health Statistics. Use of dental services and oral health: United States, 1989. DHHS Publication No. [DHS] 93-1511, Series 10 No 183. Washington DC: Government Printing Office, 1992.)

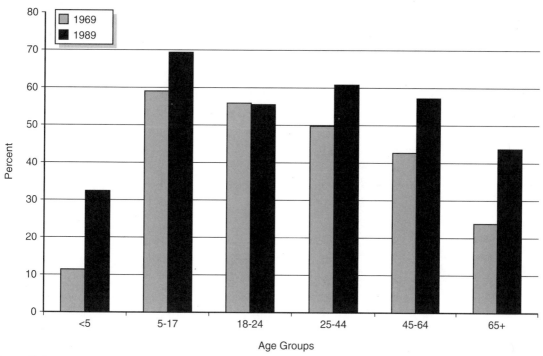

Figure 2–9. Increases in the utilization of dental services, United States, 1969 and 1989. (From US Public Health Service, National Center for Health Statistics. Dental visits: Volume and interval since last visit. United States, 1969. DHEW Publication No. [HSM] 72-1066, Series 10 No 76. Washington DC: Government Printing Office, 1972; US Public Health Service, National Center for Health Statistics: Use of dental services and oral health: United States, 1989. DHHS Publication No. [PHS] 93-1511, Series 10 No 183. Washington DC: Government Printing Office, 1992.)

older years is obvious, and increased use has also taken place among preschool-aged children.

A low use of dental services by older adults was once thought to come from loss of interest in dental health with age, but it is now clear that it is related to loss of teeth rather than interest. The difference was first pointed out in an analysis of 1983 data from the National Health Interview Survey, where it was found that among dentate people, there was little decrease in use of dental services with increasing age.[3] This analysis showed that 59.5% of dentate persons aged 65 to 74 reported a dental visit within the previous year, which was actually more than the 58.4% utilization among dentate persons aged 25 to 34. Among edentulous persons of all ages, however, annual utilization was only 12.6%. The distribution of annual dental visits for American adults aged 35 or more in the 1989 National Health Interview Survey, by age and dentate-edentulous status, is shown in Figure 2–10. When looked at this way, it is remarkable how uniform dental utilization remains with increasing age when people retain their teeth.

Socioeconomic Status

Socioeconomic status (SES) in the United States is usually measured by years of education and annual income, which not surprisingly are closely correlated. SES is directly related to use of dental services; the higher the SES, the greater the use of dental services. As with gender differences, this relationship is found consistently in all industrialized countries, even in those where the cost barrier for dental care has been removed through public financing. For the United States in 1989, utilization for adults aged 22 or more is shown by age for 4 different educational levels in Figure 2–11. The close association between use of dental services and educational levels is obvious, and the difference in the older age groups is especially marked. The majority of edentulous people, and those without dental insurance, are in the lower educational attainment groups, so those factors would be influencing the data seen in Figure 2–11. Once again, it is remarkable how uniform is the use of dental services with increasing age among college-educated people (more than 13 years of education). Persons

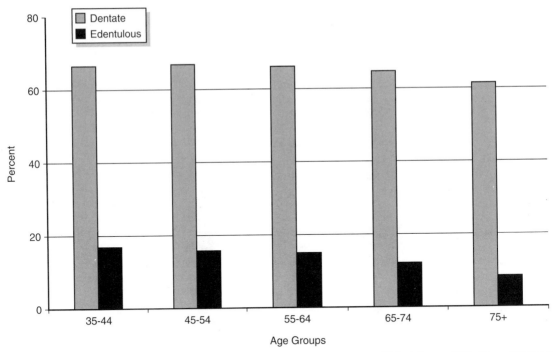

Figure 2–10. Utilization of dental services by dentate and edentulous persons. United States, 1989. (From US Public Health Service, National Center for Health Statistics: Use of dental services and oral health: United States, 1989. DHHS Publication No. [PHS] 93–1511, Series 10 No 183. Washington DC: Government Printing Office, 1992.)

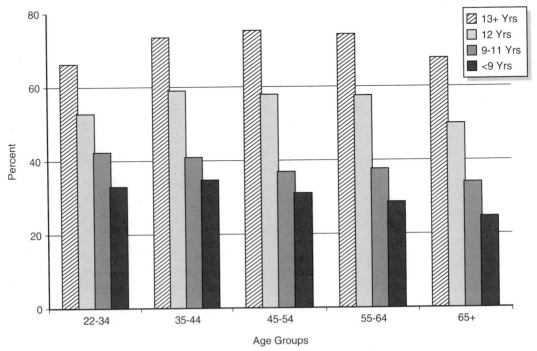

Figure 2–11. Utilization of dental services by years of education received. United States, 1989. (From US Public Health Service, National Center for Health Statistics: Use of dental services and oral health: United States, 1989. DHHS Publication No. [PHS] 93–1511, Series 10 No 183. Washington DC: Government Printing Office, 1992.)

with higher incomes also use dental services much more than do persons with lower incomes, and as noted before, income and educational level are tightly correlated in the United States and Canada.

The reasons for this consistent relationship between SES and use of dental services are more complicated than they might appear. It is easy to say that lower SES people are less interested in oral health or less aware of the value of dental care. That often-heard assertion is rather oversimplified. Values and attitudes are naturally different, and many lesser educated people are from backgrounds in which dental care was virtually nonexistent, so there is none of the middle-class culture of which dental care is a part. More obviously, lower SES groups are less able to afford care when it does exist, and because there are fewer dentists in lower-SES areas (Chapter 9) care is usually less available. Dental insurance has made some difference to the problem of affording care, but experience from a number of countries has long shown that even when the cost barrier is completely removed, there are still marked differences in use of dental services among the different socioeconomic groups.

Race and Ethnicity

In 1989, 59.3% of white Americans reported visiting a dentist, compared with 44.5% of African-Americans and 46.4% of Hispanic Americans. Among the Hispanic groups, 40.9% of Mexican-Americans reported a visit within the last year, fewer than the 53.7% of other Hispanics.[20] It is likely that SES influences this differential seen among Hispanic populations. Continuing with that same theme, utilization data are not easy to interpret because race and ethnicity in the United States are inextricably related to wealth and poverty, education, cultural values, and residential location. Hispanics and African-Americans have also suffered historically from deliberate exclusion from many care facilities, and there are relatively few dental providers from these groups.

Data on the use of dental services by American Indians and Alaska Natives are scarce. Those who live on reservations are largely treated through the Indian Health Service, an agency of the Department of Health and Human Services (Chapter 1). Use of dental services is generally not high, although it varies from one location to another.

Geographic Location

Suburbanites are the most frequent users of dental services in the United States, 60.7% of them reporting a dental visit within the last year in 1989; 54.8% of central city residents and 53.2% of people outside metropolitan areas reported a visit.[20] Almost certainly these distributions are closely related to SES, dental insurance, and race/ethnicity, and perhaps also to age and dentate status.

There are also variations by region of the country, as shown in Figure 2–12. The Northeast, Midwest, and the West show similar usage patterns, but the South has a lower level of utilization. The South has the lowest SES ranking of the 4 regions, as well as the most unfavorable dentist/population ratio, which probably are major factors in explaining this diversity.

General Health

People who consider themselves in excellent health visit a dentist more often than those who see themselves as in good or only fair health. Among those who considered themselves to be in "excellent" health, 61.9% reported a visit during 1989 compared with 51.5% who thought their health was "good," and 39.8% who thought it was "fair or poor."[20] Distributions of a similar nature were found among those who had no restriction of activity compared with those who were limited to some degree.

These findings are hardly unexpected, because people whose mobility is restricted quite naturally would find getting to a dentist more difficult. Those in poor general health may be too preoccupied, or too restricted generally, to face the dentist. These distributions also are likely to be related to age and perhaps to SES.

Dental Insurance

People with dental insurance visit a dentist more often than people without insurance. The 1989 data showed that 71.4% of those with private dental insurance visited a dentist within the last year, compared with 50.0% of those without. The contrast for all age groups is shown in Figure 2–13.

These differences are to be expected because dental insurance can substantially reduce the financial burden of dental care. It was mentioned earlier that cost is not as

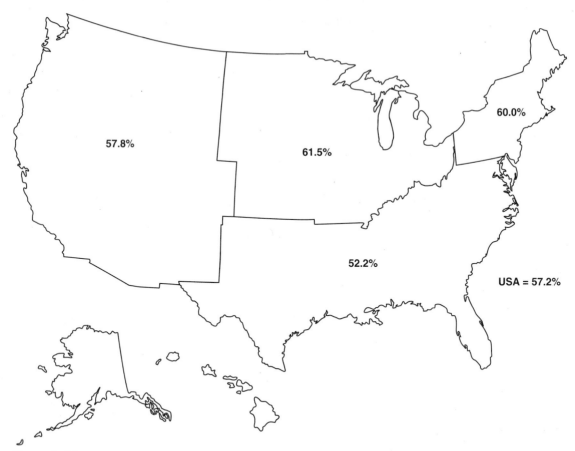

57.8%

61.5%

60.0%

52.2%

USA = 57.2%

Figure 2–12. Proportion of the United States population reporting a dental visit within the last year, by geographic region, 1989. (From US Public Health Service, National Center for Health Statistics: Use of dental services and oral health: United States, 1989. DHHS Publication No. [PHS] 93–1511, Series 10 No 183. Washington DC: Government Printing Office, 1992.)

much of a barrier to receiving dental care as is often thought; even among groups where there is no direct charge for dental treatment, there is still the relationship between receipt of care and SES. To explain the role of dental insurance, we have to look at who has it: Professionals, white-collar workers, and the larger labor unions who receive group dental care as a fringe benefit of employment. So again, there is likely to be an SES relationship, as well as some financial incentive for these groups.

FUTURE USE OF DENTAL SERVICES

Should we expect the trend of steadily increasing dental utilization to continue? If so, how far before it hits a ceiling? These questions are of fundamental importance to students and new graduates, and the data presented give us a basis for making estimates.

Apart from gender, the data show that the most powerful correlates of dental utilization are SES, dentate status, and the extent of dental insurance. Overall economic conditions are also a major factor. Prosperity provides more disposable income for people to afford dental care, permits employers to offer more generous dental insurance plans, and leads to a feeling of optimism. If economic conditions in the United States decline over the long term, however, more people will be forced out of the middle classes, and use of dental services will decline. Poor economic conditions would force many corporations to drop dental insurance, which would also reduce the use of dental services.

Increasing tooth retention (Chapter 7), especially the decline in total tooth loss among the elderly, is reason for optimism about an increase in the use of dental services for the next generation of older Americans. The data clearly show that when people are dentate,

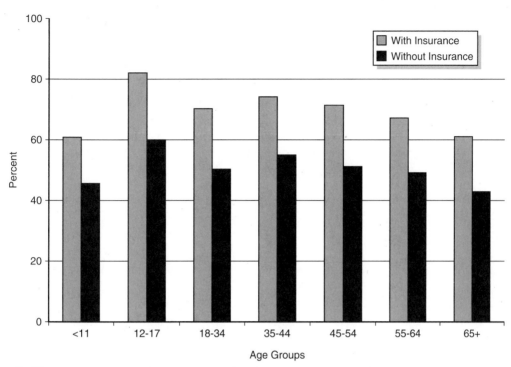

Figure 2–13. Proportion reporting a dental visit within the last year, by age and status of dental insurance. United States, 1989. (From US Public Health Service, National Center for Health Statistics: Use of dental services and oral health: United States, 1989. DHHS Publication No. [PHS] 93-1511, Series 10 No 183. Washington DC: Government Printing Office, 1992.)

they go to the dentist; when they are edentulous, they do not.

As stated earlier, population growth in the United States in recent years has been greatest in the lower SES groups, among African-Americans and Hispanics, groups with relatively low use of dental services. As these groups make up a larger proportion of the population (Figure 2–6), rigid adherence to current methods of providing dental care will lead to a decline in utilization. People in these social strata are largely outside the usual dental insurance groups, and the cuts in public health programs through the 1980s left many of them with little opportunity to receive dental care at all, let alone to adopt habits of regular attendance. Growth in the population utilizing dental services will require the introduction of the lower SES population to dental care, which in turn will require more resources in the public health sector to provide the necessary education and acculturation.

SUMMARY

The use of dental services is tied closely to economic developments and demography,

neither of which dental personnel can do much to influence. Increasing tooth retention is one factor that tends to increase utilization among older Americans. The utilization patterns of younger generations is harder to predict, and overall utilization could remain at current levels, but with a distributional shift away from younger toward older patients. Specific programs aimed at bringing today's minority groups into the dental care system will also be a major step toward improvement of the nation's oral health. Without such action, utilization of dental services could go into long-term decline.

REFERENCES

1. Gift HC. Utilization of professional dental services. In: Cohen LK, Bryant PS, eds: Social sciences and dentistry: A critical bibliography. Vol II. London: Quintessence/Federation Dentaire Internationale, 1984, pp 202–66.
2. Increasing diversity of the U.S. population. SB (Stat Bull Metropolitan Life) 1996;77:12–7.
3. Ismail AI, Burt BA, Hendershot GE, et al. Findings from the dental care supplement of the National Health Interview Survey, 1983. J Am Dent Assoc 1987;114:617–21.

4. Jeffers JR, Bognanno MF, Bartlett JC. On the demand versus need for medical services and the concept of "shortage." Am J Public Health 1971;61:46–63.

5. Spencer AJ. The estimation of need for dental care. J Public Health Dent 1980;40:311–27.

6. Tala H. Oral health in Finland. Helsinki: Finnish National Board of Health, 1989.

7. US Department of Commerce, Bureau of the Census. Statistical abstract of the United States: 1995. 115th ed. Washington DC: Government Printing Office, 1995.

8. US Department of Commerce, Bureau of the Census. Population of the United States: Trends and prospects, 1950-1990. Series P-23 No 49. Washington DC: Government Printing Office, 1974.

9. US Department of Commerce, Bureau of the Census. Current population reports: Estimates of the population of the states by age; 1971 to 1979. Series P-25 No 875. Washington DC: Government Printing Office, 1980.

10. US Department of Commerce, Bureau of the Census. Projections of the population of states by age, sex, and race: 1988 to 2010. Series P-25 No 1017. Washington DC: Government Printing Office, 1989.

11. US Department of Commerce, Bureau of the Census. U.S. population estimates by age, sex, race, and Hispanic origin: 1980 to 1991. Series P-25 No 1095. Washington DC: Government Printing Office, 1993.

12. US Department of Commerce, Bureau of the Census. U.S. population estimates by age, sex, race, and Hispanic origin: 1993 to 2050. Series P-25 No 1104. Washington DC: Government Printing Office, 1993.

13. US Department of Commerce, Bureau of the Census. Population projections for states, by age, sex, race, and Hispanic origin. Series P-25 No 1111. Washington DC: Government Printing Office, 1994.

14. US Department of Commerce, Bureau of the Census. Measuring the effect of benefits and taxes on income and poverty. Series P-60 No 186RD. Washington DC: Government Printing Office, 1994.

15. US Public Health Service, National Center for Health Statistics. Current estimates from the National Health Interview Survey, 1989. DHHS Publication No. (PHS) 90-1504, Series 10 No 176. Washington DC: Government Printing Office, 1990.

16. US Public Health Service, National Center for Health Statistics. Current estimates from the National Health Interview Survey, 1993. DHHS Publication No (PHS) 95-1518, Series 10 No. 190. Washington DC, Government Printing Office, 1994.

17. US Public Health Service, National Center for Health Statistics. Dental care: Interval and frequency of visits. United States, June 1957–June 1959. PHS Publication No 584-B14, Series B No 14. Washington DC: Government Printing Office, 1960.

18. US Public Health Service, National Center for Health Statistics. Dental visits: volume and interval since last visit. United States–1969. DHEW Publication No. (HSM) 72-1066, Series 10 No. 76. Washington DC: Government Printing Office, 1972.

19. US Public Health Service, National Center for Health Statistics. Use of dental services and dental health. United States, 1986. DHHS Publication No. (PHS) 88-1593, Series 10 No 165. Washington DC: Government Printing Office, 1988.

20. US Public Health Service, National Center for Health Statistics. Use of dental services and oral health: United States, 1989. DHHS Publication No. (PHS) 93-1511, Series 10 No 183. Washington DC: Government Printing Office, 1992.

21. Vu MT. World population projections 1984. Washington DC: World Bank, 1984.

3

Ethics and Responsibility in Dental Care

A Framework for Ethical Standards ◆ Individual and Social Responsibility ◆ Individualism in the United States ◆ The Right to Health Care ◆ Ethics in Patient Care ◆ Professional Ethics and Self-Regulation ◆ Ethical Standards in Research ◆ Dentistry's Ethical Challenge: Access to Care for Everyone

As noted in Chapter 1, professionalism brings with it the responsibility to adhere to the highest ethical standards. Even the most conscientious practitioner, however, will find that ethical dilemmas can easily arise. For example, how does a practitioner respond to a patient who wants all her amalgam restorations removed because she believes they are the cause of her chronic fatigue? What is the practitioner's obligation in treating a patient with an infectious disease? Questions like these arise frequently in dental practice, and although definitive answers are not always easy to find, some guidelines can be offered.

This chapter discusses the place of professional ethics in dental care. We discuss the framework for ethical codes, the social and cultural background against which our ethics are defined, and the role of the professional associations in defining ethical codes.

A FRAMEWORK FOR ETHICAL STANDARDS

Ethics, a branch of philosophy and theology, is the systematic study of what is right and good with respect to conduct and character.[21] The nature of moral decisions means that much of the ethics literature asks questions rather than provides answers, and this lack of a "formula" approach can be frustrat-

ing for some. Because ethics is the study of the general nature of morals and of specific moral choices, ethical decisions can vary over time and with different cultural standards.

Four basic principles have become widely accepted as guidelines for decision making in biomedical ethical dilemmas; they apply to dental professionals as they do to physicians and nurses. These principles can be summarized as follows:[4]

- *Beneficence:* which basically means to do no harm and promote good for others.
- *Autonomy:* which is respect for all persons and all points of view.
- *Veracity:* meaning honesty in dealing with others. In dental practice, this would mean pointing out the potential hazards in a course of treatment, as well as the potential benefits.
- *Justice:* providing a person with what is due. Distributive justice is the proper distribution of social benefits and burdens in the community, which makes up the core of much political debate.

For a professional organization, these principles need to be formulated as ethical standards. Standards can take the following forms:

- *Aspirational:* a broadly worded statement of ideals. No precise definitions of right or wrong behavior are given.

27

- *Educational:* which combine the principles with explicit guidelines that can assist decision-making in morally ambiguous situations.
- *Regulatory:* which go a step further and include a set of detailed rules to govern professional conduct and serve as a basis for adjudicating grievances. Such rules are assumed to be enforceable, with a range of sanctions imposed by the profession if the rules are contravened.[10]

Professions adopt ethical standards because that is part of the professional charge; a client's trust in a professional comes in part from the expectation that the professional's behavior is governed by norms prescribed by the group.[10] It is also a public expectation that ethical standards be developed and enforced by any profession with the privilege of self-regulation.

We now examine briefly some social and cultural forces that underlie ethical expectations in the United States.

INDIVIDUAL AND SOCIAL RESPONSIBILITY

Who is responsible for health? Is it society as a whole, or is health each individual's responsibility? That is a broad question, to which the answer can only be some of both.

It is well understood today that individual lifestyle choices are a major factor in determining a person's health status. Every educated person knows the rules: don't smoke, drink in moderation, eat a varied diet that is low in saturated fats and includes fiber, get enough sleep, exercise regularly, click-in the car's seatbelt, maintain friendships. What about those individuals who are unfortunate enough to have genetic predispositions to disease, or are mentally or physically handicapped through no fault of their own? Others became addicted to cigarettes at a time when such addiction was not understood, and some became alcoholic or drug-addicted in response to great social or personal pressures. For some people these conditions are compounded by their inability to pay for necessary medical care. What do we do in these instances?

If we believe that health is solely an individual responsibility, we would shrug our shoulders, say "Bad luck," and be thankful that this wasn't happening to us. But we don't do that; virtually all developed nations accept some degree of social responsibility through health and social support systems for sick people. These systems in many European countries, Canada, Australia, and New Zealand can be extensive, usually more so than their counterparts in the United States. Arguments in the United States can turn toward whether such programs should exist at all, even though many balk at suggestions that the last vestiges of a "safety net" should be removed. There is ongoing vigorous debate, however, about the extent and eligibility criteria for public financing of health and welfare, and about the right division between public and private financing for them. American attitudes toward publicly financed social systems differ from those in other developed countries, so it is worth looking at how American cultural attitudes toward individualism and social responsibility have developed.

INDIVIDUALISM IN THE UNITED STATES

Americans cherish their individual rights and freedoms; individualism has been a more powerful cultural force in the United States than in other countries.[5] Many of the settlers who first immigrated to America (voluntary settlers at least) were leaving rigid social, religious, or political systems to seek a new life where they would be free of the constraints they had left behind. An abundance of natural resources and a seemingly limitless frontier gave rise to the attitude that in America people could mold their own destinies largely by their own efforts. Although historical evidence shows that this belief is at best only partly true,[5] it still remains a powerful cultural perception.

The high point of unfettered laissez-faire capitalism in Western Europe occurred in the mid-19th century, and in the United States a generation or so later. By the early years of the 20th century, however, philosophies in Europe were turning away from individualism toward more shared responsibility for basics such as housing, education, social security, and health care. By the 1970s, national state-sponsored social programs were the norm in Europe, but less so in the United States. One reason suggested for the slower development in the United States is that America's relative isolation from external political turbulence during its formative years allowed the development of a more introspective national character than was the case in Europe.[22] Another reason, given that catastrophic events have a way of hastening social change, is that the effects of two major wars in the first half of the 20th century hastened the development of social welfare programs in Europe. The United States largely escaped the social devastation of those wars. It should be remembered, however, that the first Social Security Act in the United States was passed in 1935 in the midst of the great depression, which was a social catastrophe by any measure.

Another major contribution to individualism in American society comes from what is referred to as the *Puritan ethic,* which historians consider to have arrived with the first English colonists.[8] Many of these and other pioneers were members of nonconformist religious groups, who brought their rigid beliefs about human nature to the new land. These attitudes became part of the American national character, and remain prominent today. Essentially, the Puritan ethic is a set of beliefs and attitudes that holds that God rewards people for their honest toil in this life as well as in the next, and that individual wealth or poverty is justified and largely controllable by one's own efforts. It follows that under the Puritan ethic the accumulation of great personal wealth can be seen as a reward for virtue and hard work, just as poverty can be seen as a punishment for immorality or laziness. The Puritan ethic also produces a strong aversion to paying taxes, especially for social programs aimed at helping those seen as the "undeserving" poor.

The first serious questioning of individualism in the United States came during the widespread social distress caused by the great depression of the 1930s. Many people lost everything at that time through what was clearly no fault of their own, and the response of the federal government was a series of emergency relief measures aimed at avoiding total societal collapse. Most of these programs no longer exist, although Social Security has not only survived but has become institutionalized as a major "entitlement" that figures prominently in current political debate.

World War II (1939–1945) followed the depression, after which the next wave of social activity followed the revelations about the extent and consequences of poverty in the United States during the early 1960s. The 89th Congress (1964–1965) passed a series of legislative measures intended to improve social equity; the main measures were the Medicare and Medicaid health programs (Chapter 8), the Voting Rights Act, the Economic Opportunity Act, the Model Cities Act, and the Elementary and Secondary Education Act. The more conservative mood that set in during the 1980s, a growing awareness of limited resources, and a loss of faith in government's ability to solve complex problems slowed this trend. The 1990s brought both a general acceptance of the need to reduce the national debt and perhaps a slowly growing realization that it is not in the national interest to tolerate immense social problems such as homelessness, inadequate education, and lack of access to health care.

THE RIGHT TO HEALTH CARE

American attitudes, historically shaped by individualism and the Puritan ethic, are evolving only slowly to the belief that access to health care is a right rather than a privilege.[3, 7] The "right to health care" is an emotional and often misunderstood concept, one frequently interpreted as "the right to health." Of course, no one has a right to health. Health, an elusive entity to define, is a dynamic state influenced by such factors as genetic endowment, nutrition, housing and environment, life habits, personal attitudes and beliefs, and medical care received, probably in that order of importance. Although medical care has probably been overvalued as a determinant of health[3, 12, 14] most individuals at some time in their lives have a need for it, sometimes an urgent need.

Health care has always been rationed in one way or another. The traditional rationing method has been fee-for-service, meaning that those who can afford care get it, whereas those who cannot afford it do not. Simple enough, although there is a cost in wasted human resources. This philosophy was challenged in the United States during the 1960s, when access to health care was extended to millions of poorer citizens. As would be expected, one result of better access to care was that public expenditures on medical care increased substantially. When the public mood later swung toward emphasis on controlling medical care expenditures, managed care emerged in the 1980s and grew rapidly in the 1990s (Chapter 8). Managed care appeared to reduce the rate of increase of medical expenditures, although it did so by introducing other forms of rationing. Ethical problems have multiplied as a result.

ETHICS IN PATIENT CARE

Society has bestowed self-government on the dental profession because it recognizes that the profession conducts itself honorably in its contacts with patients. As discussed in Chapter 1, this is one of the cornerstones of professionalism. Because the professional has knowledge that the patient does not, and is in a position to evaluate the likely outcomes of treatment better than the patient, the professional carries the burden of avoiding paternalism, and sharing her knowledge and experience with the patient in such a way that the patient can make informed choices.[17] Regardless of the best of intentions, this is frequently difficult to do, especially when a patient yearns to put unqualified trust in the professional:

> Although intellectually patients—including doctors when they become patients—know that doctors are not infallible, emotionally we want to believe that they are, that they know what they are doing and are capable of doing it. The most skeptical of us longs to leave such skepticism in the waiting room.[11]

This situation can force the professional to take a paternalistic role, no matter how reluctantly, and it can sharpen the conflict between professional and proprietary values that frequently arises in dental practice.[16] Some have argued that dentistry needs well-defined standards of care to fall back on in such circumstances,[11] but the profession has never been comfortable about defining such standards because of concerns about infringing on professional judgment. The American Dental Association (ADA) has made a hesitant first step in the direction of standards with its Dental Practice Parameters, adopted by the House of Delegates in 1994 and 1995, in which broad descriptions of what constitutes acceptable procedures are preceded by statements that the clinical judgment of the dentist comes first. Ethically, it could be added that the dentist has the obligation to form her clinical judgment on the best available science rather than a personal preference or unfounded belief. Discharging this professional obligation requires the dentist to have a good grasp of what constitutes scientific study (Chapter 12) and to keep up with the literature and with continuing education. Regardless of the framework for studying ethics, the requirement to maintain professional competence is a prime ethical responsibility.[17]

PROFESSIONAL ETHICS AND SELF-REGULATION

The ADA maintains a Code of Ethics, which is reviewed and amended periodically by the association's Council on Ethics, Bylaws, and Judicial Affairs. The current version of the Code of Ethics can be found on the ADA's website. This code would be classified as educational, according to the types of standards listed earlier. This code is primarily concerned with issues related to the care of patients, although it also deals with the handling of fees, referrals, criticism of colleagues, advertising, and limitation of practice to a specialty. The code has been modified over the years as new issues arise and as societal views on particular issues evolve. It is also influenced by judicial outcomes, as evidenced by growth in the legal advisory opinions in the code. As an example, the 1982 statement on patient selection stated:

> While dentists, in serving the public, may exercise reasonable discretion in selecting patients for their practices, dentists shall not refuse to accept patients into their practice or deny dental service to patients because of the patient's race, creed, color, sex or national origin.[1]

That statement was unchanged in later versions of the code, but an advisory opinion, which dealt primarily with treating infected patients, was appended after 1988. This opinion stated:

> A dentist has the general obligation to provide care to those in need. A decision not to provide treatment to an individual because the individual has AIDS or is HIV seropositive, based solely on that fact, is unethical. Decisions with regard to the type of dental treatment provided or referrals made or suggested, in such instances, should be made on the same basis as they are made with other patients, that is, whether the individual dentist believes he or she has need of another's skills, knowledge, equipment or experience and whether the dentist believes, after consultation with the patient's physician if appropriate, the patient's health status would be significantly compromised by the provision of dental treatment.[2]

This advisory opinion is an example of an issue that causes misgivings among practitioners who do not feel it is unethical to turn away an AIDS patient on the grounds that the health of the dentist and staff would be unduly at risk if treatment were offered. Despite the facts that the human immunodeficiency virus (HIV) is extremely difficult to transmit through dentist-patient contact[19]

(Chapter 6), and that many dentists have treated asymptomatic HIV-infected individuals without knowing it, dentists' attitudes about the willingness to treat infected patients are progressing only slowly.[18]

The obligation to keep current through continuing education and reading the literature, discussed earlier in this chapter, is given only cursory mention in the ADA's professional code. Although some think that this issue should be stated more strongly, perhaps it is being overtaken by events. Minnesota was the first state to introduce mandatory continuing education as a requirement for dental relicensure in 1969, and by the mid-1990s most states had such a requirement in place. It could be argued that continuing education is therefore no longer an ethical responsibility but a legal one. It would be a pity, however, if continuing education came to be interpreted solely as a legal requirement; uncaring practitioners can always fulfill the requirements on paper without transferring the knowledge to practice. Regulations aside, the ethical responsibility still remains for practitioners to do their best to continue professional education.

Community service is also dealt with rather vaguely in the ADA code. Section 1-C of the current code (from the ADA website) states:

> Since dentists have an obligation to use their skills, knowledge, and experience for the improvement of the dental health of the public and are encouraged to be leaders in their community, dentists in such service shall conduct themselves in such a manner as to maintain or elevate the esteem of the profession.

Some dentists involved in a fluoridation campaign in the community, for example, have thought that an appearance on local television may contravene the spirit of the ethical constraint on excessive advertising, even if such an appearance would help the campaign. This unduly cautious interpretation has to be respected, although the statement in the code was never intended to preclude such obviously-public-spirited activity. Additional comments on working cooperatively with public health authorities would also be likely to result in better oral health for the public.

Dental hygienists should be familiar with the Code of Ethics approved by the American Dental Hygienists' Association (ADHA) in 1995, and available from ADHA. Aspects dealing with professional conduct and patient care are generally similar to those of the ADA. The ADHA lists as "basic beliefs" that all people should have access to health care, justly and fairly distributed, and that people are responsible for their own health and entitled to make choices regarding their health. Dentists may not give much thought to the ethical problems of hygienists, but a national survey of ADHA members in the late 1980s disclosed the three most frequent ethical issues faced by hygienists to be (a) observation of a dentist's behavior in conflict with standard infection control procedures, (b) failure of the dentist to refer patients to specialists, such as periodontists, and (c) nondiagnosis of oral disease by the dentist.[13] Although 86% of those responding said that they had some instruction in ethical theory, only 51% reported that they had received instruction in how to cope with these ethical problems. It is noted that ADHA's 1995 Code of Ethics includes a requirement for a hygienist to report inappropriate, inadequate, or substandard care to the proper authorities.

ETHICAL STANDARDS IN RESEARCH

Researchers bear the responsibility for identifying and propagating truth in matters of science. Much research involves studies with humans and human tissues, as well as with animals, and there are strict rules governing research with both.

Although codes defining what is acceptable treatment of humans in research go back a long way, the horror and revulsion that followed the disclosure of Nazi "experiments" during World War II (1939–1945) brought serious public attention to the issue. This led to the 1949 Nuremberg Code, which introduced the requirements that research subjects be able to exercise choice, have the legal and intellectual capacity to give consent, and be able to understand what they are consenting to.[15] Since its adoption, the Nuremberg Code has served as the basis for the extensive legal requirements that many countries have developed to govern the participation of humans in research. Legal requirements aside, there is always the ethical obligation of researchers to treat human research volunteers with respect and dignity. Codes for treatment of animals in research are also now well developed.

The International Association for Dental

**Table 3–1. SUGGESTED ETHICAL
CONVENTIONS FOR
RESEARCH INVOLVING
HUMAN SUBJECTS***

1. The research must be scientifically sound, with an identifiable prospect of benefit.
2. Human subjects must be selected equitably.
3. Risks to humans, and the numbers of humans involved, must both be minimized.
4. Voluntary informed consent must be obtained from all human subjects, or from their proxies, before any research is started.
5. Human research subjects must be permitted to withdraw from the research at any time, and to be assured that such withdrawal will not prejudice any ordinary treatment they may be receiving.
6. People must be withdrawn from a research project as soon as there is any indication of possible harm, physical or psychological, as a consequence of their being research subjects.
7. The privacy of research participants and the confidentiality of the data concerning them must both be protected.
8. Research results must be written honestly and accurately.

*Based on a preamble and principles for Ethics in Research adopted by the International Association for Dental Research in 1995.

Research (IADR) adopted a preamble and principles for a Code of Ethics at its annual meeting in 1995. This code is *aspirational* in nature. Research is essentially a search for truth, and this code outlines the numerous principles that govern that search. An example of the ethical requirements that could be applied to research with humans, based on the IADR preamble, is listed in Table 3–1. It has been suggested that codes of research ethics need to distinguish between two types of problematic practices: those that are clearly misconduct because they undermine the trustworthiness of science (e.g., data falsification), and those that are unethical but are better described as disrespectful of the work of others. An example of the latter kind is plagiarism, which is unethical but rarely undermines the trustworthiness of science.[6]

DENTISTRY'S ETHICAL CHALLENGE: ACCESS TO CARE FOR EVERYONE

An overriding ethical challenge to the dental professions is to meet their stated aims of bringing oral health care to all members of the public. That can only happen with the right mix of public and private care.

The vast majority of the dentist-attending public receives its dental care from private practitioners. Private practice in the United States is well suited for the healthy, employed, dentally conscious middle-class patient for whom accessibility to private care is rarely a problem, who can generally afford necessary treatment, and who practices good oral hygiene. Private practice has adapted readily to dental insurance since that payment mechanism began to grow in the 1960s, which makes private practice even more attractive. The popular expression "the best dental care in the world" is accurate enough in these circumstances.

However, not every prospective dental patient in the United States fits the category just described. As discussed in Chapter 2, many Americans are poor, and it is a major challenge for the nation to find ways of making health care accessible to the growing proportion of Americans without health insurance of any kind—17.3% in 1994.[20] (This is general health insurance, not dental insurance, for whom the proportion without is nearer 50%.) Intertwined with the world of poverty are the homeless, the unemployed and unemployable, and the homebound and chronically ill. The marginally mentally retarded, who used to reside in institutions, can have the capacity and the will to work but need the support of sheltered workshops to do so. When these are not available, these individuals can drift into dependency again. For those who remain institutionalized for mental and physical disabilities, dental care is sporadically available at best. There is also the large number of working poor, usually uninsured and in minimum-wage positions, who can find the typical private practice not only expensive but also intimidating.

These are groups for whom regular visits to the dentist occupy no place in their lives. Not only is dental care financially out of reach for the people concerned, but many practitioners can signal the message, often inadvertently, that they would prefer not to have to treat such patients. Private practice is most efficient when patients understand the need for care, know how to behave while receiving treatment, and are from the same socioeconomic group as the dentist. Disabled people take longer to treat and often require special equipment and training to be treated satisfactorily. The circumstances of poverty mean that the poor are often interested only in minimal care and often skip appointments. As a consequence, dental care for many of these groups can be delivered effectively only through public health agencies.

The need for dental public health services is self-evident, but there are still formidable practical problems in making them available. Public services in the United States, by contrast with their counterparts in Canada and Europe, are chronically underfunded. This is partly an offshoot of the individualist culture described earlier, which leads to public services being held in low esteem. The problem was exacerbated by the severe cuts in public spending for social services during the 1980s,[9] cuts that have gone even deeper in the 1990s. Even when resources are adequate, treatment for these special groups is usually less efficient than it is for patients in private practice. Oral health needs are often greater, appointments can be missed if a patient has a chance to earn some money instead of going to the dentist, and the mentally or physically disabled just take more time to treat. Many poor people change their place of residence frequently in search of jobs, thus making continuity of care impossible.

There is no simple answer to these problems, although adequate funding of public health departments would enable most of them to be dealt with in time. Adequate funding would permit better staffing and equipment levels, acceptable clinical facilities, special transport where necessary, and community outreach programs to educate the special groups on the benefits of dental care. Adequate funding for public services would assist more dentists and hygienists to receive special training than is possible at present, so that in time the care received by these diverse groups would approach that received by most mainstream Americans. Public treatment programs are not a threat to private practice, as they serve a different patient group.

The overriding ethical challenge to all in dentistry is achieving the noble goal of adequate oral health for all. The right mix of public and private services is needed for this to occur.

REFERENCES

1. American Dental Association, Council on Bylaws and Judicial Affairs. Principles of ethics and code of professional conduct. J Am Dent Assoc 1982;105:493–5.
2. American Dental Association, Council on Ethics, Bylaws, and Judicial Affairs. Principles of ethics and code of professional conduct. J Am Dent Assoc 1988;117:657–61.
3. Banta D. What is health care? In Jonas S, ed: Health care delivery in the United States. 1st ed. New York: Springer, 1977, pp 12–39.
4. Beauchamp TL, Childress JF. Principles of biomedical ethics. 4th ed. New York: OUP, 1994.
5. Billington RA. Frontiers. In: Woodward CV, ed: The comparative approach to American history. New York: Basic Books, 1968, pp 75–90.
6. Camenisch PF. The moral foundations of scientific ethics and responsibility. J Dent Res 1996;75:825–31.
7. Chapman CB, Talmadge JM. The evolution of the right to health concept in the United States. Pharos 1971;34:30–51.
8. Cooke A. America. New York: Knopf, 1974.
9. Evans CA. A national survey of public health dental services in local health departments. J Public Health Dent 1984;44:112–9.
10. Frankel MS. Developing ethical standards for responsible research. J Dent Res 1996;75:832–5.
11. Friedman JW, Atchison KA. The standard of care: an ethical responsibility of public health dentistry. J Public Health Dent 1993;53:165–9.
12. Fuchs V. Who shall live? Health, economics, and social choice. New York: Basic Books, 1974.
13. Gaston MA, Brown DM, Waring MB. Survey of ethical issues in dental hygiene. J Dent Hyg 1990;64:216–23.
14. Illich I. Medical nemesis: The expropriation of health. New York: Bantam Books, 1976.
15. McCarthy CR. Legal and regulatory considerations concerning research involving human subjects. J Dent Res 1980;59(Spec Issue C):1228–34.
16. Nash DA. A tension between two cultures. Dentistry as a profession and dentistry as a proprietary. J Dent Educ 1994;58:301–6.
17. Ozar DT. A framework for studying professional ethics. J Am Coll Dent 1991;58:4,6–9.
18. Sadowsky D, Kunzel C. Measuring dentists' willingness to treat HIV-positive patients. J Am Dent Assoc 1994;125:705–10.
19. US Public Health Service, Centers for Disease Control and Prevention. Recommended infection-control practices for dentistry. MMWR 1993;42, No RR-8.
20. US Public Health Service, National Center for Health Statistics. Health United States 1994. DHHS Publication No. (PHS) 95-1232. Washington DC: Government Printing Office, 1995.
21. Weinstein BD. Ethics and its role in dentistry. Gen Dent 1992;40:414–7.
22. Woodward CV. The comparability of American history. In: Woodward CV, ed: The comparative approach to American history. New York: Basic Books, 1968, pp 3–17.

The Practice of Dental Public Health

What is Public Health? ◆ Identifying a Public Health Problem ◆ Development of Public Health in the United States ◆ Dental Public Health ◆ Dental Public Health and the Private Practitioner ◆ Collection and Use of Data in Dental Public Health ◆ Personal and Community Health Care: Similarities and Differences

Public health is an aspect of life that most people take for granted, insofar as they think about it at all. We take it for granted that we can drink a glass of water without thinking about cholera and can buy a packet of frozen vegetables without worrying about botulism. Thoughts of scarlet fever, typhoid, and polio-myelitis simply never cross our consciousness. To many of the younger generations, dental caries is almost as distant as those infectious diseases from the past. This state of affairs has not just happened; it is the end point of years of public health research and practice.

The low profile of public health has both good and bad aspects. Although it is good that "invisible" basics like drains, sewage treatment, fluoridated drinking water, and immunizations against infectious diseases are part of the accepted institutions of modern life, it is not good that most people have so little grasp of how public health functions. Without a constituency to press for them, funding and legislation for public health can be eroded, with subsequent threats to health and the quality of life. By way of contrast, everyone is acutely conscious of their access, or lack of it, to personal health services, and that subject is a constant political issue.

This chapter examines the structure and practice of dental public health in the United States and argues that dental public health and private dental practice need to work together if the community's oral health is to continue to improve.

WHAT IS PUBLIC HEALTH?

Health is an elusive concept to define. The World Health Organization (WHO) definition[32] is often quoted: "health comprises complete physical, mental, and social well-being and is not merely the absence of disease." Noble indeed, but too idealistic to be of much practical value. A sociologist's pragmatic definition is that health is "a state of optimum capacity for the performance of valued tasks."[16] This is a more useful definition in that it presents health as a means to an end, that of maximizing the quality of life, rather than an end in itself.

Public health, too, does not lend itself to easy definition. Among the many definitions that have been formulated, Winslow's is the most widely-accepted and quoted. Winslow defined public health as "the science and art of preventing disease, prolonging life, and promoting physical health and efficiency through organized community efforts."[31] The generality of Winslow's definition has much to do with its widespread acceptance; however, it still provides little working knowledge of public health. A more businesslike definition is "the organization and application of public resources to prevent dependency which would otherwise result from disease or injury."[18] In this context, dependency is defined as a condition that requires external resources, such as an attendant or medication, to carry out the activities of daily living. Just as some definitions of public health can be vague and idealistic, this one might go too far in seeing only dependency as the outcome to be avoided. Public health should deal with quality-of-life conditions, when it is economically reasonable to do so, rather than just those that result in death or dependency.

A more recent definition of the public health mission, one that accepts health as a means rather than an end, is this: ". . . fulfilling society's interest in assuring conditions in which people can be healthy."[11] This definition seems to encompass everything from maintaining the stratospheric ozone layer to providing recreational facilities or dental care when needed. The landmark report from the Institute of Medicine, from which that last definition came, went on to describe the functions of public health agencies as the following:

- *Assessment:* The regular collection and dissemination of data on health status, community health needs, and epidemiologic studies.
- *Policy Development:* Promoting use of the base of scientific knowledge in decision making on policy matters affecting the public's health.
- *Assurance:* Assurance of the constituents that services necessary to achieve mutually agreed upon goals are provided, either directly, by encouraging other entities, or by regulation.[11]

The essence of public health practice is shown in Table 4–1, which presents a succinct definition of the mission and basic services that only public health can provide. This statement, developed by the American Public Health Association, was adopted in 1994 and has since received virtually universal acceptance.

Identifying a Public Health Problem

Ask people in the street whether they consider AIDS a public health problem, and most will give a resoundingly affirmative reply. What about deaths from traffic accidents? There will be much more equivocation, even though the number of deaths each year from road accidents is similar to that from AIDS.[28] Substance abuse similarly is seen by most as a major social and public health problem, but infant mortality would have fewer supporters, even though nearly one fourth of all expectant mothers receive no prenatal care in

Table 4–1. ESSENTIAL SERVICES IN PUBLIC HEALTH IN THE UNITED STATES

Vision
Healthy people in healthy communities
Mission
Promote health and prevent disease

PUBLIC HEALTH

- Prevents epidemics and the spread of disease
- Protects against environmental hazards
- Prevents injuries
- Promotes and encourages healthy behaviors
- Responds to disasters and assists communities in recovery
- Assures the quality and accessibility of health services

ESSENTIAL PUBLIC HEALTH SERVICES

- Monitor health status to identify community problems
- Diagnose and investigate health problems and health hazards in the community
- Inform, educate, and empower people about health issues
- Mobilize community partnerships and action to solve health problems
- Develop policies and plans that support individual and community health efforts
- Enforce laws and regulations that protect health and ensure safety
- Link people to needed personal health care services and assure the provision of health care when otherwise unavailable
- Assure an expert public health work force
- Evaluate effectiveness, accessibility, and quality of health services
- Research for new insights and innovative solutions to health problems

From American Public Health Association. Report of the Core Public Health Functions Steering Committee. The Nation's Health, Dec. 1994, p. 1, 3.

the first trimester.[28] Given that handling a public health problem demands some allocation of resources, how is a public health problem determined?

Over the years some criteria have emerged. Blackerby,[5] for example, stated that a public health problem exists if (a) there is a condition or situation that is a widespread actual or potential cause of morbidity or mortality, (b) there is a body of knowledge about this situation that could relieve the situation, and (c) this body of knowledge is not being applied. These criteria, however, are restrictive. The Black Death in the 14th century, for example, killed one third of the population of Europe in 3 years. It was certainly a public health problem, even though there was no body of knowledge with regard to managing it. Subsequent epidemics of typhoid, cholera, yellow fever, and other infectious diseases were also public health problems before there were effective means to deal with them; the same is true for some viral infections today. In the situation portrayed by Blackerby, failure to take action for a problem is a breakdown in public organization or political will.

Additional criteria can broaden the scope of what constitutes a public health problem. Public perception is one, as in the example of the human immunodeficiency virus (HIV) epidemic, the end point of which is AIDS. If enough of the public perceive a public health problem, then the mandate exists to allocate resources to deal with it. HIV is in that category (even though the only means to prevent its spread, apart from the barrier precautions in medical and dental practice, are behavior modifications). Not only public perception, but governmental perception goes far toward defining a public health problem. When a governing body assigns a problem to the public health agency for attention, virtually by definition it is a public health problem. If a president, governor, or mayor defines a public health problem by decree, then a public health problem it is, whether or not public health professionals agree. These latter two types of decision, legislative mandate and executive order, can have the advantage of ensuring immediate action and the disadvantage of disturbing the orderly process of program planning and operation.

Today, we can define a public health problem as an issue that meets the following criteria:

- There is a condition or situation that is a widespread actual or potential cause of morbidity or mortality.
- There is a perception on the part of the public, government, or public health authorities that the condition is a public health problem.

Using cigarette smoking as an illustration, the first condition has been satisfied since the first report from the Surgeon General of the United States in 1964.[29] There is no question that the second condition has also been met. These criteria have also been met with the HIV epidemic. Allocation of public resources to deal with a recognized problem is a logical consequence, although not a criterion for problem recognition. In the case of cigarette smoking, there has been considerable action through widespread public education campaigns, advertising bans, and efforts to block the sale of cigarettes to minors. On the other hand, the public is divided about condom distribution and needle-exchange programs intended to restrict the spread of HIV.

Development of Public Health in the United States

Early public health practice in the colonies on the eastern seaboard naturally reflected the English experience. The first English Poor Laws, dating from the 17th century, put the burden of caring for the disadvantaged on the local community. This was rational enough in an agricultural society in which there was little mobility. But when the Industrial Revolution took hold in Britain during the late 18th century, the Poor Laws broke down, for industrialization was really a massive social revolution.[27] Mass migration to the cities created overcrowding, disease, and epidemics. The laissez-faire economic attitudes of the time led to great wealth for some, the emergence of a comfortable middle class, and appalling squalor for many. The Poor Laws, which dealt only with the relief of destitution, were not designed for these completely new kinds of social and health problems.

The ideology of laissez-faire economics in Victorian Britain, combined with an acceptance of Malthusian theories of population growth, led to only grudging action to improve the lot of the destitute. Malthus, a 19th-century English country clergyman, wrote that unrestricted growth of population would eventually exceed the expansion of the food supply.[15] The growth of population therefore needed to be checked, either by "moral restraint" or by the inroads of starvation, disease, or other disasters, which Malthus grouped under the cheerful heading of "misery and vice." Public attitudes at the time supported Malthus' theory that terrible living conditions were not the result of uneven socioeconomic development but rather the consequence of necessary natural laws. Given these views, new public welfare programs that were as degrading as possible were perceived as being in the public interest, as well as morally justified.

Although Britain's provision of health services subsequently turned full circle to the establishment of a National Health Service in 1948, these condescending views on public health and welfare were the norm when organized public health development began in the

United States during the 19th century. It was not an environment in which public health could grow much beyond attempts to limit the spread of epidemics. Not surprisingly, 19th century industrialization produced the same pattern of social turbulence in the United States as had occurred earlier in England.[7] At a local level, similar upheavals are still seen today when the abrupt closure of an industry can blight the vacated community. These disruptions take place now in a highly mobile society, where the old Poor Laws approach that local communities should be fully responsible for public assistance is clearly obsolete. In a modern industrial society, such problems are national in scope and should be treated that way.

One reason why the modern American approach to public health and welfare differs from the current British model is that the stern Puritan views of the early European settlers have had a more sustained influence on public policy in the United States than in Britain and Europe. One expression of the Puritan ethic in the United States is that general welfare relief and payment for health care services for the indigent remained linked together longer than they did in European countries, compounding rather than disentangling the problems.[25] When added to the American culture of individualism, and the relative freedom from the wartime cycle of social disruption and reform, it is not hard to see why communal attitudes toward health and environment have never really flourished in the United States.

Dentistry did not play a significant part in the early development of public health in the United States. Oral health was of little concern at a time when the population was decimated periodically by typhoid, diphtheria, cholera, smallpox, and gastroenteric diseases. Although a few public clinics were established on a voluntary basis by dentists as early as the mid-19th century, public dental care facilities remained almost nonexistent for many years.[21] The US Public Health Service, for example, did not employ dentists on a regular basis until 1919,[22] and philanthropic dental clinics such as Eastman, Forsyth, Guggenheim, Mott, and Strong-Carter opened between 1910 and 1930.

DENTAL PUBLIC HEALTH

Dental public health is one of the 8 specialties of dentistry in the United States. The American Board of Dental Public Health adapted Winslow's definition to develop one subsequently approved by the American Association of Public Health Dentistry, the Oral Health Section of the American Public Health Association, and the American Dental Association (ADA):

> Dental public health is the science and art of preventing and controlling dental diseases and promoting dental health through organized community efforts. It is that form of dental practice which serves the community as a patient rather than the individual. It is concerned with the dental health education of the public, with applied dental research, and with the administration of group dental care programs as well as the prevention and control of dental diseases on a community basis.[2]

Implicit in this definition is the requirement that the specialist have broad knowledge and skills in program administration, research methods, the prevention and control of oral diseases, and the methods of financing and providing dental care services. Table 4–2 is the dental corollary of the public health functions listed in Table 4–1, a concise listing of the essential functions of dental public health as adopted by the Association of State and Territorial Dental Directors.

Dentists or dental hygienists have entered the field when they are employed full-time with the administration of public health programs (which can include health promotion, community prevention, and provision of dental care to specified groups); become faculty members in departments dealing with community-oriented dental practice; or when they become researchers in epidemiology, prevention, or provision of health services. Some researchers in the behavioral sciences related to dental health can also be considered "public healthers." Dentists become recognized specialists when, in addition to full-time employment in the fields mentioned, they achieve diplomate status with the American Board of Dental Public Health. Specialty certification first requires satisfying the educational requirements of the Council on Dental Education of the ADA (i.e., 2 years of accredited advanced graduate education in the specialty, plus a work experience requirement, and then completing the specialty board examinations).

Although there are fewer than 200 board-certified specialists in dental public health, the specialty's influence on the oral health of the public is greater than those numbers would suggest.[1] Dental public health profes-

Table 4–2. ESSENTIAL STATE DENTAL PUBLIC HEALTH SERVICES TO PROMOTE ORAL HEALTH IN THE UNITED STATES

ASSESSMENT

- Assess oral health status and needs so that problems can be identified and addressed
- Analyze determinants of identified oral health needs, including resources
- Assess the fluoridation status of water systems and other sources of fluoride
- Implement an oral health surveillance system to identify, investigate, and monitor oral health problems and health hazards

POLICY DEVELOPMENT

- Develop plans and policies through a collaborative process that supports individual and community oral health efforts to address oral health needs
- Provide leadership to address oral health problems by maintaining a strong oral health unit within the health agency
- Mobilize community partnerships between and among policy makers, professionals, organizations, groups, the public, and others to identify and implement solutions to oral health problems

ASSURANCE

- Inform, educate, and empower the public regarding oral health problems and solutions
- Promote and enforce laws and regulations that protect and improve oral health, ensure safety, and ensure accountability for the public's well-being
- Link people to needed population-based oral health services, personal oral health services, and support services, and assure the availability, access, and acceptability of these services by enhancing system capacity, including directly supporting or providing services when necessary
- Support services and implementation of programs that focus on primary and secondary prevention
- Assure that the public health and personal health work force has the capacity and expertise to effectively address oral health needs
- Evaluate effectiveness, accessibility, and quality of population-based and personal oral health services
- Conduct research and support demonstration projects to gain new insights and applications of innovative solutions to oral health problems

From Association of State and Territorial Dental Directors. Essential state public health services to promote oral health in the United States. Typescript, Jan. 1997.

sionals are employed by federal, state, or local health departments; are conducting research in universities and government agencies; and are administrators in professional organizations and various foundations. Dental public health practice gets away from the relative isolation of the dental office, for its programs require cooperative effort with other professionals such as physicians, nurses, engineers, social workers, and nutritionists. Among the rewards is the ability to bring about improvement of the oral health status of populations rather than single patients. Public health dentists serving in the Indian Health Service of the US Public Health Service, for example, have demonstrated, over the last generation, their ability to increase dental care for several million Native Americans from a bare emergency service to comprehensive care for many, and carried out in excellent clinical facilities. Similarly, a dental public health professional who institutes water fluoridation for a community has done more for its oral health than could be achieved in a lifetime of dental practice.

Achievements of dental public health professionals include the epidemiologic studies that established the basis for community water fluoridation, clinical trials to demonstrate the effectiveness of fluoride toothpastes and other products, and the implementation of those caries-control programs which have been fundamental to the decline in caries among children.[1, 6] Oral epidemiologists have also charted the natural progression of periodontal diseases,[4] and are beginning to assess other oral conditions about which little is known. Administrators in dental public health pioneered the concept of providing regular dental care in a logical, sequential way for large population groups,[9, 10, 30] and they demonstrated the increased productivity that efficient use of dental auxiliaries brings to patient care.[14, 17] Dental hygienists have proven their value in dental public health well beyond their traditional roles as educators. Hygienists act as directors of fluoride mouthrinse programs, members of epidemiologic survey teams, sealant teams, and in several capacities in the growing field of special programs for the elderly.

To round out this discussion of what dental public health is, it might be useful to state what it is not. It is not just "welfare dentistry," although provision of care to persons who do not fit the private practice mode is part of it. It is not just "Medicaid dentistry," although improving that creaky and inefficient program is of concern to all health professionals. It is not just conducting surveys of oral health, although monitoring disease trends and collecting data for program planning and evaluation is an integral part of public health practice. It is not just fluoridation, although dental public health has always been in the front line for that public health measure. Similarly, dental public health is not "socialized dentistry," HMOs, PPOs, OSHA regulations, infection control, quality assurance, financial support (or lack of it) for dental education, or expanded functions for dental auxiliaries. And as the Institute of Medicine report made clear, public health is not just the provider of last resort; its function goes well beyond filling the health care gaps for those whom the private sector cannot or will not treat.[11]

Simply put, dental public health is concern for, and activity directed toward, the improvement and protection of the oral health of the whole population. Narrowing the role of dental public health only to groups defined as "high-risk" or "underserved" would exclude such basic activities as the efforts to control tobacco exposure, infection control in dental practice, and water fluoridation.[8] Since organized dentistry also espouses the goal of optimum oral health for all, public and private sectors need to understand each other and work cooperatively to achieve this worthy goal.

Dental Public Health and the Private Practitioner

The personal nature of dental care means that success in practice is usually related directly to the number of people in the community who have confidence in the dental practitioner's abilities. That confidence is not limited to technical dental services but extends over a broad scope of day-to-day community affairs. In particular, people expect expert advice on community proposals for health improvement. A clear understanding of public health, rather than just a vague concept, is essential if dental practitioners are to properly fulfill their community obligations. They should be aware, for example, that a view of community oral health based on the patients in a single practice is rarely accurate. Dental patients differ from those who do not attend dentists (Chapter 2), and patients in one practice can differ markedly from those in the next. These differences emphasize the need for the public health agencies to monitor the public's oral health through periodic surveys of a cross-section of the public from time to time, an activity in which private practitioners can take an active interest.

In the previous chapter, we noted that the ethical practitioner, while acknowledging his primary responsibility to his patients, takes an interest in promoting the oral health of all members of the public. This interest can mean some exploration of local dental programs. For example, if there is an evident problem in treating the residents of the local nursing homes, private practitioners could work with the local public health agency to seek solutions. These might go so far as establishing a dental division in the local health department.

Even dental practitioners in solo practice, therefore, need to know what public health is and how they can work with it. It isn't just a one-way street; practitioners with a genuine interest in the community's oral health also find out that a well-functioning public health agency can help them with patient referrals, providing educational materials and programs, and dealing with other governmental agencies. In the American way of doing things, the partnership between public and private resources is the only way that everyone's dental needs can be met.

Collection and Use of Data in Dental Public Health

Surveillance in public health is the ongoing systematic collection, analysis, and interpretation of outcome-specific data for planning, implementation, and evaluation of public health practice.[26] In the United States, surveillance activities at state and local levels are coordinated by the Epidemiology Program Office at the Centers for Disease Control and Prevention (CDC) in Atlanta. Data sources for surveillance include vital statistics (births, deaths), notifiable diseases (plague, cholera, yellow fever, and others designated by states), registries (congenital defects, cancer), and administrative data collection systems (hospital discharge data). There is no organized surveillance system for oral conditions (apart from oral cancer, which is included in cancer registries), and this absence hampers the development of targeted approaches to improve the oral health.[8]

The role of surveillance in dental public health has been largely restricted to *surveys,* in which samples of a defined population are examined clinically or assessed by questionnaire. Surveys range in scope from large national surveys conducted by federal agencies (Chapters 18–22), to statewide surveys,[20] to surveys of the local community conducted by a state or local public health agency.[23] Important though they are, surveys can be too expensive and logistically demanding for some smaller state or local agencies. Dental public health has probably depended too heavily on surveys as its prime surveillance method and needs to explore less expensive alternatives for collecting data to be used in program development and evaluation.[19]

In the mid-1990s, the Association of State and Territorial Dental Directors (ASTDD) developed a 7-step model for state and local agencies to collect dental data by choosing from a variety of approaches to best suit local needs.[24] This model has now been used successfully by a number of state agencies. The collected data are used to identify needs and to plan programs to meet those needs. Functioning programs then need to be evaluated, and again data are needed for that. The results of evaluation can lead to plan modifications, and so the cycle continues. This ongoing process is known as the planning cycle, and is illustrated in simplified form in Figure 4–1.

The World Health Organization (WHO) has developed and systematized basic methods of data collection for surveillance of oral conditions in all parts of the world into an approach known as *Pathfinder.*[33, 34] Although not all details of these methods have received universal acceptance (Chapter 15), WHO has succeeded in promoting the collection and use of data in parts of the world where previously there was no information on oral conditions. The simplicity of the protocol for sampling and data collection permits it to be used by dental personnel with no previous training in survey methods. The data collected by the Pathfinder method are maintained in WHO's Global Oral Data Bank in Geneva.

Survey data are part of the foundation on which public policy at federal, state, and local levels is built. Some federal funding programs for dental public health, such as the Maternal and Child Health block grants, require that needs assessment and planning data be submitted each year with a state's application for funds. Agencies and foundations that fund research use oral survey data to help establish their research priorities; dental schools use them when establishing curricula; state agencies can use them in regulating the activities of dentists and hygienists; and dental insurance companies consult them when establishing benefit packages.

PERSONAL AND COMMUNITY HEALTH CARE: THE SIMILARITIES

To illustrate the similarities between the private and public health practice, we present a way of looking at them that was first described many years ago.[12]

Examination/Survey

When patients first come to a dental office, the dental professional carries out a careful examination. So does the public health practitioner, only here it is the community that must be examined. This is done by survey or some related form of needs assessment. Parallel to the general health history is a *situation analysis,* an assessment of population demographics, mobility, economic resources, and infrastructure.[33] Like the examination of a patient, a survey may be initiated by a chief complaint, such as lack of access to dental care for indigent persons. Just as regular dental attendance is recommended for a patient, community surveys at regular intervals make for efficient public health practice.

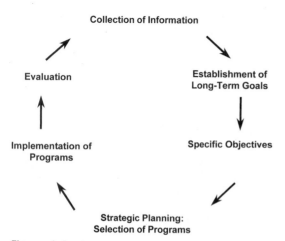

Figure 4–1. The planning cycle.

Treatment Planning/Program Planning

Treatment planning is often complex because of the many factors that must be balanced: professional judgment, the patient's interest, the cost of treatment, and the subtle dynamics of the dentist-patient relationship. Alternative methods of treatment with a range of costs often must be considered. Final outcome, whether acceptance of the dentist's ideal treatment, total rejection, or some compromise, varies among patients and depends on the balance of the factors listed.

The public health professional, like the clinician, would like to have the ideal program plan accepted with enthusiasm. However, the community's reaction to such a plan, like that of the patient, may be to reject it, to carry out only part of it, or to compromise with a less costly alternative. Like the patient in the chair, it is ultimately the community that makes the decision.

Treatment/Program Operation

A complex treatment plan may require referring the patient to specialists for certain procedures, though responsibility for coordination of these efforts rests with the patient's primary dentist. Similarly, when a specific community public health program has been adopted, a varied group of disciplines, which constitutes a public health team, may be called on for program operation. For example, if the plan is to provide dental treatment for elderly residents of nursing homes, a coordinated program involving supervisors of the homes, nurses, social workers, private dental practitioners, dental hygienists, and other health professionals will be needed.

Payment/Program Funding

Program funding in public health is often a complicated mix of local, state, and federal funds, which the dental public health professional must first know how to secure and then to manage. State funds in the package are often part of the federal appropriation through *block grants* (Chapter 8), grants to states for specified health programs. Management may demand extensive reporting requirements. Grant proposals for dental programs, submitted to local service clubs and local foundations, have proven successful in many cases.

Evaluation/Program Appraisal

The dentist or hygienist's evaluation of treatment begins during the course of treatment and is repeated at each visit. Observations made during the initial examination, such as extent of plaque and calculus deposits, are evaluated from time to time on recall. Similarly, data collected in the initial survey serve as the baseline against which an appraisal can be made to assess the effectiveness of the public health program. Public health workers are accountable to the community for a periodic appraisal of their performance, just as dental clinicians are accountable to their patients.

PERSONAL AND COMMUNITY HEALTH CARE: THE DIFFERENCES

In addition to the similarities between private and public health practice, there also are some notable differences.[13] Most practitioners do not understand the goals of public health. That is unfortunate, because both private and publicly employed dental professionals are working toward the same end: the oral health of the public. At the philosophical level, one major difference between personal care and public health is that the goals of public health are socially determined, whereas the priorities of private care are only coincidentally related to social goals.[18] Another way of looking at this distinction is to say that private care seeks to *maximize* the chance that the best outcome will occur, often unlimited by resource restraints. Public health, on the other hand, seeks to *minimize* the chance that the worst outcome will occur.[18]

The private practitioner works primarily alone. Decisions the dentist makes are in the context of his training, the legal framework for dental practice, and the dentist-patient relationship. Despite insurance carriers, quality assurance programs, and governmental requirements, the private practitioner is still a relatively independent health care provider. By contrast, the public health professional is a salaried employee who is accountable to both an immediate supervisor and to the taxpayers, represented in such forms as a board of health, an advisory council or two, and a governing body. Rarely is a major decision in public health made on one's own.

The public health professional often

works in communities with special characteristics of culture, language, socioeconomic status, and values. Public health workers often must care for those outside the mainstream, where those characteristics just mentioned make some groups of people more difficult and often more expensive to reach. The challenge in dental public health practice is that patients often do not have middle-class values with regard to brushing their teeth, keeping appointments, or regular dental attendance; but they still need care if the professional trust of working for the oral health of the public is to be preserved.

To add to the discussion on careers in Chapter 1, the rewards in public health practice differ from those of individual private practitioners. To start with, public health professionals receive a regular salary check. Although take-home pay, on average, is lower than that of private dental professionals, fringe benefits such as retirement, sick leave, insurance, and paid vacation are usually good. There are other, less tangible rewards. For example, the satisfaction from seeing the benefits of fluoridation come to a community after years of hard work is beyond measure. Knowing that one was quietly instrumental in bringing a health care program to an isolated community is another example. When private practitioners enjoy close working relationships with their public health professionals, they too can share in these intangible benefits.

REFERENCES

1. American Association of Public Health Dentistry; American Board of Dental Public Health. Dental public health: the past, present, and future. J Am Dent Assoc 1988;117:171–6.
2. American Dental Association, Commission on Dental Accreditation. Standards for advanced specialty education programs in dental health. 1996. Typescript.
3. Association of State and Territorial Dental Directors. Essential state public health services to promote oral health in the United States. Typescript, Jan. 1997.
4. Beck JD, Koch GG, Offenbacher S. Attachment loss trends over 3 years in community-dwelling older adults. J Periodontol 1994;65:737–43.
5. Blackerby PE, Jr. Treatment in public health dentistry. In: Pelton WJ, Wisan JM, eds.: Dentistry in public health. Philadelphia: WB Saunders, 1949, pp 187–221.
6. Burt BA. The future of the caries decline. J Public Health Dent 1985;45:261–9.
7. Cooke A. America. New York: Knopf, 1974.
8. Corbin SB, Mecklenburg RE. Report on the future of dental public health. J Public Health Dent 1994;54:80–91.
9. Freire PS. Planning and conducting an incremental care program. J Am Dent Assoc 1964;68:199–205.
10. Galagan DJ, Law FE, Waterman GE, Spitz GS. Dental health status of children 5 years after completing school care programs. Public Health Rep 1964;79:445–54.
11. Institute of Medicine. The future of public health. Washington DC: National Academy Press, 1988.
12. Knutson JW. What is public health? In: Pelton WJ, Wisan JM, eds.: Dentistry in public health. 2nd ed. Philadelphia: WB Saunders, 1955, pp 20–9.
13. Leavell HR, Clark EG. Preventive medicine for the doctor in his community: An epidemiologic approach. 3rd ed. New York: McGraw-Hill, 1978, pp 7–13.
14. Lotzkar SJ, Johnson DW, Thompson MB. Experimental program in expanded functions for dental assistants. Phase 3: Experiment with dental teams. J Am Dent Assoc 1971;82:1067–81.
15. Malthus TR. An essay on the principle of population. 7th ed., 1872. (reprint). New York: Kelley, 1971.
16. Parsons T. Definitions of health and illness in light of American values and social structures. In: Jaco EG, ed.: Patients, physicians, and illness. Glencoe, IL: Free Press, 1958, pp 165–87.
17. Pelton WJ, McNeal DR, Goggins JK. Student dental health program of the University of Alabama in Birmingham: VI. Chair time expended for the delivery of services. Alabama J Med Sci 1971;8:373–7.
18. Pickett G, Hanlon JJ. Public health: Administration and practice. 9th ed. St. Louis: Times Mirror/Mosby, 1990.
19. Reed SG, Tallman JA, Burt BA. Collecting state-level oral health data when resources are limited: An approach to oral health surveillance. J Public Health Dent 1993;53:253–7.
20. Rozier RG, Dudney GG, Spratt CJ. The 1986–87 North Carolina school oral health survey. Raleigh: North Carolina Department of Environment, Health, and Natural Resources, 1991.
21. Salzmann JA. Principles and practice of public health dentistry. Boston: Stratford, 1937.
22. Schmekebier LF. The Public Health Service. Baltimore: Johns Hopkins, 1923.
23. Siegal MD, Martin B, Kuthy RA. Usefulness of a local oral health survey in program development. J Public Health Dent 1988;48:121–4.
24. Siegal MD, Kuthy RA. Assessing oral health needs; ASTDD seven-step model. ASTDD, 1995.
25. Stevens R, Stevens R. Medicaid: Anatomy of a dilemma. Law and Contemporary Problems 1970; 35:348–425.
26. Thacker SB, Berkelman RL. Public health surveillance in the United States. Epidemiol Rev 1988;10:164–90.
27. Trevelyan GM. English social history. Longman Green 1942. Reprint. London: Pelican Books, 1967.
28. US Public Health Service, National Center for Health Statistics. Health United States 1994. DHHS Publication No (PHS) 95-1232. Washington DC: Government Printing Office, 1995.
29. US Public Health Service. Smoking and health. Report of the Advisory Committee to the Surgeon General of the Public Health Service. PHS Publication No 1103. Washington DC, Government Printing Office, 1964.
30. Waterman GE. The Richmond-Woonsocket studies on dental care services for school children. J Am Dent Assoc 1956;52:676–84.
31. Winslow CEA. The untilled fields of public health. Modern Med 1920;2:183–91.
32. World Health Organization. Constitution of the World Health Organization. Geneva: WHO, 1946:3.
33. World Health Organization. Planning oral health services. WHO offset Publication No. 53. Geneva: WHO, 1980.
34. World Health Organization. Oral health surveys; basic methods. 4th ed. Geneva: WHO, 1997.

5
Promotion of Oral Health

What is Health Promotion? ◆ Community-Based
Health Promotion ◆ Promoting Oral Health ◆
Goals for Oral Health ◆ Knowledge and Attitudes
About Oral Health ◆ Dental Health Education ◆
Promoting Water Fluoridation

Is any individual's health status solely her own responsibility, or does society have some part to play in it? We discussed this issue when trying to define health in Chapter 4, and concluded that both were involved. Put concisely, the individual is responsible for the conduct of her life, but society is largely responsible for the conditions of her life.[4] The achievement of health requires a set of social conditions within which the individual can then take actions that enhance health.[80]

This chapter discusses the promotion of oral health in the community and among individual patients. Issues of public policy that permit people to maximize their oral health are considered, and examples of major community-based health promotional interventions are assessed. Because cultural values strongly influence health promotion, public and professional attitudes and beliefs are also examined. As an example of how health promotional principles might be applied at community level, the role of health professionals in promoting water fluoridation is assessed. We do not go into details of educational theory in this chapter; a number of excellent texts provide such details.[35–37, 78]

WHAT IS HEALTH PROMOTION?

Although health is an elusive entity to define, we stated in Chapter 4 that it is more than the mere absence of disease and less than the idealistic definition of the World Health Organization (WHO). Greenberg[37] re-fers to health as a quality of life with social, mental, emotional, spiritual, and physical functions. He points out that too much emphasis is usually given to the physical function at the expense of the others. In effect, Greenberg is arguing for a "holistic" view of health. He defines *wellness* as a positive state, the degree to which a person has reached her potential regarding each of the components of health. Because it is the integration of social, mental, emotional, spiritual, and physical components at any level of health or illness, people can be healthy or ill and still possess a high degree of wellness.[37]

At least among the better-educated, the traditionally narrow view that equates health with the absence of disease has given way to a broader, positive concept based on Greenberg's definition. In day-to-day terms, attainment and maintenance of health are no longer just a matter of an annual medical check-up, but also include regular exercise, making wise food choices, getting sufficient sleep, having some form of spiritual belief, maintaining friendships, and indulging in a diversity of interests. Self-destructive behaviors such as smoking and drunken driving are much less socially acceptable than they were, and interest in healthy eating has never been higher. It is recognized, however, that although this positive view predominates in the white-collar world, it has not permeated other strata of society to the same extent.[29, 88] There are good reasons why. Education results in greater access to knowledge and information; even more important, it develops information-seeking attitudes and skills. In addition, better-educated people usually lead lives that give them more opportunities to develop healthy lifestyles than do those who have to spend more time and energy just making ends meet.

Community health promotion is defined as any combination of educational, social, and environmental actions conducive to the health of a population of a geographically defined area.[35] Another definition is that health promotion is a set of processes that can be used to change the conditions that affect health, so that targets are not always the people whose health is in question.[78] These definitions suggest roles for the health professional, political leaders, society as a whole, and for the individual in maximizing health status. Health education is an important part of health promotion, although it is just one part of the larger entity. Health education is defined as any combination of learning opportunities designed to facilitate voluntary adaptations of behavior that are conducive to health.[34] Health education and health promotion have been described as the mechanisms that connect prevention activities; policy development; and program implementation, maintenance, and evaluation.[27]

This concept of health promotion began to take root during the 1970s and was much influenced by a working paper by the Canadian Minister for Health at the time, Marc Lalonde. More of a visionary than many political leaders, Lalonde introduced the health field concept, a new idea at the time, as he tried to evaluate the impact of Canadian health policies.[52] Specifically, Canada had moved to a program of equal access to health care for all citizens through public financing, and Lalonde had observed that increased access to health care services did not by itself improve health status. The health field concept is a conceptual framework for the evaluation and analysis of community health needs that includes assessments of human biology, environment, lifestyle, and health care organization in more or less equal parts. Up to Lalonde's analysis, such assessments had usually been dominated by health care organization (i.e., the view was that health services = health), but today we are much more aware of the importance of other factors as well. The environmental movement is now an integral part of many health and social issues, and lifestyle choices are recognized as a major factor in health status. The wider concept of health promotion reaches up to such issues as community provision of libraries, recreational facilities, biking and walking trails, and open space, things provided by the community rather than at individual level. Although far removed from the direct provision of health services, such amenities are now considered to be integral contributions to the health of the community.

Health promotion requires active interventions at different levels and by different organizations, and the health professional organizations are certainly important components. Campaigns conducted by professional organizations themselves, however, are often a mix of health promotion and public relations. (Public relations exercises may have their place, but they should not be confused with health promotion.) The American Dental Association (ADA), for example, launched a television campaign in the mid-1980s to increase patient visits among adults over age 30, mostly by presenting the health benefits of regular dental care.[14] Although the ADA's House of Delegates voted not to finance this campaign nationally, several state associations picked it up for local use. Success of this campaign, in terms of improving oral health, is uncertain because of its narrow focus. The same could be said about Children's Dental Health Month, even though it has reached the status of an institution and is moderately broad-based. The American Dental Hygienists' Association launched its Oral Health Initiative in 1984.[73] It primarily called for professional and public educational efforts to increase demand for dental care, and it included recommendations for additional research in prevention and for legislation to increase access to preventive care. Success of this program is also uncertain.

Other suggestions for broadening the health promotional role of hygienists followed a survey on their health beliefs. The survey group concluded that hygienists were too narrowly focused on oral health. As examples of health issues that hygienists could promote they listed stress, weight problems, physical activity, fat consumption, and seatbelt use.[40] This interesting suggestion does not seem to have been adopted, perhaps because time for specific instruction in these matters would have to be found in an already crowded curriculum. The activities aimed at getting dentists more involved in smoking cessation among their patients (Chapter 29) are also a contribution toward community health promotion.

COMMUNITY-BASED HEALTH PROMOTION

The principal community-based health promotion programs in the United States have been directed at reducing the risk for cardiovascular disease. Nothing on the scale of these programs has been carried out for oral health, but there are issues in these programs from which dentistry could learn.

Four major community-based programs aimed at reducing the risk of cardiovascular disease were conducted in the United States during the 1980s. These studies were conducted in Pawtucket, Rhode Island,[7] the state of Minnesota,[43] and 2 related projects based in 5 cities in central California.[25] These projects had been completed by the 1990s, all with some degree of success, although it was qualified success in some instances. The projects had some features in common:

- The extensive use of epidemiologic data in planning. Specific data on the frequency of heart attacks in the communities concerned were added to research information on the major risk factors: hypertension, obesity, sedentary lifestyle, smoking, high-fat diets, and high blood cholesterol.
- Educational and intervention activities were based on currently accepted theories of health behavior.
- Clearly specified hypotheses, using measurable exposures and outcomes, could be readily tested to evaluate the success of the projects.

It is worth looking at one of these projects in detail. The purpose of the Stanford Five-Cities study, as an example, was to seek reductions in the cardiovascular risk factors of smoking behavior, high blood cholesterol, and hypertension. It had begun as the Stanford Three-Community study in 1972,[21] which had yielded promising results and was thus expanded to the Five-Cities study. This project was designed to test whether a comprehensive program of community organization and health education would produce favorable changes in risk factors, morbidity, and mortality in 2 treatment cities compared with 3 control cities over 6 years. The methods chosen for comparative study were mass media health education in one city, and mass

media plus personal instruction for those identified by screening to be at highest risk in the second.

This 6-year intervention was influenced by Bandura's social learning theory.[3] This theory states that reciprocal relationships exist between an individual's behavior, cognitive processes, and the external environment, and that these relationships are mediated by self-efficacy: the individual's belief in her competence to carry out specific actions. In practical terms, this theory states that the professional office environment is not conducive to learning and maintaining good health behavior; such activities are best carried out at home, at work, and in other community settings. The Stanford Five-Cities study was a sophisticated program that included community organization principles and social marketing methods and was intended to be self-sustaining after the project finished.

The Stanford study design included biennial assessments of cohorts followed over the 6 years and of independent cross-sectional samples at 2-year intervals. Results at the end of the 6 years showed that the treatment cities exhibited greater improvements in most of the risk factors being measured (cardiovascular disease knowledge, blood pressure, and smoking behavior, resting pulse) than controls.[20, 26] Mixed results were found with body mass index; improvements occurred in the cross-sectional samples but not in the cohorts,[81] which suggests less than fully effective results. Generally positive changes were found in the control cities, presumably because of the widespread publicity given to cardiovascular risk factors in the media. Although these changes were overall positive findings, these trends in the control cities had the effect of making the net changes attributable to the program rather small.

A major question after such large-scale projects is whether the good results achieved were maintained after the project ended. To answer that question, a follow-up study was conducted 4 years after the termination of the main project. Small net improvements in most risk factors measured were maintained in the treatment cities relative to the controls, although trends in body mass index were negative in both treatment and control cities.[90] This outcome was similar to the one found in the Minnesota Heart Health Program, where strong efforts at obesity control ended in failure.[46] The conclusion by the Stanford researchers was that the modest net differences suggested that new designs and forms of intervention are needed to better reach those at highest risk. Later reflections on the Stanford study in health promotion included the rather humble admission that the researchers had learned little about the factors that determine population-level change, and the lowering of risk factors in the control cities was clearly unexpected.[25]

When the combined success of the interventions in all 3 of the cardiovascular health promotion projects was assessed, trends were in the favorable direction, although most differences between treatments and controls were not statistically significant.[89] There was agreement, however, that the success of community intervention strategies of this type depended on the community organization process.[62]

Cardiovascular disease is a life-and-death matter, and the modest effects of these extensive and expensive health promotional interventions on such a potentially serious disease are sobering. At the same time, most risk factors showed a secular decline in both treatment and control cities, which is good news. It is correct to conclude that we do not know much about how to effect community-wide behavioral change. It is worth reflecting on the lessons from these cardiovascular studies for oral health promotion, given that apart from oral cancer, we do not deal with life-threatening diseases.

PROMOTING ORAL HEALTH

Governments should have policies in place that promote health and do not interfere with people's lives, but give them the freedom to make informed choices on their health behavior. As a negative example, homeless people are so preoccupied with day-to-day survival that they have little opportunity to make rational choices on matters affecting their health. The first step in promoting health among the homeless, therefore, would be the provision of decent housing, adequate food, and whatever else can reasonably be done to improve self-esteem. Harking back to the definition for health promotion, such steps represent the organizational, social/economic, and environmental supports basic to the development of healthy behaviors. Governmental action in this area often means legislation; in developed countries we are familiar with specific laws pertaining to cigarette

advertising, use of seatbelts and safety helmets, and immunizations for children. These laws, through which society accepts some constraint on absolute freedom in the interests of public health, are in addition to the public health codes covering water supplies, food preparation, and public accommodations. In the oral health area, legislation that mandates or permits water fluoridation, and the statutory basis for school dental programs in some countries, are both organizational aspects of oral health promotion.

Dentists and dental hygienists have spent a lot of time educating patients and the public on the value of good oral health. Organized campaigns such as the ADA's Children's Dental Health Month have also been conducted fairly regularly. This effort has probably had some impact, although we can't tell how much. There is little question that during the last few decades, the status of the public's oral health and its standards of oral hygiene have continued to improve. Once again, however, we do not know how much of this can be attributed directly to oral health education and how much to rising living standards and norms of personal cleanliness and grooming. We can also accept that the rising utilization of dental services (Chapter 2) is evidence of increasing public acceptance of the value of good oral health.

The mass media, especially television, are frequently used in promotional programs in oral health, but the effects are uncertain. For example, a national campaign in Finland in the early 1980s used the mass media to try to increase demand for dental services. Although the proportion of adults visiting a dentist after 1 year rose from 54% to 65%, the researchers concluded that the mass media were not effective in changing health behavior.[63] The value of the mass media in promoting dental visits and good oral health behavior was also questioned after a 1980s campaign in the Netherlands.[72] These findings were not really surprising, for researchers earlier had defined the limitations of mass media in changing health behavior.[8, 28] The Stanford Five-City cardiovascular intervention program, described previously, also reached ambivalent conclusions on intervention strategies that relied heavily on television and newspapers.

One problem in defining a role for mass media in oral health promotion is that evaluation carried out by market researchers, accustomed to dealing with commercial advertisements, is often "process" evaluation, which stops short of detecting outcomes. An example is the evaluation of a Michigan television campaign in the late 1980s. Correct description of the advertisements was given by 22% of a random sample of adults, up from 13% early in the campaign. Aided recall, meaning recall after some prompting on the nature of the content, rose from 23% to 32%; and 12% of those interviewed said they were influenced by the commercials.[51] This type of evaluatory data is relatively cheap and easy to collect by an experienced social research group, but measuring the actual impact of the campaign on oral health is more complicated. Use of more than one medium is likely to better promote health messages. One campaign that involved both television and printed material found that the television spots were the least well remembered and that the printed material, which demanded active involvement of participants at home, was more effective in improving oral health knowledge.[76]

An example of an oral health promotional campaign was seen in a sealant program conducted by the Ohio Department of Health.[77] Results of an oral health survey of children in Columbus, which showed that caries experience was greatest among poorer children, were used as the rationale for grant support that permitted continuation, and even expansion, of the sealant program in the city schools. The data served wider purposes as well. They were invaluable in "marketing" the program among influential legislators, in developing a supportive constituency among parents and school personnel, and in educating the public. The result was a preventive program that not only directly improved the oral health of the children concerned, but also had the solid support of the community because its purposes were well understood and accepted.

Goals for Oral Health

At the international level, global goals for oral health were established by the World Dental Federation (FDI) in 1982 and are listed in Table 5–1. These goals were developed after a great deal of discussion, and with the strong involvement of the WHO. As global goals, they are intended to stimulate individual countries to either adopt them as they are for their own goals, or to modify them for

Table 5–1. GLOBAL GOALS FOR ORAL HEALTH FOR THE YEAR 2000, ESTABLISHED BY THE WORLD DENTAL FEDERATION AND THE WORLD HEALTH ORGANIZATION

- 50% of 5- to 6-year-olds will be caries-free.
- The global average will be no more than 3 DMF teeth at age 12.
- 85% of the population should retain all their permanent teeth at age 18.
- A 50% reduction in present levels of edentulousness at age 35 to 40 will be achieved.
- A 25% reduction in present levels of edentulousness at age 65 and over will be achieved.
- A database will be established for monitoring changes in oral health.

From the Fédération Dentaire Internationale (World Dental Federation). Goals for oral health in the year 2000. FDI Newsletter 1982 March:5–8.

their own circumstances. The FDI followed up on these global goals with its guidelines for national dental associations to use in promoting the oral health of the public.[11]

The United States adopted national goals for health in 1980.[82] These were part of a 10-year plan for improvement of national health status by 1990. A midcourse review[85] found that some of the oral health goals in this plan had already been achieved, others would clearly not be achieved, and still others could not be evaluated because of a lack of data. In the process, it became clear that goals were not going to be met without specific programs, and that programs required funds and trained personnel if they were to have any impact. National goals for health for the year 2000 were announced in September 1990,[83] with generally favorable media publicity. Among them are 16 goals for oral health, listed in Table 5–2. Midcourse reviews found that some progress had been made toward most goals, although disparities were growing between some minority groups and the main population in some areas. As a result, new subobjectives were established for Native Americans in the reduction of edentulous persons, and for African-Americans in the prevention of oropharyngeal cancer.[84]

The goals shown in Table 5–2 are not all that could be listed in the pursuit of oral health, but are more of a consensus priority listing. Some baseline data were presented for each of them (not shown in Table 5–2); these provide the point of reference against which progress will be measured. Activities in the

Table 5–2. ORAL HEALTH OBJECTIVES FOR THE UNITED STATES IN THE YEAR 2000

HEALTH STATUS OBJECTIVES

1. Reduce dental caries so that the proportion of children with one or more lesions (in permanent or primary teeth) is no more than 35% among children aged 6 to 8, and no more than 60% among adolescents aged 15.
2. Reduce untreated dental caries so that the proportion of children with untreated caries (in permanent or primary teeth) is no more than 20% among children aged 6 to 8 and no more than 15% among adolescents aged 15.
3. Increase to at least 45% the proportion of people aged 35 to 44 who have never lost a permanent tooth due to dental caries or periodontal disease.
4. Reduce to no more than 20% the proportion of people aged 65 and older who have lost all of their natural teeth.
5. Reduce the prevalence of gingivitis among people aged 35 to 44 to no more than 30%.
6. Reduce destructive periodontal diseases to a prevalence of no more than 15% among people aged 35 to 44.
7. Reduce deaths due to cancer of the oral cavity and pharynx to no more than 10.5 per 100,000 men aged 45 to 74 and to 4.1 per 100,000 women aged 45 to 74.

RISK REDUCTION OBJECTIVES

8. Increase to at least 50% the proportion of children who have received protective sealants on the occlusal surfaces of permanent molar teeth.
9. Increase to at least 75% the proportion of people served by community water systems providing optimal levels of fluoride.
10. Increase use of professionally or self-administered topical or systemic (dietary) fluorides to at least 85% of people not receiving optimally fluoridated public water.
11. Increase to at least 75% the proportion of parents and caregivers who use feeding practices that prevent baby bottle tooth decay.

SERVICES AND PROTECTION OBJECTIVES

12. Increase to at least 90% the proportion of all children entering school programs for the first time who have received an oral health screening, referral, and follow-up for necessary diagnostic, preventive, and treatment services.
13. Extend to all long-term institutional facilities the requirement that oral examinations and services be provided no later than 90 days after entry into these facilities.
14. Increase to at least 70% the proportion of people aged 35 and older using the oral health system each year.
15. Increase to at least 40 the number of states that have an effective system for recording and referring infants with cleft lips and/or palates to craniofacial anomaly teams.
16. Extend requirement of the use of effective head, face, eye, and mouth protection to all organizations, agencies, and institutions sponsoring sporting and recreational events that pose risks of injury.

From the US Public Health Service. Healthy people 2000: national health promotion and disease prevention activities. Conference edition. Washington DC: Government Printing Office, 1990.

late 1990s were proceeding to establish health goals for the nation for the year 2010; these include goals for oral health. The nature of these goals will depend to a large extent on progress made toward the *Healthy People 2000* goals.

As mentioned, however, goals without a program to achieve them are no more than wishful thinking. Plans to reach the *Healthy People 2000* goals require a high level of agreement and coordination among federal, state, and local agencies, as well as between public and private sectors. Successful achievement of most goals is unlikely without the allocation of sufficient resources for the necessary programs. Setting the conditions to achieve these goals presents major opportunities for promotion of oral health.

Knowledge and Attitudes About Oral Health

People demonstrate a wide variety of attitudes toward teeth, dental care, and dentists.

These attitudes naturally reflect their own experiences, cultural perceptions, familial beliefs, and other life situations; and they strongly influence oral health behavior.[9, 30, 58, 91, 95]

The important role of negative attitudes as a reason for loss of teeth is described in Chapter 18. As examples, a study in the Netherlands found that the majority of decisions for full mouth extractions are made by the patient rather than the dentist,[6] and a Scottish study related total tooth loss to negative attitudes about dental care and passivity about tooth loss.[64] It is possible that these negative attitudes might be unconsciously encouraged by dental professionals if the patient does not fit the "good patient" model. Not surprisingly, dentists' profile of a "good" patient was one who shared the dentist's values on oral health, complied with advice and accepted treatment plans, was concerned about her oral health, arrived on time, and paid the bills.[66] Because the same study found that "personal warmth" was valued by dentists, it is likely that many dentists have trouble relating to a patient who does not possess these attributes.

Knowledge gaps concerning a number of preventive procedures have been found among researchers, practitioners, and patients[65]; and lack of consensus between researchers and practitioners can be a major barrier to more effective promotion of caries prevention. This unfortunate confusion can be alleviated by health promotional activities aimed at changing attitudes and practices. For example, dentists in one Indian Health Service region developed a significantly greater orientation toward preventive services after such a promotional campaign.[57] Realizing that positive attitudes toward health promotion need to be developed during student days rather than afterward, the FDI has recommended that substantial changes in the dental curriculum be implemented to give dentists the knowledge, skills, and attitudes they will need in future practice.[23] The behavioral sciences, and the control of fear and anxiety in patients, were listed among those areas needing more attention. Calls for such curricular changes date back to the 1960s,[48] although they have not been well heeded; relatively little curricular change seems to have taken place over the years. Knowledge and attitudes on oral health among other influential professionals, schoolteachers for example, also can be disappointingly poor,[33, 53, 56] which emphasizes the responsibility of the dental professions to see that trainee teachers, nurses, and others who influence public attitudes receive correct information on oral health.

Even a relatively low level of serious oral disease in the community does not always reflect positive dental attitudes. In fluoridated Hong Kong, for example, where neither caries nor periodontitis was found to be a major public health problem, ignorance and misconceptions about the most common oral conditions were widespread.[55] Poor knowledge of oral diseases is common in many countries, including the United States and Canada, as shown by reports that many people do not associate existing signs, such as calculus deposits or bleeding gums, with periodontal diseases.[32, 54] A more encouraging study in North Carolina found that patients of general practitioners were generally knowledgable about the signs, causes, prevention, and treatment of periodontal conditions.[2] Few serious misconceptions were found in this study, al-though improvement on the significance of bleeding gums was needed. When incipient disease cannot be recognized, there will naturally be inadequate self-care, and promotion of self-care is one of the major goals of oral health education.

DENTAL HEALTH EDUCATION

In the past, unless health professionals were unusually sensitive to patients' reactions, health education was often patronizing. When a health provider who believed she knew what was best for the patient "educated" a person who was tacitly assumed to know nothing, it's a safe bet that little of value eventuated. This has been called the "empty vessel" approach to health education: the patient is empty, and waiting for the health professional to "pour in" the knowledge. It was enshrined in an early WHO report[92] that recognized the need to teach educational theory and methods to student dentists so that they may successfully "motivate" their patients and the public to behave as we would like them to. It also showed itself unconsciously in terminology such as "toothbrushing drills," a so-called educational method in which children were taught to brush their teeth in a semimilitary manner. The "empty vessel" approach also dated from a time when the guild model of professionalism (Chapter 1) was accepted, a model that saw the all-knowing professional as dominant in dentist-patient relations.

In more recent years, greater acceptance has been given to the idea that the recipients of this attention might have some thoughts of their own. Item 4 in The Declaration of Alma-Ata, the outcome of a major international conference on primary health care, stated that "people have a right and duty to participate individually and collectively in the planning and implementation of their health care."[93] In a subsequent WHO report, the evolution of professional attitudes was demonstrated when it was stated that (a) participant involvement was essential for success in health education, and (b) what is taught needed to be compatible with local customs and culture as well as with scientific knowledge.[94]

It is a basic precept that everyone has a right to the best available knowledge about caring for her own health. It is crucial to remember, however, that knowledge alone does not lead to action. Many health care workers assume that when people have knowledge about health care they will act on that knowledge. It is a rational assumption, but human behavior is more complicated than that. Knowledge dissemination is a fundamental part of the mission of health professionals, but health care workers must accept that much of their effort will go unheeded.

School-based oral health education programs, by definition, are aimed at more cohesive groups rather than at the public at large. Whatever approach is to be adopted, it requires a plan of action, with appropriate involvement of all parties concerned and clear delineation of responsibilities.[42] Fundamental components of a school-based program for the promotion of oral health have been described as:

- Oral health services, meaning preventive procedures, health screening and treatment, referral, and follow-up.
- Health instruction, to include both personal and community health topics.
- A healthy environment, with attention to all aspects of the school environment that could affect the health of students or school personnel.[42]

Even though schoolchildren are more homogeneous than the public as a whole, any group of them still have a variety of beliefs and attitudes; in a multicultural society the differences can be profound.[17] Methods used in school programs, therefore, should be a mix of small-group and mass approaches, and some are clearly more successful than others. The more successful approaches, as shown by evaluations of teachers, administrators, and by the oral health of participants, use a fair degree of active involvement.[12, 13, 24, 39, 67, 79] This finding applies to all ages and social groups, for active involvement increased the effectiveness of programs conducted with employed adults[38, 69, 75] and with mothers of young children.[41] Nursing home residents who monitored their own progress toward oral hygiene goals showed improvements in psychological well-being and self-esteem, as well as in oral hygiene.[49, 50]

On the other hand, programs that involve less individual participation can increase knowledge of oral disease mechanisms and its prevention, but have less impact on attitudes, beliefs, and behavior.[60, 70, 86] The mass media, which by definition do not develop personal involvement, are generally seen as effective in disseminating basic knowledge, but their role in influencing behavioral change is less clear. The result of oral health campaigns favors the necessity of personal involvement for behavioral change, but these findings must be contrasted against the favorable results reported from use of mass media in the cardiovascular studies described earlier. When the necessary degree of sensitivity to the astonishing variety of racial and ethnic cultures present in much of modern-day America is included, designing programs for personal involvement becomes a challenge.

The most intensive form of oral health education is one-to-one instruction. Although oral health education is clearly an integral part of professional responsibility, simply passing across information does not by itself lead to desirable action; personal involvement is necessary. A study of educational outcomes among "high-plaque" patients who received instruction in oral hygiene in dental practices in Washington found that only 28% had substantially reduced their plaque scores over 6 weeks, and 13% had actually become worse. The researchers concluded that the therapists often did not follow the principles of effective instruction, although outcome also was related to patients' oral status and life situations.[87] The same study also found that educational effort was not being concentrated on patients with greatest need, but rather was being more or less equally distributed.[61] A British project found that the Community Periodontal Index of Treatment Needs (CPITN) index (Chapter 15) was a useful way of improving patient awareness of periodontal conditions.[10] FDI is encouraging greater use of CPITN (the PSR index in the United States) as a patient education tool in many countries, although a more useful side effect might be to improve periodontal awareness among some practitioners.

Many health care professionals have enormous faith in the value of dental health education. Educational programs are rarely opposed on the grounds that the resources involved might better be placed elsewhere, and educational programs are good at promoting a general "feel-good" atmosphere among all concerned. There is no question that all people have a right to the best knowledge about how to care for their health, even though they will act on this knowledge in different ways. The conclusions from a searching review of dental health education outcomes should be borne in mind by all those planning educational programs: (a) educational programs work well at improving knowledge levels; (b) they have a positive but temporary effect on plaque levels; and (c) have no discernible effect on caries experience.[47]

At a practical level, the principles of oral health education that emerge from the literature can be summarized as follows:

- People interpret health messages through the "filter" of their own values and attitudes. These need to be understood, as far as possible, if the educational process is to have any chance of success.
- The most successful education maximizes self-involvement of the participants.
- Mass media are effective in transmitting simple and consistent messages, although their value in influencing health behavior seems limited. They have been found effective in some behavior change related to cardiovascular disease, but less so for oral conditions.
- Health professionals have to accept that not all people share their values about the importance of physical health. An acceptance of all components of wellness will help in dealing with the infinite variety of human beliefs on health.
- Dental health education programs can improve knowledge and temporarily improve oral hygiene, but they have failed to demonstrate any direct effect on caries experience.

PROMOTING WATER FLUORIDATION

The issue of water fluoridation gives dental professionals the chance to promote oral health at the community level and to apply the experiences gained from other successful community-based campaigns. The ADA has a long-standing policy that dentists should work to promote fluoridation in their communities,[1] although it is recognized that the issue can provoke mixed feelings. Dentists and hygienists, accustomed to life outside the public spotlight, are often far from comfortable in the political arena. For such individuals, there are still key roles for dental professionals as low-profile resource persons.

Dentists and hygienists should at least educate their patients about what fluoridation is and who benefits from it (Chapter 24). They should aim to have patients support the measure, especially with a vote if a referendum is coming. Patients are a more-or-less captive audience, and there is evidence that dentists could do better with this particular educational role.[45] Dental professionals should know the concentration of fluoride in their own community's drinking water, information that comes from the state or local health department. Cost estimates for fluoridating a community can be obtained from a state health department or water supply division, and from the fluoridation engineers at the Division of Oral Health of the CDC. If there were previous attempts to fluoridate the community, it is useful to have a history of which individuals were involved and what happened.

At the local community level, a decision by city council to fluoridate has proven far more likely to result in a favorable outcome than a referendum. Lobbying of city councillors both answers questions and identifies the members who are for, against, and undecided, information that can help shape the further promotional effort needed. When a city council decides to place the issue of fluoridation out for referendum, the role of dental professionals becomes more overtly political. Defining this role may not be easy. A thoughtful study from the 1960s, still relevant today, found that political efforts of dentists and other health professionals in a local fluoridation campaign got unfavorable reactions for two reasons.[71] First, the community expected partisans in a political campaign to be motivated by self-interest and to conduct a propaganda campaign to further those interests. Because the health professionals supporting fluoridation were seen as political partisans, their endorsements of fluoridation were not accepted as dispassionate expert testimony. Second, their efforts to maintain professional decorum and to avoid the hurly-burly of open controversy were interpreted as arrogance. This study suggests that in a fluoridation referendum, the health professionals cannot expect to maintain a detached role, and referendum tactics must be structured accordingly.

Regardless of the nature of the political campaign, experience has shown that a successful outcome is more likely when a citizen's committee coordinates it, often as the "Citizens for Healthy Teeth" or some such name. The first task of the coordinating committee is to draw up a plan of action to guide promotional activities. Dental professionals can fill the role of technical experts in this committee, although many have the qualities to take more prominent roles. If needed, CDC and the ADA have materials to help. The composition of the citizens' committee should be as broadly based as possible, with attention to socioeconomic, age, and ethnic groupings, to:

- Represent the community and demonstrate that fluoridation has widespread political support.
- Increase the number of volunteer workers for telephoning potential voters, canvassing, and distributing materials.[59]
- Increase the base of financial support.[44]

Experience has also shown that a hired consultant in a political organization can be helpful.[19] A political expert can assist in these areas:

- Legally registering the political action committee in those states where it is required.
- Reaching the large segments of the population that ordinarily do not participate in organizations and who are not much influenced by mass media.
- Identifying the community power structure, and the key individual leaders whose support will be needed.
- Developing campaign strategy and tactics.
- Enlisting the aid of "celebrities" and "outside experts," if appropriate.

The citizens' committee should use all appropriate methods of health education and political dissemination, including advertisements and news releases. A speakers' bureau, to provide talks to civic groups, and mass mailings are usually needed. Leaflets and pamphlets should be printed in terminology and language understandable by the group to which they are directed. Newspapers, radio, and television can be powerful allies in a community debate, although they have been known to turn the debate into a hysterical public spectacle in which the real issues get lost.

Political tactics vary with each community; there is no cookbook, although there are some standard issues. For example, should an invitation to publicly debate a fluoridation opponent be accepted? A refusal can be interpreted as professional arrogance,[71] but a debate with a committed opponent cannot be "won." An opponent can imply, for example, that fluoridation is in the same category as toxic chemical waste or acid rain, and that proponents are trying to increase both unnecessary regulation and taxes. Despite the successful record of fluoridation in the courts (Chapter 24), a good speaker can still score on the "freedom of choice" issue. Even the necessary dissemination of objective facts on fluoridation can be self-defeating, for the burden of proof always falls on those advocating change.[31] Skilled opponents of fluoridation can quickly put the proponents on the defensive.

Successful referendum campaigns have been reported in the dental literature, and strategies for dealing with fluoridation in the political arena have now been well defined.[5, 15, 16, 18, 19, 44, 59, 68, 74] The common theme in these reports is that fluoridation is politics. It demands the use of the media, publicity, education, intensive door-to-door canvassing, telephone campaigns, and getting out the vote on polling day. Above all, it means consistent hard work over a long period and starting with solid preparation.

REFERENCES

1. American Dental Association, Council on Dental Health. Statement of American Dental Association on role of dentists and dental societies in the promotion of fluoridation. Am Dent Assoc Trans 1962; 103:44.
2. Bader JD, Rozier RG, McFall WT, Ramsey DL. Dental patients' knowledge and beliefs about periodontal disease. Community Dent Oral Epidemiol 1989; 17:60–4.
3. Bandura A. A social learning theory. Englewood Cliffs NJ: Prentice Hall, 1977.
4. Birn H, Birn B. Education for wellness. Community Dent Health 1985;2:51–6.
5. Boriskin JM, Fine JI. Fluoridation election victory: a case study for dentistry in effective political action. J Am Dent Assoc 1981;102:486–91.
6. Bouma J, Westert G, Schaub RM, van de Poel F. Decision processes preceding full mouth extractions. Community Dent Oral Epidemiol 1987;15:268–72.
7. Carleton RA, Lasater TM, Assaf AR, et al. The Pawtucket Heart Health program: Community changes in cardiovascular risk factors and projected disease risk. Am J Public Health 1995;85:777–85.
8. Chambers DW. Susceptibility to preventive dental treatment. J Public Health Dent 1973;33:82–90.
9. Chen MS. Children's preventive dental behavior in relation to their mothers' socioeconomic status: Health beliefs and dental behaviors. J Dent Child 1986;53:105–9.
10. Chesters RK, Dexter CH, Life JS, et al. Periodontal awareness project in the United Kingdom: CPITN and self-assessment. Int Dent J 1987;37:218–21.
11. Cohen LK. Promoting oral health: Guidelines for dental associations. Int Dent J 1990;40:79–102.

12. Craft M, Croucher R, Dickinson J. Preventive dental health in adolescents: short and long term pupil response to trials of an integrated curriculum package. Community Dent Oral Epidemiol 1981;9:199–206.

13. Craft M, Croucher R, Dickinson J, et al. Natural nashers: A programme of dental health education for adolescents in schools. Int Dent J 1984;34:204–13.

14. Decision 84: ADA's proposed paid public education program. J Am Dent Assoc 1984;108:740–8.

15. Dolinsky HB, McFadden RT, Kleinfeld L, Miller PT. A health systems agency and a fluoridation campaign. J Public Health Policy 1981;2:158–63.

16. Domoto PK, Faine RC, Rovin S. Seattle fluoridation 1973: Prescription for victory. J Am Dent Assoc 1975;91:583–8.

17. Durward CS, Wright FA. Dental knowledge, attitudes, and behaviors of Indochinese and Australian-born adolescents. Community Dent Oral Epidemiol 1989;17:14–8.

18. Evans CA, Pickles T. Statewide antifluoridation initiatives: A new challenge to health workers. Am J Public Health 1978;68:59–62.

19. Faine RC, Collins JJ, Daniel J, et al. The 1980 fluoridation campaigns: A discussion of results. J Public Health Dent 1981;41:138–42.

20. Farquhar JW, Fortmann SP, Flora JA, et al. Effects of communitywide education on cardiovascular disease risk factors. JAMA 1990;264:359–65.

21. Farquhar JW, Maccoby N, Wood PD, et al. Community education for cardiovascular health. Lancet 1977;1:1192–5.

22. Fédération Dentaire Internationale. Goals for oral health in the year 2000. FDI Newsletter 1982 March;5–8.

23. Fédération Dentaire Internationale. The impact of changing disease trends on dental education and practice. FDI Tech Rep No 30. Int Dent J 1987;37:127–30.

24. Flanders RA. Effectiveness of dental health educational programs in schools. J Am Dent Assoc 1987;114:239–42.

25. Fortmann SP, Flora JA, Winkleby MA, et al. Community intervention trials: Reflections on the Stanford Five-City project experience. Am J Epidemiol 1995;142:576–86.

26. Fortmann SP, Winkleby MA, Flora JA, et al. Effect of long-term community health education on blood pressure and hypertension control. The Stanford Five-City project. Am J Epidemiol 1990;132:629–46.

27. Frazier PJ, Horowitz AM. Oral health education and promotion in maternal and child health: A position paper. J Public Health Dent 1990;50:390–5.

28. Frazier PJ, Jenny J, Ostman R, Frenick C. Quality of information in mass media; a barrier to the dental health education of the public. J Public Health Dent 1974;34:244–57.

29. Freimuth VS, Mettger W. Is there a hard-to-reach audience? Public Health Rep 1990;105:232–8.

30. Friedman LA, Mackler IG, Hoggard GJ, et al. A comparison of perceived and actual dental needs of a select group of children in Texas. Community Dent Oral Epidemiol 1976;4:89–93.

31. Gamson WA. Commentary on "Fluoridation attitude change." Am J Public Health 1968;58:1880–2.

32. Gift HC. Awareness and assessment of periodontal problems among dentists and the public. Int Dent J 1988;38:147–53.

33. Glasrud PH, Frazier PJ. Future elementary school-teachers' knowledge and opinions about oral health and community programs. J Public Health Dent 1988;48:74–80.

34. Green LW. National policy in the promotion of health. Int J Health Educ 1979;22:161–8.

35. Green LW, Anderson CL. Community health. St. Louis: Mosby, 1986.

36. Green LW, Kreuter MW. Health promotion planning: an educational and environmental approach. 2nd ed. Mountain View, CA: Mayfield, 1991.

37. Greenberg JS. Health education. Dubuque IA: Brown, 1989.

38. Hager B, Krasse B. Dental health education by "barefoot doctors". Community Dent Oral Epidemiol 1983;11:333–6.

39. Hodge H, Buchanan M, O'Donnell P, et al. The evaluation of the junior dental health education programme developed in Sefton, England. Community Dent Health 1987;4:223–9.

40. Holcomb JD, Mullen PD, Thomson WA, et al. Health promotion/disease prevention; registered dental hygienists' beliefs and practice behaviors. Dent Hyg 1986;60:158–65.

41. Holt RD, Winter GB, Fox B, Askew R. Effects of dental health education for mothers with young children in London. Community Dent Oral Epidemiol 1985;13:148–51.

42. Horowitz AM, Frazier PJ. Effective oral health programs in school settings. In: Clark JW, ed: Clinical dentistry. Philadelphia: Harper and Row, 1986, pp 1–15.

43. Irbarren C, Luepker RV, McGovern PG, et al. Twelve-year trends in cardiovascular disease risk factors in the Minnesota heart survey. Are socioeconomic differences widening? Arch Intern Med 1997;157:873–81.

44. Isman R. Fluoridation: Strategies for success. Am J Public Health 1981;71:717–21.

45. Isman R. Effects of the dentist as the primary information source about fluoridation. J Public Health Dent 1983;43:274–83.

46. Jeffery RW. Community programs for obesity prevention: The Minnesota Heart Health program. Obesity Res 1995;3(Suppl 2):283S–8S.

47. Kay EJ, Locker D. Is dental health education effective? A systematic review of current evidence. Community Dent Oral Epidemiol 1996;24:231–5.

48. Kegeles SS. Some changes required to increase the public's utilization of preventive dentistry. J Public Health Dent 1968;28:19–26.

49. Kiyak HA, Mulligan K. Studies of the relationship between oral health and psychological well-being. Gerodontics 1987;3:109–12.

50. Knazan YL. Application of PRECEDE to dental health promotion for a Canadian well-elderly population. Gerodontics 1986;2:180–5.

51. Kochheiser T. Latest consumer research reveals "Apple Lady" ads effective. J Michigan Dent Assoc 1990;72:227–9.

52. Lalonde M. A new perspective on the health of Canadians: A working document. Ottawa: Information Canada, 1974.

53. Lang P, Woolfolk MW, Faja BW. Oral health knowledge and attitudes of elementary schoolteachers in Michigan. J Public Health Dent 1989;49:44–50.

54. Lie T, Mellingen JT. Periodontal awareness, health, and treatment need in dental school patients. I. Patient interviews. Acta Odont Scand 1987;45:179–86.

55. Lind OP, Evans RW, Corbet EF, et al. Hong Kong survey of adult oral health. Part 2. Oral health related perceptions, knowledge and behaviour. Community Dent Health 1987;4:367–81.

56. Loupe MJ, Frazier PJ. Knowledge and attitudes of schoolteachers toward oral health programs and preventive dentistry. J Am Dent Assoc 1983;107:229–34.

57. Malvitz DM, Broderick EB. Assessment of a dental disease prevention program after three years. J Public Health Dent 1989;49:54–8.

58. McCaul KD, Glasgow RE, Gustafson C. Predicting levels of preventive dental behaviors. J Am Dent Assoc 1985;111:601–5.

59. McGuire KM. Strategies for a fluoridation campaign. J Michigan Dent Assoc 1981;63:681–6.

60. McGuire MK, Sydney SB, Zink FJ, et al. Evaluation of an oral disease control program administered to a clinic population at a suburban dental school. J Periodontol 1980;51:607–13.

61. Milgrom P, Weinstein P, Melnick S, et al. Oral hygiene instruction and health risk assessment in dental practice. J Public Health Dent 1989;49:24–31.

62. Mittelmark MB, Hunt MK, Heath GW, Schmid TL. Realistic outcomes: Lessons from community-based research and demonstration programs for the prevention of cardiovascular diseases. J Public Health Policy 1993;14:437–62.

63. Murtomaa H, Masalin K. Effects of a national dental health campaign in Finland. Acta Odont Scand 1984;42:297–303.

64. Nuttall NM. Characteristics of dentally successful and dentally unsuccessful adults. Community Dent Oral Epidemiol 1984;12:208–12.

65. O'Neill HW. Opinion study comparing attitudes about dental health. J Am Dent Assoc 1984;109:910–5.

66. O'Shea RM, Corah NL, Ayer WA. Dentists' perceptions of the "good" adult patient: An exploratory study. J Am Dent Assoc 1983;106:813–6.

67. Olsen CB, Brown DF, Wright FA. Dental health promotion in a group of children at high risk to dental disease. Community Dent Oral Epidemiol 1986;14:302–5.

68. Paul BD. Fluoridation and the social scientist: A review. J Social Issues 1961;17:1–12.

69. Petersen PE. Evaluation of a dental preventive program for Danish chocolate workers. Community Dent Oral Epidemiol 1989;17:53–9.

70. Peterson FL Jr, Rubinson L. An evaluation of the effects of the American Dental Association's dental health education program on the knowledge, attitudes and health locus of control of high school students. J School Health 1982;52:63–9.

71. Raulet HM. The health professional and the fluoridation issue: A case of role conflict. J Social Issues 1961;17:45–54.

72. Reelick NF, Verbeek MH. The Dutch dental campaign. J Am Dent Assoc 1986;113:803–4.

73. Rosen J, Deck SA. The ADHA dental health initiative: more than just a pretty smile. Dent Hyg 1984;58:106–9.

74. Rosenthal DB, Crain RL. Executive leadership and community innovation: The fluoridation experience. Urban Affairs Q 1966;1:39–57.

75. Schou L. Active-involvement principle in dental health education. Community Dent Oral Epidemiol 1985;13:128–32.

76. Schou L. Use of mass-media and active involvement in a national dental health campaign in Scotland. Community Dent Oral Epidemiol 1987;15:14–8.

77. Siegal MD, Martin B, Kuthy RA. Usefulness of a local oral health survey in program development. J Public Health Dent 1988;48:121–4.

78. Simons-Morton BG, Greene WH, Gottlieb NH. Introduction to health education and health promotion. 2nd ed. Prospect Heights, IL: Waveland Press, 1995.

79. Sogaard AJ, Holst D. The effect of different school based dental health education programmes in Norway. Community Dent Health 1988;5:169–84.

80. Sogaard AJ, Koch AL. Dental health education—a question of values. J Public Health Dent 1984;44:169–71.

81. Taylor CB, Fortmann SP, Flora J, et al. Effect of long-term community health education on body mass index. The Stanford Five-City project. Am J Epidemiol 1991;134:235–49.

82. US Public Health Service. Promoting health: Objectives for the nation. Washington DC: Government Printing Office, 1980.

83. US Public Health Service. Healthy people 2000; national health promotion and disease prevention activities. Conference edition. Washington DC: Government Printing Office, 1990.

84. US Public Health Service, National Center for Health Statistics. Healthy people 2000 review 1997. DHHS Publ No (PHS) 98-1256. Hyattsville MD: Public Health Service, 1997.

85. US Public Health Service, Office of Disease Prevention and Health Promotion. The 1990 health objectives for the nation: A midcourse review. Washington DC: Government Printing Office, 1986, pp 147–61.

86. Walsh MM. Effects of school-based dental health education on knowledge, attitudes and behavior of adolescents in San Francisco. Community Dent Oral Epidemiol 1985;13:143–7.

87. Weinstein P, Milgrom P, Melnick S, et al. How effective is oral hygiene instruction? Results after 6 and 24 weeks. J Public Health Dent 1989;49:32–8.

88. White SL, Maloney SK. Promoting healthy diets and active lives to hard-to-reach groups: Market research study. Public Health Rep 1990;105:224–31.

89. Winkleby MA, Feldman HA, Murray DM. Joint analysis of three U.S. community intervention trials for reduction of cardiovascular disease risk. J Clin Epidemiol 1997;50:645–58.

90. Winkleby MA, Taylor CB, Jatulis D, Fortmann SP. The long-term effects of a cardiovascular disease prevention trial: The Stanford Five-City project. Am J Public Health 1996;86:1773–9.

91. Woolfolk MP, Sgan-Cohen HD, Bagramian RA, Gunn SM. Self-reported health behavior and dental knowledge of a migrant worker population. Community Dent Oral Epidemiol 1985;13:140–2.

92. World Health Organization. Dental health education. Tech Rep Series No 449. Geneva: WHO, 1970.

93. World Health Organization. Declaration of Alma-Ata. World Health, 1983, Sept. 24–25.

94. World Health Organization. Prevention methods and programmes for oral diseases. Tech Rep Series No 713. Geneva: WHO, 1984, pp 24–32.

95. Wright FA. Children's perception of vulnerability to illness and dental disease. Community Dent Oral Epidemiol 1982;10:29–32.

section II

Dental Practice

6

The Healthy Dental Practice: Infection Control and Mercury Safety

Infection Control—Guidelines for Infection Control ◆ OSHA and Dental Practice ◆ HIV Infection/ AIDS: the Disease ◆ Hepatitis B: the Disease ◆ Oral Manifestations of HIV Infection ◆ Public and Professional Perceptions of Infectious Diseases ◆ HIV Issues in Dental Practice and Dental Education ◆ Backflow Prevention ◆ Mercury and Dental Amalgam

In earlier days of dental practice, a blood-stained swab after a tooth extraction was simply thrown in the trash without further thought. Not any more. Today, dental offices must use universal precautions, a set of procedures based on the assumption that any patient, or any person working in the dental office, might carry a serious infection. All phases of treatment are then conducted so as to minimize the risk of cross-infection.

Some dentists look on the "old days" with nostalgia, a time when they did not have to work in gloves, mask, and eyewear; to ensure that office waste went into the appropriate container; and to worry about the latest regulations from the US Occupational Safety and Health Administration (OSHA). This nostalgic view is misplaced. It is fair to say that dentistry should have been a lot more concerned about cross-infection in the "old days" than it was. It took the jolt from the human immunodeficiency virus (HIV) epidemic to force improvement. Although some dentists, and even some of their leaders in the American Dental Association (ADA), still see OSHA's regulations on waste disposal as just another bureaucratic burden, the management of the office environment has clearly become an integral part of running a modern dental practice. Given that many more people are infected with the HIV and hepatitis B

viruses than demonstrate overt disease, the only defensible approach is to assume that any patient could be infected and to act accordingly. Dental practices today are far healthier environments than they ever were, and both the public and the professions will continue to benefit as a result.

This chapter reviews the principal infectious concerns in dental practice, HIV infection and hepatitis B (HBV infection), and reviews the issue of mercury safety as an example of an environmental concern. Both can be defined as public health issues (Chapter 4), which means that public agencies and the public at large will join the profession in determining how to deal with these issues.

INFECTION CONTROL

After the emergence of antibiotics during World War II (1939–1945), the developed nations lost much of their age-old concerns about infectious diseases. The major epidemics of the past were gone, and parents no longer feared the worst when they heard a child cough in the night. It was a short, complacent period during which some of the painful antisepsis lessons from the 19th century were forgotten in our dependence on antibiotics. This period ended suddenly in the early 1980s with the emergence of the HIV epidemic, a harsh reminder that mortal infectious diseases were still with us. In addition to being a devastating disease that shredded the social fabric in a way not seen since tuberculosis in the 19th century, the HIV epidemic is a humbling reminder that the path of biomedical advancement is not always smoothly upward.

Of course, HIV is not the only infectious disease to raise concerns about cross-infection during dental treatment. Dental professionals have always been at risk of catching the mundane colds and other upper respiratory tract infections from patients, but hepatitis B virus (HBV) infection is far more ominous than a cold, and the risk of HBV infection in the unprotected dental practice setting is higher than in most other environments. Hepatitis B was around long before HIV, but it took the impact of HIV to force adoption of those old-fashioned barrier techniques of infection control that had never been a routine part of dental practice. That has now changed to the extent that infection control is one of the major forces in shaping dental practice at the end of the 20th century.

Guidelines for Infection Control

Numerous guidelines for practicing infection control are now available to dental office personnel. The ADA had a set of rather gentle guidelines in the pre-HIV era,[7] mostly concerned with hepatitis, but the advent of HIV in the early 1980s led to a more stringent approach. Detailed guidelines have been produced by the ADA,[10] and the American Association of Public Health Dentistry,[5] although the definitive guidelines for dental practice are those from the US Public Health Service's Centers for Disease Control and Prevention (CDC).[91] CDC has also developed guidelines for field examinations for surveys or research studies.[86]

All of these guidelines are based on the concept of *universal precautions,* because their underlying philosophy is that infected patients cannot be detected from uninfected, so the prudent thing to do is to assume that all patients may be infected. They emphasize barrier procedures, meaning the wearing of gloves, masks, and protective eyewear by dental personnel, as well as routine autoclaving of instruments and means of handling potentially infectious materials. These principles hark back to the beginnings of antiseptic

medical practice, and they are effective: the incidence of HBV infection is twice as high among dentists who never wear gloves than among dentists who wear gloves routinely.[36] With universal precautions, the risk of transmission of either HIV or HBV in the dental office is extremely low.[91]

OSHA and Dental Practice

OSHA was established by Congress in December 1970 (P.L. 91-596), and some amendments to the original Act were enacted in November 1990. The mission of this regulatory agency, as laid out in the introduction to the original Act, is "to assure safe and healthful working conditions for working men and women." OSHA is responsible for establishing standards for safe and healthy working conditions for all employees, and to regulate maintenance of these standards. OSHA's standards cover almost all industries: mining, shipyards, construction, logging, food service, along with the health care industry and many others. OSHA also has standards that are specific to workers handling hazardous or potentially hazardous substances and materials, so the reach of this federal agency is considerable. A number of states have set up their own OSHA-type agencies, and OSHA is required to work cooperatively with them.

Dentists, like all other employers, are subject to occupational health and safety laws and regulations that cover a range of activities in the dental office. The OSHA regulation that has most affected dental practitioners is the Bloodborne Pathogen (BP) standard, which came into effect in March 1992 after a period of intense public debate in which the ADA was prominent. The BP standard applies to all activities in which health care workers come into contact with human blood or other bodily fluids, or are in a position where they may do so. The BP applies to hospitals and other medical facilities, paramedical and ambulance services, blood banks, research facilities, and dental offices. The BP (available in full on the OSHA website) is comprehensive and highly detailed. It requires each dental office to prepare an Exposure Control Plan, which is intended to minimize employee exposure to infection. The BP covers instrument sterilization and storage, handling potentially contaminated equipment, disposal of medical waste, and many related topics. It specifies that dentists must offer HBV vaccination to staff, and there are fastidious requirements for reporting "incidents," that is accidents during which skin has been broken (e.g., a needlestick) and hence where there is potential risk of infection. Details get down to the level of washing and storing laundry.

The ADA has not had a good relationship with OSHA through the 1990s. The ADA has complained that it was not consulted adequately before the promulgation of the BP, and that OSHA indiscriminately and inappropriately lumped dental practice in with hospitals and other facilities. The ADA considered that OSHA made no good attempt to understand dental practice, and its calls for industry-specific standards were not heeded. OSHA inspects health care facilities in response to complaints, and soon after the BP regulations went into effect the ADA began receiving complaints from dentists that some OSHA inspections of dental practices were heavy-handed and clumsy. OSHA admitted that there was some justification for these complaints, and with better communications the relations between the two organizations were improving by the mid-1990s. A major step in improved relations came when OSHA permitted dentists to respond to complaints by phone or fax rather than be subjected to a site visit; complaints from dentists on OSHA's tactics dropped sharply. Further OSHA regulations in matters affecting dental practice are likely, but consultation with the dental profession has improved.

For dentists unaccustomed to reading "federalese," the BP is a formidable document. To assist practitioners to meet the standards, manuals have been developed that give the elements of an exposure control plan, and put infection control guidelines together with OSHA guidelines in standard operating routines for the dental office.[73] (The BP relies heavily on universal precautions.)

Dentists have also complained about the cost of compliance with OSHA standards. A 1994 ADA survey concluded that the annual compliance cost per practice was $45,718, or $9.31 per patient visit,[24] much higher than OSHA's own estimates. Some of the more trivial aspects of the BP could be refined in time, which should have the effect of reducing costs, but compliance will always have some price. Who pays? Patients of course. OSHA is unlikely to go away, and in time the public will have to decide whether the cost of compliance is money well spent.

HIV Infection/AIDS: The Disease

AIDS, acronym for acquired immunodeficiency syndrome, is the end point of HIV infection. With the dominant position this condition now occupies in the lives of all health professionals, it is sobering to recall that the HIV virus was identified only in 1983.[61] The knowledge that has accumulated since then on the virology and epidemiology of the condition is the result of some impressive research, although the public hysteria that can surround AIDS is a reminder that humans have not fundamentally changed much since the Black Death of the 14th century.

The AIDS virus is the human T-lymphotropic virus type III/lymphadenopathy-associated virus (HTLV-III/LAV), a retrovirus usually called the HIV virus. It attacks the CD4+ T-lymphocytes in infected humans, thus leading to immunosuppression. As the number of CD4+ T-lymphocytes is reduced, the affected patient becomes increasingly vulnerable to opportunistic infections, which can overwhelm the patient's compromised defense systems. *Pneumocystis carinii* pneumonia is the most common serious opportunistic infection, although there are many others, including pulmonary tuberculosis. AIDS was formerly defined solely by clinical conditions, but a 1993 revision by CDC redefined the condition as stages of HIV infection in terms of 3 ranges of CD4+ T-lymphocyte counts and 3 clinical categories, set out in a 9-cell matrix.[18] These 9 categories range from asymptomatic HIV infection or persistent generalized lymphadenopathy with a CD4+ T-cell count of $500/\mu L$ or more at the mild end of the scale, to the diagnosis of one of 25 AIDS-indicator clinical conditions plus a CD4+ T-cell count of $200/\mu L$ or less at the severe end.[18] Dentally-related conditions listed in the clinical diseases that are considered part of the AIDS diagnosis include oropharyngeal candidiasis, oral hairy leukoplakia, chronic herpes simplex, and Kaposi's sarcoma.

The disease we call AIDS is the "finale in a progressive process of immunological deficit mediated by the virus."[61] It is more useful to think of it as HIV disease, rather than AIDS, because the condition has such a wide spectrum of manifestations, including a lack of symptoms. The primary epidemiology of HIV infection has been well described in terms of risk factors and modes of transmission, although much research is still needed on the dynamics of transmission and infection.[4] The average time between infection with HIV virus and the onset of AIDS-like symptoms is estimated to be 10 years,[61] which leads to the "time-bomb" implications of HIV disease.

HIV is a sexually transmitted pathogen, with birth to an infected mother or injection of substantial quantities of infected blood through transfusion or intravenous drug use the only other documented modes of transmission.[61] Principal risk groups in North America and Europe through the 1980s were male homosexuals and intravenous drug users who shared nonsterile needles, although HIV is also transmitted by heterosexual intercourse. Indeed, this is the principal mode of transmission in many parts of the world, and in the United States the number of infected women is steadily approaching that of men.[61] Despite the publicity given to the risk of certain sexual and drug use behaviors, behavioral change among the highest risk groups does not come easily. For a series of complex reasons, risk reduction is seen more through modification of behavior than through its elimination, and longitudinal studies have shown that back-sliding is common among high-risk individuals after some apparent progress.[13] However, the disease is not confined solely to these highest risk groups; by the early 1990s it was becoming more common in middle-class America.

The numbers in the HIV epidemic change rapidly. In mid-1997, the Joint United Nations Programme on HIV/AIDS recorded the global extent of the pandemic as shown in Table 6–1.

At the end of 1996, there had been 362,004 deaths from AIDS in the United States, including 4406 children under age 13. The cumulative number of cases reported was 581,429. The number of adults and adolescents living with AIDS is 223,000, an increase of 65% since 1993. No one knows how many people are infected with HIV who have not yet been diagnosed, but it is thought by CDC to be about 1 million.[18] Because of this large number, estimates on the growth of the epidemic are ominous. Vaccines are not considered likely, and the success of protease inhibitors in a drug "cocktail" appears to be in some degree of disease control rather than cure, so that control of the epidemic falls back on the toughest measure of all—education to control risky human behavior.

Table 6–1. THE GLOBAL EXTENT OF AIDS/HIV INFECTION IN 1997

- Globally, 21.8 million people, 21 million adults and 830,000 children, are estimated to be living with AIDS/HIV. (This was later upgraded to 30 million).
- In 1995, HIV-associated illnesses caused the death of 1.3 million people, including 300,000 children under age 5.
- Women are becoming increasingly affected; some 42% of HIV-infected adults are women.
- Since the beginning of the pandemic, over 9 million children under age 15 have lost their mothers to AIDS.
- If current trends continue, 60 to 70 million adults will have been affected by AIDS by the end of the year 2000.

Data from the websites for the Centers for Disease Control and Prevention and the World Health Organization.

AIDS presents some paradoxes. For example, despite the "time-bomb" implications from the extent of current infection, and thus the near certainty of the continued growth of the epidemic, the HIV virus is really quite delicate and hard to transmit. Although dental professionals are relatively more at risk than average members of the public because of their close contact with saliva and blood, they still demonstrate extremely low risk of occupational exposure.[43] A small number of health care workers have become HIV-infected through occupational exposure, but the risk of seroconversion even after needlestick exposure to HIV-infected blood is still only about 1:200.[94]

A possible case of HIV transmission from an infected dentist in Florida to a patient was reported in 1990[65]; the dentist died soon after the patient was diagnosed. In this case the patient had two maxillary third molars removed by the dentist. She reported pharyngitis 4 months later, and had oral candidiasis 17 months later. Two years after the extractions, she was seropositive for HIV antibody and was diagnosed with *P. carinii* pneumonia. The dentist was reported to have worn gloves and mask throughout the procedure, and from the patient's statement there was no evidence of exposure to the dentist's blood. There were similar DNA sequences in peripheral blood mononuclear cells of both dentist and patient, similar to those found in many cases that have been epidemiologically linked. Soon afterward, evidence emerged that 4 other patients from this practice were HIV-infected, and there were strong indications that the dentist was the source of infection for at least 2 of them.[90] The ADA responded quickly to this disclosure in early 1991 with an interim policy that HIV-infected dentists should not perform invasive procedures or should disclose their seropositive status to their patients.[55]

Hepatitis B: The Disease

Hepatitis is a far more prevalent disease than HIV, both worldwide and in the United States. The CDC estimates (data from the CDC website) that 45% of the world's population live in areas of high prevalence, 43% in areas of moderate prevalence, and only 12% in areas of low prevalence. The United States and other economically developed nations are areas of low prevalence, although there are still between 140,000 and 320,000 infections per year in the United States. Hepatitis B, primarily a disease of young adults in the United States, is the most serious and widespread of these conditions and is the variety that is of most concern in dental practice. The disease is transmitted by contact with infected blood, sexual contact, and perinatally. Although the case-fatality rate from infection is low (0.5% to 1.0%) and most infected people recover completely, a significant number of people can develop chronic infection, and the most serious sequelae are found in those people. The risk of becoming a chronic carrier varies with age of first infection. Among those first infected as young children, 30% to 90% develop chronic infection, whereas among those who were adults when first infected, only 2% to 10% do so. Approximately 24% of chronic HBV infections are acquired perinatally, and another 12% in early childhood. Chronic infection can be asymptomatic, but 15% to 25% of this group can die prematurely from cirrhosis or liver cancer. The CDC estimates that there are 140 to 320 deaths per year from acute hepatitis and 5,000 to 6,000 deaths each year from chronic liver disease.

Signs and symptoms of hepatitis B can be very general (fatigue, abdominal pain, loss of appetite, intermittent nausea and vomiting, and jaundice); hence the condition can easily be misdiagnosed. Health care workers are among those at higher risk than the general population because of their likely contact with chronic carriers. The CDC has estimated that there are 18,000 infections each year among health care workers in the United States, the majority through exposure to in-

fected blood. Blood and serous fluids have the highest concentration of the hepatitis B virus in infected persons; the concentration in saliva is a little lower. Carriers are at risk of long-term sequelae such as chronic liver disease, cirrhosis, and liver cancer, although a more common outcome than death is severe and usually lifelong debilitation. All things considered, hepatitis B is not a disease to be taken lightly.

Hepatitis viruses A, B, C, D, E, and G have now been identified, but the G virus is not yet well understood. Stringent screening of blood donors, beginning in the 1970s, resulted in a sharp decrease in hepatitis B resulting from blood transfusions. The hepatitis that still persisted after blood transfusions was recognized as a different type and was given the designation of *non-A, non-B* hepatitis. Approximately 90% of non-A, non-B is now recognized as hepatitis C. Hepatitis C has an insidious onset, and like hepatitis B it can be easily missed in its early stages; only some patients become symptomatic (symptoms are similar to those for hepatitis B). It is estimated that 4 million Americans are infected, with the disease more common in minority populations.[93] Some 85% of infected persons develop chronic infection. Transmission is bloodborne, sexual, and perinatal; and health care workers are considered to be at higher risk than the general population. Unlike for hepatitis B, there is no vaccine yet developed to treat hepatitis C, which is responsible for 8000 to 10,000 deaths from chronic liver disease annually in the United States. Without effective intervention, that number is expected to triple over the next 10 to 20 years.

Figure 6–1 shows the incidence of hepatitis B, hepatitis C, and tuberculosis in the United States from 1979 to 1993. The decline in the incidence of hepatitis B through the 1990s is thought to be due in part to the effectiveness of hepatitis B vaccine, but mostly to behavioral change among risk groups (injection drug users, the indiscriminately sexually active, and immigrants from high-prevalence areas) because of their fear of AIDS.

The most insidious aspect of HBV infection is the relative ease with which carriers can inadvertently transmit the disease to anyone with whom they come in contact. The worst reported instance of an infected dentist inadvertently transmitting HBV to his patients came from Indiana in 1984–1985. Nine patients of a dentist in a rural county devel-

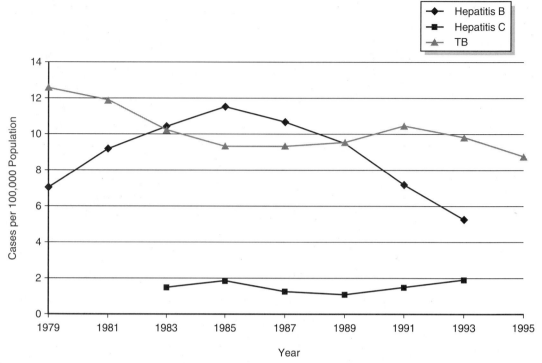

Figure 6–1. Annual incidence of hepatitis B, hepatitis C, and tuberculosis in the United States, 1979–1995. (From Centers for Disease Control and Prevention website.)

oped hepatitis B within 2 to 5 months after being treated by the dentist, a vastly higher incidence than had previously been reported there. Two of the patients died. Although the dentist had never had hepatitis symptoms, serum tests showed that he was probably a carrier.[79]

In contrast to the AIDS virus, HBV is hardy and capable of being transmitted much more readily via percutaneous and nonpercutaneous routes.[25] To heighten the contrast, it was reported in 1989 that whereas 15 health care workers had become seropositive for HIV over the last 7 years in the absence of outside risk factors, a total of between 1750 and 2100 health care providers had died from complications associated with HBV infection.[51] Because carrier states for HBV are not uncommon, with only 1 in 5 infections being recognized, the patient history can be of little value for dental practitioners.[25] The risk of contracting hepatitis B has been estimated at 3 to 10 times greater for dentists than for the general population,[3, 99] although those estimates came from the days before universal precautions were widely used. The greatest risk of infection in the dental office clearly comes from the undiagnosed carrier, whether

a patient, the dentist, or one of the office staff.[26] Hepatitis has been recognized for some time as a significant health hazard in dentistry,[101] and it was also demonstrated years ago that the proportion of HBV seropositive dentists does not vary with geographic region or size of community.[56]

The barrier precautions (gloves, masks, and eyewear) and sterilization procedures for preventing transmission of hepatitis non-A, non-B are the same as those for prevention of HBV transmission. Unlike the case with AIDS, however, there has been an effective vaccine against hepatitis B since 1982.[23] Since then, both the CDC and ADA have strongly recommended immunization against HBV for all dental office staff who contact patients, and as described earlier, OSHA regulations now require that dentists cover the cost of HBV vaccination for the office staff. Immunity status is readily tested. For most, immunization in a series of 3 injections over 6 months is required. Vaccination is specific to HBV and does not protect against non-A, non-B.[64]

Dentists have responded well to the need to ensure their immune status to hepatitis B. Among dentist participants in the ADA's health screening at the annual meeting, those reporting vaccination increased from 22% in 1983 to 84% in 1992, and those whose blood tests showed infection (i.e., presence of the hepatitis B surface antigen) dropped from 14% to 9% over the same period. Chronic carrier status (i.e., positive both to the hepatitis B surface antigen and core antigen) among dentists dropped from 0.95% in 1983 to 0.25% in 1992.[21] Even higher rates of immunization were reported from a national survey of dental personnel in Britain.[77] Vaccination is more common among younger than among older dentists, so in time virtually all dental personnel should have high levels of protection against hepatitis B.

Oral Manifestations of HIV Infection

All dental professionals should be thoroughly familiar with the oral manifestations of HIV infection. The principal signs are oral candidiasis, Kaposi's sarcoma, and oral hairy leukoplakia, although periodontal conditions are frequently severe in persons with advanced immunosuppression[100] and a number of less common pathoses are also found.[76] The details of these conditions are covered thoroughly in oral pathology texts[38] and workshop proceedings[67]; the three principal signs are described only briefly here.

Oral Candidiasis

A fungal infection, candidiasis (called candidosis in Britain) usually presents as a semiadherent white plaque on the palate, although glossitis and angular stomatitis forms are not uncommon. The plaques can be sore, and they are common among HIV-positive individuals. Pindborg[62] has described the diagnosis and treatment of oral candidiasis.

Kaposi's Sarcoma

Kaposi's sarcoma is diagnostic for AIDS and is found in 20% to 34% of AIDS patients.[31] The oral cavity may be the first or only site of the lesion; the most common intraoral site is the palate. The pathogenesis of Kaposi's sarcoma is still not well understood, nor is its interaction with HIV infection. Treatment is required because of functional impairment, pain, bleeding, or for cosmetic reasons. Radiation treatment appears to be the most practical and effective treatment procedure.[31]

Oral Hairy Leukoplakia

In a study of 375 homosexual males who either had AIDS or were considered at risk for the disease, 28% presented with oral hairy leukoplakia.[81] The lesions presented most commonly on the lateral surface of the tongue, with wide variation in the size, severity, and surface characteristics.[75] The condition is highly predictive of the future development of AIDS. In a longitudinal study of a group with oral hairy leukoplakia, survival analysis showed that the probability of AIDS developing was 48% after 16 months and 83% after 31 months.[37]

Pediatric AIDS

The particularly distressing condition of pediatric AIDS, in which the HIV virus is transmitted from an infected mother, appears to be on the increase. Recognition can be difficult because of the varied presentation of the condition, although the most common oral findings include candidiasis, parotid salivary gland enlargement, and herpetic infections.[82]

Public and Professional Perceptions of Infectious Diseases

As the public grows more accepting of the fact that there is an HIV epidemic, attitudes of dentists towards treating infected people have also matured. Not surprisingly, dentists in a number of countries have demonstrated ambivalent attitudes toward treating infected patients.[32, 69, 74, 89] Treating infected patients was reluctantly seen as a professional responsibility, and many clearly would prefer not to.[14, 44, 70] With the adoption of universal precautions and a realization that adherence to them largely reduced the risk of transmission of HIV, HBV, and HCV, rational fears on the part of dentists seem to be allayed. However, there clearly are still many irrational fears and anxieties,[14, 54, 72] especially of HIV infection, which do not abate with continuing education and evidence of extremely low risk of transmission. A general willingness to treat HIV-positive patients was expressed by two thirds of dentists in a New York City study in the early 1990s, but this proportion dropped when the patients concerned were not patients of record in the practice.[71] HIV-infected patients who used to be referred to clinics dedicated to treating them are increasingly feeling comfortable in general dentists' offices.[12] As noted earlier in this chapter, dentists do not have the legal right to turn away prospective patients who are, or who may be, HIV- or HBV-infected. By the same token, with universal precautions, there is no need for anxiety when treating such patients.

Surveys in the mid-1980s found variable adherence to infection-control procedures in the dental office[32]; some dentists were apparently slow to accept that they were at risk without them. Dental professionals who accepted that some of their patients were probably infected were more likely to adhere to the recommendations,[34] and educational programs for dental personnel were effective in improving adherence to these procedures.[29, 33] Attitudes and infection-control practices appeared to move forward considerably in the late 1980s, however, for a national survey of general dentists in 1990 found virtually universal acceptance of the need for infection control procedures in the dental office.[70] These advances in attitudes and practice have continued for dentists through the 1990s,[22, 35] although it has been pointed out that although use of universal precautions has become common, poor communication between dentists and HIV patients has changed little.[39] A study of hygienists in Mississippi also disclosed that their attitudes and beliefs had not kept pace with modern knowledge, so there is still apparently a need for continuing education on infection control.[28]

HIV Issues in Dental Practice and Dental Education

The legal implications of cross-infection continue to evolve, and all dental practitioners need to be constantly aware of them. HIV-infected dentists are in a particularly difficult position. A number of states have responded to public clamor with laws restricting the rights of infected dentists to practice.[48] Many interpret these laws as overreaction, although in states without them a dentist's legal obligation to tell patients and staff that he or a staff member is HIV- or HBV-infected is not clear. If he does, the ensuing hysteria would probably force the practice to close; if he does not, he is probably liable if a patient becomes infected.[48]

On the other hand, dentists have a clear legal obligation, under the Americans with Disabilities Act of 1990, to not deny treatment to a patient solely on the grounds of the patient's infection. This became clear in a 1997 US District Court judgment against a dentist who, it was alleged, denied treatment to a patient solely on the grounds of the patient's HIV status.[40] The dentist appealed, but the US Court of Appeals reaffirmed the District Court's decision. The case may eventually go to the US Supreme Court. The ruling is based on the evidence that universal precautions reduce the risk of transmission to extremely low levels.

Willingness to treat HIV-infected patients is an issue that organized dentistry and the dental schools in their curricula should deal with vigorously. The ADA has included in its Code of Ethics (Chapter 3) the statement that refusal to treat an HIV-infected patient, solely on those grounds, is unethical. Refusal to treat an infected person, solely on the grounds of that infection, is not only unethical but also, as stated in the previous paragraph, illegal. It is a position that also makes little sense because (a) the risk of transmission of HIV from patient to dentist, as already discussed, is extremely low when the dentist is using universal precautions and (b) many dentists will already have treated HIV-infected persons without knowing it.

The fact remains that a level of anxiety remains about treating infected patients, especially HIV-infected patients. Some dentists are adamant that they do not have an ethical responsibility to treat HIV-positive patients.[72] These dentists cite a lack of confidence in universal precautions and concerns about what will happen to their practice if it becomes known that HIV-positive patients are treated there. The majority of dentists accept the ethical responsibility to treat infected patients, although most would rather not do so if they had the choice.[14] In a 1991 national survey of senior dental students, 76% agreed with the ethical responsibility to treat infected patients, although 54% admitted to some fear in treating infected patients and 53% would prefer not to do so if given the choice.[84] AIDS clinics exist in a number of major cities, staffed by dental professionals whose commitment to equality of care for all represents the highest degree of professionalism. However, the trend in the late 1990s for treating infected patients was clearly toward "mainstreaming" (i.e., treatment in private dental offices rather than in segregated facilities).

Many issues have been raised in dental education by the AIDS epidemic and will take years to become resolved. Two questions readily arise:

- Should an HIV-positive student applicant be admitted to dental school?
- What is the dental school's obligation if a student becomes HIV-positive in the course of clinical duties?

Some experience in these matters has now been accumulated. There are several documented cases of students who were identified as HIV-positive during their studies and after they had begun treating patients,[27, 41, 88] and there is at least one documented case of a faculty member who died of AIDS.[17] In each instance, the experience was disruptive for all concerned. In the case of the students, what followed was similar in each school. The student was immediately taken away from patient contact, patients treated by the student were offered free testing and counseling, and confidentiality of the student's identity was maintained in the face of intense media pressure. Reviews were made of the student's compliance with infection control procedures and of the school's procedures for sterilizing instruments. Extensive meetings between school administration with faculty and students were held to explain actions taken and the reason for them. (None of the patients tested were seropositive.) At least one of the students concerned completed his dental degree, carrying out his remaining clinical requirements on patients known to be HIV-infected.[41]

It seems clear that dental schools should have clear policies on these issues and an established plan of action when an incident arises. There are many implications to whatever policies are adopted, but experience has shown that the worst thing to do is stick our collective heads in the sand and hope that nothing unpleasant happens with respect to HIV in dental educational settings. Almost certainly the situations described here will occur at other schools, and the schools should be ready to handle the situation. A set of principles for developing these policies, originally presented in 1989 and shown in Table 6–2,[51] is still a good starting point today.

The AIDS epidemic has already had a dramatic effect on the practice of dentistry, and it will continue to affect it in complex ways for the foreseeable future. As was said the day after the first nuclear bomb was dropped on Hiroshima in 1945, nothing will ever be the same again.

BACKFLOW PREVENTION

Cross-connection is the name given to the link by which contaminated materials may enter a public water supply when the pressure from the polluted source exceeds the pressure of the water supply. The risk of such an occurrence, already extremely low, is reduced even further when backflow prevention devices, or antiretraction valves, are used

Table 6–2. SUGGESTED PRINCIPLES ON WHICH POLICIES FOR DEALING WITH HIV-INFECTED STUDENTS, EMPLOYEES, AND PATIENTS IN DENTAL INSTITUTIONS COULD BE BASED

- People suffering from HIV-related conditions are entitled to the same dignity and respect as those who are suffering from any other illness.
- There should be an appropriate balance between public health needs and the privacy and dignity of those afflicted with HIV infection.
- HIV virus is transmitted by definable behaviors that can be changed by educational efforts.
- Requiring an HIV test does little unless behavior changes. Behavior is only changed through counseling and education.
- With regard to testing for HIV, no person should have his or her blood tested without written consent.
- Confidentiality in HIV testing is essential if we are to obtain the cooperation of risk groups. If confidentiality is inadequate, risk groups will not participate in testing or in educational programs.
- Although confidentiality is the hallmark of HIV testing, in certain circumstances test results may be divulged to: (a) the subject; (b) a spouse; (c) a legal representative; (d) a sexual partner; (e) an individual sharing hypodermic needles; (f) a health care provider and the health care team; (g) a local health officer.
- Universal precautions, that is, the wearing of gloves, gowns, masks, and other steps to prevent transmission of HIV virus, should be followed by all health care providers.
- There is a public interest in providing HIV test results on individuals and cadavers from which tissues are taken for transplant and/or blood is taken to protect the blood supply.
- Individuals and other health care providers should report all confirmed cases of HIV infection to public health authorities, and such information should be kept in confidence.

From Lundberg JF. Legal and ethical aspects of the AIDS crisis. J Dent Educ 1989;53:515–7.

to prevent back-siphonage of contaminated fluids. While a cross-connection is also theoretically possible through the high-speed handpiece and the air and water syringe, this risk, too, is extremely low and has not yet been documented. A lot of the concern expressed about backflow relates to the chance of HIV and HBV infection through this route, but this possibility is seen as near enough to zero because neither virus is transmitted through contaminated water. The use of self-contained water systems in the dental office (i.e., water systems not connected to the public water supply) is a recommended measure to reduce any possible risk even further.

MERCURY AND DENTAL AMALGAM

Amalgam restorations have been used in dental practice since the mid-19th century, and it would be impossible to calculate how many have been placed since then. Today, millions of people around the world are carrying amalgam restorations in their mouths without apparent ill effects. Amalgam has lasted so well because it is a versatile material for intraoral use, is easy to handle, and is relatively inexpensive. Even with new composite and bonding materials now in use, amalgam remains a basic restorative material in dental practice. However, the toxic properties of mercury have been known for years, and with current environmental sensitivities, some observers have charged that it is no longer appropriate to use mercury in the human mouth.

Mercury vapor is released from amalgams, and average daily intake of mercury from amalgam restorations is estimated to be 1.2 to 1.3 μg when tested subjects have 7 to 8 restorations.[52, 85] This amount constitutes 6% to 12% of total mercury intake from all sources.[53] Earlier estimates of up to 20 μg/day from amalgams[95] have been criticized as being 16 times too high because of the failure to account for the difference between the flow rate of the mercury vapor detector and that of human respiration.[53] Opponents of amalgam use, however, still insist that exposure to mercury from dental amalgams exceeds the sum of exposure from all other sources.[49]

The evidence against the use of amalgam restorations is largely circumstantial. Among patients, intraoral measurements of mercury vapor show higher readings in adults with amalgam restorations than in those without, and the differential is higher after chewing.[87, 95, 96] Computer simulations from these data have led to the estimate that long-term inhalation of mercury vapor from restorations results in an increasing mercury burden in the tissues.[97] In animal studies, deleterious effects on brain tissue and intestinal microbial flora have been reported from amalgams.[49] In humans, blood mercury levels have been correlated with the number and surface area of amalgams and have been measured as significantly lower in people without amalgam restorations.[1, 46, 85] However, raised levels of mercury in urine could not be demonstrated in children after a single session of restorative dentistry,[60] although this finding could have resulted from the relatively small amounts of amalgam used.

Measures of urinary mercury among dentists attending the ADA annual session show wide variability, but generally are higher in dentists who have greater exposure to mercury. Higher levels are thus seen in older dentists and in generalists rather than specialists, and are related to the number of amalgams placed, form of amalgam preparation, and type of heating and cooling system in the office. Dentists in the New England and mid-Atlantic regions, on average, had twice the urinary mercury levels found in West Coast dentists.[57] Swedish studies have shown higher urinary mercury levels in dental personnel compared with nondental controls, although all values were well below those set for occupational health standards.[58, 59]

Because one of the outcomes from mercury toxicity is neurologic damage, some studies had looked specifically for neurologic syndromes related to amalgam restorations. The evidence here is weak. One researcher concluded that the prevalence of multiple sclerosis was related to the use of amalgam restorations,[42] although the evidence presented was so broad that this conclusion was hard to accept. (The evidence presented was ecologic: there are more amalgams placed in the northern United States than in the South, and there is also more multiple sclerosis in the North. The prime weakness in this argument is that the people with the disease are not necessarily the people with the restorations.) Evidence for neurologic damage has been reported in some dentists with exceptionally high mercury tissue levels,[78] and there are a few reports of mental distress in dentists and patients, supposedly resulting from exposure to mercury.[80, 83] Other reports have concluded that the symptoms reported by patients who believed that amalgams were making them sick were of psychosomatic origin.[47]

Widespread media publicity has been given to the results of animal studies with amalgam. Reports on studies with sheep, for example, have concluded that mercury inhaled from amalgams placed in pregnant ewes appears in the fetal circulation within 2 days.[98] Critics contend that the sheep, a ruminant, is a poor model in which to study mercury inhalation.

The validity of a number of these studies, both with humans and animals, remains a subject for debate; firm conclusions are hard to reach. Critical reviews of the literature have concluded that mercury from amalgam restorations does find its way into human tissues,[20, 30, 45, 66] although these same reviewers consider that there is no evidence for ill effects in humans from the amounts in question. For example, no difference in lymphocyte levels could be found in comparisons between persons with amalgam restorations and those without.[53] Subsequent studies examining the potential effects of mercury from amalgam fillings on human health have all concluded that there is no association,[2, 15, 16] although on the other hand, some literature reviews have concluded that negative health effects result from amalgams.[50, 63] In a debate that sometimes has overtones of that surrounding water fluoridation (Chapter 24), not every single health hypothesis can be tested, and the question of subtle side effects requires additional research to be fully answered. The concern is whether potential public health problems might exist, given the millions of people exposed,[19] although on balance, evidence suggests that there are no public health problems resulting from routine use of dental amalgams.

By the early 1990s, the issue had become an emotional debate that spilled over from scientific discussions into the public arena. The ADA has consistently maintained its support for the use of amalgams on the grounds that there are no substantiated reports of ill health to humans resulting from their use.[45] The issue is not new in ADA circles; a 1971 review concluded that normal handling of mercury in practice does not present a threat to patients, but could present a threat to dental personnel if precautions were not taken.[68] This review led to the ADA's first set of 15 recommendations on mercury hygiene in 1974.[6] In its own review of the literature, the ADA concluded that there was no need to remove amalgams from patients, except in the rare cases of mercury allergy.[8] A second set of recommendations on mercury hygiene were issued in 1984. It was more stringent than the first edition and included reference to OSHA requirements for disposal of scrap amalgam.[9] The ADA derided the claims that removal of amalgams could improve the condition of multiple sclerosis sufferers as "a cruel hoax,"[11] and made perhaps its strongest statement with an advisory opinion in the current Code of Ethics on the ADA website:

> . . . the removal of amalgam restorations from the non-allergenic patients for the alleged purpose of removing toxic substances from the body, when such treatment is performed solely at the recommendation or suggestion of the dentist, is improper and unethical.

It is clear that research and public enquiry on this issue should continue, although as with many environmental questions, the determination of cause and effect is extraordinarily difficult. Symptoms of mercury toxicity are general in nature, similar to those for dozens of other medical conditions. Threshold limits in occupational medicine are at best broad estimates, and extrapolation from animal studies to human conditions is always difficult. Humans are also exposed to environmental mercury from other sources, such as organic mercury from seafood; it was mentioned earlier that mercury from amalgams constituted only 6% to 12% of daily intake for adults with amalgam restorations. Improvements in alternative restorative materials are nevertheless to be encouraged, and the evolution of sealants and minimum preparation restoration procedures (Chapter 26) is increasingly appropriate for restorations in children. The mercury issue will probably diminish over time as sealants replace amalgams in children, and as complex restorations in young people become increasingly uncommon.

When amalgam is used, however, all precautions should be taken to minimize exposure to mercury vapor for both patients and office staff. Guidelines for storing and disposing of amalgam scrap and for handling mercury spills need to be followed as rigidly as are those for dealing with potentially contaminated waste. As with infection control, developments in many issues related to mercury use can be expected to evolve considerably in the next century.

The US Public Health Service conducted an exhaustive review of amalgam safety in 1993.[92] The review concluded that amalgam use was declining as caries experience diminished and as other materials were used more often. However, there was an appropriate note of caution. The committee (which could hardly be accused of bias, as no member was a dentist) concluded that, although there was no good evidence of amalgam causing harm in humans apart from rare allergic reactions, the paucity of reliable studies required further studies on the issue. As with all issues in infection control and environmental safety, however, the dental profession cannot determine policy by itself. The dental profession should act as a leader, but both issues are public health issues and must be handled as such.

REFERENCES

1. Abraham JE, Svare CW, Frank CW. The effect of dental amalgam restorations on blood mercury levels. J Dent Res 1984;63:71–3.
2. Ahlqwist M, Bengtsson C, Lapidus L, et al. Concentrations of blood, serum and urine components in relation to number of amalgam tooth fillings in Swedish women. Community Dent Oral Epidemiol 1995;23:217–21.
3. AIDS less prevalent than hepatitis B virus. J Am Dent Assoc 1986;112:464–5.
4. Allen JR, Curran JW. Prevention of AIDS and HIV infection: Needs and priorities for epidemiologic research. Am J Public Health 1988;78:381–6.
5. American Association of Public Health Dentistry. The control of transmissible diseases in dental practice: a position paper of the American Association of Public Health Dentistry. J Public Health Dent 1986;46:13–22.
6. American Dental Association, Council on Dental Materials and Devices. Recommendations in mercury hygiene, February 1974. J Am Dent Assoc 1974;88:391–2.
7. American Dental Association, Council on Dental Materials and Devices and Council on Dental Therapeutics. Infection control in the dental office. J Am Dent Assoc 1978;97:673–7.
8. American Dental Association, Council on Dental Materials, Instruments, and Equipment, Council on Dental Therapeutics. Safety of dental amalgam. J Am Dent Assoc 1983;106:519–20.
9. American Dental Association, Council on Dental Materials, Instruments, and Equipment. Recommendations in dental mercury hygiene, 1984. J Am Dent Assoc 1984;109:617–9.
10. American Dental Association, Council on Dental Therapeutics and Council on Prosthetic Services and Dental Laboratory Relations. Guidelines for infection control in the dental office and the commercial dental laboratory. J Am Dent Assoc 1985;110:969–72.
11. American Dental Association, Council on Ethics, By-laws, and Judicial Affairs. American Dental Association principles of ethics and code of professional conduct. J Am Dent Assoc 1990;120:585–92.
12. Barnes DB, Gerbert B, McMaster JR, Greenblatt RM. Self-disclosure experience of people with HIV infection in dedicated and mainstreamed dental facilities. J Public Health Dent 1996;56:223–5.
13. Becker MH, Joseph JG. AIDS and behavioral change to reduce risk: A review. Am J Public Health 1988;78:394–410.
14. Bennett EM, Weyant RJ, Wallisch JM, Green G. A national survey: Dentists' attitudes toward the treatment of HIV-positive patients. J Am Dent Assoc 1995;126:509–14.
15. Bergdahl BJ, Anneroth G, Anneroth I. Clinical study of patients with burning mouth. Scand J Dent Res 1994;102:299–305.
16. Berglund A, Molin M. Mercury vapor release from dental amalgam in patients with symptoms allegedly caused by amalgam fillings. Eur J Oral Sci 1996;104:56–63.
17. Butters JM, Hutchinson RA, Koelbl JJ, Williams JN. A dental school's experience with the death of an HIV-positive faculty member. J Dent Educ 1994;58:19–25.
18. Castro KG, Ward JW, Slutsker L, et al. 1993 revised classification system for HIV infection and expanded surveillance case definition for AIDS among adolescents and adults. MMWR 1992;41(RR-17):1–19.
19. Clarkson TW. Mercury—an element of mystery [editorial]. N Engl J Med 1990;323:1137–9.
20. Clarkson TH, Hursh JB, Sager PR, et al. In: Clarkson TH, Friberg L, Nordberg GF, Sager PR, eds: Biological monitoring of toxic metals. New York: Plenum Press, 1988, pp 199–246.
21. Cleveland JL, Siew C, Lockwood SA, et al. Hepatitis B vaccination and infection among U.S. dentists, 1983–1992. J Am Dent Assoc 1996;127:1385–90.
22. Cohen AS, Jacobsen EL, BeGole EA. National survey of endodontists and selected patient samples: Infectious diseases and attitudes toward infection control. Oral Surg Oral Med Oral Pathol Oral Radiol and Endodont 1997;83:696–702.
23. Cooley RL, Lubow RM. Hepatitis B vaccine: Implications for dental personnel. J Am Dent Assoc 1982;105:47–9.
24. Cost of OSHA compliance gets mixed response. ADA News 1994 Oct 3; 25:1, 8, 10.
25. Cottone JA. Hepatitis B virus infection in the dental profession. J Am Dent Assoc 1985;110:617–21.
26. Cottone JA, Goebel WM. Hepatitis B: The clinical detection of the chronic carrier dental patient and the effects of immunization via vaccine. Oral Surg Oral Med Oral Pathol 1983;56:449–54.
27. Cottone JA, Kalkwarf KL, Kuebker WA. The assessment of an HIV seropositive student at the University of Texas Health Science Center at San Antonio Dental School. J Dent Educ 1992;56:536–9.
28. Daniel SJ, Silberman SL, Bryant EM, Meydrech EF. Infection control knowledge, practice, and attitudes of Mississippi dental hygienists. J Dent Hyg 1996;70:22–34.
29. DiAngelis AJ, Martens LV, Little JW, Hastreiter RJ. Infection control practices of Minnesota dentists: Changes during 1 year. J Am Dent Assoc 1989;118:299–303.
30. Enwonwu CO. Potential health hazard of use of mercury in dentistry: Critical review of the literature. Environ Res 1987;42:257–74.

31. Ficarra G, Berson AM, Silverman S Jr, et al. Kaposi's sarcoma of the oral cavity: A study of 134 patients with a review of the pathogenesis, epidemiology, clinical aspects, and treatment. Oral Surg Oral Med Oral Pathol 1988;66:543–50.

32. Gerbert B. AIDS and infection control in dental practice: Dentists' attitudes, knowledge, and behavior. J Am Dent Assoc 1987;114:311–4.

33. Gerbert B, Badner V, Maguire B. AIDS and dental practice. J Public Health Dent 1988;48:68–73.

34. Gerbert B, Maguire B, Badner V, et al. Changing dentists' knowledge, attitudes, and behaviors relating to AIDS: A controlled educational intervention. J Am Dent Assoc 1988;116:851–4.

35. Gibson GB, Mathias RG, Epstein JB. Compliance to recommended infection control procedures: Changes over six years among British Columbia dentists. J Can Dent Assoc 1995;61:526–32.

36. Gonzales E, Naleway C. Assessment of the effectiveness of glove use as a barrier technique in the dental operatory. J Am Dent Assoc 1988;117:467–9.

37. Greenspan D, Greenspan JS, Hearst NG, et al. Relation of oral hairy leukoplakia to infection with the human immunodeficiency virus and the risk of developing AIDS. J Infect Dis 1987;155:475–81.

38. Greenspan D, Greenspan JS, Schiodt M, Pindborg JJ. AIDS and the mouth. Copenhagen, Denmark: Munksgaard, 1990.

39. Hazelkorn HM, Bloom BE, Jovanovic BD. Infection control in the dental office: Has anything changed? J Am Dent Assoc 1996;127:786–90.

40. HIV discrimination ruled; judge says Maine dentist violated disabilities law. ADA News 1996 Jan 8, 27:1, 6, 23.

41. Heuer MA. Recent dental school experiences concerning HIV positive students: Northwestern, 1991–92. J Dent Educ 1992;56:528–35.

42. Ingalls TH. Epidemiology, etiology, and prevention of multiple sclerosis. Hypothesis and fact. Am J Forensic Med Pathol 1983;4:55–61.

43. Klein RS, Phelan JA, Freeman K, et al. Low occupational risk of human immunodeficiency virus infection among dental professionals. N Engl J Med 1988;318:86–90.

44. Kunzel C, Sadowsky D. Comparing dentists' attitudes and knowledge concerning AIDS: Differences and similarities by locale. J Am Dent Assoc 1991;122:55–61.

45. Langan DC, Fan PL, Hoos AA. The use of mercury in dentistry: A critical review. J Am Dent Assoc 1987;115:867–80.

46. Langworth S, Elinder C-G, Akesson A. Mercury exposure from dental fillings. I. Mercury concentrations in blood and urine. Swed Dent J 1988;12:69–70.

47. Lindberg NE, Lindberg E, Larsson G. Psychologic factors in the etiology of amalgam illness. Acta Odont Scand 1994;52:219–28.

48. Logan MK. Legal implications of infectious disease in the dental office. J Am Dent Assoc 1987;115:850–4.

49. Lorscheider FL, Vimy MJ, Summers AO. Mercury exposure from "silver" tooth fillings: Emerging evidence questions a traditional dental paradigm. FASEB J 1995;9:504–8.

50. Lorscheider FL, Vimy MJ, Summers AO, Zweirs H. The dental amalgam mercury controversy—inorganic mercury and the CNS: Genetic linkage of mercury and antibiotic resistances in intestinal bacteria. Toxicology 1995;97:19–22.

51. Lundberg JF. Legal and ethical aspects of the AIDS crisis. J Dent Educ 1989;53:515–7.

52. Mackert JR Jr. Factors affecting estimation of dental amalgam mercury exposure from measurements of mercury vapor levels in intra-oral and expired air. J Dent Res 1987;66:1775–80.

53. Mackert JR Jr, Leffell MS, Wagner DA, Powell BJ. Lymphocyte levels in subjects with and without amalgam restorations. J Am Dent Assoc 1991;122:49–53.

54. Manz MC, Weyant RJ, Adelson R, et al. Impact of HIV on VA dental services: Report of a survey. J Public Health Dent 1994;54:197–204.

55. Meskin LH. A letter of importance [editorial]. J Am Dent Assoc 1991;122:8–10.

56. Mosley JW, Edwards VM, Casey G, et al. Hepatitis B virus infection in dentists. N Engl J Med 1975;293:729–34.

57. Naleway C, Sakaguchi R, Mitchell E, et al. Urinary mercury levels in US dentists, 1975–1983: Review of Health Assessment Program. J Am Dent Assoc 1985;111:37–42.

58. Nilsson B, Gerhardsson L, Nordberg GF. Urine mercury levels and associated symptoms in dental personnel. Sci Total Environ 1990;94:179–85.

59. Nilsson B, Nilsson B. Mercury in dental practice. II. Urinary mercury excretion in dental personnel. Swed Dent J 1986;10:221–32.

60. Olstad ML, Holland RI, Pettersen AH. Effect of placement of amalgam restorations on urinary mercury concentrations. J Dent Res 1990;69:1607–9.

61. Osborn JE. Dispelling myths about the AIDS epidemic. In: Fransen VE, ed: Proceedings of the AIDS prevention and services workshop. Princeton NJ: Robert Wood Johnson Foundation, 1990, pp 15–21.

62. Pindborg JJ. Oral candidiasis in HIV infection. In: Robertson PB, Greenspan JS, eds: Perspectives on oral manifestations of AIDS. Littleton MA: PSG Publishing, 1988, pp 28–37.

63. Pleva J. Dental mercury—a public health hazard. Rev Environ Health 1994;10:1–27.

64. Porter SR, Scully C. Non-A, non-B hepatitis and dentistry. Br Dent J 1990;168:257–61.

65. Possible transmission of human immunodeficiency virus to a patient during an invasive dental procedure. MMWR 1990;39:489–93.

66. Reinhardt JW. Risk assessment of mercury exposure from dental amalgams. J Public Health Dent 1988;48:172–7.

67. Robertson PB, Greenspan JS, eds: Perspectives on oral manifestations of AIDS. Littleton MA: PSG Publishing, 1988.

68. Rupp NW, Paffenbarger GC. Significance to health of mercury used in dental practice: A review. J Am Dent Assoc 1971;82:1401–7.

69. Rydman RJ, Yale SH, Mullner RM, et al. Preventive control of AIDS by the dental profession: A survey of practices in a large urban area. J Public Health Dent 1990;50:7–12.

70. Sadowsky D, Kunzel C. Are you willing to treat AIDS patients? J Am Dent Assoc 1991;122:29–32.

71. Sadowsky D, Kunzel C. Measuring dentists' willingness to treat HIV-positive patients. J Am Dent Assoc 1994;125:705–10.

72. Sadowsky D, Kunzel C. Dentists' HIV-related ethicality: An empirical test. J Am Coll Dent 1997;64:27–9.

73. Schaefer ME. Infection control, OSHA, and a hazards communication program. J California Dent Assoc 1990;18:53–8.

74. Scheutz F. Dental care of HIV-infected patients: Atti-

tudes and behavior among Danish dentists. Community Dent Oral Epidemiol 1989;17:117–9.

75. Schiodt M, Greenspan D, Daniels TE, Greenspan JS. Clinical and histologic spectrum of oral hairy leukoplakia. Oral Surg Oral Med Oral Pathol 1987;64:716–20.

76. Scully C, Epstein JB, Porter S, Luker J. Recognition of oral lesions of HIV infection. 1. Candidosis. Br Dent J 1990;169:295–6.

77. Scully C, Griffiths M, Levers H, et al. The control of cross-infection in UK clinical dentistry in the 1990s: Immunisation against hepatitis B. Br Dent J 1993; 174:29–31.

78. Shapiro IM, Cornblath DR, Sumner AJ, et al. Neurophysiological and neuropsychological function in mercury-exposed dentists. Lancet 1982;1:1147–50.

79. Shaw FE Jr, Barrett CL, Hamm R, et al. Lethal outbreak of hepatitis B in a dental practice. JAMA 1986;255:3260–4.

80. Siblerud RL. The relationship between mercury from dental amalgam and mental health. Am J Psychother 1989;43:575–87.

81. Silverman S Jr. AIDS update: Oral findings, diagnosis, and precautions. J Am Dent Assoc 1987;115:559–63.

82. Silverman S Jr, Wara D. Oral manifestations of pediatric AIDS. Pediatrician 1989;16:185–7.

83. Smith DL Jr. Mental effects of mercury poisoning. South Med J 1978;71:904–5.

84. Solomon ES, Gray CF, Gerbert B. Issues in the dental care management of patients with bloodborne infectious diseases: an opinion survey of dental school seniors. J Dent Educ 1991;54:594–7.

85. Snapp KR, Boyer DB, Peterson LC, Svare CW. The contribution of dental amalgam to mercury in blood. J Dent Res 1989;68:780–5.

86. Summers CJ, Gooch BF, Marianos DW, et al. Practical infection control in oral health surveys and screenings. J Am Dent Assoc 1994;125:1213–7.

87. Svare CW, Peterson LC, Reinhardt JW, et al. The effect of dental amalgams on mercury levels in expired air. J Dent Res 1981;60:1668–71.

88. Taylor M. Recent dental school experiences concerning HIV-positive students: Creighton University. J Dent Educ 1992;56:540–7.

89. ter Horst G, Hammann-Konings GM, van Hegten

MJ, et al. AIDS and infection control: Amsterdam dentists surveyed. J Public Health Dent 1989; 49:201–5.

90. Update: Transmission of HIV infection during an invasive dental procedure—Florida. MMWR 1991; 40:21–33.

91. US Public Health Service, Centers for Disease Control and Prevention. Recommended infection-control procedures for dentistry. MMWR 1993;42(RR-8):1–12.

92. US Public Health Service, Committee to Coordinate Environmental Health and Related Programs. Dental amalgam: A scientific review and recommended Public Health Service strategy for research, education, and regulation. Washington DC: Government Printing Office, 1993.

93. US Public Health Service, National Institutes of Health. NIH Consensus Statement Online, 1997 Mar 24-26. Management of hepatitis C.

94. Verrusio AC. Risk of transmission of the human immunodeficiency virus to health care workers exposed to HIV-infected patients: A review. J Am Dent Assoc 1989;118:339–42.

95. Vimy MJ, Lorscheider FL. Intra-oral air mercury released from dental amalgam. J Dent Res 1985;64:1069–71.

96. Vimy MJ, Lorscheider FL. Serial measurements of intra-oral air mercury: Estimation of daily dose from dental amalgam. J Dent Res 1985;64:1072–5.

97. Vimy MJ, Luft AJ, Lorscheider FL. Estimation of mercury body burden from dental amalgam: Computer stimulation of a metabolic compartmental model. J Dent Res 1986;65:1415–9.

98. Vimy MJ, Takahashi Y, Lorscheider FL. Maternal-fetal distribution of mercury (203Hg) released from dental amalgam fillings. Am J Physiol 1990; 258:R939–45.

99. West DJ. The risk of hepatitis B infection among health professionals in the United States: A review. Am J Med Sci 1984;287:26–33.

100. Winkler JR, Robertson PB. Periodontal disease associated with HIV infection. Oral Surg Oral Med Oral Pathol 1992;73:145–50.

101. Withers JA. Hepatitis. A review of the disease and its significance to dentistry. J Periodontol 1980; 51:162–6.

7

The Structure
of Dental Practice

Private Dental Practice ◆ Solo and Group
Practice ◆ Open and Closed Panels ◆
Managed Care ◆ Dentistry in Managed Care ◆
Health Maintenance Organizations (HMOs) ◆
Dental Personnel in HMOs ◆ Assumption of Risk ◆
Preferred Provider Organizations ◆ Hospital Dentistry ◆
Franchised Practices and Department Store Clinics ◆
Public Programs ◆ Auxiliaries in Public Programs ◆
Primary Health Care ◆ Quality Assurance ◆
Evolution of Quality Assurance ◆ Recent Emphasis in
Quality Assurance ◆ Examples of Quality
Assurance Activities: The Dimensions of Quality ◆
Quality Assurance and Cost Control

Organized dentistry has two primary goals: to promote the oral health of the public and to preserve the autonomy and economic well-being of the profession. These goals can be in conflict, however, when dentistry's efforts to secure its own well-being are perceived as not being in harmony with the public interest, or when public efforts to improve oral health are seen by the professions as antagonistic to their self-interest. This type of conflict will continue; just and acceptable outcomes are more likely if the dental professions understand the pressures that produce them.

A delivery system is a collective health care expression that incorporates the various means by which care is provided to patients. The principal components are:

- The structure of the system, that is, the organizational arrangements by which patients and providers get together.
- The means by which the care is paid for.
- The supply of various types of health care personnel.

Other elements of a delivery system can be identified, such as physical facilities and record keeping, but the three elements listed here are the most basic. They are interdependent; a change in any one affects the others, though this book divides the subject into three chapters to give these issues adequate consideration. This chapter examines the structure of dental care provision systems in the United States, with some reference to methods used elsewhere.

PRIVATE DENTAL PRACTICE

Traditionally, dental care in the United States has been delivered by independent private practitioners. The American Dental Association (ADA) estimated that approximately 92% of all active dentists were in private practice in the mid-1990s.[17] This proportion has remained remarkably stable over the years. Indeed, an essential feature of dental care delivery in the United States is the diversity of practice modes and their constant evolution within a private practice philosophy. Adaptability in a rapidly changing world is a major strength of private practice, an attribute that ensures private practice will endure.

Private practice has a number of inher-

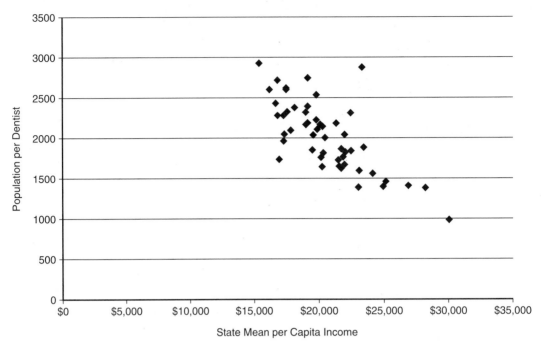

Figure 7-1. The association between mean per capita income and the population:dentist ratio. By individual states. United States, 1995. (From American Dental Association, Survey Center. Distribution of dentists in the United States by region and state, 1995. Chicago: ADA, 1997; US Census Bureau website.)

ently desirable features. One advantage to both provider and patient is flexibility. A dental practitioner can provide care for as many hours per day and for as many days per year as she chooses. When demand for care in a locality increases, private practitioners can respond if they wish by working longer hours, by increasing their productivity to meet it, by increasing their fees, or by some combination thereof. There is a built-in economic incentive to be as efficient as possible in private practice, because it represents a big investment of private capital in facilities and equipment; the return on that investment is the practitioner's profit. Choice of equipment, materials, and employees therefore is made carefully, and all can be chosen to suit the tastes of the individual dentist.

Private practice has often been equated with "free choice" of dentist by the prospective patient, and conversely, with freedom for the dentist to treat or not to treat anyone seeking care. Whether these concepts were ever fully true is arguable, but it is certain that current circumstances put some limits on these freedoms. In many inner-city communities, for example, there is often little choice of dentist because dentists are less likely to establish practices there. Because dentists in private practice are self-employed business

people, they tend to establish their practices in localities where they can be reasonably sure of demand for their services; these localities are typically higher-income suburban areas. There is a clear association between the availability of dentists and the per capita income of an area.[4, 5, 17] Figure 7–1 shows this association at the level of the states. Usually there are relatively more dentists in states with higher per-capita incomes. This same phenomenon holds for smaller geographic units such as counties and cities.

Even within communities that are well served by dentists, some groups are not readily treated in private practice. Treatment of the behaviorally difficult preschool child, for example, requires a degree of time and patience that can be uneconomical for a general practitioner, and pediatric dental specialists are not always available. Many elderly people cannot afford the care that they need, and many have difficulty traveling because of physical infirmities. In addition, there are people who are chronically ill, mentally retarded, or physically handicapped, or who have illnesses that require them to be dentally treated in a hospital. Private practice is poorly geared to care for such groups.

Poorer groups often have a double problem: care is less available to them, and when it can be found it is relatively expensive. It is hardly surprising that people in low socioeconomic areas are often thought "not to value dental care." That belief is not necessarily true; rather, the circumstances of their lives do not always permit the disadvantaged the luxury of "valuing dental care" the way that dentists would like.[32] Given this situation, "free choice" can be most accurately described as a middle-class value that may mean little in other socioeconomic contexts.

"Free choice" also cuts the other way: dentists have some freedom to reject patients (although not solely on the basis of race, ethnicity, or human immunodeficiency virus status; see Chapters 3 and 6). Some practitioners may believe that they are treating as many patients as they can manage and therefore will accept no new patients of any kind. Others may reject patients whose care is financed by public programs such as Medicaid (Chapter 8). This rejection may be based on the dentist's view that such programs offer poor compensation or have too much "red tape" or the dentist may be unable to accept the attitudes, values, and needs of low-income individuals.

From the community viewpoint, the principal advantages and disadvantages of private practice as a delivery system relate to economics. Private funds are used to build the facilities, buy equipment, hire auxiliary staff, and pay for some (although by no means all; see Chapter 9) of the expensive education of personnel. Dentists set their own fees. Dentists also have traditionally practiced "price discrimination," meaning that they charged wealthy patients higher fees than they charged poorer ones. Wealthier patients in these practices therefore subsidized the poorer ones. This once common practice, however, is discouraged under the "usual, customary, and reasonable" fee requirements of some insurers (Chapter 8).

Although the need to run a profitable business can be too readily forgotten by some critics of private dental practice, running a business is frequently incompatible with the need to provide for the dental treatment requirements of all people. Dental fees simply remain too high for some. The solo dental practitioner has certain overhead costs to meet: utilities, rent, equipment, supplies, staff payroll, equipment, and various forms of insurance. These expenses must be met regardless of whether or not patients come, or whether or not bills are collected. In addition,

the dentist is a highly trained and qualified professional and thus is deemed by American culture to be entitled to a good income. Many dentists are graduated from dental school heavily in debt[3] because of the high costs of their education and thus have a strong incentive to begin showing profits soon after they begin practice. It is interesting to compare these facts of the dental practitioner's position with that of the medical surgeon, for whom the hospital beds and hospital support staff are provided.

Solo Practice

Within the overall picture of private practice as the principal form of dental practice in the United States, the solo practitioner is the most common form of practice. The ADA estimated that in 1994 more than two thirds (67.4%) of private practitioners worked in a practice with no other dentists, about 20% worked with 1 other dentist, and just over 12% worked with 2 or more other dentists.[16] This distribution is shown in Figure 7–2.

Group Practice

The arrangements by which dentists can work together are so varied that the term *group practice* is difficult to define precisely. In fact, the ADA has adopted the term *nonsolo*

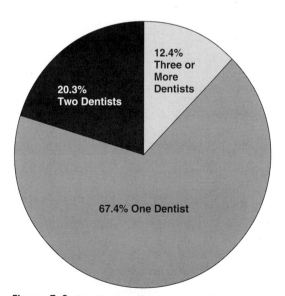

Figure 7–2. Distribution of private practitioner dentists by type of practice, United States, 1995. (Survey Center. 1995 survey of dental practice—dentists in solo and non-solo practice. Chicago: ADA, 1996.)

practice. The ADA definition states that a non-solo dentist works "in a practice with at least one other dentist. Some of these dentists may be employed by the owner dentist in the practice."[6] As demonstrated in Figure 7–2, solo practice remains the most common form of dental practice, and group practices generally are small, most of them consisting of 2 dentists. Although it is uncommon for newly graduating dentists to directly enter practice as a solo practitioner, the long-term pattern suggests that the dominance of solo and small group practices will continue, with a possible gradual shift in the balance toward small group practices.

Open and Closed Panels

Closed panels are defined by the ADA as existing "when patients eligible to receive benefits can receive them only if services are provided by dentists who have signed an agreement with the benefits plan."[8] An additional characteristic is that only a small percentage of providers in an area are available to provide care under the plan. Open panels, on the other hand, are characterized by 3 features[8]:

- Any licensed dentist may elect to participate.
- The beneficiary may receive treatment from among all licensed dentists, with the corresponding benefits being payable to either the beneficiary or the dentist.
- The dentist may accept or refuse any beneficiary.

Although these definitions do not necessarily allow precise classification of all practices, their intent is clear. A principle of great importance to the ADA is the idea that patients should be able to choose among all dentists in a community, and that any dentist should be allowed to provide care to any particular patient. The ADA does not encourage forms of practice that severely restrict the number of dentists who are approved to provide care (almost always the result of payment restrictions). Although the majority of dental practices that could be classified as closed panels are not exclusively so, perhaps the purest form of a closed panel is a practice that is set up by an employer or union for the treatment of the employees and staffed by salaried dentists who treat only the employees and their dependents.

Closed-panel clinics have aroused much emotion in the past[15, 34, 66]; it was charged that they were unethical and that they delivered care of inadequate quality. Neither the quality question nor the ethics issues were objectively shown to be true, and the question seems to be of less concern in the 1990s. This is probably because the continuing proliferation of third-party payment mechanisms and the resulting diversity of forms of dental practice have gradually widened and liberalized the perception of what constitutes a "proper" form of dental practice.

MANAGED CARE

Managed care is a term that is in widespread use, but for which there is no precise definition. The Health Insurance Association of America (HIAA) defines managed care as:

Systems that integrate the financing and delivery of appropriate health care services to covered individuals by means of arrangements with selected providers to furnish a comprehensive set of health-care services to members; explicit criteria for the selection of health care providers; formal programs for ongoing quality assurance and utilization review; and significant financial incentives for members to use providers and procedures associated with the plan.[43]

This definition is a real mouthful, and as complicated as managed care itself. Its key elements are:

- A comprehensive set of health care services
- Selected providers
- Financial incentives to use the selected providers

Simply stated, what has come to be called managed care are arrangements through which people receive (1) all or most of their health care, (2) from providers (hospitals, physicians, and other personnel) who are formally linked to the organization, (3) at an out-of-pocket cost that is substantially lower than if care is sought outside of the managed care organization.

The most common form of these arrangements are health maintenance organizations (HMOs) and preferred provider organizations (PPOs) (described later in this chapter). There are also innumerable hybrids, with more coming every day. Although these types of arrangements are not new, the movement of the medically insured population to managed care in the 1990s has been on a massive scale. It was estimated that by 1997 nearly 75% of all insured workers in the United States were in managed care plans.[44] At the same time, there was a concerted effort under way by the federal Health Care Financing Agency (HCFA) to move Medicaid and Medicare enrollees from traditional fee-for-service to managed care. The effect of these trends on medicine has been profound, for managed care has come to dominate the practicing life of most physicians.

The primary stimulus for the growth of managed care is concern over the seemingly endless increases in medical treatment costs (Chapter 8). The widespread hope is that managed care can somehow help control the costs of medical care. This hope, however, begs the question as to what is the "correct" amount of care, and it assumes that there is some way that it can be determined for each patient. The hopes for cost control also depend on the assumption that the "correct" amount of care will be less expensive to provide than what people would buy outside of managed care.

However, no one system for organizing care can be expected to solve all the underlying conflicts associated with health and health care. Although health care is sometimes judged only in terms of life and death, measuring the worth of a system is more complex. It is more sensible to look at how the system affects the quality of life, although the problem that immediately arises is that modern medicine's ability to add comfort and length to life usually comes at ever-increasing cost. Every dollar spent on health care is a dollar that is unavailable for some other purpose, which means that there is an implicit trade-off when an individual decides to spend money for more health care rather than for something else. The problem becomes especially difficult when small increases in comfort or longevity come at high dollar cost. These decisions are difficult enough when made by individuals with their own money; they are infinitely more difficult when made in a public forum with collective funds.

These tensions associated with deciding how much health care is appropriate, and for how much money, are driving the rapid evolution in the financing and delivery of medical care. That no single approach is going to be a panacea should be self-evident, because there is no single answer to the underlying question of how much health care is the right amount, and at what price. In fact, we see that even as managed care is rapidly increasing market share, there is a growing backlash against it. It cannot satisfy everyone, and its promise of controlling costs is seen as the reason for its failures when inevitably some people experience unsatisfactory health care outcomes.

DENTISTRY IN MANAGED CARE

In some ways, dentistry is inevitably caught up in this maelstrom in medicine. Virtually all of the innovations that have been, and are being, tried in medicine are evident in dentistry. Some of this has occurred because purchasing groups have demanded the same kind of system from their dental coverage that they are using for their medical coverage. Some has come from entrepreneurs, both inside and outside dentistry, who see managed care as an opportunity to move dental practice into the future, or more crassly as a way to make quick money.

On the other hand, there are important differences between medicine and dentistry that make it unlikely that managed care will play as large a role in dentistry as it has in medicine. The most important difference is that whereas about 85% of the population have medical insurance, less than 50% have coverage for dental care. Insured patients account for nearly all of the income of physicians and hospitals. If large purchasing groups want these providers to change their practices, physicians and hospitals are extremely vulnerable. With dentistry, on the other hand, there are still large numbers of patients who are not covered by dental insurance, so that dentists, individually and as a group, are far less susceptible to pressure from large purchasers.

The difference in governmental involvement in the payment for care is also important. For medical care in general, government funds account for almost one half of all expenditures, whereas government funds account for less than 4% of dental expenditures. As government struggles to control expenditures, medical care costs cannot be ignored, but dental care costs are relatively unimportant. Because it controls such a large portion of medical reimbursement, government is in a position to exert an enormous influence over providers. In the case of dental care, however, this is not the case. In the case of Medicaid, for example, with reimbursement levels well below what many dentists deem reasonable, dentists can simply refuse to participate without affecting their economic well-being. This would not be possible for many practitioners in medicine.

HEALTH MAINTENANCE ORGANIZATIONS (HMOs)

The concept of the HMO is based as much on financial arrangements as on structure, but HMOs are discussed here, rather than in Chapter 8, as a prime example of managed care.

Although the idea of HMOs is not new, its implementation was formally promoted with the passage of the Health Maintenance Organization Act of 1973 (PL 93-222). This Act made federal funds for the development of HMOs available under certain conditions. It was intended to provide an acceptable alternative to the private practice system and help restrain the costs of care.

One of the principal advantages of HMOs, as a method of providing health care, lies in their claim to reduce the cost of care for those enrolled. These savings are purportedly due to the greater emphasis on ambulatory care and consequently on reduced hospital utilization as well as on close control of costly services. "Unnecessary" hospitalization, principally for routine diagnostic tests and minor surgery, is thereby curtailed. Dental care, however, is almost exclusively ambulatory care, as few dental procedures require inpatient hospitalization. The major advantage of the HMO concept in reducing hospitalization, therefore, has little application to dentistry, but the close monitoring of utilization emphasized in HMOs is relevant.

An HMO was defined in the 1973 Act as "a legal entity which provides a prescribed range of health services . . . to each individual who has enrolled in the organization in return for a prepaid, fixed, and uniform payment."[70] Usually, but not always, an HMO looks like a large group practice with a number of services available under one roof. An HMO is described as having 5 essential elements: a managing organization, a delivery system, an enrolled population, a benefit package, and a system of financing and prepayment.[56] HMOs use a prepaid capitation system of financing medical services. Capitation means that the care provider is paid a fixed sum on a regular basis, usually monthly, for each enrolled person, whether or not the enrollee uses any care in that month.

Federal funding for the development of HMOs continued for 8 years after the passage of the HMO Act in 1973. Growth in the number of HMOs and in the number of enrollees has continued to be vigorous since the end of federal incentives, with much of the recent growth coming in the for-profit sector (HMOs are owned by both for-profit and not-for-profit corporations). From a total of 25 HMOs serving 3 million people in 1971, the number had risen to 574 by 1994, serving 51.2 million people.[43]

The 1973 Act defined certain basic services that an HMO was required to provide in order to qualify for federal support funds. Dental care, limited to preventive services (prophylaxis, topical fluoride, and prescription of systemic fluoride) for children up to age 11, was originally part of these basic services. Regulations for the 1973 Act allowed a phase-in period of 3 years for the basic services, but even before the end of that period the limited dental care required was removed and made a supplemental service. With the elimination of federal incentives, there were no specific requirements for the inclusion of dental care in HMOs. In the 1990s, only a small proportion of HMOs offered dental services. When dental services are present, they are financed through (a) the primary capitation premium, (b) a separate premium, or (c) a fee-for-service basis.

In the early days of HMOs, there was occasional opposition from dentists in the immediate area of a proposed HMO, based on fear of a perceived increased competition for patients.[29] The ADA has never directly opposed HMOs, but it was initially opposed to their federal incentives, viewing these as unfair preferential treatment.[7] With the expiration of federal incentives, this objection no longer applies. Although there is still no great enthusiasm for HMOs within the official policies of the ADA, a primary concern of organized dentistry remains preservation of the principle of freedom of choice of provider.

Dental Personnel in HMOs

Dental care can be provided in an HMO according to 1 of 4 basic organization models:

- **Staff Model:** Dentists, dental hygienists, and dental assistants are salaried employees of the HMO. The staff model is the only one of the 4 modes that affects auxiliary personnel directly, because in the other 3, the terms of their employment in dental practices do not differ from those in traditional private practice.

- **Group Model:** The HMO contracts directly with a group practice, partnership, or corporation for the provision of dental services. The group receives a regular capitation premium from the HMO.

- **Independent Practice Association (IPA):** The IPA is an association of independent dentists (or physicians in medical practice) that develops its own management and fiscal structure for the treatment of patients enrolled in an HMO. An IPA is thus not a different form of practice, but instead a legal arrangement through which individual dental offices can participate as providers to groups of patients who are enrolled in HMOs. Dentists continue to practice in their own offices. The IPA receives its capitation premium from the HMO (or other prepayment agency) and in turn reimburses the individual dentists on either a modified fee-for-service basis or a capitation basis. In many instances, the dentist is "at risk" (described in the next section) to provide the specified services. The IPA can also contract with other insurers to provide dental services to groups on a capitation basis. The ADA considers the IPA to be an open panel, as all dentists in a community are theoretically free to join. In practice, however, the IPA usually includes only a small percentage of practices in an area, thus blurring the distinction between open-panel and closed-panel practice.

- **Capitated Network or Direct Contract Model:** The network is similar to the IPA, except that the HMO contracts directly with the individual provider for provision of services. This is the most common form of capitation arrangements in dentistry. Dental insurers who wish to offer a capitation product recruit and contract with dental offices who are willing to have patients assigned to them.

Assumption of Risk

The concept of assumption of (financial) risk is important in health care. In the case of a patient who pays for her own care, the situation is uncomplicated: if the patient accepts the treatment proposed by the dentist, the patient is responsible for the necessary payment. With the advent of traditional fee-for-service insurance, the insurance companies typically agreed to assume the financial risk. In this arrangement, there are a set of covered services, usually subject to some co-payments and an annual maximum, but the insurance company is responsible to pay for the care with the money that they have collected from the premiums. The insurers carefully "rate" each group to estimate how much their care will cost, so that they can be sure to set their premiums at a level sufficient to cover the costs of care, but not to charge so much that a competitor will take the business with a lower bid. In any case, with traditional insurance, the insurance company is "at risk" for most excess costs. Acceptance of this risk is part of what the insurer is selling.

In principle, one of the main features of a capitation payment is that the assumption of risk, previously accepted by the insurer, is shifted to the provider. The essence of the capitation system of payment is that the provider receives a previously-agreed-upon sum per patient enrolled, regardless of whether or not the patient seeks care. In return, the provider agrees to provide specified services as necessary for a predetermined period.

Clearly, the concern of the provider is that the amount of money received (*known* before a contract is signed) be sufficient to cover the services needed (which are *unknown*, although they often can be reasonably estimated, especially for a large group of patients). If the cost of the services required exceeds the income received through the contract, the provider loses. Conversely, if the services required are less than the income provided by the contract, the provider gains. It follows that in some contracts there is the potential for undertreatment and discouragement of service utilization, raising concerns about both ethics and the quality of care received.[53]

It is understandable therefore that both the ADA and individual dentists are cautious about "assumption of risk." Of course, risk is assumed by an HMO when it establishes its monthly premium for its enrollees, just as it is assumed by any insurer in a prepaid care plan. Capitation, however, brings the concept of assuming risk directly to the dentist. By the 1990s, features such as patient co-payments and annual maximums had become common in capitation plans as ways to reduce the dentist's risk. These were and still are standard cost-control mechanisms in fee-for-service plans.

As of 1995, the National Association of Dental Plans (NADP) estimated that nearly 24 million individuals were enrolled in dental HMOs (sometimes referred to as DHMOs). Although this number is acknowledged to be inexact, there is an extremely broad range in what is called a DHMO. Whereas some of these capitation plans cover a comprehensive set of services under the capitation fee, some cover little more than an initial examination, with all other services the responsibility of the patient on a (sometimes discounted) fee-for-service basis.

Preferred Provider Organizations

PPOs are also considered in this chapter because they, along with HMOs, are the main managed care arrangements. PPOs typically involve contracts between insurers and a number of practitioners who agree to provide specific services for fees that are lower than the average for the area. Competition for patients is the driving force behind the willingness of some providers to discount their fees for PPO patients; a clinician who has ample demand for her services at her usual fees is not likely to be interested in a PPO agreement. PPOs differ from HMOs in that they are fee-for-service plans, so in PPOs a beneficiary can go to any participating provider for any covered service, because payment is made only when care is provided. By 1994, approximately 45 million Americans had medical coverage through PPOs.[43] The extent of dental coverage through PPOs is much smaller; the National Association of Dental Plans estimated that in 1995 14 million people were enrolled in dental PPOs.

HOSPITAL DENTISTRY

Although only a small fraction of dental care is provided in hospitals, dentists still have a substantial role in hospitals. In the mid-1980s, approximately 1000 hospitals in the United States had formally organized departments of dentistry, and about 40,000 dentists were members of the medical staff of at least one hospital.[10, 36] As of 1995, the number of dentists in the United States with hospital privileges was still about 40,000.[18]

The number of dental general practice residencies (GPRs) in hospitals grew rapidly through the 1970s, and as of 1996 there were 883 positions in residency programs.[3] The extended experience in the hospital environment that the GPR provides is likely to make it easier for these dentists to make use of hospital privileges later in their careers. Many dentists affiliated with these and other educational programs in hospitals have full-time or substantial part-time commitments to hospital-based care. Dentists in the military and with the Department of Veterans' Affairs are also commonly in hospital-based practices. A majority of dentists who have hospital privileges, however, are in private practice and provide care only occasionally in the hospital.

Dental care provided in hospitals is often for those situations in which general anesthesia and the other resources of a hospital are required, such as for treatment of very young children with rampant caries, oral surgery to remove carcinomas, cleft palate repair, and maxillofacial prosthetic treatment for victims of burns or trauma in the head and neck region. In addition, some routine dental care is provided in hospitals for patients who are suffering from serious systemic disease, and for whom the risk of being treated in the private dental office would be unacceptably high. The inclusion of the ADA on the board of the Joint Commission on Accreditation of Healthcare Organizations since 1980 helps to ensure an appropriate role for dental consultation and services within hospitals.

Beyond the traditional role of educational programs and consultative services, a major challenge for hospital dental departments is economic justification. All departments within hospitals are increasingly being pressed to show that the income that they produce is sufficient to justify their existence; and the traditional roles of teaching, consultation, and care for indigent patients do not provide high levels of revenue. On the other hand, moves by hospital-based programs to solicit insured patients through ambulatory care facilities are seen as unfair competition by some private practitioners.[36, 63]

FRANCHISED PRACTICES AND DEPARTMENT STORE CLINICS

In the late 1970s, several major department store chains, including Sears and Montgomery Ward, opened dental clinics in some of their stores and announced their intention to open more. These clinics operated during usual store hours and were perceived by the stores' management as a further step in "one-stop shopping." The stores' management viewed the dental clinics as an extra service for their customers, no different from the pharmacies and optical departments in chain stores. However, dental practices in department stores have not prospered and were few in number by the late 1990s.

The concept of franchises is common in the United States, encompassing such varied entities as motels, restaurants, automobile servicing, retail stores, and child-care services. The franchisor, for some combination of initial fees and periodic payments, provides the name plus additional services such as advertising, training, coordinated purchasing, and management services. The franchisee runs the individual business location, and except for the agreed payments to the franchisor, retains the profits from the business.

By the early 1980s, there appeared to be the beginning of an explosive growth of franchised dental practices.[9, 19, 75] The idea as applied to dental practice varied in detail among franchises, but tended to include such things as a franchise name; marketing and management services; bulk purchasing of supplies; and sometimes the design, construction, and equipping of the practice itself. The dental clinic space itself was usually leased by a dentist because most state laws do not allow dental practices to be owned by a non-dentist.

After a quick start in the early 1980s, most franchise dental organizations had fallen on difficult times by 1988[77]; all but a few were out of business or under bankruptcy protection. Reasons for this turn of events include undercapitalization, overexpansion, poor management control, unprofessional image, and high costs.[77] Fundamental conflicts between the traditional strengths of franchises and dental practice make it unlikely that franchised dental practice will ever be a major force; the standardization of process and procedures that lead to cost savings and uniform quality in many businesses is unlikely to produce cost savings in dental care. These features of franchising also run counter to dentists' desires to consider each patient individually and not according to externally imposed productivity and efficiency standards.

Despite the difficulty encountered by most of the franchise organizations, many individual practices have nevertheless continued as independent private practices. Individual private practices located in large department stores or in shopping malls, but that are not necessarily part of franchise chains, are sometimes referred to as retail or department store clinics. Other than the fact that some of these practices were at one time part of a franchise organization, most are now no different from any other large private practice. The practices in shopping malls are simply located where there is a high level of traffic by potential patients, thus maintaining a long-standing pattern in dentistry.

In the mid 1990s, there were also a few reports of dental insurers buying individual dental offices. The reason for these purchases is usually to acquire the capacity to handle managed care offerings, particularly in areas where individual dental offices are reluctant to sign on. The impact of these arrangements will take some years to be properly evaluated.

PUBLIC PROGRAMS

As stated earlier, private practice cannot meet the dental demands of all people. A number of public dental care programs therefore have been developed to meet the needs of specific groups. Some of these government-sponsored programs use a specific delivery system in addition to a funding mechanism. Some receive funding from the federal government, although many still remain under the control of state and local health departments. Many are under considerable strain because social services budgets have been severely cut over recent decades.

The oldest health care programs of the federal government are directed either at certain groups of its own employees or at other specific groups for whom it has an obligation or who would find it difficult to get care anywhere else. Each branch of the armed forces, for example, provides dental care for its own active duty personnel. Care is provided for the most part by dentists who themselves are members of the armed services and is dispensed from clinical facilities wholly owned and maintained by the service concerned.

Many of the long-established clinical programs of the US Public Health Service were described in Chapter 1. In addition to those programs, the Community and Migrant Health program of the US Public Health Service provides grants to support public and nonprofit organizations to plan, develop, and operate health care facilities, known as Community and Migrant Health Centers, in rural and urban areas where existing health care resources are inadequate. In addition to medical services, these centers are required to provide or arrange for preventive dental services. Where resources permit, restorative services are also provided. These centers are established in areas where access to private care is limited, and they employ salaried dental personnel.

Another program aimed at making care available in areas unattractive to private practice is the National Health Service Corps. This program, discussed more fully in Chapter 9, has provided incentives, including scholarships and salaries to encourage dentists to practice in remote and underserved areas.

Many states, counties, and cities have had their own dental care programs, with their own facilities and salaried personnel, operating for years. Most of these programs, which are often administered by an agency of the state or local government, have been aimed at providing care for people who are eligible to receive some form of public welfare. The services available through these programs vary widely. Many of these state and local dental treatment programs cover a portion of their costs of operation by billing Medicaid for eligible patients.

Auxiliaries in Public Programs

Auxiliary-based programs have long been the backbone of public dental care in some countries, although not the United States. The oldest and best known is the New Zealand school dental nurse plan, introduced in 1921. New Zealand is a nation of 3.6 million people in the South Pacific, 1500 miles off the eastern coast of Australia. Living standards are high, and New Zealand has been a world leader in a number of social programs: old-age pensions, visiting maternal and child health nurses, and the secret ballot at political elections. A number of these programs began in the late 19th century, about the time that social security programs were initiated in Bismarck's Germany. Given these traditions, the introduction of the school dental nurse plan was not as radical an innovation as it might seem, although there was some concern among dentists at the time.[69] The stimuli for the program were the extensive dental disease found in army recruits during World War I (1914–1918) and government intent to do something about this problem. Dentists were in short supply at the time, and treatment of young children was not as accepted in dental practice as it is now. Caries experience remained high for a long time in New Zealand.[23, 24]

When the service began, care was offered only to younger school-aged children, but eligibility now extends to all preschool-aged children and all children in primary and intermediate school (2½ to 13½ years of age). Children between 13½ and 16 are eligible for treatment by private practitioners at public expense, but beyond that age dental care is provided through traditional private practice, with some exceptions for special groups who receive public assistance. School dental clinics are attached to primary and intermediate schools throughout the country.

The dental nurses' training course is 2 years and concentrates on technical procedures. Considerable emphasis is placed on learning to recognize conditions that are beyond the nurses' competence to treat. These conditions are then referred to a private practitioner or to one of a small number of dentists employed by the School Dental Service. Dental nurses' clinical duties include oral examinations, cavity preparation and placement of restorations, pulp capping, and extraction of primary (but not permanent) teeth. They also provide extensive dental health education, both in the classroom and to individual patients.

Because each supervising public health dentist is responsible for a large number of nurses, nurses function with a high degree of independence. Many young children in New Zealand are examined and treated totally by dental nurses and never see a dentist until their teenage years. Although this fact has disturbed some American observers,[39, 61] there is no evidence that the oral or general health of the children suffers as a result. One measure of the acceptance of the service is the high degree of utilization among the target population: nearly 100% of the primary and intermediate school population are treated by the service. (By contrast, 69% of 5- to 17-year-old children in the United States reported visiting a dentist during 1989.[72])

The decline in caries experience in New Zealand, as in most developed countries, has reduced the need for restorative treatment. In addition, women are staying in the workforce longer than they used to. As a result of these influences, the intake of new trainees had to be reduced. At present only 1 training school is operating in New Zealand, down from 3 schools a few decades ago.

The New Zealand school dental nurse plan has attracted the attention of dental organizations all over the world. Other countries and jurisdictions that have adopted similar programs, with modifications to suit the local environment, include Canada (Chapter 10), Britain, Australia, Thailand, Malaysia, Singapore, Myanmar, Sri Lanka, Brunei, Hong Kong, and Indonesia.

Operating auxiliaries (Chapter 9) have been trained and employed only sporadically in public programs in the United States. This is at least partly attributable to the consistently strong opposition of the ADA.[14, 15] An attempt to introduce an auxiliary-based school dental program in Massachusetts in the mid-1950s was defeated after political action by organized dentistry.[33] Despite this history, it is well established from research, much of it ironically from the United States, that well-trained dental therapists (as the trained auxiliary of the dental nurse type is now usually called) are able to carry out many procedures as well as dentists can.[1, 2, 22, 40, 48–50, 62, 65] In most of the countries where these programs are established, children would be far less likely to be receiving any care were it not for the dental therapists.

Primary Health Care

Developing countries generally do not have the resources to train the number of dentists they need. Even if large numbers of dentists were available, the cost of care would still be beyond the reach of many. Recognition of this fact has led the World Health Organization to establish its principles of primary health care.[76] Under this concept, the focus for health care is to assist in maintaining health rather than to wait for problems to occur. In countries and localities where dentists are in short supply, much of the responsibility for first-level oral health care is assigned to a primary health care worker who resides in the community. In some places these individuals have been trained to provide dental examinations, to provide nonsurgical procedures such as calculus removal, topical fluorides, and the placement of sealants and glass ionomer restorations.[60, 76] Under such a system, much of the preventive care is provided by people who are already part of the health

care system in the community, and the more scarce and expensive personnel are used mainly as a second-level referral resource.

In circumstances of extreme shortages of trained oral health care professionals, the concept of primary health care tries to give to individuals as much practical information as possible for their own care and provides guidance for nondental health care workers when it is necessary for them to place temporary fillings or extract teeth.[27]

Dental care can be provided in ways that are markedly different from those in North America. If at first some of these alternative ways of meeting the needs of people seem unusual, it must be remembered that the system that seems right for any particular country is determined by a combination of its history, economics, cultural traditions, and its prevailing philosophies on rights and responsibilities for health care.

QUALITY ASSURANCE

Although quality assurance is a legitimate concern of dentistry, regardless of the way that care is organized, there is no question that formal quality assurance activities have received renewed attention because of concerns about managed care. Many see the prime purpose of managed care as controlling or reducing the costs of treatment, and that achievement of this goal leads to provision of inferior care.

Every dental professional wants to provide the best possible care, but defining what is meant by quality, and then reaching agreement on how to attain it, continues to be a major challenge. A typical dictionary definition of quality is "degree of excellence." Schoen[64] defined quality in dental care as "that characteristic that relates to the effective and efficient maintenance of optimum oral health when present, and improvement of oral health when needed. . . ." Although this definition gives us the general idea of quality in dental care, it leaves much room for disagreement about how quality is actually measured. Terms such as "effective and efficient maintenance" and "optimum oral health" do not have precise definitions. This ambiguity is behind the variety of approaches to quality assurance.

The term *quality assessment* is defined by the ADA as "the measure of the quality of care provided in a particular setting."[8] *Quality assurance* is in turn defined as "the assessment or measurement of the quality of care and the implementation of any necessary changes to either maintain or improve the quality of care rendered."[8] The difference in these definitions is important; quality assessment is limited to the appraisal of whether or not standards of quality have been met, whereas quality assurance includes the additional dimension of action to take corrective steps if these are needed to improve the situation.

The most frequently used approach to quality assessment and quality assurance builds on the concepts of structure, process, and outcome, as described by Donabedian.[30, 31] The model is based on the idea that although the outcome of treatment is important, and should be evaluated, a desirable outcome is more likely if the structural arrangements, such as well-designed treatment facilities, proper equipment, and appropriate and properly trained staff, meet adequate standards. A good outcome is also more likely if the processes used, such as diagnostic methods, treatment planning, record keeping, and the treatment procedures themselves, follow recognized protocols. Perhaps even more important, Donabedian argues that if a less than satisfactory outcome is detected, the search for the cause is likely to be within the process of care and the structures that support it. This means that we must have a clear understanding of process and structure of a system, even though outcome is the most desirable evaluatory measure.

Numerous dental practice assessment procedures that follow the structure-process-outcome model have been developed.[55, 64, 73] Table 7–1 lists examples of some of the dimensions that can be assessed under this approach. These many dimensions of quality can present problems, because when people of good faith focus on different dimensions they can disagree as to whether quality has been attained. Further, the same level of technical quality can be commendable in one setting and inappropriate in another.

The picture can be confusing because much of the recent literature in this area uses different terms to describe some or all of the dimensions of quality assurance and quality assessment. Some examples of different terms in the literature (Table 7–2) are quality improvement,[67] continuous improvement,[25] continuous quality improvement,[46] quality ensurance,[73] quality management,[67] total quality management,[38] outcomes management,[74] clinical practice guidelines,[71] practice parameters,[11, 12] standards of practice,[47] evidence-based clinical guidelines,[54] best practices,[45] report cards,[41] and risk prevention.[59]

Although all of these topics are not nec-

Table 7–1. EXAMPLES OF DENTAL PRACTICE ELEMENTS THAT CAN BE ASSESSED UNDER THE STRUCTURE, PROCESS, AND OUTCOME APPROACH

STRUCTURE	PROCESS	OUTCOME
FACILITIES	*MANAGEMENT*	*PATIENT SATISFACTION*
setting	practice	*ORAL HEALTH STATUS*
physical structures	personnel	oral hygiene
layout	patient	tooth loss
amenities	*RECORDS*	periodontitis
access	content	caries
EQUIPMENT	completeness	function
operatories	availability	comfort
instruments	legibility	esthetics
supplies	*DIAGNOSIS*	*COMPLETION OF TREATMENT*
sterilization	appropriateness	timely and appropriate
PERSONNEL	documentation	*RECALL PATTERN*
appropriate types	thoroughness	frequency
training	*TREATMENT PLAN*	needs at recall
licensure	written plan	
certification	sequencing	
continuing education	appropriateness	
ADMINISTRATION	*TREATMENT*	
procedures	appropriateness	
record system	timeliness	
protocols		

Table 7–2. QUALITY-RELATED TERMS IN THE LITERATURE

Quality improvement
Continuous improvement
Continuous quality improvement
Quality ensurance
Quality management
Total quality management
Outcomes management
Clinical practice guidelines
Practice parameters
Standards of practice
Evidence-based clinical guidelines
Best practice
Report cards
Risk prevention

essarily equivalent to quality assurance, they do fit easily within the broad concept. The purpose of quality assurance is to help provide the best possible health care. All of the items are potential tools to accomplish this goal, and they all fit comfortably within the structure-process-outcome paradigm. In that sense, the proliferation of terms, rather than representing competing approaches to quality assurance, represent the development and refinement of the methods to implement quality assurance.

Evolution of Quality Assurance

We could begin with the work of Florence Nightingale, who gathered hospital statistics in an effort to improve clinical outcomes.[57] An important milestone in medicine was the Flexner report,[35] which led to a major overhaul in the education of physicians in North America, which in turn affected medical practice. The publication of the Gies report on dental education[37] was a similar milestone for dentistry and dental education. One result of the Gies report was the eventual closure of proprietary dental schools in the United States and the development of a system of accreditation of dental schools that, with refinement, continues to this day (Chapter 1). An example of these continuing refinements is that since the late 1980s, the Accreditation Standards for Dental Education Programs of the Commission on Dental Accreditation has had an explicit requirement for a formal system of record review.

Activities that can legitimately be included as part of quality assurance in dentistry go back as far as the aptitude testing and scrutiny of the academic credentials of dental school applicants. The process of accreditation of the dental schools themselves is also part of quality assurance, as are the processes to acquire and periodically evaluate the faculty members who teach in these schools. The requirements for entering dental practice are also part of the quality assurance process. In most countries there is a requirement for graduation from a properly accredited dental school, and some require the passing of an independently administered set of examinations, or perhaps a period of supervised practice.

Further, requirements for periodic continuing education for renewal of licensure, the establishment of peer bodies to review and adjudicate complaints against clinicians, and, when all else fails, the use of the legal system to resolve disputes between patients and providers of care can all be viewed as part of quality assurance. The development, testing, and certification of dental materials, devices, and equipment are also important quality-related functions.

Recent Emphasis in Quality Assurance

Although a broad spectrum of activities legitimately is part of quality assurance, most of the attention to quality assurance in dentistry in recent decades has focused much more narrowly on dental practice itself. This recent emphasis on formal quality assurance activities in the United States has been attributed to the following 5 influences.[28]

- **Rapid growth of dental prepayment, with associated cost and quality concerns:** Before 1970, almost all payment for dental care in the United States was made by the individual patient. Government and third parties had little involvement. By about 1985, however, the proportion of the US population with some form of prepayment for dental care approached 50%. This rapid change brought the third parties into the dental care delivery system, and they brought collective interest in the overall cost of the insurance programs. Along with cost concerns came concerns about the quality of care.

- **Rapidly rising health care costs:** Because both government and private purchasers are increasingly involved, there was great concern when it became evident that the costs of care were increasing faster than the overall rate of inflation in the economy. It was clear that if the costs of health care were not brought into line with overall cost increases, less and less money would be available for other desired purposes.

- **Professional standards review legislation:** Dentistry has also been influenced by the general climate of increasing demands for accountability that have been imposed on medical and hospital care through legislation. Especially since the advent of Medicare and Medicaid in 1965, government funds account for a large and growing part of medical care expenditures, and as a result requirements related to quality assurance have been imposed on medical and hospital-based care. Even though government involvement in the payment for dental care in the United States is small, dentistry has been affected both directly and indirectly by this increasing climate of accountability.

- **Growth of consumer involvement:** Through the past several decades there has been an increase in the interest of consumers, as a group, in issues related to all sorts of services and products. Dentistry has been affected by this general movement, especially in the sense that it has created a climate in which providers of services are seen as being far more subject to scrutiny that had previously been the case.

- **Malpractice litigation:** Perhaps also related to the growth in consumerism, individual patients have become far more likely to seek relief through the legal system to redress perceived shortcomings in the care that they receive. One result has been the growth of quality-related activities such as risk prevention and standards of care, in an effort to reduce the likelihood that such a lawsuit will need to be undertaken.

Examples of Quality Assurance Activities: The Dimensions of Quality

The types of activities that are part of quality assurance in dentistry illustrate the wide scope of the field. The following 7 topics are representative of quality assurance approaches in dentistry.

- **Technical quality:** The assessment of technical quality of restorative procedures has perhaps the most highly detailed criteria, but is also one of the least-used forms of quality assurance in dentistry. First of all, measures of technical quality are expensive. It is time-consuming for examiners, and it is difficult to get cooperation from more than a small fraction of the patients who are selected for evaluation. Further, the results from random audits have not been encouraging, partly because of the low turnout of patients, and also because unacceptable care is so infrequently found.[26] Because of the high costs and low yield, direct assessment of technical quality has not developed into a major area of quality assurance.

- **On-site evaluation of dental practice:** On-site evaluation of dental practice is perhaps the most widely used form of quality assurance, especially for programs directed by third-party payers. Various combinations of structure, process, and outcome are measured by trained auditors who visit the dental office. Although there are numerous examples of this approach in the dental literature,[55, 64, 73] it is the subject of many concerns. For one thing, the process is expensive. It is time-consuming for a trained evaluator to visit each dental office and to conduct what is usually a highly detailed assessment. Marcus,[52] who has considerable experience with this approach to quality assurance, has stated: "I am not convinced that our quality assurance efforts have had a significant impact on improving the process of care, nor has it been effective in eliminating those providers who are unwilling to change their pattern of care delivery."

  The work of van der Wal and colleagues[73] also casts uncertainty on the validity of the process. This group was unable to find the expected associations between structural aspects and outcomes of dental care. Although there is much room to debate the validity and completeness of both the structure and outcome measures that were used in their study, it nevertheless does raise several important points. First, this study adds to the concern that the structure-process-outcome paradigm has not been empirically shown to represent accurately the "real world." It continues to be unsettling that we cannot produce good empirical evidence of the connection that is so widely believed to be present. Second, the authors suggest the possibility that the structural characteristics included in dental office evaluations are now so well known to dentists that virtually all are in compliance, so that structural indicators are no longer valid predictors of outcomes.

- **Oral health status:** If there were a simple, valid, sensitive, and easily measured index of oral health status, the job of quality assurance would be made much easier. After all, the ultimate objective of oral health care is to help patients attain and maintain the highest possible level of oral health.

While there have been noteworthy efforts to develop such indexes of oral health,[51, 58] their acceptance has been limited, and there has been little progress in this direction in the past decade. These indexes are discussed in Chapter 13.

- **Appropriateness of care:** Appropriateness of care is a dimension that has so far received little attention in dentistry. There is general agreement that the use of a technically superior restorative procedure when it is not needed is not acceptable quality. Standards for the appropriate use of dental care nevertheless continue to elude clear definition.
- **Consumer satisfaction:** Work in this area is also in its infancy, but it is currently of considerable interest, especially to purchasers of group dental insurance. One of the primary reasons for employers to purchase dental insurance for their employees and their families is to make the employee happy and loyal to the employer. Although these purchasers are certainly interested in the oral health of their employees, of considerable importance is the satisfaction of these employees with the dental benefit. As a result, purchasers are increasingly pressing for measures of consumer satisfaction.
- **Audit of dental records:** In addition to the assessment of technical quality of restorations, the record audit as a quality assurance mechanism is perhaps the most highly developed and widely used approach for institutions[20] such as dental schools and hospital dental departments.[13] In hospitals, record audits fit well with the approach that has been used for a long time in medicine for hospital accreditation. In dental schools, it fits well with the traditional teaching functions. Through the detailed review of dental records, not only can the dental care provided by the institution be assessed, but the student is also exposed to a review of the rationale and process of patient management and care.

As with several of the other approaches to quality assurance, the audit of dental records is a relatively expensive and time-consuming process. Apart from the institutional settings where they are required by external auditors, record audits are not widely used.

- **Profiling of dental providers:** With the advent of computer-based records of dental treatment, especially in insurance companies, there have been attempts to make use of these kinds of data to evaluate the quality of dental care indirectly. If successful, this approach could be much less expensive than the direct methods already discussed. The idea is that by aggregating treatment records from large numbers of providers across many patients, inappropriate patterns of care can be detected and corrective actions taken.[42, 68] At least in theory, this approach offers considerable promise. Not only can potentially inappropriate use of care be identified cross-sectionally, but patterns of care in individual patients over time also can be used to permit inferences about the effectiveness and appropriateness of the care provided.

Quality Assurance and Cost Control

In the often-heard accusations that quality assurance is being misused as a tool for cost control, there is the implication that quality and cost control are incompatible. However, an honest view of quality assurance should accept that quality assurance may result in higher costs. There is no doubt that quality assurance activities themselves are costly, and that quite often quality assurance activities identify deficiencies that cost money to rectify. Quality assurance and cost control are not only compatible, but they must be considered together for truly meaningful quality assurance.

Important to the issue of quality assurance is the fact that there is not, nor will there ever be, an unambiguous, universal, and stable formula for what constitutes quality dental care. The definition at any one time and place must be conditional on what is possible (the state of the science and art of dentistry) and what is affordable to the individual and to society. Even in the richest of societies, resources are finite. Therefore it follows that the definition of what constitutes quality dental care is a continuously variable one, and it will inevitably include consideration of cost.

Because cost considerations therefore are fundamentally part of quality, it follows that if there are 2 or more equally effective and acceptable ways of reaching a desired outcome, the least expensive one (i.e., the most efficient one) is of higher quality. Simply put, if the desired outcome can be reached with fewer resources, the excess resources can be used by the individual and society to pursue additional desired goals, and the individual and society will be better off. This philosophy illustrates that cost is fundamentally part of the quality equation.

Nevertheless, the tensions between quality assurance and cost containment are considerable. On one hand, if cost containment reduces unnecessary care, quality should increase. On the other hand, substitution of lower-cost services might reduce the quality of care. Bailit[21] has pointed out that cost containment is not likely to be as simple as reducing the so-called unnecessary services; the more expensive treatments usually do produce benefits for individual patients. Nevertheless, the same amount of money could often produce even more benefit for a large number of people if it were used for other, less expensive services.

Although it has been said that better quality care is more expensive, the converse is not necessarily true: more expensive care is not necessarily of better quality. If too much of the available funds go to a small number of the group, the overall oral health of the group may well suffer. This emphasizes a dilemma that is discussed further in Chapter 8, which is that there is no inherently "right" amount of health care. The amount of money that any individual, group, or society as a whole will want to spend for a particular health care procedure, or for health care in general, can be determined only by balancing it against other needs and desires. Implicit in this idea is that there is such a thing as too much health care, even if the use of a service can be shown to improve the medical or dental condition of a person. If the resources required to provide such a service are so large that other even more beneficial services cannot be provided, then it would be rational for individuals and society to conclude that such a procedure should not be used.

It has become more obvious with third-party payments that when there is a finite amount of money for care, priority decisions must be made as to who receives services, what services may be provided, or both. How these priorities will be set and how the inevitable trade-off between the benefit to the group versus the individual patient will be resolved will continue to be a topic of debate.

REFERENCES

1. Abramowitz J, Berg LE. A four-year study of the utilization of dental assistants with expanded functions. J Am Dent Assoc 1973;87:623–35.
2. Ambrose ER, Hord AB, Simpson WJ. A quality evaluation of specific dental services provided by the Saskatchewan Dental Plan: Final report. Regina: Government of Saskatchewan, 1976.
3. American Association of Dental Schools. Trends in dental education: 1997. Washington DC: AAADS, 1997.
4. American Dental Association, Bureau of Economic Research and Statistics. Distribution of dentists in the United States by state, region, district, and county. Chicago: ADA, 1977.
5. American Dental Association, Bureau of Economic Research and Statistics. Distribution of dentists in the United States by region and state; 1987. Chicago: ADA, 1987.
6. American Dental Association, Bureau of Economic Research and Statistics. The 1989 Survey of Dentistry. Dentists in nonsolo and solo practice. Chicago: ADA, 1989.
7. American Dental Association, Council on Dental Care Programs. Policies on dental care programs. Chicago: ADA, 1977.
8. American Dental Association, Council on Dental Benefit Programs. Current dental terminology CDT-2. 2nd ed. 1995–2000. Chicago: ADA, 1994.
9. American Dental Association, Council on Dental Practice. A brief overview of the franchise concept as applied to the practice of dentistry. J Am Dent Assoc 1983;106:518–9.
10. American Dental Association, Council on Hospital and Institutional Dental Services. Hospital dental statistics: An update. J Am Dent Assoc 1985;110:241–3.
11. American Dental Association. Dental practice parameters. Parameters for 12 oral health conditions. Adopted by the American Dental Association House of Delegates. October 1994. J Am Dent Assoc 1995;126(Suppl):1–37.
12. American Dental Association. Dental practice parameters. Parameters for 12 oral health conditions. Adopted by the American Dental Association House of Delegates. October 1995. J Am Dent Assoc 1996;128(Suppl):iS–iiS, 1S–36S.
13. American Dental Association. Directory of dental quality assessment and quality assurance programs in the United States, 1989. Chicago; Office of Quality Assurance, ADA, 1990.
14. American Dental Association, House of Delegates. Resolution 78-1972-H. Trans Am Dent Assoc 1973;114:707–9.
15. American Dental Association, House of Delegates. Resolution 40-H-1976. Trans Am Dent Assoc 1977;117:839.
16. American Dental Association, Survey Center. 1995 survey of dental practice—dentists in solo and nonsolo practice. Chicago: ADA, 1996.
17. American Dental Association, Survey Center. Distribution of dentists in the United States by region and state, 1995. Chicago: ADA, 1997.
18. American Dental Association, Survey Center. 1995 survey of dental services in hospitals. Chicago: ADA, 1996.
19. Anderson C. The arrival of franchise dentistry. J Missouri Dent Assoc 1984;64:16–8.

20. Bailit HL, Gotowka T. Guidelines for the development of a quality assurance audit system for hospital dental programs. Chicago: American Dental Association, Office of Quality Assurance, 1983.

21. Bailit HL. Is overutilization the major reason for increasing dental expenditures? Reflections on a complex issue. J Dent Pract Admin 1988;5:112–5.

22. Baird KM, Purdy EC, Protheroe DH. Pilot study on advanced training and employment of auxiliary dental personnel in the Royal Canadian Dental Corps: Final report. J Can Dent Assoc 1963;29:778–87.

23. Barmes DE. Features of oral health care across cultures. Int Dent J 1976;26:253–66.

24. Beck DJ. Dental health status of the New Zealand population in late adolescence and young adulthood. National Health Statistics Centre Special Report No 29. Wellington NZ: Government Printer, 1968.

25. Berwick DM. Continuous improvement as an ideal in health care. N Engl J Med 1989;320:53–6.

26. Boylan ME. Ongoing assessment of the quality of dental care. In: National Round Table on Quality Assurance. Summary of proceedings. Chicago: The American Fund for Dental Health, 1983:pp 121–4.

27. Dickson M. Where there is no dentist. Palo Alto: The Hesperian Foundation, 1987.

28. DeAngelis AJ. Quality assurance: Definition and direction for the 80s. J Dent Educ 1984;48:27–33.

29. Dietz J. Harvard plan growth vexes the competition. Boston Globe, 1978 Oct 9.

30. Donabedian A. Evaluating the quality of medical care. Milbank Q 1966;44:166–203.

31. Donabedian A. The definition of quality and approaches to its assessment. Vol. I. Ann Arbor: Hospital Administration Press, 1980.

32. Dummett CO. Understanding the underprivileged patient. J Am Dent Assoc 1969;79:1363–7.

33. Dunning JM. Extending the field for dental auxiliary personnel in the United States. Am J Public Health 1958;48:1059–64.

34. Feldstein, PJ. Health associations and the demand for legislation: The political economy of health. Cambridge MA: Ballinger, 1977.

35. Flexner A. Medical education in the United States and Canada: A report to the Carnegie Foundation for the Advancement of Teaching. New York: Carnegie Foundation, 1910.

36. Giangrego E. Dentistry in hospitals: Looking to the future. J Am Dent Assoc 1987;115:545–55.

37. Gies WJ. Dental education in the United States and Canada: A report to the Carnegie Foundation for the Advancement of Teaching. New York: Carnegie Foundation, 1926.

38. Goldfield N, Nash DB. Providing quality care: Future challenges. 2nd ed. Ann Arbor: Health Administration Press, 1995.

39. Gruebbel AO. A study of dental public health services in New Zealand. Chicago: American Dental Association, 1950.

40. Hammons PE, Jamison HC, Wilson LL. Quality of service provided by dental therapists in an experimental program at the University of Alabama. J Am Dent Assoc 1971;82:1060–6.

41. Harris N. Are health plans making the grade? Business and Health 1994;June:22–8.

42. Hayden WJ, Marcus M, Lewis CE. Developing population profiles from dental claims data for conceptualizing effectiveness of care. J Dent Educ 1989;53:619–28.

43. Health Insurance Association of America. Source book of health insurance data—1995. Washington DC: HIAA, 1995.

44. Jensen GAA, Morrisey MA, Gaffney S, Listen DK. The new dominance of managed care: Insurance trends in the 1990s. Health Affairs 1997;16:125–36.

45. Jensen UJ. From good medical practice to best medical practice. Int J Health Planning Management 1989;4:167–80.

46. Kritcheusky SB, Simmons BP. Continuous quality improvement: Concepts and applications for physician care. JAMA 1991;226:1817–23.

47. Leake JL, Woodward GL. Introduction to the quality assurance workshop in dentistry: Why dental educators need to learn how to develop practice guidelines. J Dent Educ 1994;58:610–2.

48. Lobene RR, Berman K, Chaisson LB, et al. The Forsyth experiment in training of advanced skills hygienists. Dent Hyg 1974;48:204–13.

49. Lotzkar SJ, Johnson DW, Thompson MB. Experimental program in expanded functions for dental assistants. Phase I: Baseline, and phase 2: training. J Am Dent Assoc 1971;82:101–22.

50. Lotzkar SJ, Johnson DW, Thompson MB. Experimental program in expanded functions for dental assistants. Phase 3: Experiment with dental teams. J Am Dent Assoc 1971;82:1067–81.

51. Marcus M, Koch AL, Gershen JA. A population index of oral health status as derived form dentists' preferences. J Public Health Dent 1983;43:284–94.

52. Marcus M. Trends in quality assurance in the dental profession. J Dent Educ 1990;54:224–7.

53. Marcus M. Managed care and dentistry: promise and problems. J Am Dent Assoc 1995;126:439–46.

54. McCulloch CAG. Can evidence-based dental health care assure quality? J Dent Educ 1994;58:654–6.

55. Morris AL, Bentley JM, Vito AA, Bomba MR. Assessment of private dental practice: Report of a study. J Am Dent Assoc 1988;117:153–62.

56. Myers BA. Health maintenance organizations: Objectives and issues. HSMHA Health Rep 1971;86:585–91.

57. Nightingale F. Notes on hospitals. 3rd ed. London: Longman, Green, Longman, Roberts, and Green, 1863.

58. Nikias MK, Sollecito WA, Fink R. An oral health index based on ranking of oral status profiles by panels of dental professionals. J Public Health Dent 1979;39:16–26.

59. Owens JA, Tennenhouse DJ, Kasher MP. Dental risk prevention. San Rafael, CA: Tennenhouse Professional Publications, 1990.

60. Phantumvanit P, Songpaisan Y, Pilot T, Frenken JE. Atraumatic restorative treatment (ART): A three-year community field trial in Thailand. Survival of one-surface restorations in the permanent dentition. J Public Health Dent 1996;56:141–5.

61. Redig DF, Dewhirst F, Nevitt G, Snyder M. Delivery of dental services in New Zealand and California. J South Calif Dent Assoc 1973;41:318–50.

62. Romcke RG, Lewis DW. Use of expanded function hygienists in the Prince Edward Island manpower study. J Can Dent Assoc 1973;39:247–62.

63. Rowe NH, Doelle PJ, Loos PJ, Herschfus L. Hospital dentistry—survival? J Michigan Dent Assoc 1985;67:507–11.

64. Schoen MH. A quality assessment system: The search for validity. J Dent Educ 1989;53:658–61.

65. Smith QM, Pennell EH, Bothwell RD, Gailbreath MN. Dental care in a group purchase plan: A survey of attitudes and utilization at the St. Louis Labor Health

Institute. PHS Publication No 684. Washington DC: Government Printing Office, 1959.

66. Soricelli DA. Implementation of the delivery of dental services by auxiliaries: The Philadelphia experience. Am J Public Health 1972;62:1077–87.

67. Spath PL, ed. Quality management in ambulatory care. Chicago: American Hospital Publishing, 1992.

68. Torchia M. Using data to improve quality. Business and Health 1994 March; nv:23–7.

69. The state dental scheme and the New Zealand Dental Association [editorial]. NZ Dent J 1921;16:145–8.

70. US Congress, Senate. Health Maintenance Organization Act of 1973; Public Law 93-222. 93rd Congress, 2nd Session. Washington DC: Government Printing Office, 1974.

71. US Preventive Services Task Force. Guide to clinical preventive services: An assessment of the effectiveness of 169 interventions. Baltimore: Williams & Wilkins, 1989.

72. US Public Health Service, National Center for Health Statistics. Dental services and oral health: United States, 1989. DHHS Publication No (PHS) 93-1511, Series 10 No 183. Washington DC: Government Printing Office, 1992.

73. van der Wal CJP, Nakahata DT, Posl WM, et al. Dental office structure and treatment outcome—related or independent? J Calif Dent Assoc 1995; 23(9):41–9.

74. Wojner AW. Outcome management: An interdisciplinary search for the best practice. AACN Clinical Issues 1996;7:133–45.

75. Wood WL, Scher AZ. Franchise dentistry. NY State Dent J 1984;50:677–8.

76. World Health Organization. Report of the International Conference on Primary Health Care, Alma-Ata, USSR, 1978 Sept. Geneva: WHO, 1978.

77. Yavner SB, Yavner DL, Douglass CW. The failure of the dental franchise industry. J Dent Pract Admin 1988;5(1):21–4.

8

Financing Dental Care

Insurance Principles and Dental Care ◆
Expenditures for Health Care ◆ Expenditures for Dental
Care ◆ Fee-for-Service Dental Care ◆
Third-Party Payment ◆ Reimbursement of
Dentists in Third-Party Plans ◆ Delta Dental
Plans ◆ Reimbursement of Dentists in Delta
Plans ◆ Percentile Fees ◆ Preauthorization ◆
Blue Cross Blue Shield ◆ Commercial Insurance
Plans ◆ Other Dental Insurance Mechanisms ◆
Prepaid Group Plans ◆ Capitation Plans
and Preferred Provider Organizations (PPOs) ◆
Direct Reimbursement Administrative
Services Only (ASO) ◆ Medical Savings
Accounts (MSAs) ◆ Controlling the Costs of Third-Party
Dental Care ◆ Public Financing of Health
Care ◆ Public Financing of Dental Care ◆
Medicare ◆ Medicaid ◆ Children's Health Insurance
Program ◆ Other Programs of Public Financing of
Dental Care ◆ National Health Insurance (NHI)

Health care traditionally has been provided on a fee-for-service basis, in which the patient pays the provider directly for services. This 2-party system is a private contract involving only the provider and the patient. Methods of financing health care in the United States, however, have progressed far beyond this traditional system since the mid-1930s, and especially since 1965. The fundamental change has been the emergence of third parties, meaning that the financing of health services is no longer a matter of a purely private contract between provider and patient. In 1995, for example, 81% of the total outlay for health services and supplies were administered through a third party, and 46% of all health care services were paid for by government agencies.[25] Dentistry's entry into the third-party system has been more recent, but third-party dental care is now a major and still-evolving part of dental practice.

This chapter reviews the various mecha-
nisms used to finance dental care, and the effects that these mechanisms have on care provision.

INSURANCE PRINCIPLES AND DENTAL CARE

To understand how dentistry fits into third-party payment, a review of insurance principles is helpful. During the years after World War II, when medical insurance was growing rapidly, dental care was one of the "fearful four" areas of health care (dental care, psychiatric care, prescription drugs, and long-term care) considered uninsurable by carriers. This reasoning was based on the assumption that the nature of dental need violated the basic principles of insurance,[12] which state that to be insurable a risk must be:

- Precisely definable.
- Of sufficient magnitude that if it occurs, it constitutes a major loss.

- Infrequent.
- Of an unwanted nature, such as destruction of a home through fire.
- Beyond the control of the individual.
- Without "moral hazard," which means that the presence of insurance itself should not lead to additional claims.

All health insurance violates some of these principles. For example, many of the benefits paid by health insurance represent relatively small amounts of money, and people with insurance are more likely to use care than those without it.[26, 30] Insurance carriers found they could get around these problems in several ways, such as:

- Having patients pay a share of the costs.
- Limiting the range of services available.
- Offering coverage only to groups.
- Including waiting periods after enrollment before benefits became payable.
- Using preauthorization and annual expenditure limits.

Requiring patients to pay part of the cost of some services is an economic disincentive to overutilization. The portion of the cost of the service that a patient pays is either a deductible or co-insurance. A *deductible* is a set amount of money that the patient must pay toward the cost of treatment before benefits of the program go into effect.[2] A familiar example of a deductible is the "front-end" payment of a claim under automobile insurance. *Co-insurance* means that the patient pays a percentage of the total cost of treatment.[2] For example, if a patient is to pay 20% of the cost of an amalgam restoration, the amount the patient must pay varies depending on the actual fee for an amalgam, but in any case will be 20% of that fee.

Insurance carriers also limit the range of health care services covered: some are available and some not, according to the plan. This is termed *coverage, covered charges,* or *schedule of benefits.* Examples of services that are rarely covered in dental policies are implants, cosmetic restorations, and extensive temporomandibular disorders (TMD) treatment. An additional cost-control mechanism, *preauthorization,* means that treatment plans for more than a specified sum must be reviewed by the carrier's dental consultants to ensure that the proposed treatment is reasonable and that the same quality of care could not be achieved at less expense.

Health insurance was at first offered only to groups because illness experience is reasonably predictable in a group, although not for an individual. The risk of *adverse selection,* which means the inclusion of too many high-risk beneficiaries, was reduced because insuring only large groups "averaged out" the risks. Although a group would likely include people with high levels of need, there would also be many who had little need for care for whom premiums would also be paid. In fact, this is the essence of insurance. The fact that the cost of care required for a few people far exceeds the premiums paid for them is irrelevant as long as the average cost of care across the group is in balance with the premium.

The probability of adverse selection was further reduced by the use of waiting periods after enrollment. The waiting period ensured that people with existing disease were not simply going to use the plan to have that disease treated and then drop out. As experience with the administration of health insurance grew, carriers were able to offer individual policies. Today, many commercial and nonprofit insurance carriers make individual policies available for hospital and major medical coverage, although premiums are considerably higher and benefits are often more limited than for group policies.

After looking at the list of insurance principles, it can be seen why dental care was for a long time considered uninsurable. Nearly everyone has some dental treatment needs. They tend to be frequent rather than infrequent, and unlike hospital care the cost of dental treatment is rarely catastrophic. Nevertheless, evaluations of some of the earliest group prepayment plans indicated that dental care indeed was insurable because cost was found to be not the only barrier to dental care[37–39]; even with the cost barrier removed, potential patients did not pour in as many had expected. Although utilization of dental service was increased, it stayed well short of 100%. In other words, although all members of the group may have needed dental care and all were paying a premium toward it, only some members were seeking treatment. Indeed, if 100% of the group sought dental care on a regular basis, it might be less expensive for them to pay for their care individually rather than through prepayment.

EXPENDITURES FOR HEALTH CARE

Expenditures for health care have risen sharply in all industrialized countries in the

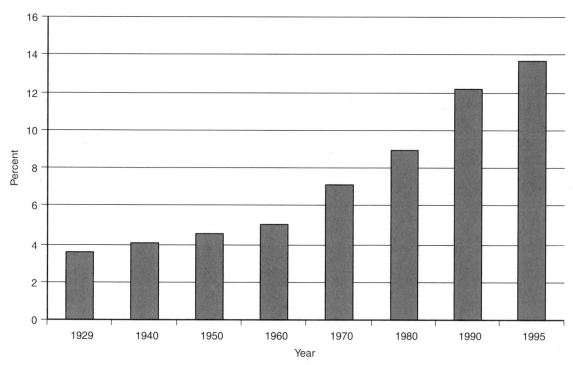

Figure 8-1. National health expenditures as a percentage of the gross domestic product, United States, selected years, 1929–1995. (From Gibson RM, Fisher CR. National health expenditures, fiscal year 1977. Soc Security Bull 1978;41:3–20; Levit KR, Lazenby HC, Braden BP. National health expenditures. Health Care Financing Rev 1996;18:175–82.)

last several decades, but nowhere has this pattern been as dramatic as in the United States. Figure 8–1 shows that in 1929, expenditures in the United States for health care (including dental care) accounted for 3.6% of the gross domestic product (GDP). Since 1929, the pattern has been steadily upward, reaching 13.6% of GDP in 1995.[16, 25] Predictions suggest that spending for health care will rise to 15% to 20% of the GDP in the next few decades,[13, 43] a level of national expenditure that is a cause for deep concern.

Figure 8–2 shows how the per capita national health expenditures have risen since 1960. From an annual average of $141 in 1960, the average cost per person had risen to $3621 in 1995. Figure 8–2 also shows that the portion of the cost of health care paid by public funds has grown since 1960. Some of the reasons given for this increase in the cost of health care in the United States are the following:

- Increasing costs: Incomes of health care workers have risen faster than the incomes for many other workers.
- Difficult economies of scale: It is harder to achieve economies of scale in health care than in many other sectors of the economy.

In many manufacturing industries, for example, it does not require 10% more workers to produce an additional 10% of a product. In health care, by contrast, increasing the amount of care provided requires a nearly proportional increase in the workforce.

- The practice of "defensive" medicine: Tests carried out to protect the provider against possible litigation, rather than to treat the patient, lead to a rise in costs.
- The aging population: An aging population causes an increase in per capita costs. Because older people use more health care services, the average cost of care will increase as the average age of the population increases. In addition, the expectation of longer life brings a greater willingness to provide heroic care for a person who in earlier days would not have been expected to live much longer even if healthy, but who today would be thought to have a reasonable chance for more years of life.
- Developments in technology: Some innovations reduce the costs of care because they are so much more effective than any available alternatives (antibiotics, for example, reduced the average length of a hospital

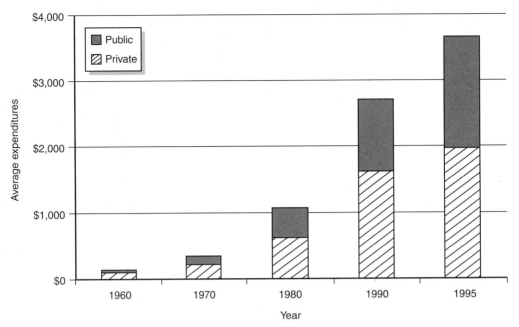

Figure 8–2. Per capita national health expenditures, showing the proportionate expenditure of private and public funds, United States, selected years 1960–1995. (From Levit KR, Lazenby HC, Braden BR. National health expenditures. Health Care Financing Rev 1996;18:175–82.)

stay when they were introduced in the 1940s and 1950s). Others, because they are providing care that was previously unavailable, can only add to aggregate costs. An example is treatment for end-stage renal disease for patients who in earlier days would have soon died. With dialysis they now live, but at a cost that was estimated to average $24,976 per patient per year in 1983.[36]

- Third-party payment: Insurance has provided large amounts of money for care that would otherwise have been unavailable. For example, many of the elderly and the poor who receive the benefits of Medicare and Medicaid would not otherwise have had the money to purchase this care. Without these programs, the total and per capita costs of care would undoubtedly be smaller. The same is true for private insurance, as many who otherwise would have faced large bills for hospitalization and other services would have been forced to do without.

The spiraling costs of health care present American society with the classic trade-off dilemma we discussed in Chapter 7. On the one hand, if people go without health care that can improve or prolong their lives, both the individual and society suffer. On the other hand, it should be evident that the proportion

of the GDP going to health care cannot continue to climb indefinitely, because as more of our available resources go to health care there is less for housing, education, recreation, and other necessities that contribute to health, wealth, and happiness. Although there is ample reason to be concerned for people who receive too little health care, there is also the possibility that a point can be reached where, at least in the aggregate, there is too much health care relative to life's other necessities. The dilemma is made even more difficult by the fact that as of 1995, nearly 40 million people in the United States have no health insurance.[43] Although there is a justifiable outcry that some form of coverage should be provided for these people, it is also obvious that to do so will further increase national expenditures.[20, 30, 52] Health care providers, in their honest desire to do the best for their patients, need to recognize that this individual-versus-social tension will always exist.

Resolution of this dilemma is made even more complex by the inclusion of government and private third-party agencies in the equation. As the total costs of care continue to climb and put more and more pressure on the economy, and with most health care costs being paid for through third parties, the pressure for collective action to control these costs will continue. No one in health care should be surprised to see a continuing stream of proposals aimed at controlling or reforming the health care system.

EXPENDITURES FOR DENTAL CARE

Expenditures for dental care, although only a fraction of the total for health care, are nevertheless substantial. Figure 8–3 illustrates that the total expenditures for dental care by Americans grew from less than $500 million in 1929 to an estimated $45.8 billion in 1995.[10, 25] This latter figure represents an average per capita expenditure for dental care of $154 in 1995.

Figures 8–4 and 8–5 present two additional views of the cost of dental care. Figure 8–4 shows that relative to the total cost of personal health care expenditures, dental expenditures have fallen steadily from the 14% reported in 1929 to 5.2% in 1995. This pattern reflects the combination of the steep rise in the overall costs of medical care against the more modest rise in the costs of dental care. Throughout most of the 1990s, however, it appears that dental care has stabilized at around 5% of total personal health expendi-

tures. Figure 8–5 presents the expenditures for dental care as a percentage of the GDP. The pattern here is especially interesting; the relative decline from 1929 to 1950 corresponds to the period of the Great Depression followed by World War II. Dental care is income- and price-elastic, so that as real income fell during the depression, and as the cost of other goods and services rose during and after the war, there was simply less money available for dental care. The rise since 1970 coincides with a period of growth in real income, and also in the extent of dental insurance. Economic theory suggests that both of these changes should result in a relative growth in dental expenditures, a phenomenon that has indeed occurred. The relative growth in dental expenditures has continued right up to the present, to just over 0.6% of the GDP in 1995, even though the percentage of the population covered by dental insurance has plateaued. This is a sign that the dental sector continues to be a robust part of the national economy.

Fee-for-Service Dental Care

Private fee-for-service payment, the two-party arrangement, is the traditional form of

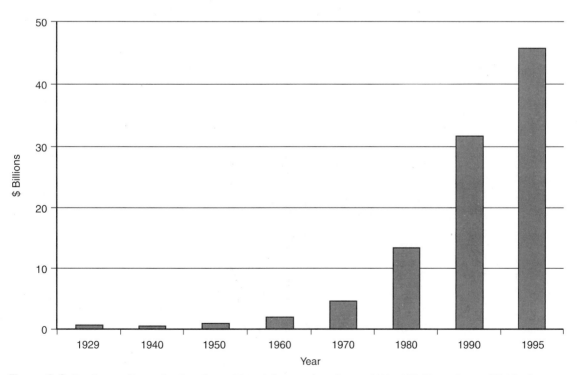

Figure 8–3. Total expenditures for dental care, United States, selected years 1929–1995. (From Cooper BS, Worthington NL. National health expenditures, 1929–72. Soc Security Bull 1973;36:3–19,40; Levit KR, Lazenby HC, Braden BR. National health expenditures. Health Care Financing Rev 1996;18:175–82.)

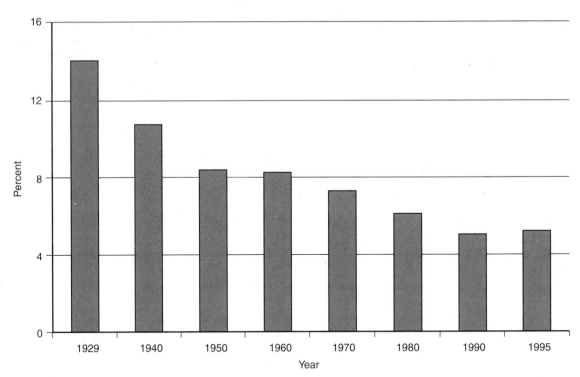

Figure 8–4. Per capita expenditure for dental care as a percentage of total health expenditures, United States, selected years 1929–1995. (From Gibson RM, Fisher CR. National health expenditures, fiscal year 1977. Soc Security Bull 1978;41:3–20; Levit KR, Lazenby HC, Braden BR. National health expenditures. Health Care Financing Rev 1996;18:175–82.)

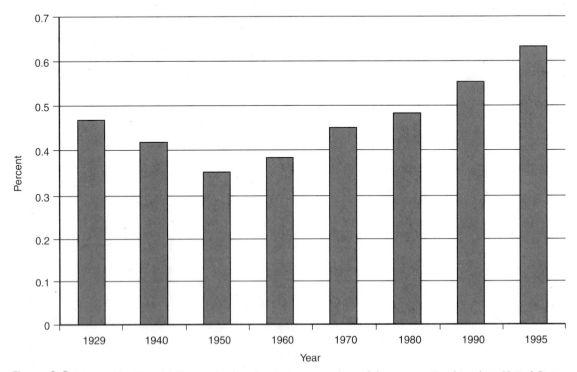

Figure 8–5. National health expenditures for dental care as a percentage of the gross national product, United States, selected years 1929–1995. (From Gibson RM, Fisher CR. National health expenditures, fiscal year 1977. Soc Security Bull 1978;41:3–20; Levit KR, Lazenby HC, Braden BR. National health expenditures. Health Care Financing Rev 1996;18:175–82.)

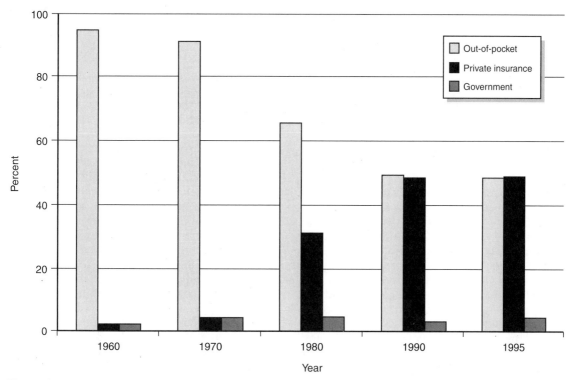

Figure 8–6. Proportions of total dental care expenditures paid by consumers out-of-pocket, by private insurance, and by government funds, United States, selected years 1960–1995. (From Levit KR, Lazenby HC, Braden BR. National health expenditures. Health Care Financing Rev 1996;18:175–82.)

reimbursement for dental services in the United States and elsewhere. Under this system, the patient decides when to visit a dentist, and the dentist suggests appropriate treatment and informs the patient of the fee for the service. If the patient chooses to follow the recommendations of the dentist and receives the services, the patient is then responsible for the fee. As recently as 1970, as shown in Figure 8–6, the vast majority of payments for dental services came directly from patients. By 1995, however, because of the substantial growth in prepayment, direct consumer payment had dropped to just under one half of all payments, virtually identical to the proportion paid by private insurance.

Third-Party Payment

In the language of contracts, the patient and dentist are the first and second parties, and the administrator of the finances is the third party, defined as the party to a dental prepayment contract that may collect premiums, assume financial risk, pay claims, and provide administrative services. Third-party payment for dental services therefore is pay-

ment to the dentist by an agency rather than directly by the patient. The third party is sometimes called the *carrier, insurer, underwriter,* or *administrative agent.* The purchaser of the plan can be an organized private group such as a union, or it can be an employer, a union-employer welfare fund, or a governmental agency. Usually, however, the term *third party,* without further qualification, refers to a private carrier such as an insurance company. When the government acts as the third party the term more commonly used is *public financing of care.*

Passage of the Taft-Hartley Act in 1947 allowed labor unions to seek fringe benefits, in addition to wages, through collective bargaining. Since then, health care insurance has been a popular fringe benefit. One of the reasons for this popularity is that the premiums paid by the employer are not usually counted as taxable income for the employee. Each dollar of earnings taken in the form of health insurance therefore buys more health care than if it is taken as cash wages, because cash wages are taxed while the insurance benefits are not. (Health insurance as a fringe benefit, with protection from tax, is popular with the insurance and health care industries, too, because it actually is a subsidy for them). There have been frequent unsuccessful attempts at the federal level to limit the amount of these health insurance premiums that are protected from taxes. It is reasonable to expect renewed attempts of this type in the future in times of budgetary difficulty. Such a "tax cap," if it were enacted, could reduce the popularity of dental insurance. It is assumed that if such a limit were to be placed on the tax deductibility of health insurance premiums, most people would apply the tax-deductible amount of their hospitalization and medical insurance. This would mean that the money paid by employers for dental insurance would be treated as taxable income, and additional wages would be deducted from each paycheck to pay this tax. Dental insurers fear that this change would cause many individuals and groups to drop their dental insurance.

By the late 1960s, with some 85% of the American population covered by hospital and surgical expense insurance,[22] coverage for dental expenses emerged as an area for negotiation by labor groups seeking additional fringe benefits. Growth of dental prepayment plans through the 1970s and 1980s therefore can be seen as an evolutionary step in the growth of employment fringe benefits.

Who actually pays for third-party care? A union that negotiates a dental plan as a fringe benefit is choosing to accept the plan rather than cash wages, so the union members pay for it in wages foregone. Ultimately, if the companies employing the union members increase the price of their products to finance the plan, the purchasers of those products pay for it. Reference to the third-party agency as the "payer for services," although common, is incorrect; nor are the union members getting "free" care, even if they do not pay directly out-of-pocket.

In private third-party plans, periodic premiums are collected to meet the costs of providing care, as well as the administrative costs of the third party. It has been argued that this arrangement should most properly be called prepayment rather than insurance, because it does not fulfill the classic definitions of insurance. Be that as it may, the term dental insurance has entered the language, and the terms *dental prepayment* and *dental insurance* as commonly used are virtually synonymous. The main difference between dental and some other forms of insurance is that traditional insurance involves a group of people making small payments in order to cover the risk of a few suffering catastrophic loss, such as the loss of a home through fire. The expectation is that few of them will ever suffer such a loss, and most, therefore, will never collect any insurance payments. Dental prepayment, on the other hand, is a mechanism to spread the financial load of dental care over a group and over time. Virtually all of them can reasonably expect to make regular and somewhat predictable use of the benefits.

For the companies who administer these plans, the methods for setting the premiums is essentially the same as it is for any other form of insurance. Based on the characteristics and previous history of a group, the actuaries estimate how much dental care will be provided to the group in the coming period of time (usually at least 1 year). The expected reimbursable cost of that care plus the administrative expenses form the basis for premium calculations. Virtually all private dental insurance in the United States is available only through group purchase; there are few individual policies. Those that are available are characterized by high premiums and limited benefits; this is the carriers' method of countering the risk of high utilization and adverse selection.

The rapid growth of prepayment since 1970 has changed the nature of dental practice. The growth is illustrated by Figure 8–6, which shows that the portion of dental care costs paid by prepayment plans increased more than 10-fold between 1970 and 1995. The number of people covered by some sort of private dental insurance increased from approximately 12 million in 1970 to approximately 100 million, or about 40% of the population, by the mid-1990s. When those eligible for care through publicly funded programs are added, approximately one half of the US population has some form of dental insurance; it is a rare dental practice nowadays that sees no insured patients at all. In many parts of the country, 90% or more of the patients in some practices have dental insurance.

Although the growth in dental insurance has been spectacular since 1970, further rapid growth in the immediate future is not likely. This is because the large unions in the major US industries are, for the most part, already covered. For dental insurance to grow, mechanisms will have to be developed to reach small businesses and individuals. A second reason why dental insurance will grow only slowly is the general climate of cost control in all aspects of business, which in turn comes from the fierce demands on the United States and Canada to be competitive in the global economy. Increased concern for worldwide competitiveness works against offering benefits to workers not already covered, and there are already some signs of cutbacks in some industries. A third factor that may work against further expansion of dental insurance is the improvement in oral health that is especially evident in young adults and children (Chapters 18–20). It may be that because people in these age cohorts have experienced little need for expensive and unexpected dental treatment they will not push as hard for dental insurance as did their elders, who had much higher levels of need for treatment.

Reimbursement of Dentists in Third-Party Plans

Control of the costs of third-party plans is essential to their success, for if the insurance plan is seen as a bottomless money-pit, the plan will have to raise premiums to higher and higher levels, making it unlikely that anyone will be willing to buy the policy. Because the implications of "control" in this context are anathema to most practitioners, methods of reimbursing dentists under third-party plans have long preoccupied the American Dental Association (ADA). The ADA sees the need for controls, but also tries to maximize the independence of the dental practitioner. The major forms of third-party reimbursement currently in use are:

• Usual, customary, and reasonable (UCR) fee
• Table of allowances
• Fee schedules
• Capitation

In line with its philosophy of maximizing practitioner independence, the ADA has consistently supported the concept of the UCR fee as a reimbursement method for dentists in prepayment plans. However, ADA resolutions that UCR fees should be the preferred method of reimbursement were rescinded on legal grounds after the US Supreme Court decision in June 1975 in *Goldfarb* v. *Virginia State Bar et al*. This decision ruled that learned professions were not exempt from antitrust laws.[1, 4, 5] In effect, the court said that each practitioner should be free to choose how he wants to be reimbursed, and that it was inap-

propriate for a professional association to suggest to its members which choice to make.

The ADA definitions of usual, customary, and reasonable fees are as follows:

• **Usual fee:** The fee that an individual dentist most frequently charges for a given dental service.
• **Customary fee:** The fee level determined by the administrator of a dental benefit plan from actual submitted fees for a specific dental procedure to establish the maximum benefit payable under a given plan for that specific procedure.
• **Reasonable fee:** The fee charged by a dentist for a specific dental procedure that has been modified by the nature and severity of the condition being treated and by medical or dental complications or unusual circumstances, and therefore may differ from the dentist's "usual" fee or the benefit administrator's "customary" fee.[2]

When third-party dental programs first began, many dentists were opposed to them on the grounds that they would be forced to adopt lower fees than those that they usually charged. The evolution of the UCR fee concept as a mechanism acceptable both to dentists and carriers has allowed third-party dental care to be provided while still permitting the individual dentist to charge what he believes his services are worth. It is reasonable to suggest that dental prepayment plans would not have been accepted by dentists to the extent they have without the UCR fee concept.

A table of allowances (or schedule) is defined as a list of covered services with an assigned dollar amount that represents the total obligation of the plan with respect to payment for such service, but that does not necessarily represent the dentist's full fee for that service.[2] For example, if a dentist's usual fee for a particular service is $20 and the plan lists a fee of $15 as payable for that service, the dentist will provide the service, collect $15 from the carrier, and may charge the patient $5 to make up the difference. Under UCR fees, on the other hand, the plan pays the dentist's usual fee in full (less any required patient co-payment), in this case the $20. The table of allowances as a method of reimbursement requires that dentists carefully explain to patients the limited nature of the insurance payment, because some patients are unaware that their plan may not cover them in full.

A fee schedule is defined as a list of the charges established or agreed to by a dentist for specific dental services.[2] A fee schedule is usually taken to mean payment in full, whereas a table of allowances, as just explained, may not. A program in which the payment is meant to represent full payment, with no additional charge to the patient allowed beyond a pre-established co-payment or deductible, is also called a service plan. Fee schedules for dental care are sometimes established by public programs, such as Medicaid in some states. Dentistry's opposition to fee schedules is based on: (a) their potential inflexibility, meaning that the fees listed can fall below customary fees, particularly in times of rapid inflation; (b) the implicit assumption that all dentists' treatment is of the same quality and therefore worth the same fee; and (c) the fear that autonomy is threatened, especially if the fee schedule is not controlled by the dentists. A potential risk with a fee schedule is that if the fees paid are too far below the usual level, few dentists will be willing to treat the covered patients. This has been cited as one reason why many dentists either severely limit the number of their Medicaid patients or refuse to accept them as patients altogether.[11, 24, 45]

Reimbursement of the dentist by capitation, as in a medical HMO, became more common during the 1980s and 1990s. The ADA defines capitation as a dental benefit program in which a dentist or dentists contract with the programs' sponsor or administrator to provide all or most of the dental services covered under the program to subscribers in return for a payment on a per capita basis.[2] A capitation fee is usually a fixed monthly payment paid by a carrier to a dentist based on the number of patients assigned to the dentist for treatment. Capitation requires that patients be assigned to specific dentists or dental practices for care, so that the capitation payment can be paid to the appropriate dentist or practice. This assignment is important because the dentist receives a fixed sum of money per head per month, regardless of whether the participants in the plan receive care in that particular month. The assumption is that while some patients will receive a lot of care and some receive none, the total amount of money paid to the dentist will be sufficient to cover the overall costs of care in the covered group.

Many dentists are resistant to capitation because of a fear that high utilization and demands for expensive forms of care could rapidly outrun the capitation fee and that dentists will thus be at an economic disadvantage. As a dissenting voice, Schoen[33-35] argued that capitation works every bit as well as fee-for-service and that with proper planning it is a highly efficient method of financing group dental care, especially for less affluent groups. But despite Schoen's claims of success with capitation in his own group practice, many dentists and the ADA remain cautious. The ADA is opposed to capitation and fee schedules as the sole forms of reimbursement in prepayment plans, arguing that where such mechanisms exist they should be on an equal footing with UCR fees so that prospective patients have a choice. In fact, by the 1990s there were very few "pure" capitation plans. Most capitation plans now include co-payments, especially for more expensive services, and annual maximums, both of which limit the economic risks that the dentist faces.

DELTA DENTAL PLANS

In June 1954, the Seattle District Dental Society in Washington State was approached by the International Longshoreman's and Warehouseman's Union-Pacific Maritime Association with a request that the society submit a proposal for a comprehensive dental care program for children up to 14 years of age. The proposal requested by the union required information on administration, fees, methods of operation, dental care provided, and control of quality; at that time there was almost no previous experience or data upon which to draw. The dental society nevertheless wished to discourage the union from setting up its own closed-panel clinics, and it developed a plan whereby the children could be treated in the offices of private dentists. Shortly thereafter, the first dental service corporation was born.[47] Within a few years dental service corporations were also formed in Oregon and California, and in subsequent years the idea of the dental service corporation spread throughout the country from the West Coast.

A dental service corporation is a legally constituted not-for-profit organization, incorporated on a state-by-state basis, that negotiates and administers contracts for dental care. The original dental service corporations, now know as Delta Dental Plans, were sponsored

Property of
High-Tech Institute of Sacramento, CA
Library/Resource Center

by the constituent dental societies in each state. Most Blue Cross and Blue Shield dental plans are now also organized as dental service corporations.

Dental service corporations, as well as the private for-profit insurance companies, are subject to the insurance laws of the state in which they operate. As the number of dental service corporations grew through the early 1960s and the size of the groups for which dental care benefits were negotiated grew, the need for a national organization of dental service organizations became apparent. Accordingly, the National Association of Dental Service Plans was formed in 1966, with staff and financial help from the ADA. The name became Delta Dental Plans Association (DDPA) in 1969,[18] and most of the member corporations became known as the Delta Dental Plan for the particular state.

DDPA has also become the vehicle through which the Delta plans in individual states compete with national insurance companies for contracts with companies with employees in more than one state. Through DDPA, an organization called Delta USA was formed to coordinate and administer these multistate contracts. By the mid-1990s, more than 100,000 participating dentists were available to Delta USA through the individual state Delta plans, accounting for approximately 70% of all dentists in practice nationwide. Collectively, Delta plans cover approximately 20 million people in the United States and account for about 25% of total claims paid annually by all dental carriers.

The underlying philosophy of the Delta Dental Plans was to permit the dental practitioners to adapt their traditional patterns of practice to meet the demand for group purchase of dental care. In this sense, Delta plans have followed the lead of the professionally sponsored Blue Cross and Blue Shield hospital and medical plans. Most Delta plans were formed for the sole purpose of providing dental prepayment, and most have retained dental insurance as their sole or major business.

Delta also pioneered specific approaches to ensure the quality of care provided and to keep a program's costs under control, although other carriers now use virtually all of these approaches as well. Quality of care is sometimes monitored by post-treatment examinations, in which a sample of individual patients who have received care through a plan is examined by a panel of disinterested dentists to ensure that (a) the care claimed and paid for was in fact provided and (b) that it is of "acceptable" quality (Chapter 7). When there are concerns about quality, referral can be made to the state's peer review mechanism if the matter cannot be resolved to the satisfaction of all involved.

Billing for services not actually provided, or other instances of noncompliance with the contract such as waiving required co-payments, are taken seriously by insurers. Although the problem with billing for services not provided is obvious, waiving of co-payment is perhaps less so. For insurers who base payments on the UCR method, the co-payment is part of the "usual" fee and often an important part of the cost-control mechanism as well. If a dentist has claimed $40 as his usual fee for a service that has a 20% co-payment, the insurer will pay the dentist $32 and expect the dentist to collect the remaining $8 from the patient. If the dentist chooses not to collect this $8, then the fee in fact is $32, not the $40 claimed, and the insurer should have paid 80% of $32 instead of 80% of $40. Further, if dentists were allowed to simply raise their filed "usual" fees so that the fee minus the co-payment equalled the fee that they really wanted, and then simply forgave the co-payment, the cost-controlling effects of co-insurance would be lost. Concern over these billing practices have led to strict laws in many states, under which these practices are considered to be felonies. Any dentist dealing with third-party payment is well advised to read and understand the rules of participation, and to make a good-faith effort to comply fully with the terms of the agreement.

Reimbursement of Dentists in Delta Plans

Because of Delta's initial close association with organized dentistry, Delta plans at first used the UCR fee-for-service concept almost exclusively, and this method of payment still dominates. Under the fee-for-service programs, the way in which a dentist is reimbursed depends on whether the dentist is participating or nonparticipating (often referred to as *par* and *nonpar* dentists) with Delta. A participating dentist is one who has entered into a contractual agreement to provide care to eligible persons.

Delta plans encourage all dentists to participate. Those who do generally agree to conditions similar to the following:

- Filing of their usual and customary fees with Delta. The accumulated fees of all participating dentists form the basis of the UCR fee system. When a dentist decides to raise his fees, he must refile the new fees. As long as the new fees are charged to all patients, they will become the fees that Delta uses for reimbursement purposes.

- Acceptance of payment for their services at an agreed-on percentile (to be described) as payment in full, which means they will not assess the patient for any further charges, other than co-payments as specified by a particular contract.

- Fee audits by auditors from Delta, who may check the office records from time to time. The purpose of these audits is to ensure that the dentists are indeed charging their Delta patients the same fees as they charge their other patients, and that co-payments are being properly billed to the patient.

- Post-treatment inspection of randomly-chosen patients, whom they have treated, by other dentists. The participating dentists agree to abide by decisions regarding quality of care rendered.

- The withholding by Delta of a small amount of each payment, usually to build up insurance reserves. Adequate reserves are required by state insurance commissioners in most states.

In the early days of dental insurance, the amount withheld was often approximately 5%. As the corporations built up sufficient financial reserves, the withhold has been reduced to as little as 0.5% in some states. Dentists who chose to become participating dentists agreed to the withhold because they supported the idea of developing a form of payment for dental care that they felt represented their interests, and in which they had some voice. In addition, the prospect of direct, prompt payment from the insurer for their services was considered by many to be well worth the small amount withheld.

Nonparticipating dentists can also treat patients covered under Delta plans and be reimbursed by Delta. They do not need to prefile their fees and are not subject to fee audits or withholding. However, nonparticipating dentists are usually paid at the 50th percentile of fees, rather than the 80th or 90th percentile typically paid to participating dentists.

Percentile Fees

The percentiles of a dataset divide the total frequency into hundredths, so that the 90th percentile is that value below which 90% of the observations lie. To illustrate how percentiles are applied to dental fees, suppose in a given area there are 1000 participating dentists who have filed their fee for a particular service. In this example, the range of fees charged for the service runs from $10 to $70. If each of these filed fees is spread out in a frequency distribution from the lowest to the highest, the result might be like that shown in Figure 8–7. About 10% charge less than $30

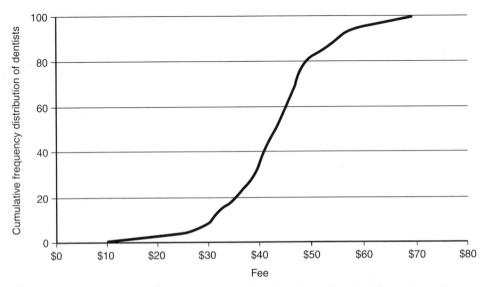

Figure 8–7. Cumulative frequency distribution of hypothetical fees for a given dental service to illustrate the 90th percentile.

for their service, 50% charge $43 or less, 80% charge $49 or less, and 90% charge $55 or less for this particular service. For this service, therefore, $55 is the 90th percentile fee. A few dentists charge more.

When payment is made at the 90th percentile, 90% of the participating dentists will receive their full fee for the service, and only 10% will be paid at less than their usual fee. Those dentists who normally charge $45 would receive $45, those who normally charge $50 would receive $50, and so on up to $55, the 90th percentile. Those who normally charge more than $55 would be paid $55. If nonpar dentists are paid at the 50th percentile, which in this example is $43, they would be paid the lower of the fee that they actually charged, or $43.

The rationale behind paying at the 80th or 90th percentile is to control payment at the top end of the scale while paying the vast majority of dentists (at least 80% or 90%) their full fee. This approach fits the definition of "customary." It is thus a cost-control mechanism usually written into Delta plan contracts.

Preauthorization

Another cost-control mechanism that is widely used by insurers is *preauthorization* (also called *predetermination, precertification, pretreatment review,* or *prior authorization*[2]). With preauthorization, when the costs of treatment are expected to exceed some limit (usually several hundred dollars), the dentist is required to submit the treatment plan to the insurer for review before the treatment begins. This review has several functions, including certification that the patient's insurance covers the planned treatment and at what level, and a review of the appropriateness of the care itself by a dental consultant who works for the insurer. These reviews reduce the cost of care directly, because some treatment plans are revised after discussion with a consultant. They also reduce it indirectly, because dentists soon learn that insurers are unlikely to allow expensive treatment when less expensive alternatives appear to be reasonable.

BLUE CROSS BLUE SHIELD

Blue Cross and Blue Shield plans for many years offered limited dental coverage as a part of their hospital-surgical-medical policies. Initially, dental coverage was usually limited only to services provided in a hospital. The "Blues" showed little enthusiasm for going any further into dental prepayment on the grounds that it was a poor insurance risk, but their attitude changed once dental prepayment was shown to be feasible.

Blue Cross and Blue Shield dental plans have adopted many of the cost-control features pioneered by Delta plans. Many now use prefiled UCR fees from dentists, either to reimburse the dentists in the same way Delta does or to establish fee profiles or fee screens for different geographic areas as a basis for reimbursement. In some states, it is difficult to distinguish Blue Cross and Blue Shield dental plans from Delta plans in terms of benefits and administration.

As is now the case with Delta plans in some states, Blue Cross and Blue Shield plans are also active in offering alternative reimbursement methods, such as capitation, including independent practice associations (IPAs), and preferred provider organizations (PPOs) to meet the demands for cost control from purchasers. These alternative provider arrangements are described in Chapter 7.

COMMERCIAL INSURANCE PLANS

More people have dental insurance from commercial insurance carriers than from any other type of carrier. Once it was clear that prepaid dental plans were viable and that they were likely to be a significant part of the health insurance market, commercial insurance companies saw dental insurance as a potentially profitable area of business. The fundamental difference between commercial insurance companies and the dental service corporations is that the commercials operate for profit. It might be expected, therefore, that commercial insurance carriers would need to charge higher premiums than would the service corporations to allow for the profit margin. In practice, however, this is not generally true, for a number of reasons.

Commercial insurance is often designed as an indemnity plan, meaning cash payments to the providers, rather than as a service benefit plan. This allows the commercial carriers to organize reimbursement differently from the way that dental service corporations usually do. Dentists in most cases do not file their UCR fees with a commercial insurance company, but rather the carrier develops fee profiles; that is, they work out the "going rate" for services from their reported experience of fees in the area, and dentists are paid at that rate. The amounts paid can vary from one insurer to another. Commercial companies are also less likely to conduct fee audits and post-treatment dental examinations, although like the service corporations, most use preauthorization, annual expenditure limits, and careful monitoring of treatment patterns.

OTHER DENTAL INSURANCE MECHANISMS

Prepaid Group Plans

Group practice, as a method of delivering dental care services, was defined and described in Chapter 7. Some specific points about financing care in group practices, however, should be reiterated here. There is no inherent relation between group practice and prepaid care, or between group practice and any other form of financing arrangements. Net income in a group practice can be divided equally or prorated according to patient load, years of service, and specialty status, and some group practices make all their dentists salaried.[33] Whereas the majority of patients who receive care through group practices do so on the usual private fee-for-service basis, larger group practices have resources and personnel that make it feasible for them to offer contracts to consumer groups on a prepaid, capitation basis, and a few do so. In fact, for a while in the early 1960s, the largest number of persons enrolled in prepaid dental care plans received their dental care services from group practices.[49]

Capitation Plans and Preferred Provider Organizations

The structural arrangements for capitation plans and PPOs were described in Chapter 7; here we talk about their financial aspects. By the mid-1990s, capitation plans were a part of many dental practices, especially where third-party payment affected a high proportion of patients. The pressure for innovative approaches to control the costs of medical care have in turn caused purchasers to demand, and insurers to provide, similar approaches for financing dental care. The basis of capitation, as previously described, is that the contracting provider, whether an HMO, group practice, IPA, or individual dentist, receives a fixed sum on a monthly or yearly basis for each eligible patient. The money is paid regardless of whether patients utilize care. In return, the patient is entitled to receive a prescribed set of services over a specified period.

Apart from the development of HMOs, other third-party carriers and even private entrepreneurs (including dentists) became involved in the marketing of capitation plans. In fact, capitation plans have sprouted, in all their permutations and combinations, at such a rapid rate that reliable information on them is hard to find. Some plans have "open enrollment," meaning that plans are not purchased by specified groups but that any individual can "buy in." Most of these dental plans available to individuals offer only limited services (such as examination, prophylaxis, radiographs, and treatment plan) and are probably more saleable to participating dentists because the risk assumed is low. In areas of the country where there is a real or perceived oversupply of dentists, some dentists find these limited capitation plans attractive because they provide the chance to recruit new fee-for-service patients. As mentioned earlier, "pure" capitation plans became an endangered species in the 1990s.

Again following the pattern established in medicine, insurers have embraced the idea of selectively directing patients to specific providers (the preferred providers in a PPO) who have agreed to provide care to the insured group on a fee-for-service basis, but at fees that are significantly lower than the usual fees for the area. The contracting dentists often agree to participate at the lower-than-usual fees to attract additional patients to their practice.

For some, the primary concern with capitation is that it might encourage undertreatment. Under "pure" capitation, the dentist receives the same payment whether or not treatment is provided, leading some to argue that this will encourage undertreatment and neglect. Others argue that this is a virtue of capitation, because the dentist is assured a predictable income and is thus able to make decisions about treatment without worrying about daily revenues if treatment need is low. Many think that that the fee-for-service system, in which dentists are paid only if they find treatment to provide, has a high potential for producing overtreatment. They see this risk as even greater in the current era of lower disease levels. PPOs may also encourage overtreatment because the agreed-on fees are discounted, thus providing an even greater incentive to provide more services. All of these concerns have led to increasing pressure on insurers to develop ways to monitor the quality and quantity of care. Purchasers and individual patients need to be assured that the care that they pay for is appropriate and of acceptable quality, regardless of the way for which it is paid.

Direct Reimbursement

Direct reimbursement is a form of payment for dental care that has existed informally for a long time. It continues to be promoted by the ADA as an alternative to the more common forms of dental insurance.[3] Direct reimbursement involves an agreement between an employer and its employees in which the employer agrees to reimburse the employees for some part of their expenses for dental care. The employee can go for care to any dentist he chooses. The patient is responsible for paying the dentist, and the dentist has no responsibility to the insurer for such things as scope of covered services or limits on frequency of services. All treatment decisions are between the patient and the dentist in a traditional two-party manner. After treatment has been provided and paid for, the patient takes the receipt to his employer and is reimbursed for his expenses according to the rules of the agreement. Reimbursement is usually on a percentage basis, and annual limits are customary.

The ADA promotes direct reimbursement because it keeps third parties out of the decisions on which services to provide, how frequently they can be provided, what the fee will be, or which dentists will provide them. It is also argued that direct reimbursement minimizes administrative costs.

Groups accustomed to the more conventional forms of third-party dental insurance have not readily embraced direct reimbursement because they have come to expect and value such things as direct payment from the insurer to the dentist, so that patients face fewer out-of-pocket expenses. Collectively, they expect the insurer to play an active role in ensuring that the type and quantity of services provided are reasonable, and that the quality of care is acceptable. Direct reimburse-

ment purposely attempts to keep third parties out of these areas, but for many purchasers the third-party involvement is an important part of what they expect from dental insurance. In any event, direct reimbursement has not become a major player in dental prepayment.

Administrative Services Only

In addition to conventional insurance coverage, where the insurer is "at risk" for the costs of care, insurers are increasingly providing for purchasers a service known as administrative services only (ASO). The distinguishing feature of an ASO contract is that the purchaser of the contract is at risk for the costs of care rather than the insurer. The purchaser pays a periodic fee that covers all of the normal administrative services associated with insurance, such as actuarial services, claims processing, preauthorization, post-treatment reviews, and processing of payments to providers. Virtually all of the types of payments to dentists that have been described, where the insurer is usually at risk, can be managed on an ASO basis. Whether the insurance company or the purchaser is at risk does not affect the way the plan appears to the patient or the dentist. ASO contracts are popular with large purchasers, because the purchasers do not have to hand over the large sums of money needed for payment to the insurance company up front. Instead, the purchasers retain control over the funds until the time payment is actually made. The earnings on large amounts of cash, even if held for relatively short periods of time, can be considerable, therefore effectively reducing the cost of the insurance to the purchaser. Although insurance companies handle much of the ASO business, companies called third-party administrators (TPAs) have arisen that do no insuring at all. TPAs handle only the administrative end of insurance, leaving responsibility for the funds to pay claims, and therefore the insurance risk, in the hands of the purchaser.

Medical Savings Accounts (MSAs)

The concept of the MSA is to allow a person to establish and add to a special savings account, protected from taxes, to be used as needed to cover medical expenses.[19] Any funds not needed for medical purposes could ultimately become part of a personal retirement fund. As usually envisioned, the MSA would cover most small and often discretionary medical expenses and would be used in combination with a high-deductible insurance policy that would cover the more expensive and infrequent expenses. The theory is that by making individual patients more aware of the actual cost of routine medical expenses, they will be more prudent users of care. The actual insurance would be reserved for those infrequent and high-cost needs that more ideally fit insurance principles. It is too early to say whether the MSA will be widely used or whether it will be effective in controlling the costs of care, but it is true that the development of the MSA concept in the 1990s is further evidence of the high level of interest in finding a way to control the costs of health care.

CONTROLLING THE COSTS OF THIRD-PARTY DENTAL CARE

Most mechanisms for controlling the costs of medical care also affect the way that dental care is provided and financed. In medicine, care provided under HMOs and PPOs is often referred to as managed care; both HMOs and PPOs provide substantial financial incentives to receive care from a participating provider (Chapter 7).

Many dental practices have a vital stake in the continued economic health of the third-party payment system because it represents a substantial share of their income. At the same time, purchasers of care are taking increasing notice of the growing cost to them of providing dental insurance.[7, 14, 31] The dental insurance companies are then on notice that they must keep the costs of the plans that they offer under control, which in turn affects dentists' incomes. A number of such mechanisms have been described and are in common use; others are continually under development. If cost controls are not routinely and successfully incorporated, individual dental plans will simply not succeed in the marketplace. The challenge is to find ways of keeping the costs of dental care within the range that purchasers are willing to pay, while at the same time providing a level of care that both dentists and patients find acceptable. Although dentists may have difficulty accepting the idea that not every patient should have all of the care that money can buy, purchasers of care for large groups are increasingly unwill-

ing or unable to pay the insurance premiums needed to support such extensive benefits.

The expression *cost control* to many dentists is synonymous with harassment, red tape, and poor quality of care. However, appropriate methods of cost control do not demand the use of inferior materials or techniques. Instead, cost control should be based on a concept of cost-effectiveness: how can a purchasing group best spend the available money in order to gain maximum dental health benefits for its members?

Third-party plans do not remove the cost barrier to dental care; they merely change its nature. The amount of care a plan can finance is still finite; the object of controls is to try to use the available financing to best advantage.[6] The more that dentists are able to accept this philosophy, the better they will be able to work with purchasers and administrators to devise mutually acceptable methods of cost control.

PUBLIC FINANCING OF HEALTH CARE

The federal government has been involved in the direct financing of health care almost from the time of its inception. Congress in 1798 established the Marine Hospital Fund, the forerunner of the US Public Health Service, to provide medical care for merchant seamen. The federal government gradually accepted responsibility for providing health care to other groups: the care received by military and Coast Guard personnel; American Indians, Alaska Natives, and inmates of federal penitentiaries is financed with federal funds and often provided at federal facilities. This limited and carefully-defined role of the federal government was seen for a long time as its right and proper function in health care provision.

The relation between the various levels of government in the United States was permanently changed in 1935 with the passage of the first Social Security Act. This act was passed in the midst of the great depression, when there were unprecedented problems caused by mass unemployment and widespread destitution. The Act created a system financed from compulsory employee-employer contributions to provide income maintenance for the elderly. The Old Age Insurance (OAI) provisions of the original Act of 1935 became extended to the Old Age and Survivors Insurance (OASI) in 1939, and then to the Old Age, Survivors, and the Disabled Insurance (OASDI) in 1960.[40] All provisions of the Social Security System until then were related to income security, rather than to the financing of health care. In addition, public welfare payments at that time were made directly to the recipients only. These payments were so low that most individuals could afford only limited emergency health care, and the choice was left to the recipient about whether to buy health care or something else. It is perhaps not surprising that recipients of public welfare tended to seek health care only when they perceived themselves or a member of their family to be seriously ill.

The Social Security Act of 1935 provided no funds expressly for the provision of health care. During the great depression, however, peoples' inability to purchase health care in the traditional way was recognized as a major social problem. The system of *grants-in-aid* was thus developed as a method of using federal finances for needed health care services without disturbing the traditional federal-state separation. Grants-in-aid were monies allocated to the states according to specified formulas. To receive these grants, the states had to expend their own funds for the same objectives as those supported by the grant-in-aid, often in the ratio of $1 from state or local sources to $2 from federal sources.[15] Grants-in-aid during this period were available only for support of specific categories of needy individuals, such as the blind, dependent children, permanently and totally disabled, and the aged.

A significant change in methods of federal financing for health care came with the passage of the Kerr-Mills bill in 1960. This legislation, supported by both the ADA and the American Medical Association, linked health care needs to the general welfare of the aged indigent by a program known as Medical Assistance to the Aged. Although the effects of this program were relatively disappointing,[40] the Kerr-Mills bill introduced the use of vendor payments, meaning payments directly to those who provided service rather than to the recipients of care. This procedure ensured that allocated funds could be used only for health care.

Growing public awareness in the early 1960s of the problems of poverty and ill health set the stage for the 1965 amendments to the Social Security Act. These amendments were in their own way as landmark a piece of legislation as the original Act 30 years earlier. Title XVIII, known as Medicare, provided for the receipt of health care services by all persons aged 65 and over, regardless of their ability to pay, and Title XIX, known as Medicaid, was intended to bring access to health care to the indigent and medically indigent segments of the population. The term *medically indigent* refers to those who are not dependent on public welfare to meet the basic necessities of life, but who do not have sufficient income to purchase health care through the usual private practice channels. (This concept of course is meaningless, as costly new developments in the diagnosis and treatment of previously untreatable diseases can make anyone but the super-rich medically indigent should they be unfortunate enough to get the wrong disease.)

In 1997, the Social Security Act was further amended through Title XXI, which created a State Children's Health Insurance Program. This program commits $47 billion in federal funds over a 10-year period to help states provide health insurance for the approximately 10 million American children estimated to be without such insurance.

Public Financing of Dental Care

By the mid 1990s, just under 4% of all dental expenditures were from public funds, compared with more than 45% of total health expenditures.[25] Figure 8–8 shows the proportionate expenditures between public and various types of private payments for different areas of health care in 1995. It can be seen that payment for dental care is just about evenly split between private insurance and out-of-pocket patient payments. Government, plus other sources such as charity, account for less than 5% of dental payments.

The proportion of total public expenditures on health care services in 1995 that went to dental care was also very small, less than 0.5%. More than half of all public expenditures for health care went toward hospital care; the other major areas of public expenditures were physicians' services, nursing home care, research, and the construction of health care facilities.[25]

North Carolina established the first state dental division in 1918, and many other state-level dental public health programs developed between 1935 and 1965. A great variety of dental care programs were instituted, financed, and administered by state and local

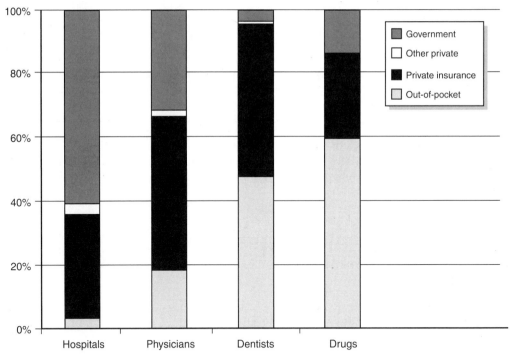

Figure 8–8. Proportionate expenditures on various categories of health services by type of payment, United States, 1995. (From Levit KR, Lazenby HC, Braden BR. National health expenditures. Health Care Financing Rev 1996;18:175–82.)

communities during this period, frequently with the help of federal monies through grants-in-aid. Many state-level dental public health programs, focusing on maternal and child health populations, got their start via such grants-in-aid through what was then the Children's Bureau. These programs vary highly from state to state. Although some are strong and active, in most states these programs are small and inadequately financed.

Medicare

Title XVIII of the Social Security amendments of 1965 is the program known as Medicare. As originally conceived, it removed financial barriers for hospital and physician services for persons age 65 and over, regardless of their financial means. Medicare also covers some people who are disabled, as well as people with permanent kidney failure. Expenditures on the Medicare program in the first few years of operation were considerably higher than estimated, and it was not long before some financial constraints were introduced. By the mid-1970s, Medicare had two parts: Part A, hospital insurance, and Part B, voluntary supplemental medical insurance.

Both parts contain a highly complex series of service benefits, and both parts also require some payment by the individual.

Medicare was brought into being because the voluntary health insurance system was unable to provide adequately for people over age 65. The health insurance industry primarily operates for profit, and the risk of adverse selection in those over 65 is high. In addition, because the income of persons aged 65 and older is usually considerably less than for those in the employed population, they have limited funds to spend on health care. Hence, there were twin problems of high health care needs and low income.

The uproar from the health professions that surrounded Medicare's birth in 1965 ("socialized medicine") subsided as the public realized that it filled a necessary gap in the financing of health care. Data from the website of the Health Care Financing Agency (HCFA) show that by 1996, more than 38 million Americans, 13.8% of the population, were enrolled in Medicare. Federal expenditures for the program were estimated to be approximately $194 billion in 1996, or $5100 per enrollee. The dental segment of Medicare is limited to those services requiring hospitalization for their treatment, usually surgical treatment for fractures and oral cancer, and hence constitutes a negligible part of the program.

Medicaid

Medicaid, Title XIX of the Social Security Amendments of 1965, differs from Medicare in several important ways. Whereas Medicare is funded wholly from federal funds, Medicaid costs are shared jointly by the federal and state governments. Data from the HCFA website show that in 1997 the federal government provided from 50% to 77% of the funds used by each state. Federal allocations are made according to a formula based on the ratio of the state's per capita income to the national per capita income.[50] The original intent of Medicaid was to provide funds to meet the health care needs of all indigent and medically indigent persons. Eligibility standards vary widely from state to state, as do the expenditures on authorized services. In 1995, for example, the average Medicaid expenditure per recipient nationally was approximately $3300, but in some states it was more than $7000 and in others less than $2000.[46]

Expenditures for the overall Medicaid program have shown a steady growth through the decades, as shown by Figure 8–9. Even after adjustment for inflation, the pattern shows a steady increase over time. Medicaid expenditures for dental care, however, follow a quite different pattern, as shown in Figure 8–10. Constant-dollar expenditures for dental care increased until about 1977, then declined through the 1980s, but have again shown an increase in the 1990s.[42, 43]

The pattern of a relative decline in dental expenditures within Medicaid is further substantiated by Figure 8–11, which shows that the proportion of the total Medicaid budget going to dental care has fallen steadily from nearly 3% from 1972 to 1977 to less than 1% in the late 1990s. Small as this fraction is, it still represents the bulk of public expenditures for dental care. This decline is made more severe by the rise in the number of recipients of dental services through this time from 2.4 million in 1972 to well over 6 million in 1995.[42, 43] The result is that the expenditure per dental recipient has fallen even more dramatically through the period, as shown in Figure 8–12. Expressed in constant 1967 dollars, payments dropped from nearly $57 per

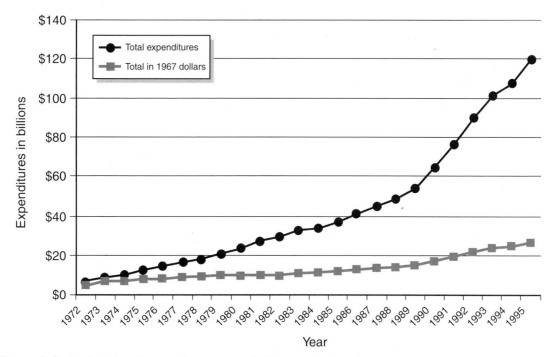

Figure 8–9. Total Medicaid expenditures, in actual dollars and adjusted to constant 1967 dollars, United States, 1972–1995. (From US Department of Health and Social Services. Social Security Administration. Social Security Bulletin annual statistical supplement, 1989. SSAB Publication No. 13-11700. Washington DC: Government Printing Office, 1989; US Department of Health and Human Services, Social Security Administration. Social Security Bulletin annual statistical supplement, 1996. SSA Publication No. 13-11700. Washington DC: Government Printing Office, 1996.)

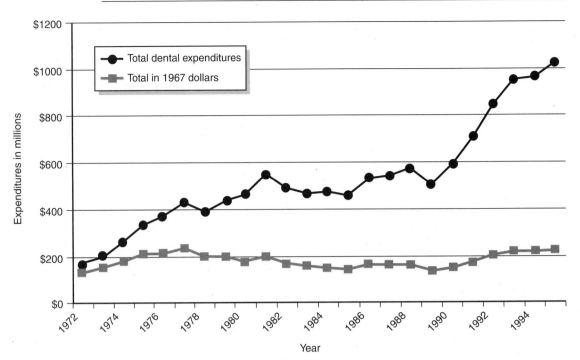

Figure 8–10. Medicaid expenditures for dental care in actual dollars, and adjusted to constant 1967 dollars. United States, 1972–1995. (From US Department of Health and Social Services. Social Security Administration. Social Security Bulletin annual statistical supplement, 1989. SSAB Publication No. 13-11700. Washington DC: Government Printing Office, 1989; US Department of Health and Human Services, Social Security Administration. Social Security Bulletin annual statistical supplement, 1996. SSA Publication No. 13-11700. Washington DC: Government Printing Office, 1996.)

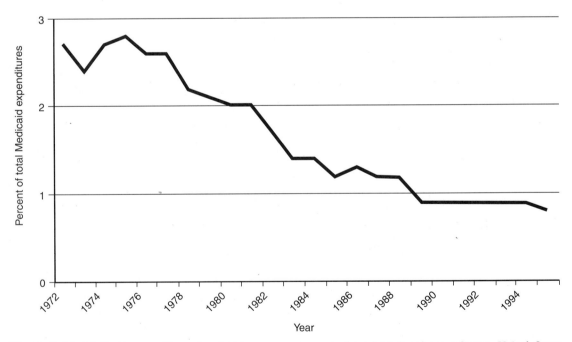

Figure 8–11. Medicaid expenditures for dental care as a percent of total Medicaid expenditures. United States, 1972–1995. (From Social Security Administration. Social Security Bulletin annual statistical supplement, 1989. SSAB Publication No. 13-11700. Washington DC: Government Printing Office, 1989; US Department of Health and Human Services, Social Security Administration. Social Security Bulletin annual statistical supplement, 1996. SSA Publication No. 13-11700. Washington DC: Government Printing Office, 1996.)

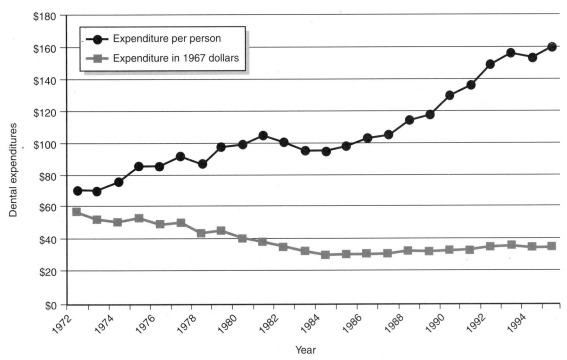

Figure 8–12. Medicaid expenditures for dental care per dental recipient, in actual dollars and adjusted to constant 1967 dollars, United States, 1972–1995. (From Social Security Administration. Social Security Bulletin annual statistical supplement, 1989. SSAB Publication No. 13-11700. Washington DC: Government Printing Office, 1989; US Department of Health and Human Services, Social Security Administration. Social Security Bulletin annual statistical supplement, 1996. SSA Publication No. 13-11700. Washington DC: Government Printing Office, 1996.)

recipient in 1972 to $35 in 1995. In the mid-1990s, only approximately 17% of Medicaid recipients received dental care under the program (Fig. 8–13).

To qualify for the federal government's share of Medicaid financing, every state Medicaid program is required to cover a set of basic services for everyone receiving federally supported financial assistance. In addition, amendments to the Medicaid program instituted in 1968 required that states offer early and periodic screening, diagnosis, and treatment (the so-called EPSDT program) to needy children through age 20. Medical, dental, vision, and hearing services are mandatory under the EPSDT program.

Unfortunately, the EPSDT program continues to be a long way from fulfilling its promise. Of slightly more than 21 million children under the age of 21 who were eligible for EPSDT services in 1993, just over 4 million (under 20%) received preventive dental services.[45] These numbers are consistent with 1995 Medicaid data, which show that among 39 million Medicaid-eligible individuals, 22 million of whom are under 21 years of age, just over 6 million received any dental

services.[43] Reasons for this situation include the initial slowness of the federal government in publishing regulations to govern program administration, and the unwillingness of some states to add to rapidly growing Medicaid costs.[28] As a result, few states actually offered the full set of services required by EPSDT, and for those actually offered, the level of payment was often so low that few dentists would accept Medicaid patients. Many children thus went without needed dental care.[41] Additional regulations in 1979 attempted to boost compliance by increasing the penalty for noncompliant states. This penalty initially was a reduction in the federal share of Aid to Families with Dependent Children (AFDC) payment to states.[27] In 1981, the pressure was increased by making adherence to the EPSDT provisions a condition for federal funding of Medicaid. As of 1990, however, despite the clear record of noncompliance by many states, no record of penalty was found by the US Congressional Office of Technology Assessment.[41]

Although Medicaid has reached a large number of people, there clearly are gaps. Despite the fact that nearly 40 million people in

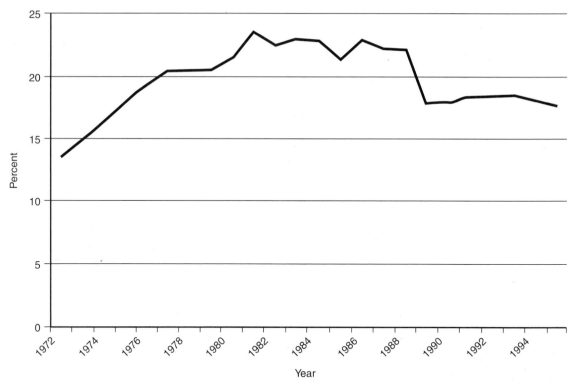

Figure 8–13. Dental Medicaid recipients as a percent of all Medicaid recipients, United States, 1972–1995. (From Social Security Administration. Social Security Bulletin annual statistical supplement, 1989. SSAB Publication No. 13-11700. Washington DC: Government Printing Office, 1989; US Department of Health and Human Services, Social Security Administration. Social Security Bulletin annual statistical supplement, 1996. SSA Publication No. 13-11700. Washington DC: Government Printing Office, 1996.)

the United States are without health insurance,[21] there have been and continue to be efforts to limit Medicaid expenditures.[8] The economic recessions of the 1970s and 1980s sharply increased the number of people eligible for Medicaid, and because this happened during periods of rapidly increasing medical care costs, the higher costs of the Medicaid program were seen as excessive by many states. As a result, some states cut back on eligibility, reducing the availability of services and the levels of payment to providers. Unfortunately, dental services are often included among the first of these cutbacks. Many dentists, frustrated by rapidly changing eligibility standards for prospective patients, reductions in available services, changes in percentile fees paid, and delays in payment for services rendered, have refused to treat new patients under Medicaid.[11, 24, 29, 51]

The future of Medicaid in the 1990s remains clouded. For one thing, the pressure to reduce government spending at both the federal and state levels is substantial. Medicaid is a prime target for reductions, partly because it does not have a vocal consistency. While the over-65 population is a powerful, articulate, and a growing force in support of Medicare, the Medicaid-eligible population is not. Although the federal government continues to push responsibility for Medicaid toward the states, the states already feel overburdened by Medicaid costs and are resisting. Whatever the outcome, the most likely losers are the Medicaid recipients, who are threatened with loss of access to health services provided by private practitioners.

The philosophy of shifting social welfare programs from the federal government to the states will cause continuing loss of needed services if funding is not also made available to already stretched state budgets. The development of block grants, in which previously categorical federal funds (evolved from the grant-in-aid days) are lumped together to be allocated to specified programs at a state's discretion, is causing difficulties for dentistry. The total sum of federal funds received by the state is reduced, and there are heavy political pressures to use the funds for health-related purposes other than dental care. The immediate future for traditional public health programs does not look optimistic, although philosophies may change if large numbers of people are unable to get the care they need. Dentistry clearly suffers from the lack of a vocal constituency in this arena.

Looking for positives, the nearly $1 billion paid by Medicaid for dental services in 1996, although undoubtedly far short of what was needed, has still allowed dentists to treat many patients who would otherwise not have received care. It should also be remembered that numerous public and philanthropic dental programs derive a substantial portion of their operating revenues by billing Medicaid for services that they provide to eligible individuals, and in this way Medicaid plays a part in sustaining and enlarging these programs. Nevertheless, it is troubling that virtually all state Medicaid programs are out of compliance with the requirements for Medicaid and EPSDT, that this noncompliance is well known by all involved parties,[41] and that no enforcement is carried out. A vocal dental constituency is needed to force action.

In an effort to help control the costs of both Medicare and Medicaid, there has been a major effort by government to encourage enrollment in managed care plans. Although there has been some success in moving beneficiaries to managed care, especially for Medicaid where there is in some states no other option, it is still too early to tell whether costs will actually be controlled in the long run and whether access and other quality measures will be satisfactory.

Children's Health Insurance Program

The Children's Health Insurance Program (CHIP), enacted in 1997 under Title XXI of the Social Security Act, is intended to encourage states to provide health coverage to the estimated 10 million uninsured children in the United States. Although this legislation does not mandate dental services, dental coverage is permitted, and it is expected that some states will include it. However, given the continuing difficulties with dental coverage under Medicaid, it seems unlikely that dental coverage under CHIP will be any more successful. The federal allocation for CHIP for 1998 was $4.275 billion, and the required state contributions equal $1.822 billion. Considering the estimate of 10 million eligible uninsured children, this total averages about $610 per eligible child. Even with additional funds from premiums that many states will choose to collect from eligible children, the funds available are likely to be well below the $1200 per child spent by Medicaid in the early 1990s.[44] These numbers indicate that the administrators of this new program will be severely challenged to provide comprehensive medical coverage to these children, and that in many states it will be decided that there are simply not enough funds to include dental benefits.

Other Programs of Public Financing for Dental Care

In addition to Medicaid and a small number of dental services under Medicare, a number of other smaller programs in the Department of Health and Human Services either directly or indirectly provide dental services for certain populations in the United States.

The Indian Health Service (IHS) is responsible for medical and dental care for American Indians and Alaska Natives who are members of federally-recognized tribes. The Dental Services Branch of the IHS is responsible for the direct care through its own clinics, and contract care through private dental offices for a large portion of this population. Dentists who are commissioned officers in the US Public Health Service are also assigned to provide dental care for US Coast Guard personnel and inmates in federal prisons.

As of 1996, there were approximately 1600 Community and Migrant Health Centers, which are joint state-federal projects designed to bring health care to people who live in rural and high-poverty urban areas. Many of these centers provide dental services and preventive education. A substantial part of the federal Maternal and Child Health Services block grants ("Title V" funds) are also used by individual states for dental care, and funds are available for dental care through Head Start for prekindergarten and kindergarten children from deprived backgrounds who are otherwise not eligible for Medicaid. Other programs with federal involvement that have a dental care component are Health Care Services for the Homeless and the Hemophilia Projects, which provide a wide range of services for hemophiliacs.

Rehabilitative care for children born with cleft lips and palates has long been financed cooperatively by state funds and federal grants-in-aid because it was recognized that just about everybody is "medically indigent" when it comes to treatment of cleft lip and palate. All states have some resources available for team treatment of this condition; dental personnel should be aware of resources available in or near their community.

Unfortunately, public financing for the dental care of people with other handicapping conditions, for example those with cerebral palsy, mental retardation, paraplegia, or quadriplegia, has never been as forthcoming. Although some states do have reasonable programs for the treatment of children with these conditions, few have any kind of financing available for their dental treatment when they become adults. The dental treatment of chronically ill and homebound adults has also been neglected almost completely, despite a successful demonstration program of providing dental care to the homebound.[48]

The Department of Veterans Affairs (formerly the Veterans Administration, or VA) program provides some dental care to eligible veterans through its more than 160 facilities nationwide. The VA dental program employed slightly more than 800 dentists in 1996. As previously noted, the various branches of the military also provide direct care for active duty personnel; and a voluntary dental insurance program, which requires the participants to pay part of the premium, is available for dependents of military personnel. Similar voluntary insurance programs are available for military retirees and members of the reserve forces (National Guard). For these latter programs, the entire premium is paid by the beneficiary. For all of these programs for other than active duty personnel, care is provided through private dental offices, with payment partially paid according to the insurance coverage.

National Health Insurance (NHI)

Although the idea of NHI in the United States is not new,[9] the fact that serious proposals for some form of it periodically resurface testifies to the persistence of the dual problems of (a) large numbers of people who have no insurance, and (b) the unrelenting increases in the costs of health care services.

However, if NHI is perceived as simply a financing mechanism without any restructuring of the care system, the rate of cost increases is not likely to diminish.[17, 23] Indeed, the rate of increase in direct expenditures would far exceed present levels. The characteristics of the system that have fueled the continuing rise in the proportion of GDP that goes to health care would be magnified by an additional large infusion of funds. The trade-offs required to balance need against costs will present challenges for which American society seems unprepared.[32] This realization, added to concerns about a balanced federal budget and strong opposition from medicine, dentistry, and private health care interests, is responsible for the hesitancy in enacting NHI.

Although proposals for universal and comprehensive publicly-financed health insurance have been consistently swept aside, the record clearly shows that government involvement in health care financing has been steadily increasing over the long term. Especially since 1965, when the federal government got involved in the direct payment for care in a big way with Medicare and Medicaid, we have seen slow expansion of groups covered. Given the relative success and popularity of Medicare, which covers essentially all the over-65 population, and the expansion of the Social Security Act (Title XXI) in 1997 to include many uninsured children, there is the possibility of some level of government-assured health care coverage for all but the working-aged population. There remain the dual concerns whether on the one hand the funding for these programs is adequate, especially with Medicaid and the Children's Health Insurance Initiative, and on the other hand whether taxpayers are willing to support what look to be ever-growing programs. Further, coverage for dental services continues to be a small part, at best, of these government health programs. For the foreseeable future, most Americans who receive regular dental care will continue to pay for it with private insurance or their own funds. Those unable to pay will continue to be far less likely to receive regular care.

REFERENCES

1. American Dental Association, Council on Dental Care Programs. Policies on dental care programs. Chicago: ADA, 1977.
2. American Dental Association, Council on Dental Benefit Programs. Current dental terminology CDT-2. 2nd ed. 1995–2000 Chicago: ADA, 1994.
3. American Dental Association, Council on Dental Care Programs. Policies on dental care programs. Chicago: ADA, 1991.

4. American Dental Association, House of Delegates. Resolution 9-1966-H. Trans Am Dent Assoc 1966;107:311.

5. American Dental Association, House of Delegates. Resolution 30-1968-H. Trans Am Dent Assoc 1968;109:305–6.

6. Bailit HL. Is overutilization the major reason for increasing dental expenditures? Reflections on a complex issue. J Dent Pract Admin 1988;5(3):112–5.

7. Bailit HL, Bailit JL. Corporate control of health care: impact on medicine and dentistry. J Dent Educ 1988;52:108–13.

8. Chang D, Holahan J. Medicaid spending in the 1980s; the access-cost containment trade-off revisited. Urban Institute Report 90-2. Washington DC: Urban Institute Press, 1990.

9. Chapman CB, Talmadge JM. The evolution of the right to health concept in the United States. Pharos 1971;34:30–51.

10. Cooper BS, Worthington NL. National health expenditures, 1929–72. Soc Secur Bull 1973;36(1):3–19,40.

11. Damiano PC, Brown ER, Johnson JD, Scheetz JP. Factors affecting dentist participation in a state Medicaid program. J Dent Educ 1990;54:638–43.

12. Faulkner EJ. The role of health insurance. In: Gregg DW, ed: Life and health insurance handbook. Homewood IL: Irwin, 1959:523–32.

13. Fuchs VR. The health sector's share of the gross national product. Science 1990;247:534–8.

14. Garrison J. Purchasers and payers: Who's driving the market? J Dent Educ 1996;60:356–9.

15. Gerrie NF. Grants-in-aid in federal-state dental public health program relationships. J Am Dent Assoc 1957;54:182–8.

16. Gibson RM, Fisher CR. National health expenditures, fiscal year 1977. Soc Secur Bull 1978;41(7):3–20.

17. Gleicher N. Expansion of health care to the uninsured and underinsured has to be cost-neutral. J Am Med Assoc 1991;265:2388–90.

18. Goetz J. The plan name and symbol. J Am Dent Assoc 1969;78:706–9.

19. Goodman JC, Musgrave GL. Patient power: Solving America's health care crisis. Washington DC: Cato Institute, 1992.

20. Hadley J, Steinberg EP, Feder J. Comparison of uninsured and privately insured hospital patients. Condition on admission, resource use, and outcome. JAMA 1991;265:374–9.

21. Health Insurance Association of America. Source book of health insurance data, 1990. Washington DC: HIAA, 1990.

22. Health Insurance Institute. Source book of health insurance data, 1977–78. Washington DC: HII, 1978.

23. Jonas S. National health insurance. In: Jonas S, ed. Health care delivery in the United States. 1st ed. New York: Springer, 1977:434–66.

24. Lang WP, Weintraub JA. Comparison of Medicaid and non-Medicaid dental providers. J Public Health Dent 1986;46:207–11.

25. Levit KR, Lazenby HC, Braden BR, et al. National health expenditures, 1995. Health Care Financing Rev 1996;18(1):175–202.

26. Manning WG, Bailit HL, Benjamin B, Newhouse JP. The demand for dental care: Evidence from a randomized clinical trial in health insurance. J Am Dent Assoc 1985;110:895–902.

27. Medicaid requirements for state programs of early and periodic screening, diagnosis, and treatment of individuals under 21. Fed Register 1974 May 18;44:29420–7.

28. Murray JB. Whatever happened to EPSDT? J Am Dent Assoc 1975;90:545–8.

29. Nainar SM, Tinanoff N. Effect of Medicaid reimbursement rates on children's access to dental care. Pediatr Dent 1997;19:315–6.

30. Oberg CN, Lia-Hoaberg B, Hodkinson E, et al. Prenatal care comparisons among privately insured, uninsured, and Medicaid-enrolled women. Public Health Rep 1990;105:533–5.

31. Olsen ED. Dental insurance: A successful model facing new challenges. J Dent Educ 1984;48:591–6.

32. Russell LB. Some of the tough decisions required by a national health plan. Science 1989;246:892–6.

33. Schoen MH. Group practice owned by a partnership using some salaried dentists and contracting directly with purchasers of group dental care. J Am Dent Assoc 1961;62:392–8.

34. Schoen MH. Group practice and poor communities: dental care. Am J Public Health 1970;60:1125–32.

35. Schoen MH. Methodology of capitation payment to group dental practice and effects of such payment on care. Health Serv Rep 1974;89:16–24.

36. Smith DG, Harlan LC, Hawthorne VM. The charges for ESRD treatment of diabetics. J Clin Epidemiol 1989;42:111–8.

37. Smith QE, Mitchell GE, Lucas, GA. An experiment in dental prepayment: The Naismith Dental Plan. PHS Publication No 970. Washington DC: Government Printing Office, 1962.

38. Smith QE, Pennell EH. Service requirements in dental prepayment: Predictability and adverse reaction. Public Health Rep 1961;76:11–8.

39. Smith QE, Pennell EH, Bothwell RD, Gailbreath MN. Dental care in a group purchase plan: A survey of attitudes and utilization at the St. Louis Labor Health Institute. PHS Publication No 684. Washington DC: Government Printing Office, 1959.

40. Stevens R, Stevens R. Medicaid: Anatomy of a dilemma. Law and Contemporary Problems 1970; 35:348–425.

41. US Congress, Office of Technology Assessment. Children's dental services under the Medicaid program: background paper. OTA Publication No OTA-BP-H-78. Washington DC: Government Printing Office, 1990.

42. US Department of Health and Human Services, Social Security Administration. Social Security Bulletin, annual statistical supplement, 1989. SSA Publication No 13-11700. Washington DC: Government Printing Office, 1989.

43. US Department of Health and Human Services, Social Security Administration. Social Security Bulletin, annual statistical supplement, 1996. SSA Publication No 13-11700. Washington DC: Government Printing Office, 1996.

44. US Department of Health and Human Services, Health Care Financing Administration. Medicaid: An overview. HCFA Pub No 10965. Baltimore, MD, 1995.

45. US Department of Health and Human Services. Office of Inspector General. Children's dental services under Medicaid. Access and utilization. Pub No OEI-09-93-00240. Washington DC: Government Printing Office, 1996.

46. US Department of Health and Human Services, Social Security Administration. Health Care Financing Review. Medicare and Medicaid Statistical Supplement, 1996. Publication No 03386. Baltimore MD: Health Care Financing Administration, October 1996.

47. US Public Health Service. The dental service corpora-

tion; a new approach to dental care. PHS Publication No 570. Washington DC: Government Printing Office, 1961.

48. US Public Health Service, Division of Dental Public Health and Resources. Dental care for the chronically ill and aged; a community experiment. Washington DC: Government Printing Office, 1961.

49. US Public Health Service, Division of Dental Resources. A dental society reports on budget payment. Washington DC: Government Printing Office, 1960.

50. US Public Health Service, Health Care Financing Administration. Medicare and Medicaid data book, 1988. HCFA Publication No 03270. Washington DC: Government Printing Office, 1989.

51. Venezie RD, Vann WF Jr. Pediatric dentists' participation in the North Carolina Medicaid program. Pediatr Dent 1993;15:175–81.

52. Weissman J, Epstein AM. Case mix and resource utilization by uninsured hospital patients in the Boston metropolitan area. JAMA 1989;261:3572–6.

9

Dental Personnel

Types of Dental Personnel ◆ The Supply of Dentists in the United States ◆ Dental Specialists ◆ Distribution of Dentists ◆ Effect of Dental Education on the Supply of Dentists ◆ State Practice Acts and Dentist Distribution ◆ Shortage or Surplus? ◆ Estimating the Number of Dentists Required ◆ Dental Auxiliaries in the United States ◆ Dental Hygienists ◆ Independent Contractual Practice of Dental Hygiene ◆ Independent Practice ◆ Dental Assistants ◆ Expanded Function Dental Auxiliaries (EFDAs) ◆ The ADA and EFDAs ◆ Dental Laboratory Technicians ◆ Denturists ◆ Legislative Influences on Dentist Supply and Distribution ◆ National Health Service Corps ◆ Subsidies to Dental Schools and Dental Students

The vision of the dental team is one of various people in dentistry with different roles, functions, and periods of training, all working together to treat patients. Although it has been promoted for years by the World Health Organization,[113] the dental team remains a concept rather than a precise term. In the United States, the dental profession has long recognized that several different categories of personnel are fundamental to the efficient provision of care. Virtually all dentists employ at least one nondentist staff person; more than 90% of general practitioners employ at least one full- or part-time chairside assistant, and more than 70% employ at least one full- or part-time hygienist.[20]

This chapter defines the various types of personnel involved in the provision of dental services and assesses the factors that influence their supply and distribution.

TYPES OF DENTAL PERSONNEL

A *dentist* is a person who is permitted to practice dentistry under the laws of the relevant state, province, territory, or nation. These laws are intended to ensure that a prospective dentist has satisfied certain requirements such as (a) completion of a specified period of professional education in an approved institution, (b) demonstration of competence, and (c) evidence of satisfactory personal qualities. Dentists are concerned with the prevention and control of the diseases of the oral cavity and the treatment of unfavorable conditions resulting from these diseases, from trauma, or from inherent malformations. They are legally entitled to diagnose and treat patients independently, to prescribe certain drugs, and to employ and supervise auxiliary personnel. The mechanisms for fulfilling these requirements differ among nations. In the United States and Canada, for example, professional education is separate from the additional testing required for licensure. In many other countries, these two functions are combined under the authority of the educational institutions.

Dental auxiliary is a generic term for all persons who assist the dentist in treating patients. It includes the categories of dental hygienist, dental assistant, hygienist or assistant with expanded functions, dental laboratory technician, receptionist, and secretary. Auxiliaries can be classified as operating and nonoperating,[114] depending on whether they carry out any intraoral procedures in the direct treatment of patients.

With rare exceptions, auxiliaries of all types operate under varying degrees of supervision by dentists. Even those auxiliaries who appear to operate more-or-less independently, such as the school dental nurse of New Zealand (Chapter 7), work under some degree of supervision. Defining the extent of supervision required for various types of dental auxiliary can be confusing, because bodies concerned with supervision continue to modify their stance and definitions. As of 1996, the American Dental Association (ADA) acknowledged four levels of supervision of auxiliary personnel as shown in Table 9–1.

The ADA policy statement on this issue states: "General supervision is not acceptable to the American Dental Association because it fails to protect the health of the public.[17]" This issue is important for public health programs, because without general supervision, it is far more expensive for dental hygienists to provide care in schools, nursing homes,

Table 9–1. LEVELS OF SUPERVISION OF AUXILIARY PERSONNEL AS DEFINED BY THE AMERICAN DENTAL ASSOCIATION IN 1998

- **Personal supervision:** The dentist is personally operating on a patient and authorizes the auxiliary to aid treatment by concurrently performing supportive procedures.
- **Direct supervision:** The dentist is in the dental office or treatment facility, personally diagnoses the condition to be treated, personally authorizes the procedure and remains in the dental office or treatment facility while procedures are being performed by the auxiliary and, before dismissal of the patient, evaluates the performance of the dental auxiliary.
- **Indirect supervision:** The dentist is in the dental office or treatment facility, has personally diagnosed the condition to be treated, authorizes the procedures and remains in the dental office or treatment facility while the procedures are being performed by the auxiliary, and will evaluate the performance of the dental auxiliary.
- **General supervision:** The dentist is not required to be in the dental office or treatment facility when the procedures are provided, but has personally diagnosed the condition to be treated, has personally authorized the procedures, and will evaluate the performance of the dental auxiliary.

Exerpted from American Dental Association, House of Delegates. Comprehensive Policy Statement on Dental Auxiliary Personnel. Copyright 1998 American Dental Association. Reproduced by permission.

and other institutional settings. Where general supervision is permitted, dentists in private practice can allow a hygienist to provide recall prophylaxis while the dentist is away from the office.

These policies of the ADA have no direct control on the practice of dentistry because the regulation of dental practice in the United States is determined by state boards, not by the professional organization. Each state has its own definition of supervision requirements and scope of practice, and there is considerable diversity among them. The ADA has some influence, but no direct control. The moves by the ADA to restrict the scope of auxiliaries' practice are occurring as dental hygienists are working for a greater degree of autonomy, so conflicts are to be expected.

A *dental hygienist* is an operating auxiliary licensed to practice dental hygiene under the laws of the appropriate state, province, territory, or nation. In nearly all jurisdictions, in order to be licensed, hygienists, like dentists, must satisfy certain qualifications such as (a) completion of an approved period of education in an approved institution (only Alabama permits on-the-job training of hygienists[85]), (b) demonstration of competence, and (c) demonstration of satisfactory personal qualities. Hygienists are recognized auxiliaries in a number of countries in which their duties and deployment are essentially similar.[62]

Dental hygienists have traditionally been concerned with prophylaxis (or "cleaning" teeth), the health of the supporting structures of the teeth, and prevention of further diseases by direct clinical procedures and by the education of individual patients and groups. In most places, hygienists work under the supervision of dentists, either in private dental practice or in institutional settings such as health departments, nursing homes, or school dental programs.

The *expanded-function dental auxiliary* (EFDA), or expanded-duty dental auxiliary (EDDA), is a more recent development in operating auxiliaries in the United States and Canada. An EFDA is usually a dental assistant, or a dental hygienist in some cases, who has received further training in duties related to the direct treatment of patients, though still working under the direct supervision of a dentist. Not all states in the United States recognize EFDAs, and the duties permitted by those that do vary considerably.

A *dental assistant* is a nonoperating auxiliary who assists the dentist or dental hygienist in treating patients but who is not legally permitted to treat patients independently. Traditionally, their duties include immediate chairside assistance in the handling of dental equipment and materials used by the dentist or dental hygienist in treating patients.

Voluntary certification programs for dental assistants exist in many countries. *Certification* is the process by which a nongovernmental agency or association grants recognition to an individual who has met certain predetermined qualifications specified by that agency or association.[91] A dental assistant is not required, however, to be legally certified, registered, or to have completed any particular duration or amount of education. The vast majority of the world's dental assistants are trained on-the-job. However, to provide certain services, such as the exposure of radiographs, a growing number of American states require either some form of formal education or certification.

The *dental laboratory technician* is a nonoperating auxiliary who fulfills the prescriptions provided by dentists regarding the extraoral construction and repair of oral appliances. *Denturist* is a term applied to those dental laboratory technicians who are permitted in some American states, some provinces of Canada, and some other countries to fabricate dentures directly for patients without a dentist's prescription. These denturists must be licensed. Illegal denturists are also known to operate in other jurisdictions; the term has strong political overtones in jurisdictions where denturists have not achieved legal recognition.

Dental nurse and *dental therapist* are more-or-less synonymous terms that describe an operating auxiliary, who in some countries is legally permitted to treat special population groups, usually children, with little direct supervision from a dentist. The extent of their duties varies from one system to another, as does the degree of supervision required; but all dental nurses and therapists require specific training, licensure, and registration. Preventive dental nurses/therapists are trained in some countries to provide preventive services only, usually in a school dental service. Because their period of training is shorter than the training for dentists and their duties limited, these auxiliaries can provide preventive services to specified groups at lower cost than can dentists or hygienists.

THE SUPPLY OF DENTISTS IN THE UNITED STATES

Table 9–2 shows the dentist:population ratios in several countries to give a perspec-

Table 9–2. NUMBER OF DENTISTS PER 100,000 POPULATION FOR 15 COUNTRIES AT VARIOUS STAGES OF ECONOMIC DEVELOPMENT

COUNTRY	DENTISTS PER 100,000 POPULATION
Norway	119
Finland	91
Denmark	89
Argentina	69
France	67
Sweden	61
United States	59
Canada	54
Switzerland	48
Ecuador	46
Chile	40
Turkey	18
Thailand	3
India	1
Kenya	1

Note: Rounded to the nearest whole number.
From World Health Organization. World health statistics annual. Geneva: WHO, 1994; US Department of Health and Human Services, Public Health Service, Health Resources and Services Administration. Factbook—Health personnel United States. Washington DC: Government Printing Office, 1997.

tive on the relative availability of dentists in the United States. The range is wide, especially between developed and developing countries, and even within the more economically developed countries the range is considerable. The numbers are given as the number of dentists per 100,000 population. Another common way of presenting the same data is as population:dentist ratios; the 59 dentists per 100,000 people in the United States is equivalent to 1695 persons per dentist.

Producing counts of dentists and other dental personnel is not as straightforward as it might at first appear. Membership lists from professional associations and licensing lists are the most common source of counts, but these are seldom completely accurate. For example, some dentists maintain association membership even when they are retired or otherwise not actively engaged in professional practice; others are not members of a professional association. Dentists can hold a license in more than one jurisdiction, leading to overcounting. As a result, it is well to realize that virtually all enumerations of dental personnel are estimates, and that in an attempt to be more precise, the counts will often be qualified as all dentists, active dentists (those actually engaged in some activity related to dentistry), or practicing dentists (which often excludes dentists in full-time teaching, research, or administration). Numbers obtained from different sources therefore can differ because they are based on different subgroups. This nomenclature is by no means standard and is often not clearly defined in source documents. Usually the differences are not of great consequence, as in the comparison across countries in Table 9–2, but when making interpretations within countries, and in small geographic areas, the differences can be important. For example, in a community where there is a dental school or a government agency that employs a number of dentists in nonclinical positions, a count of all dentists for that community could greatly overestimate the availability of dental care.

As of the mid-1990s, it was estimated that the number of active dentists in the United States was between 153,000 and 160,000.[4, 106] Approximately 5000 of these dentists were in the armed forces and other federal agencies, and according to the ADA, 141,396 of these dentists were in private practice in 1995.[22] These figures represents at least a 60% increase in the absolute number of dentists since 1970.

From 1920 until the early 1980s, 1%–3% of dentists were women,[75, 94] but since the early 1980s this percentage has increased. In 1995, approximately 11% of dentists were women.[22] In 1969–1970, women constituted only 1.3% of first-year enrollment in dental schools,[52] but by 1980–1981 the first-year class was 19.8% female.[53] By the mid-1990s it was approaching 40%.[4]

Not all observers agree on the implications of the growing proportion of female dentists.[11, 65, 71, 75, 93, 95, 108, 109] Although it is too early to be sure about trends, there are indications that women dentists are more likely to practice part-time and to interrupt their practice for an extended period of time, thus spending fewer actual hours in practice during a career. Any differences between men and women in retirement patterns will also affect productivity, and it will be several decades yet before these can be observed. Further, it is likely that the practice patterns followed by those women in decades past, when women in the profession were rare, may be of little help in predicting the future practice patterns of the women now becoming dentists. Although any substantial shift in the average productivity of dentists would affect

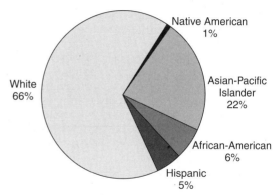

Figure 9–1. Dental school enrollment in the United States by race/ethnicity, 1996–97. (From American Dental Association. Survey Center. 1996/97 survey of predoctoral dental educational institutions. Academic programs, enrollment, and graduates, Vol 1. Chicago: ADA, 1997.)

the adequacy of the dentist supply, it is at present not clear how the increasing proportion of female dentists is affecting productivity.

In addition to the increasing numbers of women, dentistry is becoming more ethnically diverse. Although approximately 90% of dentists in practice as of 1995 reported themselves to be white non-Hispanic,[22] the picture for dental students indicates a decided shift. Dental school enrollments for the 1996–1997 academic year are shown in Figure 9–1; one third of students are members of minority groups.[21]

Foreign-trained dentists, in contrast to foreign medical graduates, have never been present in large numbers in the United States. Graduation from an accredited US or Canadian dental school is a prerequisite for licensure in most states. Information from the ADA website shows that about half of US dental schools have programs to which foreign-trained dentists can be admitted with advanced standing.

Dental Specialists

The early development of dental specialists was informal and did not require certification.[58] Varying patterns of formal training and certification developed as each specialty grew and matured relatively independently. Examining boards that certified specialty competence came into being, as well as specialty societies, such as the American Academy of Pedodontics (now Pediatric Dentistry) and the American Association of Orthodontists, that maintained educational and experiential qualifications for membership. In addition, some states established specialty licensure following examination by the state board of dental examiners.

Under guidelines originally set by the ADA House of Delegates and the Council on Dental Education, and now maintained by the Commission on Dental Accreditation, examining boards have been established in 8 areas of specialty practice: dental public health, endodontics, oral pathology, oral and maxillofacial surgery, orthodontics, pediatric dentistry, periodontics, and prosthetics. Minimum criteria for those entering a specialty are full-time limitation of practice, plus either the completion of at least 2 years of approved advanced study or specialty licensure by a state board. Certification as a diplomate by one of the specialty boards is not a prerequisite for limitation of practice. The stated purpose of specialty boards is to provide leadership in elevating standards for the practice of the specialty and, through examination and certification, to recognize those individuals who have demonstrated unusual competence. Numerous additional dental specialty groups are not officially recognized by the ADA, and the ADA actively discourages the announcement of practice limited to any area other than one of the 8 recognized specialties.

Unlike the situation in medicine, in which more than 60% of practitioners by 1990 were practicing in a specialty outside of primary care, more than 80% of dentists are general practitioners.[22, 105] Since the early 1970s, the number of first-year positions in specialty training programs has remained stable at approximately 1200. More than 50% of all specialists are orthodontists or oral surgeons, the 2 longest-established specialties.

There has been strong sentiment in dentistry for some time that a further increase in the number of specialists would not benefit either the profession or the public.[57] This view was based on the contention that one of the chronic problems in the American health care system is fragmentation, the dispersal of many medical specialists and the frequent absence of coordination among them. The growth of General Practice Residency (GPR) and Advanced Education in General Dentistry (AEGD) programs is a reflection of this emphasis on the general practice of dentistry. As of 1996 there were 883 first-year GPR and 406 first-year AEGD positions.[4]

Distribution of Dentists

In 1995 there were approximately 59 active dentists per 100,000 people in the United

Table 9–3. THE FIVE STATES WITH THE HIGHEST NUMBER OF DENTISTS, AND THE FIVE STATES WITH THE LOWEST NUMBER OF DENTISTS PER 100,000 POPULATION, UNITED STATES, 1994

STATE	DENTISTS PER 100,000 POPULATION
New York	82.7
Hawaii	81.0
Massachusetts	80.9
New Jersey	80.1
Connecticut	79.5
North Carolina	41.7
New Mexico	41.4
Arkansas	40.9
Nevada	39.7
Mississippi	37.7

From US Department of Health and Human Services, Public Health Service, Health Resources and Services Administration. Factbook—Health personnel United States. Washington DC: Government Printing Office, 1997.

States.[106] These dentists, however, were not, evenly distributed throughout the country, as seen in Chapter 7 (Fig. 7–1). This situation is not unique to dentistry as a health profession nor to the United States, for it is found wherever there is relatively free choice of practice location. Table 9–3 provides data for the 5 most favorable and 5 least favorable states in terms of availability of dentists in 1994. The figures range from 82.7 dentists per 100,000 people in New York to 37.7 per 100,000 in Mississippi.[106]

There are a number of reasons for this uneven distribution of dentists. The first and most fundamental is the relative freedom a dentist has in choosing a practice location. Dentists make this choice much as other people do, that is, for personal preference: attachment to a home town, good schools, or convenience to social, cultural, or recreational facilities.[9] Second, the location of dental schools also influences distribution, and the 55 American dental schools are located in only 32 states (plus the District of Columbia and Puerto Rico). Most dental schools are in state universities, where tuition for state residents usually is less than for out-of-state residents. A third reason is market response, meaning that the availability of dentists reflects demand for services. Areas of high income and education where demand for services is highest, such as affluent suburbs, have more dentists than do poorer areas.

Effect of Dental Education on the Supply of Dentists

Dentists were first enumerated separately in the 1850 Census. It listed 2900 dentists serving a population of 23 million,[96] or 12.6 dentists per 100,000 population. With the growth of dental schools during the latter part of the 19th century, the supply of dentists in 1900 increased to 39 dentists per 100,000 population. By 1930, there were 57.7 dentists per 100,000 population.[100] This steady increase was caused principally by changes in dental education. Although many dentists in the second half of the 19th century were still being trained under an apprenticeship system, proprietary dental schools grew rapidly as a response to demand (see Chapter 1). The number of dental graduates continued to grow until the closing of the last proprietary school in 1929.[70]

In the United States, the federal government has no direct jurisdiction over education, and there are considerable differences among states in the priority given to education. This is notably different from most other countries, where the national government directly determines how many practitioners, and of what type, will be produced. For these and related reasons, accreditation evolved as a voluntary, self-regulatory means of establishing and maintaining nationally acceptable standards of educational quality.[87] *Accreditation* is the process by which an agency or organization evaluates and recognizes a program of study or an institution as meeting certain predetermined qualifications or standards.[88, 89] The Commission on Dental Accreditation of the ADA currently serves as the accrediting body for dental and auxiliary training schools and graduate programs in dentistry. The Commission is a broad-based agency of the ADA; its membership includes auxiliaries, public members, and students in addition to dentists.

Enrollment in dental schools is obviously a prime influence on the future supply of dentists. During the 1960s and early 1970s, there was a widely held perception that there was a need for more dentists, and that a critical shortage was inevitable if strong actions were not taken. Although the federal government in the United States has no direct control over dental education, it can provide incentives to increase supply. During the 1960s and 1970s, incentives were offered to dental schools to build new facilities and to increase the number of graduates at existing dental schools. The results were impressive, as shown in Figure 9–2. The increased applications and enrollments through the 1970s also coincided with the time that the "baby boom" generation was deciding on careers. Applications to dental schools reached all-time highs during this period; the number of applicants per first-year position was 2.7:1 in 1974 and 1975. Applications began to decline in 1976; first-year enrollments began to decline in 1979. The federal incentives to dental education were reduced during this period, and the demographic bulge passed beyond college age.

The low point in applications and enrollments in the late 1980s coincided with a slow period in the US economy, and again with a public perception that there was an oversupply of dentists. During this period, dental schools made a remarkable adjustment in their capacity. Through a combination of closing of 6 dental schools and the reduction of class size in most others, the first-year capacity declined from its peak of 6301 in 1978 to approximately 4000 by 1990. Since 1990, applications have again grown steadily, although dental schools have been cautious about increasing their enrollments.

By the late 1990s, evidence suggested that the economic prospects for dentists, relative to physicians, were quite favorable. A 1994 report, analyzing the return on educational investment among several professions, projected that dentistry would provide a higher rate of return than primary care medicine and a virtually identical return to specialty medicine.[111] A more recent report suggests, perhaps because of the pressures on physicians from managed care, that in some parts of the country dentists average higher incomes than primary care physicians.[26] These favorable reports of dentists' economic prospects may have been a factor in the growing numbers of applicants to dental schools from the mid-1990s.

Fluctuations in dental school enrollments take considerable time to show their effect on the supply of dentists, and overall supply also is affected by other factors. First, with approximately 150,000 dentists in practice in the United States, a change of a few hundred graduates in any one year does not make a large difference overall. Further, a major fac-

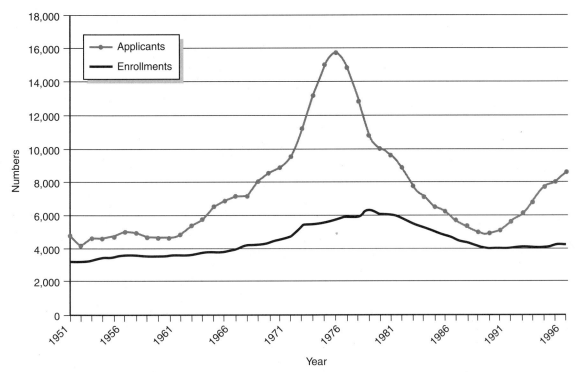

Figure 9–2. Applicants and first-year enrollees to dental schools in the United States, 1951–1996. (From American Association of Dental Schools. Deans' briefing book: Academic year 1988–89. Washington DC: AADS, 1989; American Dental Association, Survey Center. 1996/97 survey of predoctoral dental educational institutions. Academic programs, enrollment, and graduates. Vol 1. Chicago: ADA, 1997.)

tor on the overall numbers is the number of dentists retiring in any one year, which is itself a function of how many dentists graduated 40 or more years earlier. Choice of retirement age is highly variable. If demand for care is strong, a dentist may wait longer to retire than when there is an ample supply of younger dentists to take over. Finally, the population growth of the country is an additional variable. As the population grows faster, more and more dentists will be required to keep the supply constant.

The combination of these factors has resulted in a gradual increase of the supply of dentists in the United States between 1970 and the mid-1990s, from 47 to 60 dentists per 100,000 population.[106] Much of this general increase in the relative number of dentists is the result of the large number of graduates through the 1970s and most of the 1980s. Virtually all projections at the end of the century suggest, however, that the relative supply of dentists is at its peak and is likely to decline for the next several decades. This projected decline will be the product of lower enrollment levels than in earlier decades, combined with continuing population growth and pro-

jected retirement levels of dentists. It is anticipated that the relative supply of dentists will decline especially sharply between 2010 and 2020, when many of the large cohort of dentists who graduated in the 1970s and 1980s are expected to retire. By 2020, it is expected that there will be about 55 dentists per 100,000 population, back to levels of the early 1980s.

State Practice Acts and Dentist Distribution

The requirement to hold a state license to practice inhibits the movement of dentists (and also licensed auxiliaries) from one state to another.[38, 64, 70] In addition, it has been suggested that certain states adopted deliberately restrictive policies in their licensing examinations in an effort to prevent what they saw as too many dentists, or dentists "of the wrong kind," from practicing in the state.[38, 45, 64, 70] Results of state board examinations show a wide disparity among states in the proportion of applicants who fail.[6, 38, 54] Dentists in specialty practice also report difficulty in moving to states that do not have specialty licenses. In these instances, a specialist who may not have practiced general dentistry for many years is often required to take a clinical examination based on restorative procedures.

The ADA supports licensure by credentials to alleviate some of these problems. Under this concept, dentists who pass a licensing examination in a state present their credentials to another state to which they want to move; if the credentials meet the criteria the board grants a license. The actual process and requirements vary widely, but generally include requirements for some minimum time in practice and no evidence of existing or pending disciplinary or legal actions. The ADA website shows that in 1997, 32 states plus the District of Columbia allowed some form of licensure by credentials. Encompassed within this concept is reciprocity, by which two or more states agree to honor each others' licenses.

Views differ on the value of licensure by credentials. Some say that the existence of individual state practice acts, and what is seen as parochial jealousies in their administration, is a major cause of maldistribution and that the problem would be greatly alleviated by licensure by credentials. Others argue that licensure by credentials could make maldistribution worse, as large numbers of dentists would then move to desirable locations.

Movement between states has been made somewhat easier, at least for the young dentist, by the development of regional examining boards. There are four regional boards (Northeast, Southern, Central, and Western), and a dentist passing the clinical licensing examination in any participating state can apply, usually within 5 years of the original examination, for license in any state in the same region without having to take another clinical examination. By 1997, 40 states and the District of Columbia were involved in one or more of these four regional examining boards.

Whenever licensure and the assessment of dentists' competence are mentioned, the topic of mandatory continuing education as a requirement for license renewal also arises. If the competence of a dentist who moves from one state to another has to be tested, why should there not also be concern for those who stay in one place for many years? Although there is no clear evidence that mandatory continuing dental education (CDE) improves dentists' competence, by the mid-1990s most states had some form of periodic educational requirement for license renewal,

and the trend suggests that more states are likely to follow.[69] There is a similar trend toward mandatory CDE for renewal of a license to practice dental hygiene.[85] As is the case with other regulatory matters, these requirements vary widely among states and change rapidly.

Shortage or Surplus?

The meaning of the relative increase in the number of dentists between 1970 and the mid-1990s, followed by the projected decline over the next several decades, has aroused considerable discussion.[30, 45, 49, 50, 80, 91, 103] For many years after World War II, both the dental profession and the public accepted that a shortage of dental personnel was imminent if not actual. It was expected that significant increases in demand, stemming from rising affluence, rapid increases in population (the postwar "baby boom"), and a presumed increasing prevalence of caries, would outstrip the ability of the dental profession to provide all the care expected. The influential 1961 report *The Survey of Dentistry*[58] recommended marked increases in the number of dental graduates and auxiliaries and made projections of future personnel shortages.

In 1963, the ADA referred to "the impending shortage of health personnel" as "probably the most critical problem in the health field today,"[24] and again foresaw shortages in 1965.[7] These views were still in evidence in 1971, when the ADA's Task Force on National Health Programs stated as a basic assumption: "The United States faces a shortage of dental personnel in the next 20 years and the shortage will occur whether or not there is a national dental health program."[23] By the mid-1970s, however, many in dentistry no longer accepted the existence of a personnel shortage.[35, 50] The double-barreled effect of a large increase in the numbers of graduates, chiefly as a result of increased federal support of dental schools, plus the abrupt drop in the rate of population growth, led to the increase in the relative supply of dentists. The ADA agreed in 1973 that the relative supply of dentists was going to increase considerably by 1985,[8] a notable reversal from its position of only 8 years before.[7]

With the benefit of hindsight, it is fair to say that the massive support given by the federal government to dental education from 1963 to about 1980 was at least partly misdirected.[45] But no one in the early 1960s could foresee the dramatic drop in fertility rates with the consequent lowering of the rate of population increase, nor was the caries decline (Chapter 19) expected. A further projection in 1977 indicated that the supply of dentists would slightly exceed demand by 1990.[101] Assumptions in this projection were that population growth would continue at the 1977 rate, that 43%–50% of the population would be covered by dental insurance, and that the number of dental graduates would peak at 5460 in 1982 and then remain stable through 1990. Of course, we now know that the number of graduates fell as low as 3778 in 1993, substantially lower than any of these projections, and based on first-year enrollments, we can say that the number of dental graduates through the early 21st century will not be much more than 4000 per year. This whole episode is a further lesson that predictions are a hazardous business.

It now seems likely that the dentist:population ratio will slowly decline for the foreseeable future. What is not clear is the consequence of this trend on the practice of dentistry or the oral health of the public. There is no "correct" ratio of dentist:population; what may have been the "right" number of dentists in one decade is not necessarily right in the next. Although the caries decline is already reducing the need for treatment in younger Americans,[43] substantial need will remain for restoration and repair of the restorations placed in earlier generations.[30, 40, 84] This trend will be magnified by increasing tooth retention (Chapter 18). More adults will have relatively complete dentitions that they expect to maintain throughout life and will thus require restorative and periodontal care. It seems likely that the adult population will have substantially reduced need for care several decades from now, but the lessons from the recent past should be sufficient warning that speculation about the distant future should be treated as tentative at best. Even so, getting the personnel numbers "right" for the future demands policy now. Policies such as the Health Professions Education Act of 1963 and its successors take at least 10 years for their effects to be seen: schools built, faculty established, the first new classes graduated. Figure 9–2 shows that the 1963 act began to have real impact on the number of practicing dentists in the years 1970–1975, and the effect of these graduates will be with us at least through 2020.

Skeptical about what they see as govern-mental ineptitude, many leaders in dentistry (and some in government) would prefer to leave the matter of personnel numbers to market forces. Although market forces may work well to regulate some aspects of the economy, health care presents a special challenge. Market forces attract or deter dental students on conditions as they are now, and conditions can be very different in 20 years' time. In its recent comprehensive report on the future of dental education, the Institute of Medicine (IOM) gave the issue of the dental workforce careful consideration.[46] In the face of the many uncertainties already cited, the IOM recommended keeping the first-year enrollment levels at about 4000 for the foreseeable future. The dentist:population ratio has peaked and will decline slowly over the coming decade, yet one hesitates to assert that the resulting number of dentists will be enough, too few, or too many—and judged by whose standards?

ESTIMATING THE NUMBER OF DENTISTS REQUIRED

The supply of dentists traditionally has been measured by the dentist:population ratio. Apart from the problem of determining whether active, practicing, or all dentists are being counted, this measure is simple, usually easy to compute with a fair degree of accuracy, and is useful for comparative study. Ratios of other health professionals to population have been used to set national policy (e.g., the Health Professions Education Act of 1963), and they were also used to define National Health Service Corps shortage areas.[99]

It is nevertheless well recognized that crude dentist:population ratios must be interpreted with caution. If it can be assumed that need for care is equivalent between two places and that the ability and desire of the people to receive care are also the same, it is reasonable to assume that the number of dentists that is adequate in one place would also be adequate for the other. These are broad assumptions, however, so it is not surprising that there is dissatisfaction with ratios as a measure of personnel needs.[15, 73] First, dental need is not evenly distributed in a population; age, socioeconomic status, sex, race, and other demographic variables are associated with disease (see Chapters 18–22). As these characteristics are unevenly distributed between areas, so is dental need. Second, demand for care is affected by education, income, dentate status, geographic location, and availability of insurance. Where there are substantial differences in these characteristics between areas, use of dental care will also be unequal, regardless of dental need and availability of care. Finally, ratios assume constant productivity of dentists, quality of care, and mix of personnel. In fact, all three measures are dynamic, making a dentist population ratio that was appropriate at one time and place unsuitable in another.

The two other most commonly-used approaches to estimating personnel needs are demand-based and need-based models. The demand-based approach comes from economic theory and aims to make forecasts of the quantity of dental care that people will actually consume. The price and supply of services are key components of these models. Demand-based models have been used by the Health Resources and Services Administration of the US Department of Health and Human Services and by the ADA for their workforce forecasts.[78, 103, 104] Through such models, it is possible to estimate how issues such as changes in insurance coverage, number of dentists, and population growth are likely to affect the use of dental care.

Need-based approaches to personnel requirements come from a philosophically different direction. Need-based models start from measurements of oral need in a population, from which estimates are then derived of how much treatment would be required to meet those needs. The time required for treatment is added across the entire population, and from that an estimate of the number of required provider-hours of care can be determined.[116] A problem with the need-based approach is that both the accumulated backlog of need and estimates of future disease must be included. Other inherent difficulties are that dentists can treat the same condition in different ways, and that demand is often poorly related to need. Demand for some types of care, cosmetic restorations for example, is difficult to predict, which complicates the need-based approach even further.

Two additional approaches that combine elements of both need and demand are microsimulation[33, 34, 76] and system dynamics.[47] Although both require large quantities of data, a detailed understanding of the processes that underlie need and demand, and considerable computing resources to work

well, they have the potential to add to our understanding of the dynamics of dental care. Whatever approach is used, however, value judgments are still needed to weigh the uncertainties in the forecasts and to reach decisions on what the goals should be and how they should be achieved.[37, 46]

DENTAL AUXILIARIES IN THE UNITED STATES

Dental Hygienists

In 1997, there were estimated to be approximately 100,000 active dental hygienists in the United States, nearly a 7-fold increase since 1970.[102] Table 9–4 shows the growth in the number of active hygienists from 1950 to 1995 and in particular the extremely rapid growth since the early 1970s (see Chapter 1). Even with this large increase in the number of hygienists, there are still some concerns about a shortage.[39, 60, 110] After declines in enrollment through the late 1980s, roughly parallel to the enrollment declines in dentistry, dental hygiene enrollments rebounded by the mid-1990s to near-record levels. The majority of dental hygiene programs are in community colleges, and in the 1995 total of 215 programs, only 28 were in dental schools and 20 others in 4-year colleges.[4]

The duties of a dental hygienist are similar in most countries where they are part of the dental team.[61] These duties, usually carried out under the supervision of a dentist, are associated with the preventive aspects of dental care: scaling and polishing teeth, applying fluorides and other preventive agents, and educating patients to practice sound dental habits. Expanded duties for hygienists have been developed in some states in the United States, where the training of hygienists is extended to teach them to carry out additional duties in the dental office. Since 1975, however, the ADA House of Delegates has repeatedly gone on record as being opposed to delegation of expanded functions for hygienists and other auxiliaries,[10, 13, 14, 16] despite research evidence showing that trained hygienists could perform these duties competently. (There is a fuller discussion of expanded-function auxiliaries later in this chapter.)

Outside of the armed services, dental hygiene traditionally is an almost completely female profession. Even if this trend contin-

**Table 9–4. DENTAL HYGIENIST STATISTICS FOR THE UNITED STATES:
SELECTED YEARS, 1950–1995**

YEAR	NUMBER OF ACTIVE HYGIENISTS*	ACTIVE HYGIENISTS PER 100 ACTIVE DENTISTS	TRAINING PROGRAMS IN DENTAL HYGIENE	FIRST-YEAR ENROLLMENT
1950	3190	4.0	26	862
1955	4160	4.9	33	1100
1960	8800	9.8	37	1440
1965	11,600	12.1	56	2070
1970	15,100	14.8	121	3265
1975	26,900	24.0	174	5337
1980	38,400	30.4	200	5619
1985	55,000	43.0	198	4866
1990	75,000	55.6	202	5419
1995	100,000	64.5	215	5669

*Number of active hygienists is an estimate, because of the relative ease of movement into and out of active practice, and the frequency of part-time practice for more than one employer.
From references 3, 4, and 99.

ues, the traditional passiveness of hygienists has changed. Hygienists, licensed and regulated by state boards of dentistry, have shown their dissatisfaction at not having a voice in their own licensing, and there continues to be considerable activity on the part of hygienists in many states to gain more control over their profession. Attempts continue, and some have succeeded, to develop separate licensing boards for dental hygiene, to increase the representation of hygienists on examining boards, to relax supervision requirements, to allow direct third-party reimbursement to hygienists, to permit expanded functions, and to allow independent practice.[56] Not surprisingly, the ADA is firmly opposed to these moves, arguing that the only appropriate role for a hygienist is provision of care under the supervision of a dentist.[16, 17]

Independent Contractual Practice of Dental Hygiene

Dental practice acts in every state except Colorado require hygienists to work under the supervision of a dentist, with direct supervision often implied if not actually stated. This pattern was challenged in 1976 when a California hygienist opened her own office next door to that of two dentists whose patients she was treating on a contractual basis. Her action was based on their interpretation of the state dental practice law. Following the lodging of a complaint, the California Board of Dental Examiners ruled in 1978 that hygienists may not practice independently in their own offices. In agreeing to the Board's

ruling, the hygienist accepted that her office would be considered an extension of the setting in which the dentists practiced, and the case appeared settled. This hygienist continued to practice adjacent to her supervising dentists and stated that "appropriate supervision, whether general or direct, is well provided for with this arrangement."[59]

This California case pioneered independent contracting, in which the hygienist has a formal agreement regarding supervision with a specific dentist or dentists and often a financial arrangement. Hygienists may practice in a dentist's office or adjacent to it, paying their own overhead costs and collecting their own fees from patients. Because the dentist is a "supervisor," at least the letter of most state laws is preserved.[112] Although it is not known how many hygienists are functioning as independent contractors, the number in the 1990s was not thought to be high.

Independent Practice

An even greater departure from tradition is independent practice, in which the hygienist selects a site, rents or purchases space, secures equipment and supplies, and treats patients directly. In 1986, Colorado became the first state in the United States to permit the independent practice of dental hygiene. The legislation, however, did not permit a full range of hygiene services; a dentist's supervision was required for a dental hygienist to take radiographs, remove live tissue, perform root planing, and to inject local anesthetic.[107] As soon as the bill was signed into law, the

ADA filed suit to block independent practice, but the court ruled that the ADA had no standing in the case. This ruling was upheld in appellate court.[85]

It is difficult to know how many dental hygienists have established independent practices in Colorado, because the law does not require them to register that fact. Nevertheless, as of 1998, the number was small, possibly fewer than 20.[25] The costs of establishing and maintaining an office, the limited scope of services permitted, and the reluctance of insurers to reimburse hygienists for services appear to have been major barriers to further development,[85, 103] although by 1997 insurers in Colorado were required to reimburse dental hygienists for covered services. The limited evidence from Colorado, and from an experiment in independent practice in California, indicates that independent dental hygiene practices appear to compare favorably to dental offices on several measures of practice quality.[25, 48, 79] The future of independent practice for hygienists remains uncertain, but the overall trend seems to be a slow expansion of the autonomy of dental hygiene practice, fought out on a state-by-state basis.

Dental Assistants

Dental assistants are the most numerous of all dental personnel groups in the United States and, along with dental laboratory technicians, are the most long-established auxiliaries. They began to be employed with regularity in dental practices toward the latter part of the 19th century. The first assistants were trained on the job by their dentist-employers to aid in receiving patients and performing "housekeeping" chores and office clerical procedures. Many assistants today still follow this same pattern, because formal training for dental assistants who perform only the "traditional" extraoral functions is not required in any licensing jurisdiction in the United States.

The ADA estimated that in the mid-1990s, there were more than 200,000 active dental assistants in the United States, or approximately 130 per 100 active dentists. The ADA's 1995 *Survey of Dental Practice* stated that 91.6% of dentists in practice employed at least one chairside assistant.[20] The number of assistants increased sharply during the 1970s and early 1980s, rising from an estimated 91 per 100 active dentists in 1965.[102] Some of the increase may be attributable to training

programs in dental schools, originally encouraged by federal funds, in which dental students were taught how to use assistants effectively. Another measure of increased utilization of assistants can be seen in the same 1995 survey,[21] in which more than 50% of dentists reported employing two or more assistants.

During the 1980s, there was a decline in training-program enrollments, which paralleled those in dentistry and dental hygiene. The peak first-year enrollment of 8386 in 1979 fell to 5388 in 1988,[2] but then rose to 5669 in 1995.[4] In 1995, 230 institutions offered training programs, nearly double the number in 1968, although down from the peak of 296 in 1980.

In most states, dental assistants are now legally allowed to carry out more than their traditional duties; many state laws and regulations have been changed to allow "expanded functions" of assistants. A bewildering and constantly changing variety of tasks is permitted from one state to another.[18, 32, 51, 63] In some states, no certification or licensure is required; in some, certification is required; and in still others, testing and registration are required. Voluntary certification for dental assistants has been available since 1948 through the Certifying Board of the American Dental Assistants Association, now known as the Dental Assisting National Board (DANB), and this certification is accepted in some states as qualification to practice the expanded functions defined in its dental practice act.

Expanded Function Dental Auxiliaries (EFDAs)

Although dental assistants were used in the 19th century, it was not until the shortage of civilian dentists during World War II, owing to the enlistment of many dentists in the armed services, that serious consideration was given to their more efficient use.[62] The introduction of the air-turbine dental handpiece in the 1950s removed much of the drudgery from cavity and crown preparation and made greater productivity much more achievable. Development of "four-handed dentistry," with the dentist and assistant both seated, was a natural consequence. With it came sweeping changes in design of dental chairs, operating equipment, access to instruments, and layout of the dental office.

Continued developments in equipment,

materials, and procedures are constantly making the role of the dental assistant more complex; the four-handed assistant in a busy office must know instruments and understand procedures well for this type of practice to work. In the interest of greater operating efficiency, it was inevitable, therefore, that assistants began to do more and more intraoral procedures. Research has shown that both hygienists and assistants are capable of carrying out a wide range of extra duties at a good level of quality when adequately trained,[1, 27, 31, 55, 66-68, 92] and that the productivity and income of dentists can be greatly improved as a result.[28, 72, 74, 77, 86]

Moves toward utilization of EFDAs were given impetus during the 1960s, when a critical shortage of dental personnel was seen as imminent. If the country was to be short of dentists, the reasoning went, at least let those in practice be as productive as possible. Federal funds became available for dental schools to operate Dental Auxiliary Utilization (DAU) programs, which trained dental students in four-handed dentistry, and later for Training in Expanded Auxiliary Management (TEAM) programs, which taught dental students to work with auxiliaries who carried out an even wider range of functions, including packing and carving amalgams in cavities prepared by the students.

The studies with EFDAs were carried out in a variety of special institutional settings, although considerable effort was made to simulate the characteristics of the private office. Limited studies in private offices also have been conducted,[41, 72, 74, 82] and despite some difficulties in adjusting office routines, they confirmed that EFDAs can be successfully used there. EFDAs are also routinely used in the Indian Health Service and military and VA facilities, and by some private practitioners in states where they are permitted.[51, 63, 72, 74] Examples of the kinds of duties defined as expanded duties in various state dental practice acts are shown in Table 9–5.

Government's interest in promoting EFDAs is in increased productivity and in the subsequent presumed lower cost of care to the public. In fact, the US General Accounting Office, in a 1980 report, urged states to develop practice acts that permitted expanded functions, and recommended that all federal programs make wider use of EFDAs.[97] This recommendation has not been well heeded, however, and few states now permit a wide range of expanded functions. It is not known

Table 9–5. EXAMPLES OF DUTIES PERMITTED TO BE CARRIED OUT BY EXPANDED-DUTY DENTAL AUXILIARIES IN THE UNITED STATES IN THE LATE 1990s

- Applying topical fluorides
- Applying desensitizing agents
- Applying pit-and-fissure sealants
- Placing, carving, and polishing amalgam restorations
- Placing and finishing composite restorations
- Placing and removing matrix bands
- Placing and removing rubber dams
- Monitoring of nitrous oxide
- Taking impressions for study casts
- Exposing and developing radiographs
- Removing sutures
- Removing and replacing ligature wires on orthodontic appliances

Data from references 18, 25, and 81.

how many dentists are employing EFDAs, but in the late 1990s it seemed to be relatively few.

Although the research literature makes it clear that auxiliaries can function as well as dentists in providing these expanded services, an appropriate cautionary note has been sounded.[32] A careful reading of the literature shows that even though the candidates for the demonstration projects were carefully screened and selected and participated in rigorous training programs, not all candidates were able to perform successfully and were dropped from the programs. These selective and rigorous training programs are quite different from the requirements for expanded functions in many states, some of which require no formal training or evaluation at all. Caution is needed because the evidence that carefully trained auxiliaries can function at high levels when adequately trained does not necessarily mean that the same outcome can be assured in the absence of such training.

The ADA and EFDAs

A complicating factor in the legal status of EFDAs in the United States has been the position of the ADA, which although it does not directly or legally control state boards, clearly has influence. During the mid-1960s, ADA policy encouraged experimental projects. By the early 1970s, however, when many became concerned about the possible oversupply of dentists, ADA policy reversed itself to oppose such experimentation. As one health economist noted, an increase in EFDAs at the same time as an increase in dentists would clearly have a negative impact on the dentists' willingness to employ them.[44]

Because most of the research studies on the use of EFDAs were based in dental schools, some dental educators became irritated at what they perceived as the ADA's efforts to interfere with academic freedom. The ADA's mood continued to become more opposed to experiments with EFDAs, however, and since 1975 the House of Delegates has passed a series of resolutions to that effect. They are opposed to (a) delegation of many of the procedures now permitted in some states, such as the taking of final impressions, placement or adjustment of appliances, intraoral restorative procedures, and the use of local anesthetics; and (b) independent or unsupervised practice of any auxiliary personnel.[13, 16, 17] These discrepancies between the ADA's position on the one hand, and some state laws and the activism of some dental auxiliary groups on the other, continue to create tensions within dentistry.

Despite all of these activities with expanded functions over the last three decades, there has been a notable absence of suggestions to develop operating auxiliaries like the New Zealand dental nurse (Chapter 7). Part of the reason may be that in the late 1940s, an attempt was made to establish such a plan in Massachusetts, but it was stopped by swift and effective political action by organized dentistry.[42]

A possible additional reason for reduced enthusiasm about expanded-duty dental auxiliaries is the change in the types and level of restorative need that has accompanied the decline in dental caries. The greatest benefits in increased productivity with EFDAs came in the production of routine restorative care. Several decades ago it was quite common for children to require multiple restorations at each dental visit, and with the use of EFDAs, the process of "quadrant" and "half-mouth" restorative care was common. Today, however, there is evidence that the number of restorations placed per patient has declined substantially,[19, 43] and therefore the potential efficiency of EFDAs may also have declined.

Dental Laboratory Technicians

The dental laboratory technician, like the dental assistant, has been a part of dentistry for a long time. The technician's task is to fabricate crowns, bridges, dentures, and orthodontic and other appliances on the prescription of a dentist. Many of these tasks require high precision, and the technician's skill weighs heavily on the ultimate success of the treatment. Although many laboratory technicians are trained on the job, the approximately 34 dental technology programs in the US are accredited by the ADA's Commission on Dental Accreditation. Technicians also may become Certified Dental Technicians (CDT) in one or more of the areas of complete dentures, partial dentures, crowns and bridges, ceramics, and orthodontics.

Traditionally, technicians were directly employed by dentists and worked in a laboratory in the same suite of offices as the dentist. Over time, however, this arrangement became uneconomical for most dentists. In addition, some technicians have become "specialists," whose skills are properly at the disposal of many dentists. Most technicians now are employed by independent commercial laboratories, which provide their services to dentists. In the ADA's 1995 *Survey of Dental Practice*, only 5.9% of responding dentists directly employed a laboratory technician either full- or part-time.[20]

The ADA estimated that in 1997 there were about 60,000 active technicians in the United States, or 40 per 100 active dentists. The enrollment levels in accredited programs have declined from a peak of 1665 first-year enrollees in 1981 to 908 in 1990 and 652 in 1995.[2, 60] These continuing declines in enrollments are causing some concern[90, 109] that it will become increasingly difficult for many dentists to find competent laboratory services. Factors that affect the national staffing picture are relatively low hourly wages in the industry, growth in the use of dental laboratories overseas in low-wage countries, and a general decline in the need for some laboratory services because of changing patterns of disease in the population.

Denturists

During the 1970s and early 1980s, some dental laboratory technicians tried to change state dental practice acts to allow them to treat the public directly for the fabrication of dentures. These technicians call themselves denturists and their occupation denturism. This activity came at approximately the same time as similar movements in Canada (see

Chapter 10). By the mid-1990s, denturists were legally recognized in most Canadian provinces and a few states in the United States. The requirements for licensing vary among states, but usually include some educational component.

The ADA has vigorously opposed the denturist movement. The Association's principal argument is that denturists are unqualified to treat patients and that poor quality care and even actual harm could result to patients. The ADA defines denturism as "the fitting and dispensing of dentures illegally to the public,[12]" a definition both clear and brief, even if no longer accurate for some states. Although the soundness of the ADA's argument may be evident in dental circles, it may be less so to the public and to legislators. This fact became painfully clear in the 1978 Oregon elections. Supporters of denturism had put the subject on the election ballot through the statewide initiative process, which meant that if it succeeded, the measure automatically became law. Not only was it successful, but the 3-to-1 margin of victory stunned organized dentistry. The conclusions of the ADA's postmortem analysis were:

- The public viewed denturism as a consumer issue, not a health issue.
- The public believed that dentistry's campaign was spurred by economic self-interest.
- Some votes were based on sympathy for the elderly.
- Denturism provided consumers with freedom of choice.
- The media campaign organized by dentistry through a public relations firm was widely perceived as tasteless and unprofessional.[5]

The issue seems to have quieted from its peak in 1980, perhaps because in those states where denturists practice legally there appears to have been no major rush by patients to seek their care. With declining edentulism in the United States (see Chapter 18), the importance of the issue should continue to fade.

LEGISLATIVE INFLUENCE ON DENTIST SUPPLY AND DISTRIBUTION

Federal programs to provide financial aid to training institutions and to students between 1963 and 1980 were first intended to increase the *supply* of certain types of graduates. Legislation in the 1970s then attempted

to alleviate the *maldistribution* of health personnel. What should be done about maldistribution, however, continues to be a subject of debate. Some believe that a sufficient supply of dentists will permit free-market forces to sort out any problems. Some redistribution through the free movement of dentists undoubtedly does occur, but it also takes time and may be only partially effective. Others believe that only significant changes in the dental care system will solve the problem. If dentists are left as free as they now are to choose a practice location, so this argument goes, maldistribution will continue.

National Health Service Corps

One federally sponsored program aimed directly at easing maldistribution of health care providers is the National Health Service Corps (NHSC), the result of 1971 legislation.[83] The NHSC is designed mainly for physicians, but dentists and dental hygienists are also eligible. Although initially based on volunteers, the program has at various times provided scholarships and loan forgiveness for recent graduates to encourage them to practice in designated shortage areas.

After reaching a peak in 1980, when 6409 scholarships were awarded (both medical and dental), the program came under considerable strain. Severe budget cuts were enacted during the 1980s; by 1989 the scholarship program had ceased. Through the same period, a growing problem developed with defaults on student loans. The usual requirement was that each year of educational tuition and living expense support would be repaid by 1 year of practice in a shortage area, but by 1987 more than 1300 scholarship recipients were in default by having refused to serve in a shortage area.[36]

The phasing-out of the scholarship program led to a rapid decline in the number of dentists going to shortage areas, which itself suggests that the scholarship program was achieving its goals. Community health centers (Chapter 7) were particularly hard hit, because a high percentage of their staff had come from the scholarship programs. The program continues mainly through a loan repayment system, and as of 1997, a qualifying practitioner practicing full-time in a federally designated Health Professional Shortage Area (HPSA) was eligible for loan repayment of up to $25,000 per year for the first 2 years, and up to $35,000 per year for subsequent years.

Subsidies to Dental Schools and Dental Students

Before and since the NHSC, governmental programs to increase the supply of dental personnel existed in the form of financial incentives to dental schools and subsidies to dental students. Most dental schools are constructed and largely supported by state governments. Their object is to supply dentists for the state concerned, as indicated by the standard practice of charging higher rates of tuition for out-of-state residents.

Although some federal money has gone into dental schools for decades, the proportion of federal money supporting dental schools rose dramatically in the years up to the early 1970s. The Health Professions Education Act of 1963 was designed to alleviate the perceived shortage of health personnel, including dentists. This legislation subsidized existing schools, provided funds for new construction and renovation, and provided direct aid to students, all with few strings attached. An intended effect of this legislation was the sharp increase in dental graduates (Fig. 9–2).

The Comprehensive Health Manpower Act of 1971 continued financial aid to schools, but with some stricter provisions for the use of the money attached. This Act was followed by a period of financial recession, inflation, slower population growth, and growing belief in some dental circles that the perceived shortage of dentists had been alleviated and was tending toward an oversupply. The Health Professions Educational Assistance Act of 1976 was thus enacted in a different atmosphere from that of 1963; it concentrated on improving the distribution of primary-care personnel rather than on simply increasing numbers. Part of the Act's requirements were that dental schools could only qualify for federal support funds if they either (a) increased enrollment of first-year students by a specified proportion, or (b) provided "off-site" training for dental students. Some dental schools declined the federal aid rather than accept these conditions.

Between the mid-1970s and mid-1980s, there were substantial reductions in federal support to dental education. The institutional support grants that dental schools had come to rely on were eliminated. As a source of school operating revenue, federal funds fell from nearly 30% in 1973 to just over 10% by the early 1980s, where it remained through the 1990s. The result was intense financial pressure that continued through the 1980s and early 1990s, reflected in higher tuition costs, because few states were able to fill the financial gap left by the loss of federal funds. To make matters more difficult, the reduced number of applicants put limits on how high tuition could go, and how much of the budget it could cover.

It is worth remembering that student tuition, high as it is and with an average indebtedness of $81,688 per graduate in 1997,[4] represents well under half of the cost of a dental student's education. At public dental schools in 1994, only 12% of operating revenue came from tuition; in private schools it was just about 50%.[3] The combination of these pressures led to the decision during the late 1980s and early 1990s by 6 dental schools (all private) to close. In the fall of 1997, however, a new private dental school (Nova Southeastern) opened in Florida, the first new dental school to open in several decades. There may be more changes as dental education struggles to adjust to the new realities of extremely high costs of dental education, generally stagnant levels of governmental support, and potential pressure on academic health centers, brought on by the demands of managed care, to reduce costs.[29] These negative forces may be balanced, however, by the generally favorable economic picture for dentists in the late 1990s,[26, 111] and the substantial increase in the number of applicants to dental schools.

REFERENCES

1. Abramowitz J, Berg LE. A four-year study of the utilization of dental assistants with expanded functions. J Am Dent Assoc 1973;87:623–35.
2. American Association of Dental Schools. Deans' briefing book: Academic year 1988–89. Washington DC: AADS, 1989.
3. American Association of Dental Schools. Deans' briefing book; academic year, 1994–95. Washington DC: AADS, 1995.
4. American Association of Dental Schools. Trends in dental education: 1997. Washington DC: AADS, 1997.
5. American Dental Association, Bureau of Economic and Behavioral Research. The Oregon lesson: Results of postelection research. J Am Dent Assoc 1979;98:749–54.
6. American Dental Association, Bureau of Economic and Behavioral Research. Facts about states for the dentist seeking a location. Chicago: ADA, 1979.
7. American Dental Association, Bureau of Economic Research and Statistics. Number of dental graduates required annually to 1985. J Am Dent Assoc 1965;71:697–8.
8. American Dental Association, Bureau of Economic

Research and Statistics. Growth in population and numbers of dentists to 1985. J Am Dent Assoc 1973;87:901–3.

9. American Dental Association, Bureau of Economic Research and Statistics. Survey of recent graduates. II. Factors related to selection of a practice location. J Am Dent Assoc 1973;87:904–6.

10. American Dental Association, Council on Dental Education. American Dental Association statement on expanded function dental auxiliary utilization and education. Trans Am Dent Assoc 1976;117:234.

11. American Dental Association, Council on Dental Practice. A comparative study of male and female dental practice patterns. Chicago: ADA, 1989.

12. American Dental Association, House of Delegates. Resolution 97-1973-H. Trans Am Dent Assoc 1973;114:743–4.

13. American Dental Association, House of Delegates. Resolution 50-1975-H. Trans Am Dent Assoc 1975;116:701–2.

14. American Dental Association, House of Delegates. Resolution 33-1976-H. Trans Am Dent Assoc 1976;117:836.

15. American Dental Association, House of Delegates. Resolution 77-1984-H. Trans Am Dent Assoc 1984;125:537–8.

16. American Dental Association, House of Delegates. Resolution 10-H-1988. Trans Am Dent Assoc 1988;129:464–8.

17. American Dental Association, House of Delegates. Comprehensive Policy Statement on Dental Auxiliary Personnel. Trans Am Dent Assoc 1996;739–42.

18. American Dental Association, Survey Center. Facts about states 1995. For the dentist seeking a location. Chicago: ADA, 1995.

19. American Dental Association, Survey Center. The 1990 survey of dental services rendered. Chicago: ADA, 1994.

20. American Dental Association, Survey Center. The 1995 survey of dental practice. Employment of dental practice personnel. Chicago: ADA, 1996.

21. American Dental Association, Survey Center. 1996/ 97 survey of predoctoral dental educational institutions. Academic programs, enrollment, and graduates. Volume 1. Chicago: ADA, 1997.

22. American Dental Association, Survey Center. Distribution of dentists in the United States by region and state, 1995. Chicago: ADA, 1997.

23. American Dental Association, Task Force on National Health Programs. Dentistry in national health programs: a report with recommendations. J Am Dent Assoc 1971;83:569–600.

24. Association testifies in support of Educational Assistance Act. J Am Dent Assoc 1963;66:389–91.

25. Astroth DB, Cross-Poline GN. Pilot study of six Colorado dental hygiene independent practices. J Dent Hyg 1998;72:13–22.

26. Average dentist income nears or tops physician's. Managed Dental Care 1997;3(2):6–7.

27. Bader J, Mullins R, Lange K. Technical performance on amalgam restorations by dentists and auxiliaries in private practice. J Am Dent Assoc 1983;106:338–41.

28. Baird KM, Purdy EC, Protheroe DH. Pilot study on advanced training and employment of auxiliary dental personnel in the Royal Canadian Dental Corps: final report. J Can Dent Assoc 1963;29:778–87.

29. Bailit H. Managed care and dental education and research: should academicians be concerned? Crit Rev Oral Biol Med 1997;8:129–35.

30. Beazoglou TJ, Guay AH, Heffley DR. The economic health of dentistry: Past, present, and future. J Am Dent Assoc 1989;119:117–21.

31. Bergner M, Milgrom P, Chapko MK, et al. The Washington state dental auxiliary project: Quality of care in private practice. J Am Dent Assoc 1983;107:781–6.

32. Boyer EM. A second look at expanded functions research: Unintended outcomes for the public's safety. J Dent Hyg 1996;70:35–42.

33. Brown LJ, Caldwell SB, Eklund SA. Microsimulation of dental conditions and dental service utilization. In: Anderson JG, ed: Proceedings of the 1992 Simulation in Health Care and Social Services Conference. San Diego: The Society for Computer Simulation, 1992.

34. Brown LJ, Caldwell SB, Eklund S. How fee and insurance changes could affect dentistry: Results from a microsimulation model. J Am Dent Assoc 1995;126:449–59.

35. Butts HC. Dental manpower shortage? [editorial]. J Am Dent Assoc 1976;93:507.

36. Can volunteers save the health service corps? Medicine and Health 1989;43(36):Special Insert.

37. Capilouto E, Capilouto ML, Ohsfeldt R. A review of methods used to project the future supply of dental personnel and the future demand and need for dental services. J Dent Educ 1995;59:237–57.

38. Chambers DW. Who is qualified to practice dentistry? Contact Point 1987;65(3):8–15.

39. Dental leaders discuss recruitment, retention of the dental team. J Missouri Dent Assoc 1989;69(6):18–19, 21, 23–25, 27.

40. Douglass CW, Furino A. Balancing dental service requirements and supplies: Epidemiologic and demographic evidence. J Am Dent Assoc 1990;121:587–92.

41. Douglass CW, Moore S, Lindahl RL, Gillings DB. Expanded duty dental assistants in solo private practice. J Am Coll Dent 1976;43:144–63.

42. Dunning JM. Extending the field for dental auxiliary personnel in the United States. Am J Public Health 1958;48:1059–64.

43. Eklund SA, Pittman JL, Smith RC. Trends in dental care in insured Americans: 1980 to 1995. J Am Dent Assoc 1997;128:171–8.

44. Fein R. Health manpower: Some economic considerations. J Dent Educ 1976;40:650–4.

45. Feldstein PJ. Financing dental care: an economic analysis. Lexington MA: Heath, 1973.

46. Field MJ, ed: Dental education at the crossroads: challenges and change. Washington DC: National Academy Press, 1995.

47. Forrester JW. Urban dynamics. Cambridge MA: MIT Press, 1969.

48. Freed JR, Perry DA, Kushman JE. Aspects of quality of dental hygiene care in supervised and unsupervised practice. J Public Health Dent 1997;57:68–75.

49. Furino A, Douglass CW. Balancing dental service requirements and supplies: The economic evidence. J Am Dent Assoc 1990;121:685–92.

50. Goodman SE. The dentist shortage that never was. Dent Management 1976;July:33–8.

51. Govoni MM. Mandatory education and credentialing for dental assistants: Is it the answer to the manpower crisis? Dent Assist 1990;59(4):9–12.

52. Graham J. Dental education: summary of the 1977–1978 annual report of the Council on Dental Education. J Am Dent Assoc 1978;96:767–71.

53. Graham J. Dental education 1980–1981. J Am Dent Assoc 1981;102:832–5.
54. Guarino RN. Licensure and certification of dentists and accreditation of dental schools. J Dent Educ 1995;59:205–33.
55. Hammons PE, Jamison HC, Wilson LL. Quality of service provided by dental therapists in an experimental program at the University of Alabama. J Am Dent Assoc 1971;82:1060–6.
56. Harrison B, West B. Rules & regs: Who needs them? J Am Dent Assoc 1991;122(1):155–7.
57. Hillenbrand H. The necessity for trained advanced dental professionals. J Dent Educ 1981;45:76–87.
58. Hollinshead BS, director. The survey of dentistry: The final report. Washington DC: American Council on Education, 1961.
59. Interview with Linda Krol. RDH 1981 May–June;30–4.
60. Is shortage waning? ADA News 1991;22:1, 8.
61. Johnson PM. Dental hygiene practice: International profile and future directions. Int Dent J 1992;42:451–9.
62. Klein H. Civilian dentistry in war-time. J Am Dent Assoc 1944;31:648–61.
63. LeGallee-Byle BL. Trends in dental assistant utilization: a comparative study. Part I. Dent Assist 1989 58(1):17–25.
64. Licensure by credentials: Is it working? J Am Dent Assoc 1985;111:18–32.
65. Linn EL. Professional activities of women dentists. J Am Dent Assoc 1970;81:1383–7.
66. Lobene RR, Berman K, Chaisson LB, et al. The Forsyth experiment in training of advanced skills hygienists. Dent Hyg 1974;48:204–13.
67. Lotzkar SJ, Johnson DW, Thompson MB. Experimental program in expanded functions for dental assistants: Phase 1, baseline, and phase 2, training. J Am Dent Assoc 1971;82:101–22.
68. Lotzkar SJ, Johnson DW, Thompson MB. Experimental program in expanded functions for dental assistants. Phase 3: Experiment with dental teams. J Am Dent Assoc 1971;82:1067–81.
69. Mandatory CDE gaining support in states. ADA News 1990;21:12.
70. Mann WR. Dental education. In: Hollinshead BS, director: The survey of dentistry: The final report. Washington DC: American Council on Education, 1961:239–422.
71. Martens L, Glasrud PH, Burton KL. A profile of Minnesota's younger women dentists [abstract]. J Dent Res 1985;64:205.
72. Milgrom P, Bergner M, Chapko MK, et al. The Washington state dental auxiliary project: Delegating expanded functions in general practice. J Am Dent Assoc 1983;107:776–80.
73. Moen BD. Realism in maintaining the present population ratio in the next seventeen years. J Am Coll Dent 1959;26:146–8.
74. Mullins MR, Kaplan AL, Bader JD, et al. Summary results of the Kentucky dental practice demonstration: A cooperative project with practicing general dentists. J Am Dent Assoc 1983;106:817–25.
75. Niessen LC, Kleinman DV, Wilson AA. Practice characteristics of women dentists. J Am Dent Assoc 1986;113:883–8.
76. Orcutt GH, Caldwell S, Wertheimer R. Policy exploration through microanalytic simulation. Washington DC: Urban Institute, 1976.
77. Pelton WJ, Overstreet GA, Embry OH, Dilworth JB. Economic implications of adding one therapist to a practice. J Am Dent Assoc 1973;86:1301–9.
78. Perich ML. American Dental Association manpower projections. J Dent Educ 1987;51:219–23.
79. Perry DA, Freed JR, Kushman JE. The California demonstration project in independent practice. J Dent Hyg 1994;68:137–42.
80. Pew Health Professions Commission. Critical challenges: Revitalizing the health care professions for the twenty-first century. San Francisco: UCSF Center for the Health Professions, 1995.
81. Pontecorvo DA. Expanded duties: Results of ADAA's nationwide survey. Dent Assist 1988;57(4):9–13.
82. Redig D, Snyder M, Nevitt G, Tocchini J. Expanded duty dental auxiliaries in four private dental offices: The first year's experience. J Am Dent Assoc 1974;88:969–84.
83. Redman E. The dance of legislation. New York: Simon and Schuster, 1973.
84. Reinhardt JW, Douglass CW. The need for operative dentistry services: projecting the effects of changing disease patterns. Operative Dentistry 1989;14:114–20.
85. Reveal M. Dental hygiene regulation and practice. J Public Health Dent 1989;49:228–30.
86. Romcke RG, Lewis DW. Use of expanded function hygienists in the Prince Edward Island manpower study. J Can Dent Assoc 1973;39:247–62.
87. Santangelo MV. A review of dental school accreditation: development and current philosophy. J Dent Educ 1977;41:233–8.
88. Santangelo MV. The dental accrediting process. J Dent Educ 1981;45:513–21.
89. Selden WK. Study of accreditation of selected health educational programs. Part one: Working papers. Washington DC: National Commission on Accrediting, 1971.
90. Shortage of qualified dental technicians. Gen Dent 1993;41:288, 290.
91. Solomon ES. Errors in federal report on dental health personnel presents problems. J Dent Educ 1990;54:499–501.
92. Soricelli DA. Implementation of the delivery of dental services by auxiliaries: The Philadelphia experience. Am J Public Health 1972;62:1077–87.
93. Talbot NS. Why not more women dentists? J Dent Educ 1960;60:114–22.
94. Tillman RS. Women in dentistry—a review of the literature. J Am Dent Assoc 1975;91:1214–20.
95. Tillman RS, Horowitz SL. Practice patterns of recent female dental graduates. J Am Dent Assoc 1983;107:32–5.
96. US Department of Commerce, Bureau of the Census. Historical statistics of the United States: Colonial time to 1957. Washington DC: Government Printing Office, 1960.
97. US General Accounting Office. Increased use of expanded function dental auxiliaries would benefit consumers, dentists, and taxpayers. HRD-80-51. Washington DC: Government Printing Office, 1980.
98. US Public Health Service. Health manpower shortage areas: criteria for designation. Appendix B. Criteria for designation of areas having shortages of dental manpower. Fed Register 1980;45:76003–5.
99. US Public Health Service, Bureau of Health Manpower. Dental manpower fact book. DHEW Publ No (HRA) 79-14. Washington DC: Government Printing Office, 1979.

100. US Public Health Service, Division of Dental Health. Manpower supply and educational statistics for dentists and dental auxiliaries. Bethesda MD: Division of Dental Health, 1972.

101. US Public Health Service, Division of Dentistry. Projections of national requirements for dentists 1980, 1985, and 1990. DHEW Publ No (HRA) 77-48. Washington DC: Government Printing Office, 1977.

102. US Public Health Service, Health Resources and Services Administration. Sixth report to the President and Congress on the status of health personnel in the United States. DHHS Publ No HRS-P-OD-88-1. Washington DC: Government Printing Office, 1988.

103. US Public Health Service, Health Resources and Services Administration. Seventh report to the President and Congress on the status of health personnel in the United States. DHHS Publ No HRS-P-OD-90-1. Washington DC: Government Printing Office, 1990.

104. US Department of Health and Human Services, Public Health Service, Health Resources and Services Administration. Health Personnel in the United States. Eighth report to Congress 1991. DHHS Publ No HRS-P-OD-92-1. Washington DC: Government Printing Office, 1992.

105. US Department of Health and Human Services, Public Health Service, Health Resources and Services Administration. Factbook—Health personnel United States. Washington DC: Government Printing Office, 1993.

106. US Department of Health and Human Services, Public Health Service, Health Resources and Services Administration. Factbook—Health personnel United States. Washington DC: Government Printing Office, 1997.

107. Vernon TM. The licensure of dental hygienists in Colorado: An update. J Public Health Dent 1989;49:234.

108. Waldman HB. Female dentists: A factor in determining the available future dental work force. J Am Coll Dent 1985;52(4):22–7.

109. Waldman HB. Pediatric dentists: Evolving demography. J Dent Child 1990;57:111–3.

110. Waldman HB. Will there be enough trained dental auxiliaries? Illinois Dent J 1992;61:253–6.

111. Weeks WB, Wallace AE, Wallace MM, Welch HG. A comparison of the educational costs and incomes of physicians and other professionals. N Engl J Med 1994;330:1280–6.

112. Woodall IR, Bentley M. Independent contracting as an alternative financial arrangement. RDH 1981 June;46–50.

113. World Health Organization. Report of an expert committee on auxiliary dental personnel. Tech Rep Series No 163. Geneva: WHO, 1959.

114. World Health Organization. Inter-regional seminar on the training and utilization of dental personnel in developing countries, New Delhi, India, Dec 1967. WHO Doc DH/68.2. Geneva: WHO, 1968.

115. World Health Organization. World health statistics annual. Geneva: WHO, 1994.

116. World Health Organization. Health through oral health. Guidelines for planning and monitoring for oral health care. London: Quintessence, 1989.

10

Dental Care in Canada

Amid I. Ismail

National Structure ◆ Population ◆ The Canadian
Health Care System ◆ Financing Health Care in
Canada ◆ Supply of Dental Personnel ◆ Dentists
Certification and Licensure ◆ Dental Hygienists
Dental Therapists ◆ Denturists ◆ Dental Assistants
Utilization of Dental Care ◆ Costs of Dental Care ◆
Oral Health Status ◆ Provision of Public Dental Care ◆
North York Public Health Department ◆ The Nova
Scotia Childrens' Oral Health Program ◆ Provincial
Dental Public Health Programs ◆ Federal Dental Public
Health Programs ◆ Medical Services Branch (MSB),
Health Canada ◆ Other Federal Dental Programs ◆
Future Developments

There are many similarities, and also differences, between Canadian and US dental care systems. The Canadian health care system, however, is structured in a significantly different manner from that of the United States. This chapter presents an overview of how dental care is provided in Canada. In addition to providing details of specific programs, the chapter gives a perspective on dental public health in a social climate that differs from that in the United States. When finances are given as part of program details, all money is expressed in Canadian dollars unless stated otherwise.

NATIONAL STRUCTURE

Canada is one the largest countries in the world, with a land mass of 10 million square kilometers (about 6250 million square miles). Its political development has been relatively peaceful. Although the aboriginal people of Canada and French and British colonists had been there for centuries, the nation was officially born with the British North America (BNA) Act of 1867. This established Canada as a self-governing nation in what was then the British Empire, and Canada has been a parliamentary democracy ever since. There are now 5 main political parties (Liberal, Reform, Bloc Québecois, New Democrats, and Progressive Conservatives) in the House of Commons, where voting usually follows party lines more closely than is customary in the United States Congress. Ostensibly, Canadian politics are less influenced by lobbyists and special interests than is American politics, although the 1990s have shown that Canadian voters can be volatile. As examples, two parties with focused regional interests, the Reform Party and Bloc Québecois, have both made gains during the 1990s.

Canada is a federation of 10 provinces and 2 territories, with shared responsibilities between the provinces and the federal government. The provinces have jurisdiction over health and postsecondary education, although the federal government makes transfer payments to the provinces to cover the federal obligation to health, postsecondary education, and other social programs. Transfer payments to the less wealthy provinces are made disproportionately higher than those to the richer provinces, the goal being to ensure that, as far as possible, all Canadians enjoy the same health and education benefits. This equalization policy in transfer payments has been generally successful in allowing the poorer provinces to meet national standards in health programs and post-secondary education. Although this financing system is in line with traditional Canadian values, it generated some political regionalization and frictions during the 1990s that may take some time to resolve.

POPULATION

Over the 130+ years of its history, Canada's population has grown from 3.4 million to about 30 million.[21] The country has one of the lowest population densities in the world, about 5 persons per square mile. Economically, Canada is one of the world's richest countries and is a major exporter to the United States.

Its 2 official languages, French and English, recognize the 2 founding European nations, although in 1991, 4 million Canadians reported a language other than English or French as their mother tongue.[21] There were indigenous people in Canada before European colonization, and today more than 1 million Canadians claim aboriginal ancestry. Of these, 626,000 identify themselves as members of the three aboriginal groups recognized by Canada's Constitution Act of 1982: North American Indians, Inuit, and Métis.[21] The aboriginal peoples actively seek recognition of their demand for self-government and acceptance as one of the founding nations, claims that not all provinces have yet accepted. Aboriginal peoples in Canada are now generally referred to as the First Nations and Inuit.

As mentioned previously, Canadian social philosophy seeks equality of opportunity among its many diverse cultures. In pursuit of that philosophy, Canadians expect that their government should play an active role in benefiting the lives of its citizens. This contrasts with the predominant philosophy in the United States, where a view of limited government is the rule. Canadians expect that government has a fundamental responsibility to its citizens to provide many services and benefits, most of which are viewed as rights. For example, many Canadians contend that health care is a right that government must provide for them, and in some regions social assistance is considered to come with citizenship. "The government owes it to me" is a frequently used phrase to refer to these rights. (The development of American social attitudes in these issues is discussed in Chapter 3.)

THE CANADIAN HEALTH CARE SYSTEM

Given its history and societal values, it is not surprising that Canada's health care system has developed along different lines from those in the United States. It has become a major unifying factor in the country,[24] and the general desire to preserve it is very strong. No political party in Canada has called for dismantling the system, or even for serious adjustments.

The Canadian health care system has its roots in the BNA of 1867, which described the provincial responsibility to establish and maintain "Hospitals, asylums, charities . . . in and for the Province, other than Marine Hospitals." From that time until 1957, the provinces had full jurisdiction over health care. The role of the federal government was restricted to financial assistance and health programs for members of the armed forces, veterans, prisoners, and merchant seamen.

Several developments led to the first Canadian Hospital Insurance and Diagnostic Act of 1957. The province of Saskatchewan, from early in the 20th century, had implemented programs whereby taxes were levied to pay for medical care insurance in rural areas, an approach generally regarded as successful. This evolved into provincial legislation that allowed municipalities to combine into hospital districts to provide hospital insurance. In the meantime, during the 1940s, the provinces and the federal government were involved in legal disputes over the constitutional jurisdictions each had regarding health care. As a result, several provinces in the early 1950s used the Saskatchewan model to initiate their own tax-supported hospital insurance plans.

In 1957, the federal and provincial governments finally agreed on a national program to provide hospital and diagnostic services for all Canadians. This agreement paved the way for the Medical Care Act of 1966, which covered in-office physician care. As a result, Canadians today have a health care system that is comprehensive, accessible, universal, portable, and publicly administered by nonprofit organizations (Table 10–1). National health insurance covers basic health care

Table 10-1. PRINCIPLES OF THE UNIVERSAL SINGLE-PAYER CANADIAN HEALTH CARE SYSTEM (MEDICARE)*

PRINCIPLE	CONDITIONS
Public administration	The health insurance plan of a province must be administered and operated on a nonprofit basis by a public authority accountable to the provincial government.
Comprehensiveness	The plan must insure all medically necessary services provided by hospitals and physicians. Insured hospital services include inpatient care at the ward level (unless private or semiprivate rooms are medically necessary) and all necessary drugs, supplies and diagnostic tests, as well as a broad range of outpatient services. Chronic care services are also insured, although some payment in respect of accommodation costs may be required by patients who are more or less permanently resident in the institution.
Universality	The plan must entitle 100% of the insured population (i.e., eligible residents) to insured health services on uniform terms and conditions.
Accessibility	The plan must provide, on uniform terms and conditions, reasonable access to insured hospital and physician services without barriers. Additional charges to insured patients for insured services are not allowed. No one may be discriminated against on the basis of income, age, health status, etc.
Portability	Residents are entitled to coverage when they move to another province within Canada or when they travel within Canada or abroad. (All provinces have some limits on coverage for services provided outside Canada, and may require prior approval for nonemergency out-of-province services.)

*The Canada Health Act stipulates the criteria that provincial health insurance plans must meet in order for a province to qualify for its full federal transfer payments. The 5 criteria are known as the "principles" of Canada's national health system.
From Health Canada. Health System and Policy Division website, 1997.

needs regardless of age, gender, race, employment, education status, and residence.

The 1966 Act was followed by the 1977 Federal-Provincial Fiscal Arrangements and Established Programs Financing Act, and in 1984 by the Canada Health Act. These later iterations redefined the financial arrangements between the provinces and the federal government and introduced extended health care services and new guidelines for the health insurance system. Most notably, the federal government required that no extra billing be allowed by a physician for a service covered by the provincial health care program. This requirement was challenged by physicians in Ontario in the late 1980s, but the courts upheld the federal government's policy of not permitting extra billing.

In the 1990s, the federal government convened a National Health Forum of experts in health care to determine the future directions of the Canadian health care system (which is generally known as "Medicare"—not to be confused with the United States Medicare program discussed in Chapter 8). The Forum identified 4 themes to determine the future directions for the Canadian health care system: determinants of health, evidence-based

decision making, values, and striking a balance. The Forum issued its recommendations in February 1997, stating that "Canadians will not support changes to the system unless the essence of Medicare is preserved." Canadians clearly value the single-payer model and the 5 principles of the Canada Health Act (Table 10-1). The Forum recommended that preservation of the Medicare system be achieved by (a) reallocating existing funding among different programs where appropriate; (b) investing in children, communities and working people to achieve the lowest possible unemployment; and (c) developing an evidence-based health care system. Although the Forum recommendations have not yet been implemented, they provide guidelines for change as Canada approaches the 21st century.

In 1995, the federal government passed the Canada Health and Social Transfer Act, which combined federal transfer payments for health and social services to the provinces under one block grant. This gives the provinces more flexibility in allocating resources among their health and social programs. Also under this act, the federal government changed its funding formula and reduced its contribution to health and social programs.

Financing Health Care in Canada

According to Health Canada (the federal department of health), the total expenditure on health care in 1996 was $75.2 billion, or $2510 per capita (approximately $1800 US). The total expenditures on health care in Canada in 1996 accounted for 9.5% of the Gross Domestic Product (GDP), down from the peak of 10.2% in 1992. The annual rate of increase on health expenditures in Canada was cut to 1.2% in 1996, compared with 1.8% in 1994 and 1995. On average, the expenditures on health care account for about one third of the provincial budgets. About 70% of the expenditures on health care come from public financing, and the remaining 30% are financed through private insurance or out-of-pocket payments. In the 1990s, the cuts in federal transfer payments to the provinces resulted in a 1% decrease in public spending on health care and a 5.5% increase in private spending.

Canada's single-payer system is administratively simpler for both patients and physicians than the polyglot arrangements in the United States, and it provides a simple and effective method for controlling expenditures through administrative and system management. As an example, several health departments have negotiated lower fees for physicians or dentists and have limited the expansion of health facilities. Of course, not everyone sees this power as a virtue of the system; several provinces rolled back or froze payments to physicians and dentists during the early 1990s. Any carefully controlled system like Canada's will have strengths and weaknesses. In Canada's case, the control comes from government, whereas in the United States it has been coming from private managed care organizations.

According to Health Canada, the major cost centers in the health care system are hospitals, which absorbed 34.2% of the total funds spent on health care in 1996. Physicians and drugs each cost 14.4% of the $75.2 billion that was spent nationally on health care in 1996. Expenditures on public health programs accounted for only 5% of the total health budget in 1996.

The provinces and territories have considerable power to manage health care spending. The provincial governments pay for hospitals' operating costs and capital expenditures, which gives them direction over operating expenses, organization, and even the survival of hospitals. As a result, the expansion of hospitals and the acquisition of expensive technology in Canada are more tightly regulated than in the United States.

THE SUPPLY OF DENTAL PERSONNEL

Dentists

In 1997, there were 15,896 registered dentists in Canada, with 39.8% of them in Ontario and 24.3% in Québec. Between 1991 and 1997, the number of dentists increased by 10.3% from 14,402 to 15,896. The dentist:population ratio was estimated to be 53.0 per 100,000 in 1997, and 51.2 per 100,000 in 1991.

Details of the supply of dentists are shown in Table 10–2. They show a trend of

Table 10–2. LICENSED DENTISTS IN CANADA BY PROVINCE IN 1991 AND 1997

PROVINCE	NUMBER OF LICENSED DENTISTS		
	1991	1997	% CHANGE
Newfoundland	150	149	−0.7
Prince Edward Island	48	49	2.0
Nova Scotia	457	430	−5.9
New Brunswick	231	243	5.2
Québec	3341	3855	15.4
Ontario	5873	6336	7.9
Manitoba	528	534	1.1
Saskatchewan	364	355	−2.4
Alberta	1400	1435	2.5
British Columbia	2002	2443	22.0
Northwest Territories	5	56	1020.0
Yukon Territories	3	11	266.7
Total	14,402	15,896	10.3

From Canadian Dental Association, 1997.

migration of new dentists from the eastern provinces, where the number of licensed dentists did not increase between 1991 and 1997, to British Columbia, Northwest Territories, and the Yukon. There are several reasons for these trends, the main one being the uneven economic developments in different parts of the country. The Maritime Provinces, on the Atlantic coast, experienced tough economic conditions during the 1990s because of the reduction in federal transfer payments and the crisis in the fishing industry. There is only 1 dental school in Atlantic Canada (Dalhousie University), which graduates about 30 dentists annually. Only a few of these new graduates remain in that region. Québec has 3 dental schools, and had twice the rate of increase in dentists as did Ontario with its 2 dental schools. The main province of choice for new dental graduates in the late 1990s was British Columbia, which had experienced significant economic development and waves of immigration from Hong Kong during the previous 10 years. Relaxed licensing requirements in British Columbia may also have helped attract dentists, for dental graduates are not required to take clinical examinations in that province if they were graduated within the previous 5 years from any accredited dental school in Canada.

Overall, the rate of increase of new dentists in Canada between 1991 and 1997 was 10.3%, down from the 29.7% increase between 1980 and 1990. This change resulted from the 20% reduction in the number of Canadian dental students, begun in 1988, which was intended to reduce the supply of dentists in Canada. This policy, however, had the unintended effect of sending hundreds of Canadian students to study dentistry in the United States.

Certification and Licensure of Dentists in Canada

The National Dental Examination Board (NDEB), established by an Act of Parliament in 1952, is the organization responsible for examination and certification of all dental graduates in Canada. Its mandate calls for establishing and maintaining qualifying conditions for a national standard of competence of dentists in Canada. The NDEB issues a certificate for those who pass its examinations and meet the criteria it sets for certification. Licensure is a provincial responsibility; some accept the NDEB certificate as a sole require-

ment for licensure, whereas others add additional requirements. Ontario, for example, requires that candidates pass a written examination set by the provincial dental board in addition to securing the NDEB certificate, and dentists seeking licensure in Québec must demonstrate fluency in French.

Before 1994, all graduates from the 10 accredited dental schools in Canada were automatically issued a NDEB certificate upon graduation. The NDEB participated in the process through its representatives on accreditation surveys of dental schools, and by appointment of a member to the Canadian Dental Association Commission on Dental Education. Graduates from all non-Canadian dental schools were required to take written preclinical and clinical examinations, and this requirement at that time included graduates of accredited dental schools in the United States. Subsequent events, however, forced change.

After the cut in intake of new dental students in 1988, a large number of Canadian students enrolled in dental schools in the United States. In the 1990s, the validity of the NDEB's examination for graduates from non-Canadian dental schools came under intense scrutiny when a large group of these Canadian graduates failed the old NDEB examinations. The resulting political pressure from dental organizations and from government led to several changes. Canadian graduates from Canadian dental schools after 1994 were required to take the NDEB's written test and the Objective Structured Clinical Examination (OSCE). After 1997, all graduates of American dental schools wishing to practice in Canada, regardless of their citizenship, were required to complete the same written and OSCE tests that the Canadian graduates take to receive an NDEB certificate. For graduates of nonaccredited dental schools (i.e., those outside Canada and the United States), the NDEB requires that, after January 2000, they enroll in a qualifying program and then take the same NDEB examinations as the local graduates.

The cycles that the NDEB certification process have passed through in the 1990s clearly show the difficulties associated with administrative decisions intended to control the number of dentists practicing in a country. In Canada, the 1988 policy to reduce the intake of dental students had significant ramifications that were not even contemplated at the time the decision was made.

Dental Hygienists

There were about 13,000 dental hygienists in Canada in 1997. Between 1990 and 1997, there was a 47% increase in the number of dental hygienists, and the output of new dental hygienists did not change in the 1990s despite the decreased graduation rate of new dentists. The employment status of all dental hygienists in Canada is unknown. Licensing of dental hygienists is now carried out by either the dental boards or by newly established dental hygiene boards or colleges in provinces where dental hygienists are self-regulating (Ontario, British Columbia, Alberta, Saskatchewan, and Québec). The major issue facing dental hygienists in Canada is their status as members of the oral health team. Dental hygienists would like to be recognized as primary care providers; however, dentists challenge that claim. As a result, the relationship between the Canadian Dental Hygienists' Association and the Canadian Dental Association remains cool.

Dental Therapists

In 1990, there were approximately 335 registered dental therapists or dental nurses in Canada, all trained in 1 of the 2 dental therapy training schools in Saskatchewan. One of these schools has since closed. The remaining school, the National School of Dental Therapy (NSDT) in Prince Albert, which joined the Saskatchewan Indian Federated College (SIFC), trains therapists to provide dental care for the First Nations and Inuit peoples. About 20 new students are accepted annually in the NSDT program. The change in the location of the NSDT from the University of Toronto to the SIFC took place in 1995 and follows the decision of the federal government to transfer the management of health care services to the First Nations and Inuit. Currently, the NSDT program is recruiting more aboriginal students and adding cultural components to the program while ensuring that the students graduate with a high level of technical expertise.

The NSDT was established in 1972 by the federal government to train dental therapists. The model followed was that of the New Zealand school dental nurse (Chapter 9). The objective was to bring basic dental care to remote communities of the Northwest Territories, mainly populated by aboriginal people. Dental therapists are trained to provide prevention and education, restorations, and uncomplicated extractions of primary and permanent teeth. Students are accepted at the NSDT after graduating from high school. The NSDT program has trained therapists from other countries such as Mozambique, Dominica, and Nepal as part of international development programs sponsored by the federal government. The NSDT is also exploring developing partnerships with countries from south and central Africa.

Nearly 90 dental therapists are currently working in northern Canada among the First Nations and Inuit populations. In Saskatchewan, 101 licensed dental therapists work throughout the province. Most therapists currently work for Tribal Councils, Regional Health Boards, and tribes, as well as the federal and territorial governments. They work primarily with school-aged children, and with adults generally seen for emergency treatment only. However, some communities have hired additional therapists to provide dental care for adults in the community. The therapists work as part of the community's health team to target specific problems such as early childhood caries (Chapter 19) and generally to help promote healthy lifestyles.

The Canadian dental therapy program is still not widely known and recognized by organized dentistry and dental hygiene in Canada. It has largely operated outside the Canadian dental establishment because of its protected federal status and the target population it serves.

Denturists

Throughout the 20th century, dental technicians known as denturists have provided denture services in Canada.[10] Denturists were first legally recognized in 1961, and they are now recognized by every province in Canada except Prince Edward Island. There are now about 2000 denturists in Canada.

The Denturist Association of Canada defines denturists as professionals who provide removable dentures directly to patients. Denturists provide their services without any supervision or evaluation by a dentist. They are trained in community colleges or technical institutes to:

- provide visual/tactile oral examination and evaluation
- obtain a complete dental and medical history from a patient

- make impressions and necessary jaw relation records
- select artificial teeth
- design, fabricate, and insert dentures in the mouths of patients
- repair or reline or adjust removable appliances
- supervise auxiliary personnel in the performance of related duties

Students are accepted in the colleges of denturism after completing 2 years of university studies, preferably in science. There are currently 5 regular educational programs and 2 distance education programs in Canada. Denturists are licensed by denturists' boards in every province except Prince Edward Island, and they have their own national association (The Denturist Association of Canada). There is also a Canadian Council of Denturist Educators and an accreditation process for educational programs.

Denturists provide services to elderly and low-income Canadians and have always asserted that their services are less expensive than those provided by dentists. However, a recent review of the fee guides of the Ontario Dental Association and the Denturist Association of Canada found only a minimal difference between dentists' and denturists' fee guides.[1] In Alberta, a province with a universal publicly financed dental program for residents 65 years or older and their dependents, denturists provide about 22% of all new complete dentures.[8] Denturists in Alberta replaced dentures of new patients more often than dentists (20%–21% vs 7% to 8%, respectively).[9] Denturists obtained their legal status by lobbying directly to the public and to provincial legislatures, and it is hardly surprising that their role as members of the oral health team has not yet been endorsed by the 2 main dental organizations in Canada.

Dental Assistants

The current number of dental assistants practicing in Canada is unknown. Certification is not required. In 4 provinces that responded to a survey conducted specifically for this book, there was significant variation in the percentage increase in licensed dental assistants in the 1991–1997 period. In New Brunswick, their numbers increased from 108 to 274, whereas in Prince Edward Island, the increase was only from 116 to 124. In Nova Scotia, the number increased from 482 to 574

and in Saskatchewan from 735 to 842. In addition to their traditional duties, dental assistants are also allowed to take impressions. In Nova Scotia, the dental practice act was amended to allow them to perform rubber cup polishing.

UTILIZATION OF DENTAL CARE

The political and organizational differences between the Canadian and American health care systems were discussed briefly at the beginning of the chapter. Given the availability of universal medical insurance for residents of Canada, income plays only a minor role in determining the likelihood of physician visits.[20] By contrast, however, income plays a more significant role in determining the likelihood of a dental visit.[20] In 1994–1995, about 38% of low-income (lower-quartile) Canadians aged 15 years and above reported visiting a dentist in the previous year, compared with about 70% of Canadians with high income (upper quartile). These findings are generally similar to those in the United States (Chapter 2). Dental insurance coverage also influences dental visits, as does the province of residence (Table 10–3). Gender and age are weakly associated with dental visits.

Dental checkups and "cleanings" were the main reasons reported (96%) for visiting a dentist[22]; the second most commonly-reported reason was tooth filling or extraction. Ten percent of Canadians reported in 1990 that they visited a dentist to receive a crown or bridge in order to replace, repair, or maintain missing or damaged teeth. The percentage who visited a dentist for crown or bridge treatment was higher among high-income Canadians (13%) than among those with low income (7%). These findings too are as expected. Periodontal treatment was the reason for a dental visit for 7% of 45- to 64-year-old Canadians in 1990, and only 4% of Canadians aged 15 years and above had received orthodontic care. Only 7% of Canadians reported visiting a dentist as a result of a dental emergency.

COSTS OF DENTAL CARE

In 1992, the average annual expenditure on dental care by families and "unattached individuals" was $187.[19] This represented a 17.6% increase since 1986.[18] The average ex-

Table 10-3. PROPORTION OF THE DENTATE POPULATION AGED 15 AND ABOVE WHO REPORTED AT LEAST ONE DENTAL VISIT IN THE YEAR PRECEDING THE SURVEY, BY PROVINCE AND DENTAL INSURANCE STATUS, CANADA, 1990

| PROVINCE | VISITED A DENTIST BY DENTAL INSURANCE COVERAGE | |
	INSURED	NOT INSURED
Newfoundland	58	29
Prince Edward Island	54	37
Nova Scotia	59	32
New Brunswick	66	44
Québec	51	37
Ontario	74	56
Manitoba	66	49
Saskatchewan	52	47
Alberta	77	52
British Columbia	68	44
All Canada	66	46

From Stephens T, Fowler Graham D (eds). Canada's Health Promotion Survey, 1990. Technical report. Ottawa: Ministry of Supply and Services, 1993:211–22.

penditure on dental care by Canadian families and unattached individuals was higher than the reported average expenditure on physician care ($109) for services not covered by the national health insurance program. Out-of-pocket payments on dental care represented about 50% of the total expenditures on dental care in Canada.

For group dental insurance plans, the Canadian Life and Health Insurance Association estimated that the total direct claims paid to dentists by private dental insurance companies was $1127 million in 1997. Group private dental insurance covered about 6.7 million beneficiaries (employees and their dependents) in 1996. Payments to dentists by group dental plans increased by 63% between 1988 and 1996. For Administrative Services Only (ASO see Chapter 8) plans, the total benefit payments in 1996 were $1148 million. ASO plans covered 2.8 million employees and 4.1 million dependents (6.9 million beneficiaries). Payment to dentists by ASO plans increased by 138.5% between 1988 and 1996. After several decades of steady growth, enrollment in private dental insurance plans plateaued in the late 1990s, as employers sought to find ways to reduce the costs of their benefit packages for employees.

The cost of dental care increased only modestly in the 1990s after more significant increases in the 1970s and 1980s. Most of the claims (40%) paid by private dental insurance companies in 1992 were for diagnostic and preventive services. The percentage of claims paid for restorative services (25%) did not change between 1973 and 1995. Claims for periodontal care increased from only 4% of the claims in 1973 to 20% of the total claims paid in 1993, whereas claims for dentures declined from 24% to 10% of the total paid to dentists between 1975 and 1993. These data presumably reflect improving oral health status.

Because of the financial pressures on Canadian employers and employees in the 1990s, the cost of dental care has come under some public scrutiny. Some companies either canceled their dental insurance coverage or offered their employees a flexible benefit plan where each employee could decide on the benefits they would like to include (e.g., vision, dental, medical, or long-term disability) in the fixed financial benefit package offered by the employer. Managed dental care plans on the United States model (Chapter 8) have not yet widely penetrated the Canadian dental market. The Canadian and provincial dental associations strongly oppose the concepts of managed care, reduced fees, or flexible benefit plans, although this policy stance may have little effect on eventual developments in dental care financing.

ORAL HEALTH STATUS

Most oral health data available are for Canadian children. Whereas dental caries experience declined during the 1980s in Canada,[14] a slight increase in caries prevalence and severity was observed in Ontario.[17] Ontario is the most popular Canadian province for immigrants, and it is likely that the relative increase in the number of immigrants from developing countries into Ontario during the 1990s contributed to this change. Children of new immigrants have a higher prevalence of dental caries and a lower level of oral health knowledge.[3] There is evidence that dental caries prevalence among children in Québec is higher by about 40% than that in the United States.[13] Levels of tooth loss are similar to those found in the United States (Chapter 18).

PROVISION OF PUBLIC DENTAL CARE IN CANADA

Unlike medical care, dental care in Canada is not part of the universal health care system (except for major oral surgical services provided in hospitals). The dental care system generally parallels the organization, structure, and standards found in the United States. Most dental care is provided by independent private dental practitioners and, as described previously is almost exclusively financed by personal resources or group dental prepayment plans.

Nearly all provinces have dental public health programs, many of which were initiated in the 1970s. There is considerable variation among the provinces in terms of program goals and operation, as well as resources allocated. A constant theme, as in many countries at the end of the 20th century, is that public budgets for public health are shrinking, and programs must be efficient to survive. Before individual provincial plans are described, one local program and one provincial program that have adapted to resource cuts are discussed.

North York Public Health Department

North York is just north of Toronto. The North York dental program, which now serves a population of 560,000, began in 1939 when a plebiscite calling for provision of dental treatment for children was approved. Dental clinics were established in elementary schools in North York, and the program started with 2 dentists providing emergency dental care. An incremental treatment program was also developed and preventive services were added (fluoride and dental health education). In 1975, the programs employed 45 dentists and 9 dental hygienists. From that time, the program reached almost 100% of all targeted schoolchildren. The improvements in the oral health status of the children led to staff reductions, and by 1992 the program had 29 dentists, 5 hygienists, and 8 educators. In 1991–1992, about 24,000 children used the program as their main source of dental care.

The North York program entered a new phase in the 1990s, a time when Ontario enacted severe budget cuts in health care and education. The resulting further staff losses demanded innovations if the same level of service was to be provided with fewer resources. The North York dental leadership collaborated with the Department of Community Dentistry at the University of Toronto to obtain a grant from the Ontario government that supported a quality assurance and research program. This collaborative program sponsored reviews of programmatic outcomes and went on to develop evidence-based program guidelines. This approach permitted the North York dental department to continue to provide care for children even after the 1992 budget cut of 25%.

Another innovation was the introduction of the "gatekeeper" approach for identification of children at high risk of dental disease. In this program, dental hygienists act as gatekeepers to screen out the 60% of the children who are free from new carious lesions or other conditions requiring immediate treatment. Hence, the program in North York has moved from universal and routine provision of care for all children to targeted provision of preventive and treatment services to children with disease. The gatekeepers screen students first and categorize them into three groups: no care required, prevention-only required, and treatment required. For those children who need preventive care, children are categorized into those who need sealants, fluoride, or scaling, or any combination of these services. In the treatment group, students are categorized into those who need regular or urgent care. In 1992, the program provided care for about 45% of all children in North York. The program provides dental care for children whose parents do not have private dental insurance or cannot afford the cost of dental care.

Using the evidence-based methodology developed by the Canadian Task Force on the Periodic Health Examination,[25] several new program guidelines were developed.[2] These guidelines sought to identify dental procedures that provided uncertain benefits but contributed significantly to treatment costs. These included professional fluoride applications, universal sealants (rather than targeted sealant placement), space maintainers, and ill-timed restorations. Additionally, the program identified the most appropriate staff to provide each service; fluoride and sealants now are provided exclusively by dental hygienists in the North York program. The shift of care provision from dentists to hygienists resulted in a reduction in the number of dentists hired and the hours of work for dentists. Staff reorganization into multidisciplinary teams yielded further efficiencies.

As a result of these changes, preventive services are provided to approximately 15%–20% of the children and sealants to about 10% of the screened population. The cost savings are significant and allow the program to provide an extensive safety net, even in an age of uncertain public budgets. Evaluation of the target population found no decline in oral health status after the new program was introduced.

The Nova Scotia Children's Oral Health Program

Nova Scotia (population 937,800) has had a universal publicly financed dental insurance program for children since 1974. Under this program, private dentists could provide care for all children and bill the provincial government directly for their services. That program is now considered a "right" for residents of Nova Scotia, and the provincial dental association has succeeded in promoting the view that it is an efficient way to meet children's dental care needs. However, the Nova Scotia experience raises questions about economic efficiency in public programs of this type.

When the Nova Scotia dental program was established in 1974, it covered children up to their ninth birthday, and its total cost in its first year was $846,632. In 1976–1977, the dental examination schedule was changed from once to twice per year, resulting in a 10% increase in the base budget of $2 million. Through the 1970s and early 1980s, fees paid to dentists increased by about 10% annually. In 1982–1983, the age of eligibility was increased to include adolescents up to their 16th birthday, and the total budget of the program reached more than $10 million. Also in 1982–1983, frenectomies were included as a covered benefit, followed by space maintainers in 1984–1985. In 1985–1986, limited extraction of primary teeth to prevent orthodontic problems was covered. In 1987–1988, sealants were denied inclusion on the grounds that there was little information on cost-benefit ratios. Program cuts began during the 1990s. In 1990–1991, the eligibility age was reduced from the 16th to the 14th birthday, and space maintainers were excluded from the plan. In 1991–1992, the eligibility age was cut back further to end at the 12th birthday. All of these programmatic decisions were more or less arbitrary; no evaluation of the efficacy of the various services included and excluded, nor of the ages of eligibility, was conducted.

In 1994–1995, the Nova Scotia Department of Health conducted an evaluation of the program.[12] The review identified the following:

- The average cost of care per child did not change between 1983–1984 and 1993–1994 after adjusting for inflation.
- Between 1983–1984 and 1993–1994 there was an increase in the utilization of diagnostic and preventive services and a decrease in the provision of restorative services.
- About 80% of the children older than 4 years in the province visited a dentist in 1993–1994, but dental attendance of children between birth and 3 years of age is low (7%, 20%, 60% at the ages of 1, 2, and 3 years, respectively).
- More than $2 million was paid in 1993–1994 for diagnostic services. About 78% went for examinations and 21% for radiographs. Nearly three-quarters of payments were for children receiving routine recall examinations.
- 96% of all fluoride applications were preceded by a dental prophylaxis. The total cost of these services exceeded $2 million.
- 70% of all restorations were amalgams.
- In permanent teeth, pits and fissures were the most commonly restored sites.
- In primary molars, mesial and distal surfaces were the most commonly restored sites.

With severe budget cuts looming, a new program was designed after a critical literature review of various dental procedures and extensive consultations with several stakeholders. In this new program, dentists remained the primary care providers because of the opposition to the use of North York-style "gatekeepers." All children were covered up to the 10th birthday. The program paid for an annual examination and for preventive services where needed. Rubber cup polishing was covered only for children with heavy calculus accumulations or staining. Two annual fluoride applications were permitted only for children who had smooth surface caries (the definition of high-risk children). Treatment services were covered for children with severe caries; for those with medical, physical, or mental challenges; or for children whose parents declared financial hardship. In addition to the dental care program, 14 dental hygienists continued to be employed to provide education, to supervise the fluoride rinse programs in schools in high caries areas, and to organize an education and prevention program for health care professionals and caregivers who work with mothers and infants.

After the new program was announced, the dental profession strongly opposed it even though its representatives were involved in all stages of its development. Opposition centered on the elimination of rubber cup polishing as a universal service, and the restriction of treatment only to children with high caries experience, medical-physical-mental challenges, or families with financial hardships. There was also opposition to asking patients to complete the form for declaration of financial status.

After significant lobbying by the dental profession, the program was modified in 1997 to cover children with any treatment need, not just high-risk children. A new procedure was introduced that was defined as a "Caries Preventive Service" and that was assigned the same fee as polishing of teeth, but dentists could provide any of the following services during a 15-minute window: plaque disclosure, flossing and tooth brushing instruction, or selective polishing. Sealants were retained. Although guidelines for fluoride application remained unchanged, dentists did not use the opportunity for a second fluoride application for high-risk children. Of the 14,000 children who met the fluoride application guidelines during the first 9 months of 1997, only 200 received a second fluoride application.

PROVINCIAL DENTAL PUBLIC HEALTH PROGRAMS

Water fluoridation was adopted in Canada at about the same time as in the United States. In 1986, when the last national census of water fluoridation was carried out, 39.2% of Canadians on treated water systems received fluoridated water.[7] Québec and British Columbia were the least fluoridated provinces in Canada (11.6% and 12.7%, respectively), and Ontario had the highest percentage of its population receiving fluoridated water (63.4%). A Nova Scotia study found that 15% of its water wells had fluoride levels between 0.3 and 0.7 ppm, 5% had levels at 0.7 to 1.2 ppm, and 2% had levels above 1.2 ppm.[6] There has not been much change in the proportion of population receiving fluoridated water through the 1990s, and, as in the United States, there are sporadic local successes and failures.

All provinces, as mandated by the Canada Health Act, cover hospital-based oral surgical care for all people. Some provinces also provide for medically-necessary extractions, or complicated third molar extractions. In addition, most provinces have dental programs for patients with cleft lip and palate that not only cover the cost of plastic surgery but also dental treatments.

Ontario

The province of Ontario now has a population of more than 11 million. Local health department personnel regularly screen schoolchildren, and the findings form the basis for targeted educational and preventive programs. The screenings also identify children who have high treatment needs, defined by the presence of large carious lesions, infection, trauma, pathology, or irreversible periodontal disease (Children in Need of Treatment, or CINOT). Private dentists may also refer children to the local health department dental clinics for assessment when CINOT criteria are met. The treatment program is offered to children from birth to 15 years. The parents of the children with high treatment needs are so informed, and if the family meets the standards for financial hardship, the children are eligible for a one-time coverage for all necessary care. The dental services are provided either by salaried dentists employed by local health departments or by contracted private dentists. If the parents have private dental insurance or they do not wish to declare financial hardship, they are legally responsible for getting the necessary dental care for their child. The total cost of the CINOT program in Ontario was about $11 million in 1994.

The Ministry of Health also sponsors a surveillance program of 5- to 14-year-old students by annual surveys of the dental status of children in the odd-numbered ages. Data from these surveys are used for targeting of services.

Other programs in Ontario include the Hospital Cleft Lip and Palate program that covers major oral surgery for all children with these conditions. Educational programs for parents and day-care centers are also offered to promote oral health early in life.

Prince Edward Island Dental Program

In contrast to the nearby Nova Scotia dental program, the Prince Edward Island (population 136,100) Dental Program was designed in 1971 to provide care through school-based dental clinics and salaried dentists. At the time of the program's inception, dental caries was highly prevalent, and only 20% of the children visited a dentist regularly. The shortage of dentists on the island at that time led to the development of a school-based dental clinical program. The program started by targeting 6-year-old children and expanded incrementally.

Between 1971 and 1977, dental services were delivered by teams consisting of a salaried dentist, extended-duty dental hygienists who were trained in placing and finishing restorations, a receptionist, and dental assistants who were trained to provide preventive services. By the early 1980s, the program expanded to include children 13 to 16 years old. In 1983, the upper age eligibility limit was reduced to 12 years because of government budget cuts, although the full program was reinstated in 1986. Pit-and-fissure sealants were introduced in 1978 and have had a major impact on the reduction of occlusal dental caries in the province.[16]

Owing to budget cuts and political considerations, the policy of exclusive reliance on salaried dentists to provide all the care to the children gradually changed to one using contracted private dentists. In 1996, approximately three-quarters of the children were treated by private dentists, although salaried public health dental teams continue to provide preventive services. The program has an 80% utilization rate by eligible children. The services offered by the program are summarized in Table 10-4.

Funding is provided from general revenues of the province and from an annual registration fee of $15 per child, with a maximum of $35 per family. The collection of the annual registration fee from patients attending private dental clinics is the responsibility of the dentists, and this amount is deducted from the claims submitted once a year. The fees paid to the private dentists are negotiated and published annually, and dentists are not permitted to extra-bill patients for covered services. They can bill patients for noncovered services.

Table 10-4. DENTAL SERVICES PROVIDED IN THE PRINCE EDWARD ISLAND DENTAL CARE PROGRAM

CATEGORY	LIST OF SERVICES
Diagnostic	One annual examination Annual bitewing radiographs (2 only) Emergency examinations Periapical radiographs (when necessary)
Preventive	Topical fluoride application Oral hygiene instruction School classroom dental education Cleaning and polishing Dietary counseling Pit and fissure sealants
Treatment	Dental restorations Emergency treatment Extractions Acrylic partial denture to replace maxillary anterior teeth Endodontics treatment on anterior teeth
Orthodontic	Preventive and interceptive orthodontic treatment, where it can be provided, using simple removable orthodontic appliances

From Maze B. Dental Director, Prince Edward Island's Queen's Region Health and Community Services Agency, 1997.

The program is popular and is politically well supported. Its success can be largely attributed to data collection by the program that permitted sound evaluation of its success. These data showed that the average decayed, missing, and filled permanent teeth (DMFT) (see Chapter 14) of 12-year-old children decreased from approximately 3.5 to 1.7 in the 10 years between 1985–1986 and 1995–1996, and the percentage of caries-free 12-year-old children increased from 25% to 40% during the same period. This improvement was achieved without increasing the budget of the program. The precise impact of the program on the oral health status of children cannot be determined because of the lack of a control group, but that is true when evaluating any public health program. A public program is not a clinical trial (see Chapter 12).

Starting in 1990, a new dental program was introduced for residents of long-term facilities whereby they are screened by a dentist for signs of dental pain, infection, or other pathology. Simple preventive or treatment services (such as denture cleaning or labeling) are provided, and in-service sessions on the provision of preventive dental care are provided for the resident care workers.

Québec

Québec (population 7,334,000) has invested since the early 1970s in school-based dental public health programs, as well as a dental insurance program for children in which publicly funded care is provided by private dentists. Both programs were significantly reorganized in the early 1990s. At present, dental hygienists and public health dentists located in regional health centers provide screening and preventive care to school-children. Sealants are not yet offered to the children because of a dispute over the level of supervision for hygienists working for the health department. The dental insurance program pays for diagnostic and treatment services to children up to the ninth birthday. It covers an annual examination, bitewing radiographs, anesthesia, fillings and crowns, pulp therapy, and extraction. Preventive services are not included because they are offered by the public health program.

Newfoundland

Newfoundland (population 575,400) maintains a publicly financed dental insurance program for children. It is administered by the department of health and private dentists provide the care. The program covers children from birth to 12 years of age and includes an annual examination, radiographs, rubber cup polishing, and fluoride application starting at the age of 6 years. The program also covers restorations, pulp therapy for anterior teeth, extractions, and emergency care. There is a $5 co-pay for restorations and extractions. There is no other dental public health program in Newfoundland.

New Brunswick

There is no public health dentist or dental hygienist working for the province (population 760,100). The only program is dental health education, integrated with other health education and organized by community health nurses. The oral health status of the children in New Brunswick is not known.

Manitoba

Budget cuts destroyed an extensive children's dental program in 1993, when Mani-toba (population 1,137,000) cancelled the treatment component and reduced the program staff from 70 to 2.[5] The community dental health program now consists only of oral health education as part of the core educational program.

Saskatchewan

Saskatchewan (population 1,015,600) achieved considerable attention in the 1970s with its extensive school-based program in which care was provided by dental therapists trained on the model of the New Zealand school dental nurse. However, this program was cut by a conservative government in 1987, with children's dental treatment transferred to private dental practitioners between 1987 and 1993. All remaining dental programs were cut in 1993, except the one in northern Saskatchewan, which provides dental care for 3–16 year-olds. It had previously been reduced in 1985, when the treatment component was transferred to private practitioners and the staff reduced from 400 to 18.

Alberta

Alberta (population 2,747,000) is unusual in dental public health circles in that it never had a dental program for children, but instead developed the "largest universal dental plan for the elderly in North America."[8] Alberta's Extended Health Benefits (EHB) dental plan, which covers all residents 65 years or older and their dependents, began in 1973. The plan also covers the dental care provided to low-income widows and widowers aged 55–64 years. The plan has no premium and is funded entirely by the provincial budget. Although the dental benefits are broadly defined, there are restrictions on services provided and on total payments. In 1995, reductions in the annual budget from $29 million to $17 million led to the discontinuation of fluoride applications, crowns, bridges, prophylaxis, tooth bleaching, and orthodontics.[11]

Private dentists and denturists provide the dental care for elderly individuals. In 1990–1991, the average annual payment was $26,000 to dentists and $9800 to denturists.[8] In 1997, fees paid for services represented only 35% of the Alberta Dental Association fee guide. Dentists and denturists are allowed to bill patients directly for the balance of the usual fee, a practice referred to as "balance billing," provided that the patients are so informed before treatment.

In 1991–1992, 44% of eligible residents had a dental claim submitted on their behalf. An evaluation of the plan showed that between 1978–1979 and 1991–1992 there was a decline in restorative and surgical services provided by dentists from 24% to 19%. Preventive services grew modestly (12% to 16%), and periodontal services grew from 3% to 22% of all services provided by the dentists.[23]

In addition to the EHB program, regional departments of health organize school-based preventive and educational programs. Calgary and Edmonton have dental clinical programs, provided by the local health departments, which care for low-income residents. Some regions have fluoride rinse or sealant programs, and some health units provide fluoride supplements.[11]

British Columbia

British Columbia (population 3,766,000) may hold the record for a short-lived dental program, having begun a dental insurance program that was terminated after 1 year. Currently, the province has a "health passport" program in which infants and toddlers are eligible for 1 free dental check-up before the age of 3 years.[11] There is also a screening program for 5–6 year-olds carried out by a dental assistant. Children are classified into groups based on past caries experience; parents are informed of the findings, but no treatment is covered. The province pays for urgent dental care of children whose parents are classified as "working poor," although this program covered only 4% of eligible children in 1995.[11]

British Columbia also has a school-based program targeting 20% of the schools whose children have "high caries" prevalence. The program provides education and oral hygiene instructions.

FEDERAL DENTAL PUBLIC HEALTH PROGRAMS

Medical Services Branch (MSB), Health Canada

This unit was established in 1962 by Health Canada, the federal department of health, to provide dental services to members of the First Nations and Inuit communities. The services provided were intended to be "analogous to those available to other Cana-

dians living in similar geographic areas." The program has 3 types of providers: salaried, contract, and fee-for-service. The salaried dentists provide clinical, preventive, and administrative services. The staff usually includes a Regional Dental Officer, community-based dental therapists, dental assistants, and clerks. In 1997, about 90 salaried dental therapists worked in the program.

Contract providers include dentists or dental assistants, working in nursing stations or health centers, who provide services on a per diem and fee-for-service basis. The program also contracts with denturists, orthodontists, oral surgeons, and pediatric dentists to provide dental care. Reimbursement of these providers is generally based on a fee-for-service arrangement, and the contractual component provides per-diem rates and travel expenses. Total contractual expenditures in 1997 were approximately $9 million.

A fee-for-service dental insurance program covers members of the First Nations and Inuit tribes living in any part of Canada, including urban areas where private dentists are available. This program covers all regular dental care services. The program budget in 1996–1997 was about $95 million.

The MSB program experienced an increase in utilization between 1990 and 1995 from 32% to 39%, as well as a 43% increase in the volume of services provided. The dental program budget was thus increased by 67%. The major increases in services through the mid-1990s occurred in periodontics (92%) and orthodontics (178%). Like the North York and Nova Scotia dental insurance programs, the MSB dental program is now evaluating the scientific basis for covered services and treatment outcomes,[4] which means that changes may be made in this program.

Other Federal Dental Programs

The federal government, through its block funding to the provinces, shares the cost of dental care for recipients of social assistance. Local municipalities administer this dental program, which mostly covers basic dental or emergency care for children, adults, or seniors on social assistance. In some provinces, an age limit and a low annual maximum ($400–$500) are set for dental care. Dental care provided under the social assistance program therefore is limited.

The federal government also pays for the dental care, provided by contract dentists, of inmates in its correctional facilities. Dental care for the Royal Canadian Mounted Police is covered by a group dental plan administered by a third party.

The Canadian armed forces have had a dental corps since 1915.[15] The high prevalence of dental caries among recruits, especially during both world wars, led to the expansion of the corps and the services it provides. In the 1990s, private dentists were contracted to provide care on military bases in Canada, and a smaller force of dental officers was retained to serve in the United Nations' Peace Keeping Forces and to be ready for active duty. Utilization of the armed forces dental services is high.

FUTURE DEVELOPMENTS

The health care system developed in Canada has several interesting characteristics: equal access to health care, simplicity of administration, and lower cost as a percentage of the GDP compared with the United States. Canadians deeply value their health care system, and they consider it a right for all residents regardless of employment status. Dental care, unfortunately, is not part of the national health care system. Nonetheless, some community-based dental care programs have been leaders in adapting to the lean budgets of the 1990s. With the 21st century, however, the survival of many community oral health programs is threatened. The severe cuts of the last decade, added to the lack of support from organized dentistry and the dental schools, have the potential of returning Canada to a period in which dental care is a luxury enjoyed only by the well-to-do.

The Canadian experience with universal publicly financed dental insurance programs for children has shed light on the pitfalls associated with dental care systems that do not conduct rigorous self-evaluation, and whose delivery of care is routine, redundant, and without clear, measurable outcomes. These are lessons for public health programs anywhere in the world.

The future of dentistry in Canada depends on the economic health of the country. This in turn depends on how Canada will deal with the strong regional political agenda (Québec, British Columbia, and Alberta) and the environment of political uncertainty about the status of the federation and the survival of some its provinces. In Canada, as elsewhere, dental public health units are losing their traditional independence and are merging with the rest of community health units. Community-based dental care will survive if dental public health personnel can make that adaptation.

ACKNOWLEDGMENTS

The authors would like to thank the following individuals and organizations for providing data that were used in writing this chapter: Dr. Patricia Main, North York Public Health Department; Dr. Steven Wolfson, National School of Dental Therapy, Saskatchewan; Dr. Barry Maze, Prince Edward Island Dental Program; Ms. Joanne Clovis, School of Dental Hygiene, Halifax; Dr. Pauline Murphy Sutow, Nova Scotia Medical Services Insurance; Dr. Jack D. Gerrow, National Dental Examining Board of Canada; Ms. Alice Freeburn, Canadian Life and Health Insurance Association Inc.; Dr. Peter Cooney, Medical Service Branch, Health Canada; Canadian Dental Association; Dental Council of Prince Edward Island; Saskatchewan Dental Board; Provincial Dental Board of Nova Scotia; and Provincial Dental Board of New Brunswick.

REFERENCES

1. Abrams SH. Denturists: Do they really provide more affordable care in Ontario? J Can Dent Assoc 1997;63:771–4.
2. Brothwell DJ. Guidelines on the use of space maintainers following premature loss of primary teeth. J Can Dent Assoc 1997;63:753–66.
3. Clarke M, Locker D, Jokovic A. The oral health of grade 8 students in North York: A comparison between Canadian-born and immigrant adolescents. Toronto: Community Dental Health Services Research Unit, Faculty of Dentistry, 1996.
4. Cooney PV, Lavelle CC. Do regional differences preclude a national dental insurance program? A strategic analysis. Can J Community Health 1996;11:13–20.
5. DesMarias B. News from Western Canada. Can J Community Dent 1995;10:6–7.
6. Dingle J, Underhill K, Ismail AI, MacInnis WA. Fluoride analysis of Nova Scotia domestic water. Can J Community Dent 1997;12:31–7.
7. Health and Welfare Canada, Health Canada. Fluoridation census as of December 31, 1986. Ottawa: Department of National Health and Welfare, 1987.
8. Lewis DW, Thompson GW. Utilization in Alberta's Universal Dental Plan for the elderly, 1974–91. J Public Health Dent 1992;5:259–63.
9. Lewis DW, Thompson GW. Denture replacement during a 14-year period in Alberta's universal dental plan for the elderly. J Prosthet Dent 1995;74:264–9.
10. Macentee MI. Denturists and oral health in the aged. J Prosthet Dent 1994;71:192–6.

11. Main P. Dental public health programs across Canada. Can J Community Dent 1995;10:12–4.
12. Nova Scotia Department of Health. Review of children's dental health services. Halifax: Nova Scotia Department of Health, 1994.
13. Payette M, Brodeur JM, Lepage Y, Plante R. Enquete Santê Dentairé Québec. Montreal: Le Centre de Coordination de Santé Communautaire, 1991.
14. Payette M, Brodeur JM. Comparison of dental caries and oral hygiene indices for 13- to 14-year-old Québec children between 1977 and 1989–1990. J Can Dent Assoc 1992;58:921–33.
15. Protheroe DH. Seventy-five years of military dentistry in Canada. J Can Dent Assoc 1990;56:265–8.
16. Romcke RG, Lewis DW, Maze BD, Vickerson RA. Retention and maintenance of fissure sealants over 10 years. J Can Dent Assoc 1990;56:235–7.
17. Speechley M, Johnston DW. Some evidence from Ontario, Canada, of a reversal in the dental caries decline. Caries Res 1996;30:423–7.
18. Statistics Canada. Family expenditure in Canada, 1986. Ottawa: Statistics Canada, 1989:36.
19. Statistics Canada. Family expenditure in Canada, 1992. Ottawa: Statistics Canada, 1994:30.
20. Statistics Canada. National Population Health Survey Overview, 1994–95. Ottawa: Statistics Canada, 1995:14.
21. Statistics Canada. Canada Yearbook 97. Ottawa: Statistics Canada, 1997:33, 83–4, 448.
22. Stephens T, Fowler Graham D, eds. Canada's Health Promotion Survey, 1990. Technical report. Ottawa: Ministry of Supply and Services, 1993:211–22.
23. Thompson W, Lewis DW. Changes in utilization of dental services of Alberta's Universal Dental Plan for elderly. J Can Dent Assoc 1994;60:403–6.
24. Wilson DM. The Canadian health care system. Edmonton: Donna Wilson, Faculty of Nursing, University of Alberta, 1995:95.
25. Woolf SH, Battista RN, Anderson GM, et al. Methodology. In: Goldboom RB, ed: Canadian Task Force on the Periodic Health Examination. The Canadian guide to clinical preventive health care. Ottawa: Minister of Supply and Services Canada, 1994:xxv–xxxviii.

11

Reading the Dental Literature

Textbooks and Peer-Reviewed Journals ◆ Judging the
Quality of a Journal ◆ Critical Reading: Evaluating a
Published Report ◆ A Hierarchy of the Quality of
Information ◆ Criteria for Judging the Quality of a
Report ◆ Finding the Reports You Need in the Literature

The *literature* is the generic name given
to the body of writing in books, journals,
reports, and other sources that makes up the
sum of knowledge in a branch of science. In
dentistry's case we refer to the *dental literature.* The literature, however, is more than
just our compendium of knowledge and our
scientific base; it is our very identity. It defines who we are and what we do; it charts
the progress of dentistry to its present status
and provides guidelines for future directions.

Technologic and social developments in
dentistry are proceeding at a speed that can
be bewildering. Although dental and dental
hygiene graduates learn enough in professional school to begin practice, "keeping up"
is absolutely essential for professional
growth. Attendance at continuing education
courses is one way to do so (indeed such
attendance is required in many states), but
the literature is the primary source of new
knowledge. Electronic information sources
are developing rapidly, but it will be a long
time before the professional journal, in its
current form, becomes obsolete. It follows,
therefore, that dentists and hygienists must
keep familiar with those sections of the literature that most concern them if they are to
function properly. To do this, they need to be
able to locate the literature they need and to
read it critically, they need to distinguish
front-line from mediocre journals and to be
aware of how to distinguish good from poor
research. Acquiring these skills requires some
time and practice, but confidence with them
will pay off in helping practitioners use their

time efficiently while they grow professionally. This chapter describes how to locate
needed information and how to read the literature efficiently.

Professional training, unfortunately, does
not usually include critical reading. The usual
progression begins with accepting the veracity of reports unquestioningly and without
conscious thought, because "if it wasn't true
it wouldn't be printed." After being misled a
few times, readers can become increasingly
skeptical. In extremes, they can move full circle from believing everything they read to
believing nothing. The ideal course is between the two extremes, somewhere between
blind acceptance and blanket distrust.

TEXTBOOKS AND PEER-REVIEWED
JOURNALS

Textbooks are the most familiar source
of information for students. Although good
books may be the first source to be consulted
on a subject, books can soon become dated.
The copy a student buys from the bookshop
may be new, but if it was published 10 years
ago then at least parts of it risk being obsolete. All books have some degree of built-in
obsolescence, for the material when delivered
to the publisher can be several years old, and
the publication process often takes another
year before the book appears on the shelves.
That proviso accepted, the best textbooks
present the state-of-the-science, at least at the
date of publication.

Journals are the basic source of current

information in any field, dentistry included. The number of journals in dentistry, as in most other fields, has proliferated in recent years. It is virtually impossible for anyone to keep up with all journals, so selectivity is needed. There are good journals and poor ones, and there are some clues to picking which is which. The most basic is that good journals are all peer-reviewed.

Peer review means that manuscripts, when first received by the journal editor, are sent out to be reviewed by several experts in the field of study covered in the manuscript. Usually two reviewers are selected, sometimes more. The identity of the reviewers is not known to the authors. Some journals, although not all, also mask the identity of the authors from the reviewers in an effort to remove any bias from the reviewers' judgment. The reviewers' task is to assess the manuscript critically for scientific method, logic, manner of presentation, and any other feature that might reflect on its value in the literature. Poor-quality manuscripts can be rejected outright at this stage or returned to the authors for revision if the problems are less severe. Most journal papers are returned to the authors for revisions at least once before acceptance. Many prestigious journals, such as the *New England Journal of Medicine*, reject far more manuscripts than they publish; reviewing standards are rigorous. The top dental journals publish well under half of the manuscripts they receive.

Peer review is a system that has evolved down the years, and there is no question that it has served to greatly elevate the standards of published material. Like all human institutions, however, it is not perfect. For example, peer review can suffer when inappropriate reviewers are chosen, either because they are not sufficiently expert in the field of study or because their own prejudices get in the way of an objective review. More common, perhaps, are reviewers who simply do not give a manuscript the attention it deserves. An inherent problem is the tendency of the peer-review process to inhibit original research or creativity, to push imaginative thoughts into a safe middle ground. Overall, however, the still-evolving system of peer review has served to elevate the quality of the literature.

Judging the Quality of a Journal

The first step in judging a journal's quality is to find out whether it is peer reviewed.

Some say so in their sections on instructions to contributors (which often only appear at the beginning or end of volume numbers), although many do not mention the topic. If 3 or more copies of a manuscript are requested, it is likely that some level of peer review takes place, but it may take a phone call to find out.

The second thing to find out is the journal's sponsorship: who puts it out? Here are 4 broad categories of sponsorship:

A Learned Society: These societies frequently present the best and most important research papers; they are formed for the purpose of promoting and disseminating research findings. Some, like the International Association for Dental Research (IADR), promote dental research in all fields; others are for research in specialized or semispecialized areas. Journals from learned societies are invariably peer-reviewed, usually with a strong emphasis on scientific rigor. These journals are characterized by a straightforward format with relative absence of advertising, a strong editorial board, and explicit instructions to contributors. Unfortunately, a relatively small circulation often makes them expensive as well.

A Professional Organization: The best journals in this category, such as *The New England Journal of Medicine* and the *Journal of the American Medical Association*, rank among the most prestigious in biomedicine. The majority of journals in this group are peer-reviewed. In contrast to the journals from learned societies, there can be more bias shown in choice of publications: there can be a tendency to publish papers favorable to the organization's views, and to not publish papers with contrary views, regardless of their quality. These journals can carry a fair amount of advertising, which together with wide distribution to the association's membership keeps the price moderate. In the better journals, advertising material has to pass editorial scrutiny for factual content and taste.

A Reputable Scientific Publisher: Some journals from publishers of medical and dental texts are produced to fill a need: *Community Dentistry Oral Epidemiology,* and *Journal of Periodontal Research*, both published by Munksgaard in Copenhagen, Denmark, are examples. The best journals in this group are rigorously peer-reviewed and generally are the equal of those from learned societies in quality of publications.

A Commercial Publisher: These journals

comprise a category often referred to as "throwaways," and some can be more accurately described as magazines rather than journals. They carry a lot of advertising, which often permits them to be distributed free of charge, and their articles are often written by professional in-house staff. Some do take contributed papers, but peer review is unusual. The scientific quality of this group of journals is usually not high, for that is not their intention. These journals fill a niche, so long as readers recognize them for what they are.

The third step in quality determination is to look for a list of an editorial board, advisory board, or list of consultants. These terms can be used loosely and interchangeably, and the functions of these groups can vary widely from taking an active role in journal policies to being little more than window dressing. The presence of such a list, however, suggests that the journal is at least trying to maintain standards.

As the fourth step, a reader should be able to judge the nature of the papers from a quick perusal: research reports, opinion pieces, reviews, political commentary. Most important, the reader should be able to tell which is which. Looking over the editorials, in those journals that carry them, can give a feeling for any particular political stance the journal may carry.

The fifth step can be to scan the advertising for the products and services presented, and the advertising style. Better-quality journals either have no advertising, or a reasonably restrained style. Look for some statement of advertising policy, such as is found in the advertising index of each issue of the *Journal of the American Dental Association.*

Finally, the production standards should be checked. Typographical errors, lack of consistency, and inadequate citations in references can make a reader wonder what else is wrong that may be less readily apparent.

CRITICAL READING: EVALUATING A PUBLISHED REPORT

A Hierarchy of the Quality of Information

As far as possible, knowledge on which our treatment procedures and other actions are based should come from the results of carefully structured research designs, free of bias, minimizing random error, and carried out with human subjects. That is inherently impossible in some instances and simply lacking in others, so a reader needs to judge the source of information carefully when assessing the state of knowledge on any subject. The quality of source information on human studies can be expressed in a hierarchy from excellent to weak, as shown in Table 11–1.

Other hierarchies for grading the quality of scientific information have been developed—for example, that used by the US Preventive Services Task Force[2] to assess the scientific basis for preventive interventions. The US Task Force approach was itself based on a hierarchical scale developed earlier in Canada[1] to grade the evidence for various tests used in the routine physical examination. Table 11–1 is a slightly expanded but philosophically similar version of these scales.

The categories listed are broad, and there are many gray overlapping areas. In addition, many questions in dentistry are just not amenable to testing in randomized trials, either for ethical reasons (are amalgams harmful to human health?) or inherent difficulties (is group practice more efficient than solo practice?). In such instances, evidence from less-rigorous study designs simply must suffice. Case studies can be helpful in guiding appropriate treatment, but their outcomes are too subject to the vagaries of the doctor-patient relationship to count as firm scientific evidence. The opinion of an acknowledged expert is always worth listening to, but by itself it is not evidence for a particular relationship between 2 or more factors.

In many areas of basic science, animal studies and other laboratory experiments are a major source of information applied to humans. The fundamentals of trials with rats, hamsters, guinea pigs, dogs, monkeys, and other animals used in studies are the same as those for trials with humans. The reader should be sensitive to the special complications in animal studies: was the strain of rat used susceptible to the disease? Were the results potentially biased by an undue number of deaths in one group?

An ever-present difficulty with animal studies is the extent to which results should be applied to humans. The same concern applies to all laboratory procedures: does the dental enamel in the test tube react the same way as it does in the mouth? Are the bacteria produced from pure culture the same as those found in the oral environment? The ideal oc-

Table 11–1. A HIERARCHY OF THE QUALITY OF SCIENTIFIC SOURCE INFORMATION IN HUMAN STUDIES (BEGINNING FROM THE BEST QUALITY AND WORKING DOWN TO THE WEAKEST)

1. Experimental studies, or clinical trials in humans, in which all criteria described under *Experimental Study Designs* (Chapter 12) are observed.
2. Experimental trials in humans that employ concurrent controls, but in which other factors described under *Experimental Study Designs* are missing. The more that these factors are missing or inadequately satisfied, the greater the threat to validity.
3. Rigorously-controlled cohort and case-control studies.
4. Clinical trials without concurrent control groups, such as before-and-after designs. The better examples here can be considered equal to item 3.
5. Retrospective cross-sectional studies without controls, in which a group's oral health status is matched against some past exposure to suspected disease-causing or disease-preventing agents.
6. Descriptive surveys, where present oral health is surveyed and there is informed speculation on the influences which led to the observed status.
7. Case reports.
8. Personal opinion, subjective impressions, anecdotal accounts.

From the scales used in: (a) Canadian Task Force on the Periodic Health Examination. The periodic health examination. J Can Med Assoc 1979;121:1193–1254. (b) US Preventive Services Task Force. Guide for clinical preventive services. 2nd ed. Washington DC: US Department of Health and Human Services, 1996.

currence for reaching conclusions is when results from laboratory studies are confirmed in humans, but again this happy circumstance is often not possible.

In reaching a conclusion on a subject from reading the literature, the quality of the evidence must be considered. So too must the quantity. A good number of high-quality studies, all reaching more or less the same conclusions, allows a judgment to be reached quite easily. Sometimes, however, evidence is more mixed: few studies of any kind, many studies but variable quality, or many studies but variable quality and mixed results. The literature on many issues can be equivocal to some extent, and an association between one factor and another is usually not taken as documented unless the weight of evidence in the literature strongly favors it.

Criteria for Judging the Quality of a Report

There are essentially 3 kinds of papers published in journals: (a) research reports, meaning reports of original clinical, basic, or epidemiologic research; (b) reviews of the literature to summarize knowledge in a particular area; and (c) commentaries, where some documented facts are used as a basis for urging program development, methodological procedures, or some other kind of action. Combinations of 2 or 3 of these are common. The qualities that characterize good examples of each kind can be listed as follows.

Research Reports

The essential features to look for when reading the literature can be presented in semichecklist form. The list may seem rather long at first, but with practice readers will soon apply these criteria quickly, almost unconsciously in some instances. The goal in fact is that their application will become an automatic feature of reading the literature.

General Issues

1. Nature of the journal in which the report appeared (see discussion on journals earlier in this chapter).
2. Qualifications of the authors. Is at least one a well-known researcher? If not, is there evidence of research training among them? Are they affiliated with a reputable institution?
3. Research funding. If the research was commercially funded, is there any reason to believe that the sponsors might have influenced the results?
4. Date of publication. Knowledge in some fields is moving rapidly, less so in others. Is the report likely to have been superseded by more recent work?

Research Specifics

1. Is the research question, purpose of the paper, and a hypothesis succinctly stated?
2. Although the review of current knowledge must often be brief in a research report, is it a balanced summary of previous work? (The "selective" review to support a particular point of view is unfortunately not unknown).
3. Are the measurement variables and other terms specifically defined? If standard terms and measures are being used, are refer-

ences given for their definition? If new measures are being introduced, is it made clear why existing ones cannot be used? (These questions all are aimed to check validity).

4. Assuming the study is with humans, is the population studied appropriate in view of the stated purposes? Does the report give the numbers of people approached, those who agreed to begin the study, and those who remained at the end? Are there adequate details of the sampling plan or group allocation procedures?

5. Is the research design appropriate to test the hypothesis and thus answer the underlying question?

6. Are the materials and methods clearly detailed? Are measurements being applied as described? Have the researchers taken steps to ensure that the measures are being recorded as reliably as possible? This latter point means that if there are several examiners in an epidemiologic study, are they experienced in such research, or have they been trained and calibrated for this project? Are there any checks made to ensure reliability?

7. Is the statistical analysis appropriate for the types of data collected? Have the authors presented sufficient data in the way of tables or graphics to permit the reader to check this question? Are tests of significance, confidence limits, regression analyses, or any other statistical tests used appropriate for testing the hypothesis?

8. Does the discussion look critically at any limitations of the methods used? Are appropriate comparisons made with previous work and reasons discerned for similarities or differences? Is a fair assessment of the relevance of the work made, with some specifics given for the next steps?

9. Are the conclusions clear and warranted by the results of the research? Have the authors made suitable distinction between statistical significance and clinical importance?

10. Is the paper clearly and concisely written? Does the abstract give a clear profile of the study?

11. Have the issues of informed consent and ethical research been dealt with adequately?

Reviews of the Literature

When well done, reviews can be among the most influential and valuable works in the literature. Particular features to check are as follows:

1. Is the subject of the review clearly stated, and are its boundaries delineated?

2. As far as you can find out, is all appropriate work included in the review?

3. Is there a fair but critical analysis of the reports reviewed, or does the author(s) seem to be emphasizing only one side of an issue?

4. Does the review critically assess the value of different research reports, or are they all taken at face value and given equal merit? Lack of critical assessment weakens a review.

Commentaries

These reports present a case or argue an issue, sometimes with data and sometimes without. They can vary greatly in quality from beautiful insights to hopelessly biased diatribes. Again, look for author's affiliations and qualifications, description of the issue, and other related aspects. Here are some particular issues in commentaries:

1. Has the author used whatever factual basis is available to develop the case? (Hard data should always be used as far as possible, even though some conclusions must be reached with less information than is desirable).

2. Is there respect for various points of view?

3. Are conclusions warranted by the argument made, or is there a sense of preconceived conclusions?

A few other characteristics are common to all papers in the literature. They should have a concise yet informative title, allowing the reader to recognize the content and to assist electronic retrieval. A good abstract permits readers to identify quickly the basic contents of the paper. An abstract should (a) state the objectives and scope of the investigation, (b) describe briefly the methods used, (c) summarize the findings, and (d) state the main conclusions. Some journals require that an abstract be written strictly to that format. Abstracts should not contain information or conclusions not stated in the body of the report. Brevity (no more than 250 words helps electronic storage and retrieval) requires that abstracts be objective, straightforward, and free of opinion or speculation.

FINDING THE REPORTS YOU NEED IN THE LITERATURE

Practitioners often have a need to find information about a subject: What is this material which a supply house salesman is pushing? Do sealants work on primary teeth? Has this new cavity liner been adequately tested? The list is endless. Dental professionals need to know how to search the vastness of the literature efficiently to find the information they need to let them reach a conclusion. Fortunately, the rapidly developing electronic methods for searching the literature make this task much less arduous than it once was.

A useful start is the reference lists at the end of textbook chapters, although the earlier caveats on obsolete material in textbooks also pertains to the references. In addition to the risk of being dated, such reference lists are often not complete, reflecting an author's bias or incomplete grasp of a subject. These reference lists can be a good start, although usually more is needed. Good reviews of the literature in a related topic can be useful. Although the conclusions of the review may be enough for some purposes, some readers may want to follow up on some of the papers cited in the review.

The main repository of biomedical literature is the *Index Medicus,* a vast compendium managed by the National Library of Medicine (NLM), located on the campus of the National Institutes of Health in Bethesda, Maryland. The dental literature is housed in the *Index to Dental Literature,* also managed by NLM. The *Index* contains nearly every dentally related article published in journals anywhere in the world, including non-English publications, letters to the editor, and news items. In the hard-copy volumes of these indexes, reports are grouped under subject headings for the searcher who wants to see what was published in a particular subject over the years, and there is also an author index. Libraries of dental schools all have the *Index* available.

Searching the literature beyond these traditional approaches is today more and more a computerized operation, involving a search of electronic databases and the World Wide Web. All biomedical literature since 1966 handled by NLM is now available on-line through MEDLINE, and practitioners anywhere in the world need only a personal computer, appropriate software, and a modem to gain access to it. It is difficult to present instructions to practitioners on use of MED-LINE, since there are growing numbers of commercial on-line services that carry it, and the dissemination technology itself is moving so fast. The best advice is to check with dental or medical school librarians for methods of tapping into the MEDLINE database.

When use of MEDLINE first begins, the effect can be overwhelming: a tidal wave of information gushes over the user, often far more than can be readily digested. Sometimes this reflects reality; there is just so much more published on an issue than the user may have imagined. Sometimes though it means the search is too broad and a lot of inappropriate material will be included. Practice with use of key words, and increasing familiarity with the MeSH (Medical Subject Headings) terminology makes searching much more efficient. It takes a surprisingly short time for a user, who need not be particularly adept with computers, to learn to conduct a highly efficient search. A dental practitioner, for example, with a computer in the back room of the practice, can easily search an issue over a lunchtime sandwich and refine the search to a usable number of relevant references. Abstracts now accompany the reference in most journals, making the search even more efficient, and full-text paging is becoming more common (this means that the full article, complete with photos, is available from the Web in an increasing number of biomedical journals). On-line subscriptions to specific journals are also becoming common.

The result of a search is a stream of references, most with abstracts, that flow across the screen; unless they are captured and stored the search is a transitory thing. So along with the development of electronic searching procedures, there is excellent bibliographic database software now available, plus linking software to download the search into the storage database. Do the search, select the references needed from those perused, download them into the database, and then they are on hand permanently. Indexing with the databases is efficient; even when thousands of references are stored it only takes a moment to call up those needed. Once a user gets accustomed to this way of searching the literature, it is difficult to know how we ever got along without it. Eventually, it seems certain that NLM will no longer publish the hard copy of the *Index to Dental Literature* and will rely on the electronic databases instead. However, no one really knows when "eventually" might be.

The amount of useful information on the World Wide Web is growing at a staggering rate. We are assuming that readers are familiar with the Web to some extent; for those who are not, the World Wide Web is a means of storing text, graphics, and audio material in a computer server in such a way that anyone in the world with Web-browsing software can pick it up. Although the Web in the mid-1990s is a delightfully anarchic affair, there is a lot of useful information to be found in it. An example was given in Chapter 3, where the ADA's Principles of Ethics are now located through the ADA home page rather than published in print. "Downloading," or printing material located on the Web, is also becoming simpler. A vast amount of health-related information is to be found in the websites for the ADA, National Institutes of Health, Centers for Disease Control and Prevention, and the World Health Organization.

The only snag in these developments is that papers located in the search still have to be read! Photocopying is getting easier and cheaper, and dental school librarians will obtain a needed journal from inter-library loan if necessary. Even photocopying from a journal may become largely obsolete as full-text electronic storage grows. When full-text storage develops completely, practitioners in the most remote geographic location will need only a computer and modem to have the entire dental literature at their fingertips, literally! The technology for all this is in existence now; developments will depend on sorting out the legal and economic ramifications. We can be certain that progress in this area of keeping up with the literature will continue to be rapid, and that scientific knowledge will become increasingly available.

REFERENCES

1. Canadian Task Force on the Periodic Health Examination. The periodic health examination. J Can Med Assoc 1979;121:1193–1254.
2. US Preventive Services Task Force. Guide to clinical preventive services. 2nd ed. Washington DC: US Department of Health and Human Services, 1996.

section III

The Methods of Oral Epidemiology

12

Research Designs in Epidemiology

Causality and Risk ◆ Nonexperimental Study
Designs ◆ Experimental Study Designs

Epidemiology is defined as the study of health and disease in populations, and of how these states are influenced by heredity, biology, physical environment, social environment, and ways of living. Epidemiologic studies can first be classified as *descriptive*, meaning that data are collected without a specific hypothesis in mind to be tested, and *analytic*, meaning studies in which the data collection and analysis are designed to answer a particular question. The clinical trial, an experimental design to test the efficacy of an agent or procedure in humans, is an aspect of analytic epidemiology sometimes classified separately as *experimental* epidemiology. Some designs in health services research can also fit this category.

Good research demands careful, sometimes exhaustive planning. Every study, no matter how modest, needs a *protocol*, which is a written plan encompassing the purpose and the detailed operation of the study. The essential elements of a protocol are listed in Table 12–1.

A protocol demands carefully thinking through a project, a process that helps its design and also helps the researchers to anticipate potential problems. It also simplifies the writing of a final report because the protocol forms the basis of the report.

CAUSALITY AND RISK

Risk is the probability that a specified event will occur (e.g., that an individual will exhibit a disease or die within a stated period or by a particular age).[13] Analytic studies, in contrast to descriptive studies, have the gen-

eral aim of seeking out cause-and-effect associations. An analytic study cannot always go directly to cause-and-effect, so some of them seek to quantify the degree of risk of disease in specified circumstances. Causality, meaning that a certain factor results in a particular outcome, can only be demonstrated unequivocally within the experimental study design of a clinical trial (discussed in the next sec-

Table 12–1. THE ESSENTIAL FEATURES OF A PROTOCOL FOR RESEARCH WITH HUMANS

1. A precise definition of the research problem, the reasons for undertaking the research, and a review of pertinent literature.
2. Objectives of the study, or hypotheses to be tested. A hypothesis is a conjecture cast in a form that will allow it to be tested and refuted.
3. Population to be studied, including its selection, source, size, method of sampling, and method of allocation to groups (if a clinical trial).
4. Data to be collected, describing each item needed to accomplish the objectives or to test the hypotheses.
5. Procedures to be carried out, giving details of exactly how the needed data will be obtained from the participants in the study, and by whom.
6. Data collection methods, with examples of all data collection forms or computer methods of data collection, and a list of all necessary supplies, equipment, and instruments.
7. Plans for data processing and analysis, including how the data gets from field collection to computer, computer file organization, and statistical distributions to be examined.
8. Time schedule for planning, obtaining informed consent from study subjects, data collection and analysis, and report writing.
9. An assessment of any ethical issues involved in the study and obtaining the necessary institutional human subjects clearance.

Table 12-2. CRITERIA FOR CAUSALITY: CONDITIONS TO BE SATISFIED BEFORE IT CAN BE SAID THAT A PARTICULAR EXPOSURE IS THE CAUSE OF A DISEASE

1. **Consistency of Association:** If there is a good number of studies on whether an exposure is a cause of a disease, and if all of them produce fairly similar positive results, it is more likely that the factor is causal.
2. **Strength of Association:** In valid studies, the stronger the association between exposure and outcome, the more likely it is that the association is causal.
3. **Degree of Exposure (Dose-Response):** If an exposure is causal, then the risk of disease should be related to the degree of exposure: a dose-response relationship.
4. **Time Sequence of Events:** To be causal, an exposure must precede the occurrence of the disease. Demonstration of this temporal sequence requires longitudinal study.
5. **Biologic Plausibility:** The association must make biologic sense from our knowledge of the disease. It follows that the better-understood a disease is, the more stringent this criterion can become.

tion). Because clinical trials are not possible for many topics for both practical and ethical reasons, causality in the study of disease usually has to be inferred from studies with nonexperimental designs. Criteria by which a conclusion of causality can be reached from nonexperimental epidemiologic studies have evolved over the years and are summarized in Table 12-2.

The criteria listed in Table 12-2 are fairly strict, and there are often factors that both researchers and clinicians think play a role in causing a disease that do not satisfy all these criteria. If researchers then had to proceed with only the dichotomous judgment of whether a factor is or is not involved in causing a disease, our knowledge of disease causation and development would be seriously hindered. The concept of a risk factor permits quantification of the degree of importance that a particular factor brings to the development of a disease; some causal factors are more important than others.

A *risk factor* is defined as an attribute or exposure that increases the probability of disease occurrence. Although there is some lack of uniformity in the use of the term *risk factor* in the literature, modern usage ascribes a strong causal role to a risk factor. It is either

part of the causal chain, or is something that brings a person into contact with the causal chain.[2] (An example of the latter situation is an occupation that requires handling toxic materials. The occupation itself is not a risk factor for toxicity, but because it brings a person into contact with toxic materials, which are the risk factors, it does increase the chance of disease). Part of the concept of a risk factor is that it can be modified; people can stop smoking, lose weight, change to a healthier diet, or improve their oral hygiene.

A risk factor for a disease needs to be demonstrated longitudinally.[2] Three general criteria need to be met before we can suggest that something is a risk factor for a particular disease, and only longitudinal study designs are capable of disclosing them. These criteria are listed in Table 12-3. The ultimate test of a risk factor is that if it is taken away, the risk of the disease diminishes. As an example, quitting smoking reduces the risk of a heart attack.

What if a suspected risk factor cannot be confirmed because the necessary longitudinal studies are impractical or unethical? It may be classed as a *risk indicator*, defined as a factor shown to be associated with a disease in cross-sectional data and assumed, on theoretic grounds, to play some causal role.[15] Research experience has shown that risk indicators that emerge from cross-sectional studies can disappear in a more rigorous longitudinal analysis; without longitudinal assessment, a risk indicator may or may not be a true risk factor. Longitudinal studies permit the ordering of the time sequence of exposure and

Table 12-3. CRITERIA TO BE MET IN ORDER TO ACCEPT A GIVEN EXPOSURE AS A RISK FACTOR FOR A PARTICULAR DISEASE

1. **Statistical Association:** The exposure must co-vary with the disease, meaning that the frequency of the disease must be observed to differ by category or value of the exposure.
2. **Time Sequence:** The exposure must precede the occurrence of the disease.
3. **Absence of Error:** The observed association must not be the result of error, whether that be bias, sampling error, analytic errors, or the intrusion of other extraneous factors.

Adapted from Kleinbaum DG, Kupper LL, Morgenstern H. Epidemiologic research: Principles and quantitative methods. Belmont, CA: Lifetime Learning Publications, 1982:25–34.

outcome (Table 12–3) in a way that cross-sectional designs usually cannot, hence the statement given in the previous paragraph that risk factors need to be confirmed in longitudinal studies. As would be expected, there are many more risk indicators for oral diseases than there are true risk factors.

A *risk marker* is an attribute or exposure associated with the increased probability of disease, although not considered part of the causal chain. A risk marker can also be called a *risk predictor* when included in predictive statistical models. Some immutable characteristics of a person or group, namely age, gender, and race/ethnicity, can influence disease occurrence, progression, or outcome. These attributes do not fit the concept of a risk factor because they are not modifiable. Although they can be useful in statistical models designed to predict disease occurrence, they clearly are of no use when considering disease prevention based on controlling risk factors. The literature is unfortunately muddled about what to call these attributes; we suggest the term *demographic risk factors* to refer to these immutable influences. In addition to age, gender, and race/ethnicity, socioeconomic status is usually considered a demographic risk factor.

NONEXPERIMENTAL STUDY DESIGNS

The process of collecting descriptive data from a population is called a *survey*. Surveys record the *prevalence* of various conditions, meaning the number or proportion of persons in the population who exhibit a condition at any one time. (Data from national surveys in the United States are cited in Chapters 18–20, 22). Although surveys are important in assessing trends in health and disease, the field of oral epidemiology encompasses much more than surveys. We discourage the use of the term *epidemiology* to refer only to survey data.

At the most basic level, epidemiologic study designs are *cross-sectional*, *longitudinal*, or *retrospective*. A *cross-sectional* study is one in which the health conditions in a group of people, who are, or are assumed to be, a sample of a particular population (a "cross section") is assessed at one time, whereas a *longitudinal* study is one in which the same group of people is studied on two or more occasions. A survey collects cross-sectional data. Comparison of trends by examining the

results of a sequence of surveys, even if the same study protocols are used in all of them, is still a cross-sectional comparison because different people are examined in the different surveys.

Analytic studies in epidemiology look at people with and without the disease in question (the *effect* or *outcome*), and with and without exposure to the putative influences that may increase the risk of disease (the *exposure*). The identification of risk factors for a disease then allows the potential for prevention by removing or modifying the risk factors. As examples, smoking is a risk factor for lung cancer; poor oral hygiene is a risk factor for gingivitis. In both instances, removing or modifying the risk factor reduces the risk of disease, although neither exposure is a sole cause of the subsequent disease.

Longitudinal studies require at least two series of measurements among the same people at different times to determine the progress of the condition over the specified time period. Such a study is also an *incidence* study; *incidence* being defined as the number of new cases of a condition over a given time.[13] Sometimes an analytic study can be cross-sectional, such as when several cross-sectional studies are made over a period for analytic purposes. An examination of mortality trends, for example, must be cross-sectional (obviously it cannot be the same people who die on different occasions). A comparison of the prevalence of dental caries in today's sixth-graders with that of 10 years ago must be a cross-sectional study, although it could also be an analytic one; again it is obvious that different persons are studied each time. However, if all the children originally in first grade in a school system are studied periodically until they finish sixth grade some years later, the study would be longitudinal because the same children would be seen on several occasions.

Analytic studies can also be *prospective* (looking forward) or *retrospective* (looking back). *Prospective* studies collect information on an exposure of interest and compare eventual outcomes, whereas retrospective studies begin with the outcome of interest and probe back for exposure information. A *cohort* study is one prospective design, a cohort being a group of people from whom data are collected longitudinally. A cohort is often characterized by some particular characteristic in common, such as age; thus an expression such as "the 1955 birth cohort" means all persons born in 1955. A prospective or cohort study is defined as one in which a subset of a population is studied who are, have been, or in the future may be exposed or not exposed, or exposed to varying degrees, to a factor hypothesized to influence the probability of occurrence of a given disease.[13]

It has long been conventional to view retrospective studies as being inherently of poorer quality than prospective studies. This view is unjustified, however, because many unusual conditions, or conditions that develop over a long period of time, can be studied realistically only through retrospective designs. Indeed, the noted epidemiologist Rothman[20] considers the development of the retrospective study design one of the major advances in epidemiologic methods over recent years. A retrospective study is a design in which inferences about exposure to putative causal factor(s) are derived from data relating to characteristics of the persons under study, or to events or experiences in their past.[13] The principal retrospective design is the *case-control* study, in which people with a condition ("cases") are compared with people without it ("controls"), but who are similar in some other characteristics. Hypothesized causal exposures are then sought in the past of the participants. Case-control studies need to be planned thoughtfully, because characteristics by which the groups are matched (e.g., ethnic group) cannot be compared, and thus are ruled out as possible etiologic factors. Case-control studies can demonstrate risk indicators for a disease, but the retrospective design means that risk *factors* cannot be confirmed this way. Risk factors for a disease can be confirmed only through cohort or experimental study designs.

An *ecologic* study is an analytic study in which data for both exposures and outcomes come from the population level rather than from individuals. For example, studies addressing the question of whether water fluoridation is related to hip fracture experience (i.e., suggesting that fluoridation is a risk factor for broken hips) have used community data for both water fluoridation (the exposure) and for hip fractures (the outcome) to derive a relationship.[10, 21] Such studies are relatively quick and inexpensive because they avoid sampling, interviewing, and clinical examinations or access to individual medical records. Their weakness, however, is that they cannot be certain that the people with the outcome condition (in this case the hip frac-

ture) are the same ones who had the exposure (drank fluoridated water). This weakness is often called the *ecologic fallacy.* Ecologic studies can be useful, but they usually are not definitive. They have a clearer role when a variable under consideration, for example community income level, is by definition a group measure rather than an individual one.

All of these study designs are nonexperimental, meaning that they study conditions as they occur rather than manipulate conditions in the manner of a classic laboratory experiment. There are experimental designs in epidemiology, however, that are usually used to test the efficacy or effectiveness of a therapeutic drug, a preventive material, or a treatment regimen.

EXPERIMENTAL STUDY DESIGNS

In medical terminology, *clinical* trials are carried out among patients, frequently hospital inpatients, and *field* trials are carried out with people in the community who may not necessarily be patients. This medical model does not transfer well to dentistry, where the definition of a patient is less clear-cut. The term *clinical trial* tends to be loosely applied in dentistry to both types of study, so we will use it in this chapter when describing research principles common to both strict clinical trials and to field trials. We will use the term *field trial* (sometimes called a community trial, or an effectiveness study) only when specific reference to a field trial is needed.

A clinical trial is a controlled experimental study of group comparison, based on epidemiologic principles and designed to test the hypothesis that a particular agent or procedure favorably alters the natural history of a disease. The group receiving the agent or regimen under study is the *test* group, sometimes called the *experimental* or *study* group, whereas the comparable group not subject to the agent or regimen is the *control* group. Clinical trials compare 2 or more segments of a single population, divided into groups that are essentially similar (in distribution of age, sex, race, socioeconomics, disease experience). The aim is to make the only difference between the groups the fact that the test group receives the agent under study and the control group does not.

Much of the basis for preventive procedures in dentistry has come from clinical trials, although the quality of trials described in the dental literature varies from excellent to poor. The reader can judge the validity of a trial by determining how closely the report adheres to certain principles in its conduct.

Choice of Population in Which the Trial Will Be Conducted

This should be determined by the purpose of the trial. If the purpose is to test the *efficacy* of a particular agent (i.e., whether it works), then it deserves the most favorable conditions to show that it does work. For that reason, the project should be conducted with subjects who are selected for their susceptibility to the disease. This means that a population of a specific age range is usually chosen deliberately, as many oral diseases are age-associated (Chapters 18–22). Sex, race, socioeconomic status, and geographic location are other factors that can be included in the choice of a study population for efficacy trials. If the purpose is to assess the *effectiveness* of an agent under everyday conditions, however, then broad community populations, those with varying degrees of the disease under study, should be chosen.[16] Confusing the purposes of trials can lead to the error of generalizing from efficacy trials with special populations with unusual disease distributions, such as some institutionalized people, to the general population.

Adequate Numbers of Subjects

Loss of subjects during a prospective clinical trial is a fact of life and must be planned for. If the numbers of subjects in the groups are not big enough to begin with, at the end of the trial the researcher will be left with too few subjects to be able to show, by statistical logic, whether it is likely that an observed difference between the groups is real or a chance result. The result may then be that a real difference cannot be detected, and an agent that in fact is effective will not seem to be so. This issue relates to data analysis and the conclusions from the trial and is discussed more fully a little later. Sampling is discussed in Chapter 13.

Comparability of Study and Control Groups

The randomized trial, always the most elegant design,[3] is one in which group similarity is achieved by random allocation of subjects to the study and control groups. *Random allocation* means that each subject has an equal chance of being assigned to either study or control group. Statistical probability is such that the assumption can then be made that the groups differ from each other only in terms of the agent under study. Uncontrolled variables influencing the outcome are likely to affect subjects in both groups equally.

The principle of random allocation is simple, although it is a carefully planned and controlled procedure. Random allocation is not haphazard assignment or one based on volunteering or self-selection. A statistician can further improve the probability of establishing comparable groups by *stratification,* which means that before allocation the base population can be separated by those factors known, or thought, to influence disease occurrence (usually age, sex, race, socioeconomic status, or previous disease experience). Subjects from each stratum are then randomly allocated to study and control groups.

Nonrandomized trial designs are not uncommon in the dental literature.[18, 19] Although they are weaker than randomized designs, sometimes practical considerations dictate their use. For example, a school system taking part in a caries preventive trial may insist that there be no control group because school administrators want all participating children to receive a benefit. In such cases a *before-and-after* design (sometimes called historical controls) can be used. In this design, children are examined at the beginning of the trial, the agent or regimen is applied, and then cross-sectional groups of children of similar ages are examined periodically until the completion of the trial. Differences between caries status at the beginning and the end of the trial are then judged for children of similar age or grade levels. The weakness in this design is that uncontrolled change could take place during the trial to invalidate results. For example, in a trial of a fluoride mouthrinse, children in sixth grade at the completion of a 3-year trial may have brushed with a fluoride toothpaste more often than did the sixth-graders examined at the beginning. Without a true control group, it is impossible to tell if beneficial outcomes were due entirely to the mouthrinse or at least in part to the additional toothpaste use. Before-and-after trials are more properly called *demonstrations,* intended to "demonstrate" the value of accepted preventive measures.[11] Presenting a case for the scientific validity of demonstrations can get complicated,[8, 9] although it is worth noting that the pioneering Grand Rapids fluoridation trial used this design (Chapter 24). The greatest threat to the validity of a before-and-after design comes from sociodemographic change in the population under study during the period of the trial.

Some studies have used a *comparison group,* defined as any group to which the study group is compared, and a term that is often used synonomously with *control group.*[13] It is less confusing, however, if the term *control group* is reserved for randomized controls, and *comparison group* is used for nonrandomized comparisons. Examples of comparison groups are the control communities used in fluoridation field trials (Chapter 24). Some comparison groups can be similar to study groups and thus permit valid comparisons, but others have been so far removed from the study group that they serve little purpose.

Certain types of trials can use a *crossover* design, where subjects serve as their own controls. Each subject receives an active treatment for a specific time and a placebo (or no treatment) during a control period. Crossover designs are unsuitable for studies of caries prevention because the period required for lesions to develop is too long. Crossover designs are useful in short-term trials (weeks or months, rather than years) for preventing reversible conditions such as gingivitis or calculus accumulation. The principal advantage of a crossover design is that it avoids variations in response among participating subjects. Crossover designs are not appropriate for regimens that have a carryover effect because the effects of the treatment phase could influence responses during the nontreatment phase. Crossover designs are also inappropriate when the tested regimen may produce a permanent effect, when test agents may be retained at the site of action for prolonged periods, or with conditions that may naturally undergo a rapid change in prevalence, incidence, or morbidity.

In studying efficacy trials, readers should take care not to confuse the need to carefully *select* the study population with the necessity to *randomly allocate* the individuals in that population to the study and control groups.

Use of a Placebo in the Control Group

A *placebo* is a material or formulation like the test product but without the active ingredient, such as a toothpaste that feels and tastes like a fluoride toothpaste but contains no fluoride. The purpose of using a placebo in a trial is to have subjects unaware of whether they are in the test or control group (a *blind* study), so that their dental health behavior will not be consciously or unconsciously affected by group allocation. *Bias,* systematic although usually unconscious error, also can affect examiners. Examiners who expect a product to be effective may unconsciously apply stricter criteria for caries in a control group if they know which children are in which group. When neither participants nor examiners know the group allocations, the trial is *double-blind.*

A placebo is inherently impossible in some instances, such as trials of water fluoridation (where the fluoridating community is a matter of public record), fissure sealant (where sealant visibility determines the outcome), or dental health education (where the control at best is a comparable group which receives no program, a *passive control*). Placebos raise ethical issues; it is usually considered unethical to deny established beneficial products to trial participants. If a manufacturer wants to test a fluoride toothpaste with a stronger formulation than is standard, for example, the control group does not use a nonfluoride toothpaste but rather a standard-strength product. This is called a *positive control*; the results then compare the effects of the new product against the old one. Because the difference between these two groups would be expected to be less than if a placebo were used, the trial would need larger numbers of subjects to permit any true difference to be shown.

Control of Operational Procedure

An efficacy study, designed to answer the question of whether a particular agent or regimen works, has to give the test agent every chance. Susceptible populations are chosen for the trial, but in addition, the researchers need to be sure that the agent is used as prescribed. If it is a professionally applied agent or a treatment regimen, the protocol must specify precisely how the agent will be used, for how long, how often, at what concentration, and by whom. A placebo, or positive control, would be applied the same way. If a self-applied agent is being tested, such as a mouthrinse, the protocol should call for the agent to be used under professional supervision. It is the researchers' task to ensure that the protocol is adhered to throughout the course of the study.

In an effectiveness trial, the agent/treatment can be used as it normally would. That means that professionals are given instructions in use of a procedure, or participants are given the rinse to take home and use as instructed. There is less certainty in an effectiveness trial that the material has been used as intended, but part of the aims of an effectiveness trial is how the material works under "real life" conditions. In operational control, as in other aspects of a trial, the purpose of the study must be kept in mind.

Reliability in Diagnosis

Examiners in trials must record disease (at the second and subsequent examinations) that has developed over a relatively short time. This requirement forces the examiner to diagnose disease at an early stage of its development, which increases the risk of error. In caries trials, the most troublesome form of error is that a lesion classed as carious at the first round of examinations may be classified as sound in subsequent examinations, a *negative reversal*, more commonly referred to just as a *reversal*. Reversals are virtually unavoidable in any form of sequential diagnosis,[17] although they should remain a fairly small proportion of all diagnoses. The ways of dealing with reversals in data analysis are discussed in Chapter 14.

The validity of trial results depends heavily on the reliability of the examiner. This factor is usually referred to as *intraexaminer reliability*, the ability of an examiner to record the same conditions the same way over time. Most examiners with training and experience develop an acceptable degree of intraexaminer reliability. Reliability between different examiners, *interexaminer reliability*, is often more difficult, even when they train together from the same written criteria. Ideally it is best to use one well-qualified examiner, but large-scale studies often require that more than one examiner be used. In such cases, the examiners should undergo a period of training to bring their diagnostic standards as close together as can possibly be managed. This training procedure is referred to as *standardization*. Where one of the group is the "gold standard" examiner and the training is to enable other examiners to record similarly, the term *calibration* more accurately describes the exercise.

Radiographs can be helpful in a trial, but the same issues of examiner reliability are present. Diagnostic criteria must be established, and intraexaminer and interexaminer reliability maintained with radiographic interpretation just as with clinical examinations. When logistic and ethical issues are added in, radiographs are usually not recommended in field trials.[7] Clinical trials in a dental school setting, where patients may be radiographed anyway in the course of treatment, may be different.

Duration of the Trial

Clinical trials must be continued long enough to permit detection of new disease or extension of lesions already present during the period of the trial. For caries trials, the minimum duration is usually 2 to 3 years, although precise timing depends on the purposes of the trial.[6] The longer the trial, the more expensive, so trade-offs are required. The Fédération Dentaire Internationale (FDI) suggested in 1977 that trials of plaque-inhibiting agents could be as short as 8 to 21 days,[5] but that guideline was for plaque measurements only. The American Dental Association requires plaque-inhibiting agents that seek the association's seal of approval (Chapter 28) to demonstrate gingivitis reduction as well; it requires such trials to be at least 6 months long.[1] The FDI,[5] in its 1977 report, also recommended that studies of calculus-preventing agents should last 90 days for supragingival calculus and longer for subgingival calculus.

Statistical Analysis

It is not our purpose to cover the methods of statistical analysis in this text, for numerous excellent biostatistics textbooks are available. One particularly recommended for its clarity and its use of dental examples is *Biostats* by Weintraub and colleagues.[22] One particular analytic issue that can bother readers of the literature, however, is that of the relations between statistical significance and clinical importance. This issue is worth some discussion here.

A clinical trial to test a preventive agent or treatment regimen begins with a *null hypothesis* (i.e., the proposition that there is no difference in disease experience between the test and control groups). When large differences between test and control groups are expected, the groups can be smaller than when small differences are expected. Groups must be large enough so that observed differences in disease increment between test and control groups can be reasonably tested for *statistical significance,* which is the probability that the observed results are due to chance rather than to the efficacy of the tested product or regimen. *Chance* in this context means the possibility that the random allocation procedure went awry and loaded one group with disease-susceptible or disease-resistant individuals. (It does not mean the probability of a chance result because of poor design or sloppy conduct of the study!) Such differences are not always apparent when the groups are compared following allocation, and the trial therefore proceeds. (If it is apparent immediately after allocation that the groups differ in some important respect, the groups can be disbanded and the allocation procedure repeated).

When comparing the observed results in a clinical trial, it has been traditional to accept 5%, or 0.05, as the outer limit of acceptable statistical significance. This statement $p = 0.05$ thus means that the risk of accepting the observed difference between the groups as real, when actually it is due to chance, is 5 in 100. In this case, the 5% chance of falsely accepting that a regimen is effective is termed *type I error* and the Greek letter α (alpha) is the probability of making a type I error. To offer greater assurance that an observed difference is real, investigators may set α at 1% ($P = 0.01$), although the trade-off here is that larger group sizes will be necessary.

The selection of a small α-level, however, does not protect investigators from the possibility of *failing* to identify an effective agent or regimen. If the group size is too small, it is possible to conclude mistakenly that a treatment has no effect, when in fact it does. This latter mistake is known as *type II error,* with the probability of making a type II error signified by the Greek letter β (beta).

In a well-conducted study, type I errors usually arise from the random allocation process going astray, resulting in imbalance in group composition. In an otherwise well-conducted study, type II errors typically come from inadequate group sizes, too small to permit demonstrating statistical significance when clinical differences are apparent. Imprecise diagnosis can also lead to type II error. In a trial where there has been no random allocation, the assumptions underlying the statistical probability tests have been violated, so that the *p*-values presented in such reports have little value.

The chance of detecting a true effect, if it exists, is denoted as the *power* of the test and is defined as 1-β. Power is dependent on (a) the magnitude of the difference observed between the two treatments, (b) the number of study subjects in each group, (c) the population variance, and (d) the α level chosen.[22] If the findings from a study are negative (meaning that the null hypothesis cannot be rejected), the power of the test indicates how confident one can be that the findings are truly negative. The goal in considering power when calculating group sizes is to enhance the chances of finding effects if they really do exist.

The power of a test is critically important in trials using a positive control, for example testing a higher-concentration fluoride toothpaste against the positive control of a standard fluoride product. Differences in caries increments between the groups are likely to be slight. If the investigators judge that differences as small as 15% between groups are clinically meaningful, they will need to be able to demonstrate that differences this small are statistically significant. The group sizes then have to be extremely large.[4] Otherwise, with smaller groups, the researchers may falsely conclude that the regimens were equivalent because they failed to demonstrate statistical significance, when in fact the chance of demonstrating such significance, or the power of the test, was small to begin with.

Overcoming problems of sample size requires more care than simply making study groups as large as possible. The reason for that is that when groups are large, the most trivial difference in disease increment between them will reach statistical significance. This can be misleading if there is no clinical importance in the difference observed, for therapeutic importance cannot be concluded simply because statistical significance has been determined.

In trials with positive controls, or more than one test group, the investigators should report the power (1-β) of the investigation. They should describe the statistical test used and state, for example, that there was an 80% chance (1-β) of correctly rejecting the null hypothesis at an α-level of 5%, if a true difference of 15% among groups existed.

Ethical Considerations

Humans taking part in clinical trials must give informed consent, which means a written acceptance that the participant understands the conduct of the trial and the nature of any risks involved. Authors should certify that the study protocol has been accepted by their institution's Institutional Review Board (IRB), which any institution conducting research is required to maintain. If the study includes vulnerable populations (e.g., children, illiterate or mentally retarded people), then extra explanations are usually required. Additional explanation for how the rights of participants have been safeguarded may also be needed if the study is conducted in a developing country that does not have the rigorous standards for human subject protection that developed nations have.

REFERENCES

1. American Dental Association, Council on Dental Therapeutics. Guidelines for acceptance of chemotherapeutic products for the control of supragingival plaque and gingivitis. J Am Dent Assoc 1986;112:529–32.
2. Beck JD. Methods of assessing risk for periodontitis and developing multifactorial models. J Periodontol 1994;65:468–78.
3. Cochrane AL. Effectiveness and efficiency; random reflections on health services. London: Nuffield Provincial Hospitals Trust, 1971:20–5.
4. Conti AJ, Lotzkar S, Daly R, et al. A 3-year clinical trial to compare efficacy of dentifrices containing 1.14% and 0.76% sodium monofluorophosphate. Community Dent Oral Epidemiol 1988;16:135–8.
5. Fédération Dentaire Internationale, Commission on Classification and Statistics for Oral Conditions. Principal requirements for controlled clinical trials in periodontal diseases. Int Dent J 1977;27:62–76.
6. Fédération Dentaire Internationale, Commission on Oral Health, Research and Epidemiology. Principal requirements for controlled clinical trials of caries preventive agents and procedures. Int Dent J 1982;32:292–310.
7. Horowitz HS. Ethical considerations of study participants in dental caries clinical trials. Community Dent Oral Epidemiol 1976;4:43–50.
8. Horowitz HS, Meyers RJ, Heifetz SB, Driscoll WS. Eight-year evaluation of a combined fluoride program in a nonfluoride area. J Am Dent Assoc 1984;109:575–8.
9. Horowitz HS, Meyers RJ, Heifetz SB, et al. Combined fluoride, school-based program in a fluoride-deficient area: Results of an 11-year study. J Am Dent Assoc 1986;112:621–5.
10. Jacobsen SJ, Goldberg J, Cooper C, Lockwood SA. The association between water fluoridation and hip fracture among white women and men aged 65 years and older. A national ecologic study. Ann Epidemiol 1992;2:617–26.
11. Klein SP, Bohannan HM. The first year of field activities in the National Preventive Dentistry Demonstration Program. Rand Report No R-2536/1-RWJ. Santa Monica CA: Rand Corporation, 1979.
12. Kleinbaum DG, Kupper LL, Morgenstern H. Epidemiologic research: principles and quantitative methods. Belmont, CA: Lifetime Learning Publications, 1982:25–34.
13. Last JM, ed: A dictionary of epidemiology. 3rd ed. New York: Oxford University Press, 1995.
14. Lilienfeld AM, Lilienfeld DE. Foundations of epidemiology. 2nd ed. New York: OUP, 1980:289–318.
15. Locker D, Leake JL. Risk indicators and risk markers for periodontal disease experience in older adults living independently in Ontario, Canada. J Dent Res 1993;72:9–17.
16. O'Mullane DM. Efficiency in clinical trials of caries preventive agents and methods. Community Dent Oral Epidemiol 1976;4:190–4.
17. Radike AW. Examiner error and reversals in diagnosis. In: Proceedings of the conference on the clinical testing of cariostatic agents. Chicago: American Dental Association, 1972:92–5.
18. Ringleberg ML, Conti AJ, Webster DB. An evaluation of single and combined self-applied fluoride programs in schools. J Public Health Dent 1976;36:229–36.
19. Ripa LW, Leske GS, Levinson A. Supervised weekly rinsing with a 0.2% neutral NaF solution: Results from a demonstration program after two school years. J Am Dent Assoc 1978;97:793–8.
20. Rothman KJ. Modern epidemiology. Boston: Little Brown, 1986:3.
21. Suarez-Almazor ME, Flowerdew G, Saunders LD, et al. The fluoridation of drinking water and hip fracture hospitalization rates in two Canadian communities. Am J Public Health 1993;83:689–93.
22. Weintraub JA, Douglass CW, Gillings DB. Biostats: Data analysis for dental health care professionals. 2nd ed, revised. Chapel Hill, NC: Quintiles, 1985.

13

The Measurement of Oral Disease

Epidemiology: An Introduction ◆ Early Studies ◆
Epidemiology and the Practitioner ◆ The Concept of
Measuring Disease ◆ The Human Populations
Studied ◆ Methods of Measuring Oral Diseases ◆
Examiner Reliability ◆ Assessment of Disease Risk

Why do some patients have serious periodontitis, whereas apparently similar patients do not? Why does a child who seems to eat candies all day not get caries? Frequently there is no obvious answer. That branch of scientific inquiry which seeks to find order among these apparently haphazard patterns of disease is known as *epidemiology*. Epidemiology is defined as the study of health and disease in populations, and the way these states are influenced by heredity, biology, physical environment, social environment, and ways of living.

Epidemiologic studies require that disease be measured quantitatively. This chapter describes the approaches and procedures in measuring oral diseases and conditions. The methods are fundamental to the conduct of research, although they are also valuable for practitioners in monitoring their patients.

EPIDEMIOLOGY: AN INTRODUCTION

Although there are commonalities in the philosophy of all scientific research, biologic laws tend to be less universally true than are physical laws. The set of circumstances that leads to a heart attack in one person will not necessarily do so in another person of the same age, sex, and race. Biologic variation, meaning the different disease susceptibility between individuals, leads the epidemiologist to seek patterns among people who can be grouped by particular characteristics. To use the characteristics listed in the definition of

epidemiology given previously, these patterns may be related to heredity (e.g., genetic endowment), biology (e.g., age, sex, race), physical environment (e.g., sanitation levels, food and water supply, air quality, occupational hazards), social environment (e.g., educational attainment, cultural beliefs and practices), or lifestyle (smoking, exercise, dental attendance, sugar consumption, toothbrushing habits). Heredity has seen a rush of recent development with the rapid growth of *molecular epidemiology*, meaning the application of the techniques of molecular biology to epidemiology. DNA typing has been used to identify the genotype of pathogenic microorganisms, and viral DNA can be measured in host cells and their genome.[18] Molecular epidemiology holds enormous potential for disease control during the 21st century.

This is not the first time in history that there has been great optimism about prospects for disease control. In the late 19th century, when the bacterial agents in many infectious diseases were being identified, the "end of disease" was confidently being predicted. The concept of disease at the time was dominated by infections with a single bacterial agent, with little thought given to chronic conditions. Today we are more aware that disease is *multifactorial*, meaning that multiple causative circumstances can be defined for just about any disease. Heart disease, the leading cause of death in the United States, is associated with genetics, stress, diet, exercise, smoking, blood pressure, and blood cholesterol levels. So what is the "cause" of heart disease? Dental caries is of bacterial origin, but is also associated with sugar consumption, fluoride exposure, saliva quality and quantity (which are likely to be genetically determined), and family education and income. So what is the "cause" of dental caries? Within the multifactorial tangle, epidemiology attempts to identify the risk factors (Chapter 12) associated with a disease, and to determine which of them are the most important for prevention and control.

Early Studies

Epidemiology was learned and practiced empirically long before it was named. For example, people have known for ages that malaria is a disease of wet lowlands, so they avoided living in such places, but there was little true understanding about conditions that led to disease. The periodic epidemics of plague that swept Europe from the Middle Ages until fairly recent times, for example, were often seen as religious signs rather than a result of squalid living conditions. It was from the more rational study of these epidemics that epidemiology evolved to its present form. Samuel Pepys, who wrote vivid chronicles of life in 17th-century London, used the Bills of Mortality, the forerunner of modern death certificates, to measure the onset and decline of a plague epidemic in London in 1665. Percival Pott's *Treatise of the Chimney Sweep's Cancer*, in 1775, described the unusually high occurrence of scrotal cancer among chimney sweeps, which is one of the first scientific descriptions of an occupational hazard.

In 1854, John Snow, a medical practitioner in the Soho area of London, went so far as to control an outbreak of cholera by the application of his epidemiologic conclusions. His investigation took place some years before the germ theory of disease was understood, so Snow began by trying to identify the features common to those who died from the disease. After mapping out the residences of those who had died (Fig. 13–1), his subsequent enquiries disclosed that all of the victims had used water from the same source. That source, in the days before indoor plumbing, was a pump in Broad Street (now Broadwick Street, where the site of the pump is now occupied by a public toilet). Snow reached the rational conclusion that something in the water was responsible for the spread of the disease. Snow's method of con-

trolling the epidemic, still without knowing its cause, was to persuade the authorities to remove the pump handle. The epidemic soon subsided.

Snow's subsequent investigations on the relations between cholera and the source of water supply are epidemiologic classics. The results of the patiently executed research of 19th-century workers such as Snow still benefit present-day society. Their investigations led to gradual but profound improvements in sanitation, personal hygiene, and the development of the public health codes for housing, water supply, and food processing that are now taken for granted. That infectious diseases such as cholera, typhoid, yellow fever, plague, and relapsing fever are now rare in developed countries is largely due to the pioneering work of these early epidemiologists. Their work continues today: the understanding of the mode of transmission of the human immunodeficiency virus, and its translation into public health education to prevent AIDS, followed remarkably quickly on the first identification of the virus in 1983.[28, 39] That, too, is epidemiology.

The types of study design used in epidemiology were described in Chapter 12 and the various applications of the epidemiologic method in research are shown in Table 13–1.

Epidemiology and the Practitioner

Epidemiology joins the basic sciences and clinical studies to increase our understanding of diseases. The practitioner can factor her knowledge of risk factors into diagnosis and treatment planning decisions, meaning that a patient is more likely to exhibit a particular disease if she exhibits certain characteristics. For example, a man who smokes may or may not get lung cancer, but he certainly runs more risk of developing lung cancer than if he did not smoke. Similarly, an elderly man who both smokes and drinks heavily is more at risk of oral cancer than one who does not.

Another immediate use of epidemiology to the practitioner is application of the results from clinical trials, which have given dentistry its scientific basis for preventive procedures. Although not every member of a test group in a clinical trial necessarily benefits from the tested procedure, the probabilities are high that a given patient will benefit from a procedure that has been successfully tested.

Biologic variation also applies the other

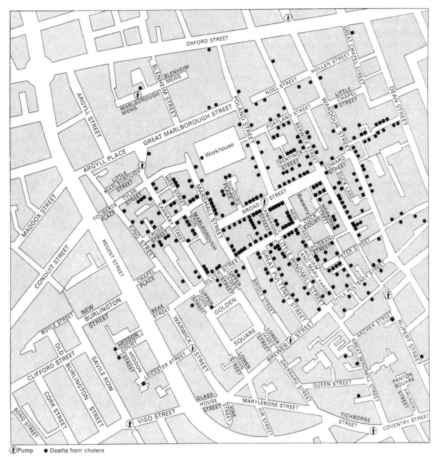

Figure 13–1. John Snow's map of the Soho area of London, showing deaths from cholera during the epidemic of 1854. (From Longmate N. Alive and Well: Medicine and Public Health from 1830 to the Present Day. Harmondsworth: Penguin, 1970. Reprinted by permission of Penguin Books Ltd.)

way. A practitioner cannot generalize from the results of an individual patient's treatment to the population at large. Successful treatment can result from a practitioner's personality, from serendipitous characteristics of the particular patient, or from outside influences, as well as from the treatment itself. Only with controls and the appropriate design can effective prevention and treatment be determined.

The Concept of Measuring Disease

The good clinician thinks in qualitative terms. During a diagnostic examination, the dental practitioner not only looks for existing disease, but also tries to look ahead for the possibility of future disease. Measuring oral disease in a population, however, requires a more standardized and objective approach. Specific diagnostic criteria, written explicitly

for clinical, radiographic, microbiologic, or pathologic examination, replace the judgment of the practitioner. These *criteria*, meaning objective standards on which diagnostic judgment can be based, are applied to judge the condition of the oral tissues as they are at examination time, not on how they might be in the future. This objective application of diagnostic criteria is the most important philosophical difference between the epidemiologic examination and that carried out for treatment planning.

Measurement, the quantifying of observations, is the crux of science. Measurement variability is inherent in all fields of science; it is one reason why experiments are repeated before their findings can be accepted. In studies of oral disease, a true count of lesions in a population is almost never achieved; a repeat examination of the same group of patients nearly always results in a different total num-

Table 13–1. THE USES OF THE SCIENCE OF EPIDEMIOLOGY

1. **Description of normal biologic processes.** Examples are height at various stages of growth, blood groups, and times and order of tooth eruption.
2. **Understanding the natural history of diseases.** Observations of disease progression and outcome in populations have enabled investigators to distinguish those diseases that are fatal or disabling from those that will resolve uneventfully.
3. **Distribution of disease in the population.** By age, gender, race, geographic region, and socioeconomic status. Comparisons of cross-sectional surveys conducted at different times demonstrate trends in disease prevalence and distribution. The comparison of survey results in the early 1980s first clearly showed that caries experience had declined among children of the United States (Chapter 19).
4. **Identifying the determinants of disease.** Within the multifactorial causes of disease referred to earlier, specific study designs (Chapter 12) can identify the risk factors and risk indicators associated with a disease. Even if the causal pathway of a disease is not fully understood, knowledge of risk factors can lead to intervention strategies for prevention and control.
5. **Testing hypotheses for disease prevention and control.** Agents, regimens, or procedures for the prevention and control of disease can be experimentally tested in clinical trials (Chapter 12). As a dental example, the various uses of fluorides to reduce caries incidence have been subject to numerous field trials in human populations (Chapters 24 and 25).
6. **Planning and evaluating health care services.** Data that describe (a) the distribution of disease, both treated and untreated, in the population under study; (b) the population's utilization of health care services; and (c) the availability and productivity of health care services can all be used to assist planning decisions on services and types of personnel required. Related applications are in validating the effectiveness of treatment techniques, both new and traditional, and in determining the quality of treatment provided.

ber of lesions. Any one count of disease in a group is therefore an estimate of conditions, rather than absolute truth. So long as criteria are applied consistently, however, valid estimates will still result because diagnostic "drifts" in one direction will be balanced by drifts the other way.

Acute diseases, such as measles, are characterized by a sudden onset of symptoms, so that the patient rapidly progresses from a state in which the disease is clearly absent to one in which the disease is clearly present. Remission of the acute phase of the disease is equally rapid, so there is little time spent in the "gray areas." Chronic diseases, however, are usually characterized by a much slower

time of onset. It is difficult to establish exactly when arthritis, alcoholism, mental illness, dental caries, and periodontitis become definitely established; there is a considerable "gray area." This problem is handled by counting as lesions only those that meet specific criteria.

The Human Populations Studied

If the intent of a survey is to project results from a sample back to the base population from which the sample was drawn, the sample should closely represent the population.

An example of representative sampling is found in national surveys of the United States. Obviously no study can examine or ask questions of all 260 million people, so sampling is required. The process itself is complicated and requires specialized training, but sampling precision is such that the 109,671 persons interviewed in the 1993 National Health Interview Survey[34] could adequately represent the whole country. This is a *probability sample*, meaning that the chance of each person being chosen in the sample is known. The probability of being chosen in a national sample is not necessarily the same for everyone. A greater proportion of older people than younger people, for example, may be sampled to compensate for poorer response in older people. What is important is that the sampling probability is known. With probability samples, the degree of sampling error can be calculated. *Sampling error* is the error that results from the sample not perfectly representing the base population, and with modern statistical methods it can be remarkably small.

When a nonprobability sample is used for a survey, however, interpretive problems arise because sampling error cannot be calculated from nonprobability samples. As an example, the National Survey of Oral Health in US Employed Adults and Seniors in 1985–1986[35] sought to obtain a profile of oral health in American adults by examining employed adults and seniors who visited senior centers. This was a practical and budget-conscious way of getting a reasonable profile, but the restricted sampling most likely introduced bias into the results. For example, the survey found that only 4.2% of persons under age 65 were edentulous, but this is almost certainly an underestimate because the unemployed, persons in agriculture and mining, the military, the self-employed, and persons not employed outside the home were excluded from the sampling frame,[35] meaning that they had no chance of selection in the sample.

Analytic studies in epidemiology, however, usually do not require probability samples. In fact, case-control and cohort studies, as well as clinical trials (Chapter 12), are usually conducted with groups carefully chosen for required attributes such as age, accessibility, presence of both the disease and the exposures under study, and willingness to participate. In analytic study designs, the critical issue is the selection and categorization of participants as cases or controls; in clinical trials, it is the allocation of participants to test or control group.

More than one analytic study is usually required to confirm the identification of risk factors, or before the results of a clinical trial can be generalized. If a weekly fluoride mouthrinse is found to reduce dental caries by 22% over 30 months among 12-year-old children in fluoridated Des Moines,[6] what does that mean for the children of the United States? Even assuming experimental conditions could be identical (which they never are), results need not necessarily be the same for children of different ethnic background, living in different climatic zones, and with differing exposure to fluoridated water. When additional studies are carried out by different researchers in different places with fairly similar results, then the weight of evidence increases the liklihood that the observed effect is real.

METHODS OF MEASURING ORAL DISEASES

Counts: The simplest form of measuring any disease is by a count of the number of cases of its occurrence. Simple counts of cases are most useful with unusual conditions of low prevalence; they become less useful as prevalence increases.

Proportions: A count can be turned into a proportion by adding a denominator, thus determining prevalence. The count of cancers in males aged 55 to 64 can be divided by the population of the group to give prevalence: 22 cases in a population of 845 men aged 55 to 64 yields a prevalence of 0.026, or 2.6%. Proportions do not include a time dimension, the figure just given would include newly

diagnosed cases, as well as long-standing ones.

Proportions can also be useful in expressing the prevalence of caries among schoolchildren, the prevalence of total tooth loss in adults, or other conditions whose occurrence is somewhere between common and rare.

Rates: A rate is a proportion that uses a standardized denominator and includes a time dimension. Infant mortality, for example, is the number of deaths of newborn infants within the first year of life per 1000 live births, usually stated for particular calendar years to illustrate trends. In the United States, the infant mortality rate for white children dropped from 9.2 per 1000 live births in 1985 to 6.9 in 1992; for African-American children the same measures were 19.0 and 16.8, respectively.[33]

Rates have actually been little used in oral disease measures, except in caries incidence over a period of time in clinical trials[6] and in annual rate of loss of periodontal attachment in longitudinal studies.[21] Proportions or index values are often mistakenly referred to as rates in the literature.

Indexes: The individual who suffers from caries in only 2 of 32 teeth clearly has a much lower intensity of disease than does the person who has carious lesions in 16 of 32 teeth. Simple prevalence does not discriminate between these two degrees of intensity, which is usually determined in oral epidemiology by use of an index (the plural form we will use is *indexes*, although the word *indices* is also used).

An index is a graduated, numerical scale with upper and lower limits, with scores on the scale corresponding to specific criteria. Index scores can be expressed for an individual; populations can be characterized by distributions or mean scores. The properties of an ideal index are listed in Table 13–2. Index scores frequently are clinical abstractions (e.g., a Plaque Index score of 1.2), which only make sense when used for comparisons between individuals or groups measured in a similar way. In the literature, the word *index* is often used broadly to mean any form of disease quantification, including proportions and rates. We encourage confining its use to scales meeting the definition here. The criteria for assigning a particular score to a condition are an integral part of the description of any index.

There are several kinds of scale for measuring the intensity of a condition. An *ordinal*

Table 13–2. PROPERTIES OF AN IDEAL INDEX

1. **Validity.** The index must measure what it is intended to measure, so it should correspond with clinical stages of the disease under study at each point.
2. **Reliability.** The index should be able to measure consistently at different times and under a variety of conditions. The term *reliability* is virtually synonymous with *reproducibility, repeatability,* and *consistency,* meaning the ability of the same or different examiners to interpret and use the index in the same way.
3. **Clarity, simplicity, and objectivity.** The criteria should be clear and unambiguous, with mutually exclusive categories. Ideally, it should be readily memorized by an examiner after some practice.
4. **Quantifiability.** The index must be amenable to statistical analysis, so that the status of a group can be expressed by a distribution, mean, median, or other statistical measure.
5. **Sensitivity.** The index should be able to detect clinically-relevant but small shifts, in either direction, in the condition.
6. **Acceptability.** The use of the index should not be unnecessarily painful or demeaning to the subject.

scale lists conditions in order of severity without attempting to define any mathematical relation between the categories. A *nominal* scale is even less rigidly defined; it simply gives names to different conditions and therefore is not strictly a scale at all. An *interval* or a *ratio* scale is one in which the numbers used in the measuring scale purport to have a mathematical relation to each other. The difference between ratio and interval scales is that a ratio scale has a true zero point, such as measures of height and weight, whereas an interval scale does not. Fahrenheit and Celsius temperatures are interval scales, where zero degrees does not mean absence of all heat, whereas the Kelvin scale is a ratio scale.

The majority of indexes used in oral epidemiology are ordinal scales, although many are treated statistically as though they were interval or ratio scales. This statistical impropriety can be a bit academic, however, for such deviations from orthodoxy usually do not give seriously misleading results.

Other terms, such as *reversible* and *irreversible*, are used in the literature to describe indexes. An irreversible index measures cumulative conditions that cannot be reversed: dental caries, for example, which has resulted in tissue loss (restored or unrestored), or tooth loss itself. Gingivitis, however, is a reversible inflammatory condition, so an index of gingivitis is considered reversible.

A final general point about disease measurements is that there are no generic, all-purpose scales that meet every need. Choice of measurement scale in any situation, whether for a practitioner monitoring a patient's progress or for a highly sophisticated clinical trial, is dictated by the needs. The first response to the often-asked question of "What index should I use?" is "What is the question you want to answer?" The process a practitioner goes through to select a measure by which to monitor the oral hygiene progress of a middle-aged periodontal patient is little different from that followed by the researcher in a complex study. Both have to determine why they are using that particular measure, how to handle it reliably, and what they want to demonstrate.

EXAMINER RELIABILITY

When measurements made are over time, conclusions reached are based on the comparison between one set of results and another. It follows that the diagnostic criteria must be applied the same way at different times; if they are not, the comparisons have little value. This is the issue of reliability of diagnosis. Assuming that the index is inherently reproducible, the ability of one examiner to record the same conditions the same way over time is *intraexaminer reliability*. This quality can be developed by most with some training and experience, but it needs to be demonstrated in certain research studies. Intraexaminer reliability can be assessed by an examiner recording conditions in a group of 10 to 20 persons, and then repeating the process a few hours to a few days later. The time between first and second examinations should be long enough for memory to fade, but short enough so that real change will not occur. Reaching agreement between 2 or more examiners, *interexaminer reliability*, is usually more tedious. It requires initial agreement on interpretation of diagnostic criteria, and then a period of training with repeated patient examinations to ensure that examiners are comparable. Interexaminer reliability is rarely perfect, but where examinations from 2 or more examiners are being pooled, evidence of interexaminer reliability training should be provided.

The issue of examiner reliability can

make people uncomfortable, for to have one's inconsistencies exposed for the world to see can be humbling. (We stress that this issue is totally unrelated to clinical skills or ability to care for patients.) In the literature, it is sometimes vaguely dismissed with a statement like "the examiners achieved 96% agreement," which by itself is of little value because of its uncertain meaning (it usually seems to mean that 96% of the scores are the same between examiners). In addition, such a comparison does not account for decisions requiring little diagnostic judgment (e.g., inclusion of many obviously sound lower incisors in the denominator), nor, more important, does it account for agreement that would be expected by chance alone.[10] The measure most frequently used at present for expressing interexaminer consistency is the kappa statistic, a value between zero and 1.0, and based on a comparison of expected and observed comparability from one examination to another, which allows for chance agreement.[10, 17] Correlation statistics and percent agreement, along with kappa, give a good picture of interexaminer reliability in a cross-sectional study.

Reversals can be a plague in longitudinal studies, notably clinical trials. A *reversal*, more properly called a *negative reversal*, is a change of diagnosis in an illogical direction over a period long enough for real change to have taken place. For example, when a surface scored as carious-into-dentin at the first examination is scored sound 1 year later, this is an illogical change. In a clinical trial, the examiner has to record disease that developed over a relatively short time; hence much of it is at incipient stages. Diagnosis of marginal lesions as caries inevitably results in some degree of negative reversals, so reversals are an inherent part of any clinical trial.[30] What has to be remembered about reversals, however, is that if the examiner is consistent, negative reversals will be balanced by positive reversals, which are changes in a logical direction made in error. In a caries trial this means a lesion diagnosed as sound at the first examination is marked as carious a year later, when the diagnosis really should have been sound-sound or carious-carious. The snag, of course, is that positive reversals cannot be separated from normal disease progression. That is where a demonstration of reliability is important. Even if the examinations are all of incipient lesions in first molars, where many reversals would be expected, a consistent examiner will have negative reversals balanced by positive reversals. Net results therefore should be analyzed without "subtracting out" the negative reversals.

Reversals are illustrated in Figure 13–2, which uses 10 tooth surfaces being measured for caries to illustrate the point. Surfaces A to C have progressed from sound to decayed, but D and E (shaded) show negative reversals. The remaining teeth have not changed in diagnosis between examinations. The net result is that the 4 "D" lesions at baseline have become 5 lesions 1 year later. How is

Surface	Baseline		1-Year
A	S	⟶	D
B	S	⟶	D
C	S	⟶	D
D	D	⟶	S
E	D	⟶	S
F	S	⟶	S
G	S	⟶	S
H	S	⟶	S
I	D	⟶	D
J	D	⟶	D

Figure 13–2. Representation of positive and negative diagnostic reversals in a longitudinal study.

this analysis affected by the negative reversals in D and E? Reversals at best can be disturbing (indeed, if the reliability examinations cast doubt on the examiner's reliability, then the entire set of data is suspect). If, however, the examiner is acceptably reliable, it can be assumed that the 2 negative reversals in D and E are random errors and will be balanced by 2 positive reversals among A, B, and C. There could also have been random error in the diagnoses for surfaces F to J, but as there are no changes in diagnosis, such error is not apparent. The net result of 4 decayed lesions progressing to 5 therefore is retained and the 1 additional lesion is referred to as the *net caries increment*.

Reversals in longitudinal studies of periodontitis are especially troublesome because reattachment has been demonstrated by experienced examiners.[20] A measure of loss of periodontal attachment (LPA) of 6 mm at one examination, which is then recorded as 5 mm a year later, could be examiner error, or it could be reattachment. A demonstration of examiner reliability in diagnosis is especially important in these circumstances. Reliability in periodontal examinations has been improved with the advent of pressure-sensitive and computerized probes,[11, 29] although the use of these instruments is largely restricted to clinical research studies.

Note the difference between an examination to check reliability and the occurrence of reversals. A reliability check consists of repeat examinations only hours apart, too close together for real change to have occurred. Different diagnoses therefore are all examination variation. Reversals occur over a period of time long enough for real change to have occurred, so there can be examiner variation mixed in with real change. In a reliability check, the duplicate examinations do not form a part of the dataset, whereas reversals are detected from the study data.

ASSESSMENT OF DISEASE RISK

Diagnostic tests in medicine are numerous and well established. An ideal test should be simple, inexpensive (relative to the direct or social cost of the disease), acceptable to the patient, valid, and reliable. A test should also be *sensitive*, meaning that a high proportion of those with the disease test positive, and *specific*, meaning that a high proportion of those without the disease test negative. Few tests meet all of these criteria, and clinicians and public health administrators often have to choose between degrees of imperfection. For example, the choice may be whether to use a test that is highly sensitive but not very specific (which would capture a lot of false-positives), specific but not sensitive (which would fail to identify some true-positives), or not to test at all. The issues of sensitivity and specificity are discussed at length in many texts on biostatistics and research design; *Biostats*[38] is an excellent example. Figure 13–3 summarizes the way in which sensitivity, specificity, and other predictive values can be derived from the results of tests and subsequent disease outcome.

In dentistry, various predictive tests have been developed through the years, especially for caries. A 1977 conference at Niagara Falls

TEST RESULT	DISEASE	NO DISEASE	TOTAL
Positive	TP	FP	TP + FP
Negative	FN	TN	TN + FN
Total	TP + FN	FP + TN	ALL

Sensitivity: Proportion of people with disease who test positive: **TP/(TP + FN)**

Specificity: Proportion of people without disease who test negative: **TN/(FP + TN)**

Positive Predictive Value: Probability that a person who tests positive will have disease: **TP/(TP + FP)**

Negative Predictive Value: Probability that a person who tests negative will not have disease: **TN/(FN + TN)**

False-Positive Rate: Proportion of people with positive tests who do not have disease: **FP/(FP + TN)**

False-Negative Rate: Proportion of people with negative tests who have disease: **FN/(TP + FN)**

Figure 13–3. Information that can be derived from the results of a predictive test related to disease outcome. *TP*, true positive; *TN*, true negative; *FP*, false positive; *FN*, false negative.

concluded that there was little at that time in the way of bacteriologic, enzymatic, or other biologic tests that predicted caries with a sufficient degree of reliability. The best predictor of future caries was past caries experience,[4] a result consistently found in more recent studies.[9, 19]

Research aimed at predicting future susceptibility to severe periodontitis has developed more recently and still has some way to go.[1, 12] Clinical signs such as gingivitis, plaque deposits, suppuration, and bleeding on probing have demonstrated poor positive predictive value; and even a pocket depth of 4 mm or more is a poor predictor of disease activity.[8] Some promise is emerging with identification of inflammatory mediators in the gingival crevicular fluid,[27] although this area requires refinement before practical everyday tests eventuate. Some modest progress has been achieved by exploring risk factors that have not figured prominently in previous research, such as stress and anxiety, tobacco use, and recent illnesses.[2]

The idea of predictively identifying caries-susceptible individuals was given renewed emphasis with the decline in caries experience during the 1980s (Chapter 19). Most cases of caries and severe periodontitis are now concentrated in relatively small groups, which logically leads to the concept of targeting preventive programs toward these susceptible individuals. Simply put, *targeting* means that it is thought to be more efficient for both practitioners and public health administrators to focus prevention efforts toward the susceptible minority rather than apply them broadly (water fluoridation is an important exception to this philosophy). The concept is logical, although the absence of practical predictive tests has precluded its thorough testing. (Targeted prevention is often assumed to be more cost-effective than a whole-population strategy, although this has not been demonstrated. When administrative costs and the costs of the predictive tests themselves are added in, targeting may not always be the most efficient approach.)

Most research into caries prediction has probably been in microbiology, with tests based on the assumption that high counts of *Streptococcus mutans* and lactobacilli indicate high risk of subsequent caries.[16, 31, 32] Although the causative role of these bacteria in caries is unquestioned,[22] the direct association between bacterial counts and caries incidence is found only with groups, rather than in any one individual.[13] Bacteriologic tests, in general, have high negative predictive values,[36] meaning that a low *S. mutans* count accurately predicts low caries experience, but they have less positive predictive value, meaning that a lot of persons who test positive with high *S. mutans* counts will not develop subsequent caries.

Efforts have also been made to predict caries susceptibility in the permanent dentition from caries experience in the primary dentition. Although some researchers have found correlations, others have not, so this approach cannot be recommended.[37] Reasons for the variable correlations are probably that the caries-etiology factors during young childhood differ from those in later years.

As caries experience continues to decline in the economically developed world, it becomes more difficult to predict the susceptible minority in a population.[14] It is also likely that the cost-effectiveness of public health efforts to identify susceptible individuals will diminish as the proportion of such individuals diminishes.[15] A combination of tests is more effective than any single test,[3] but the more tests used the higher the cost. Because one rationale for identifying the highly susceptible is to improve cost-effectiveness by focusing on preventive programs, if it becomes too expensive to identify susceptible persons then that rationale collapses. This is a vexing dilemma in the prediction area.

From current knowledge, it seems unlikely that the much-desired inexpensive and simple tests to predict future disease susceptibility will emerge; researchers are increasingly accepting that prediction with the necessary power will come only from the right combination of tests.[7] If that combination is too expensive or impractical, prediction at the individual level will continue to be uncertain. The philosophical base for research which equates high-disease status with high risk, can also be debated, for outcome cannot be used to determine risk,[25] and deterministic models do not allow for random effects.[24] Research in disease prediction still has a long way to go. In the meantime, evidence suggests that socioeconomic status is as good a predictor of group susceptibility to caries as currently exists[5, 26] for public health programs.

REFERENCES

1. Beck JD. Methods of assessing risk for periodontitis and developing multifactorial models. J Periodontol 1994;65:468–78.

2. Beck JD, Koch GG, Offenbacher S. Incidence of attachment loss over 3 years in older adults—new and progressing lesions. Community Dent Oral Epidemiol 1995;23:291–6.

3. Beck JD, Weintraub JA, Disney JA, et al. University of North Carolina Caries Risk Assessment Study: Comparisons of high risk prediction, any risk prediction, and any risk etiologic models. Community Dent Oral Epidemiol 1992;20:313–21.

4. Bibby BG, Shern RJ, eds: Methods of caries prediction: proceedings of a workshop conference. Washington DC: Information Retrieval Inc, 1978.

5. Clark BJ, Graves RC, Webster DB, Triol CW. Caries and treatment patterns in children related to school lunch eligibility. J Public Health Dent 1987;47:134–8.

6. Driscoll WS, Swango PA, Horowitz AM, Kingman A. Caries-preventive effects of daily and weekly fluoride mouthrinsing in a fluoridated community: Final results after 30 months. J Am Dent Assoc 1982;105:1010–3.

7. Fédération Dentaire Internationale, Commission on Oral Research and Epidemiology. Review of methods of identification of high caries risk groups and individuals. FDI Tech Rep No 31. Int Dent J 1988;38:177–89.

8. Haffajee AD, Socransky SS, Goodson JM. Clinical parameters as predictors of destructive disease activity. J Clin Periodontol 1983;10:257–65.

9. Hausen H, Seppa L, Fejerskov O. Can caries be predicted? In: Thylstrup A, Fejerskov O, eds: Textbook of clinical cariology. 2nd ed. Copenhagen: Munksgaard, 1994:393–411.

10. Hunt RJ. Percent agreement, Pearson's correlation, and kappa as measures of interexaminer reliability. J Dent Res 1986;65:128–30.

11. Jeffcoat MK, Jeffcoat RL, Jens SC, Captain K. A new periodontal probe with automated cemento-enamel junction detection. J Clin Periodontol 1986;13:276–80.

12. Johnson NW. Detection of high-risk groups and individuals for periodontal diseases. Int Dent J 1989;39:33–47.

13. Kingman A, Little W, Gomez I, et al. Salivary levels of Streptococcus mutans and lactobacilli and dental caries experiences in a US adolescent population. Community Dent Oral Epidemiol 1988;16:98–103.

14. Klock B, Emilson C-G, Lind S-O, et al. Prediction of caries activity in children with today's low caries scores. Community Dent Oral Epidemiol 1989;17:285–8.

15. Koch G. Importance of early determination of caries risk. Int Dent J 1988;38:203–10.

16. Krasse B. Biological factors as indicators of future caries. Int Dent J 1988;38:219–25.

17. Landis JR, Koch GG. The measurement of observer agreement for categorical data. Biometrics 1977;33:159–74.

18. Last JM. A dictionary of epidemiology. 3rd ed. New York: OUP, 1995.

19. Leverett DH, Proskin HM, Featherstone JD, et al. Caries risk assessment in a longitudinal discrimination study. J Dent Res 1993;72:538–43.

20. Lindhe J, Haffajee AD, Socransky SS. Progression of periodontal disease in adult subjects in the absence of periodontal therapy. J Clin Periodontol 1983;10:433–42.

21. Löe H, Ånerud A, Boysen H, Morrison E. Natural history of periodontal disease in man. Rapid, moderate and no loss of attachment in Sri Lankan laborers 14 to 46 years of age. J Clin Periodontol 1986;13:431–40.

22. Loesche WJ. Role of Streptococcus mutans in human dental decay. Microbiol Rev 1986;50:353–80.

23. Longmate N. Alive and well: Medicine and public health from 1830 to the present day. Harmondsworth: Penguin, 1970.

24. Manji F, Fejerskov O, Nagelkerke NJ, Baelum VA. Random effects model for some epidemiological features of dental caries. Community Dent Oral Epidemiol 1991;19:324–8.

25. Manji F, Nagelkerke N. What can variations in disease outcome tell us about risk? Community Dent Oral Epidemiol 1990;18:106–7.

26. Milen A. Role of social class in caries occurrence in primary teeth. Int J Epidemiol 1987;16:252–6.

27. Offenbacher S, Collins JG, Yalda B, Haradon G. Role of prostaglandins in high-risk periodontitis patients. In: Genco RJ, Hamada S, Lehner T, et al, eds: Molecular pathogenesis of peridontal disease. Washington DC: American Society for Microbiology, 1994:203–13.

28. Osborn JE. Dispelling myths about the AIDS epidemic. In: Fransen VE, ed: Proceedings of the AIDS prevention and services workshop. Princeton, NJ: Robert Wood Johnson Foundation, 1990:15–21.

29. Polson AM, Goodson JM. Periodontal diagnosis: Current status and future needs. J Periodontol 1985;56:25–34.

30. Radike AW. Examiner error and reversals in diagnosis. In: Proceedings of the conference on the clinical testing of cariostatic agents. Chicago: American Dental Association, 1972:92–5.

31. Sëppa L, Pollanen L, Hausen H. Streptococcus mutans counts obtained by a dip-slide method in relation to caries frequency, sucrose intake and flow rate of saliva. Caries Res 1988;22:226–9.

32. Stecksen-Blicks C. Lactobacilli and Streptococcus mutans in saliva, diet and caries increment in 8- and 13-year-old children. Scand J Dent Res 1987;95:18–26.

33. US Public Health Service, National Center for Health Statistics. Health United States 1994. DHHS Publ No (PHS) 95–1232. Washington DC: Government Printing Office, 1995.

34. US Public Health Service, National Center for Health Statistics. Current estimates from the National Health Interview Survey, 1993. DHHS Publ No (PHS) 95–1518, Series 10 No 190. Washington DC: Government Printing Office, 1994.

35. US Public Health Service, National Institute of Dental Research. Oral health of United States adults; national findings. NIH Publication No 87–2868. Washington DC: Government Printing Office, 1987.

36. Van Houte J. Microbiological predictors of caries risk. Adv Dent Res 1993;7:87–96.

37. Van Palenstein Helderman WH, ter Pelkwijk L, Van Dijk JWE. Caries in fissures of permanent first molars as a predictor for caries increment. Community Dent Oral Epidemiol 1989;17:282–4.

38. Weintraub JA, Douglass CW, Gillings DB. Biostats: Data analysis for dental health care professionals. 2nd ed. Chapel Hill, NC: Cavco, 1985.

39. Yankauer A. AIDS and public health [editorial]. Am J Public Health 1988;78:364–6.

14

Measuring Dental Caries

The DMF Index ◆ Criteria for Diagnosing Coronal
Caries ◆ Root Caries ◆ Caries Treatment Needs

This chapter describes the methods for measuring dental caries in human populations. Those devised in the early 20th century included the proportion of first molars lost through caries[19, 20] and the percentage of permanent teeth affected.[1, 37] Both of these methods were useful when there was little information about the disease, but they lacked sensitivity. At the other extreme, Bodecker's index of surfaces affected by caries, described in 1931,[10] was sensitive but complicated. Dean and colleagues[13] used a systematic approach to counting the numbers of teeth in the mouth visibly affected by caries in their pioneering studies of the caries-fluoride relationship. The first description of what is now known as the DMF index is attributed to Klein, Palmer, and Knutson[29] in their studies of dental caries in Hagerstown, Maryland, in the 1930s. Since then, the DMF index has received practically universal acceptance and is the best known of all dental indexes.

THE DMF INDEX

The DMF, an irreversible index, is applied only to permanent teeth. As originally described, D was for decayed teeth; M, teeth missing due to caries; and F for teeth that had been previously filled. Filled teeth were assumed to have been unequivocally decayed before restoration. The DMF score for any individual can range from 0 to 32, in whole numbers. A mean DMF score for a group, being the total of individual values divided by the number of subjects examined, can have fractional values. The DMF index can be applied to whole teeth (designated as DMFT) or

to surfaces (DMFS). Modifications can be made to the index for such factors as secondary caries, crowned teeth, bridge pontics, and any other particular attribute required for a study. To save time in a large survey, DMF can be used half-mouth, applied to opposite diagonal quadrants and the score doubled, an approach that assumes that caries is bilateral.

The DMF index, for permanent teeth, is always signified by uppercase letters; the equivalent index for the primary dentition is the *def* and its modifications.[17] As originally defined, *d* stood for decayed teeth, *e* meant indicated for extraction, and *f* was filled teeth. In the def index, teeth missing for caries are not recorded because of complications with exfoliation, and not knowing whether such teeth were carious before exfoliation. Modifications of this index are (a) dmf for use in children before ages of exfoliation, (b) dmf applied only to the primary molar teeth, and (c) the df index. Values for df and def should be numerically the same; def allows for two grades of caries, and neither index counts missing teeth. Both def and df, therefore, may understate the true extent of the carious attack, although the greater reliability gained by ignoring missing teeth is usually seen as a net benefit.

Other methods of measuring dental caries have been suggested with a different philosophical base from that of the DMF index. One is Grainger's hierarchy, an ordinal scale designed to simplify the recording of the caries status of a population, which uses 5 zones of severity of the carious attack.[16] It appears to be valid,[26, 28, 41] but has received little use, probably because of low sensitivity. More recently, "composite" indicators have been suggested that attempt to measure health rather than disease by weighting healthy restored teeth differently from missing or decayed teeth.[42] The first of these is the FS-T, which adds the sound and healthy restored teeth. Another is T-Health, which seeks to measure the amount of healthy dental tissue and ascribes descending numerical weights for a sound healthy tooth, a filled tooth, and a decayed tooth. These are conceptually sound approaches to measuring dental health and function (rather than disease), and they probably deserve more attention than they have received.

The DMF index has actually received remarkably little challenge over 60 years of life, probably because it is simple and versatile. It does have limitations, the principal ones being:

- DMF values are not related to the number of teeth at risk. A DMF score for an individual is a simple count of those teeth that in the examiner's judgment have been affected by caries; it has no denominator. A DMF score thus does not directly give an indication of the intensity of the attack in any one individual. A 7-year-old child with a DMF score of 3.0 may have only nine permanent teeth in the mouth; thus one third of these teeth have already been attacked by caries in a short space of time. An adult may have a DMF score of 8.0 from a full complement of 32 teeth; thus over a longer time only one fourth of the teeth have been affected. DMF scores therefore have little meaning unless age is also stated.
- The DMF index gives equal weight to missing, untreated decayed, or well-restored teeth. Common sense suggests that this philosophical basis is faulty for many purposes.
- The DMF index is invalid when teeth have been lost for reasons other than caries. Teeth can be lost for periodontal reasons in older adults, and for orthodontic reasons in teenagers. Decision rules, which go along with criteria, are required to determine how to deal with these instances.
- The DMF index can overestimate caries experience in teeth with "preventive restorations." In an epidemiologic survey, such teeth must be included in the F component of DMF; although had they not been filled in the first place, they might have been diagnosed as sound teeth. DMF scores will

thus be inflated.[5] Composite restorations judged to have been placed only for cosmetic reasons likewise should not be included in DMF counts.
- DMF data are of little use for estimating treatment needs (see Caries Treatment Needs).
- DMF cannot account for sealed teeth. Sealants did not exist in 1938. Here is where the DMF index shows its age. Sealants and other composite restorations for cosmetic purposes have to be dealt with separately.

There are two reasonable approaches for dealing with sealants in the DMF index. One says that the sealed tooth is not restored in the classic sense and therefore should be considered sound. The other says that it has required hands-on, one-to-one dental attention, and so should be considered a filled tooth. Probably the best way to deal with sealed teeth is to put them in a category by themselves, S for sealed. The DMFS index would then become DMFSS. Depending on the study's purpose, the S teeth can be left separate, included with F, or regarded as sound. The examiners have to set decision rules on how to score deficient sealants.

The DMF index can be used for measuring root caries, although this is not recommended. If it is so used, scores for coronal caries should be kept separately from those for root caries because teeth with root lesions often already have coronal lesions (see Root Caries). This can make data interpretation awkward.

With modern preventive and restorative technology, the DMF index is becoming outdated as a measure of caries attack; it may be more valid as a measure of treatment received. The unquestioned assumption at the time of its inception was that restored teeth represented unequivocal caries, an assumption we cannot make so readily today. It is philosophically questionable to use an index for a disease that is so dependent on the treatment judgments of many practitioners for its quantification. A measure of caries activity would be preferable for many purposes, but until such a measure is created DMF will continue to be used. The results of its use, however, should always be interpreted thoughtfully.

CRITERIA FOR DIAGNOSING CORONAL CARIES

There is no global consensus on the criteria for diagnosing dental caries, despite a vast

Table 14–1. CRITERIA FOR DIAGNOSING CARIES THROUGH THE FULL RANGE OF LESION DEVELOPMENT (THE "D1–D3" SCALE), SHOWN TO CONTRAST WITH THE CRITERIA FOR DIAGNOSIS AT THE DENTINAL-LESION STAGE ONLY (THE "DICHOTOMOUS" SCALE)

DIAGNOSIS THROUGH THE FULL RANGE OF CARIES (THE "D1–D3" SCALE):

0. **Surface Sound.** No evidence of treated or untreated clinical caries (slight staining allowed in an otherwise sound fissure).
D1. **Initial Caries.** No clinically detectable loss of substance. For pits and fissures, there may be significant staining, discoloration, or rough spots in the enamel that do not catch the explorer, but loss of substance cannot be positively diagnosed. For smooth surfaces, these may be white, opaque areas with loss of luster.
D2. **Enamel Caries.** Demonstrable loss of tooth substance in pits, fissures, or on smooth surfaces, but no softened floor or wall or undermined enamel. The texture of the material within the cavity may be chalky or crumbly, but there is no evidence that cavitation has penetrated the dentin.
D3. **Caries of Dentin.** Detectably softened floor, undermined enamel, or a softened wall, or the tooth has a temporary filling. On approximal surfaces, the explorer point must enter a lesion with certainty.
D4. **Pulpal Involvement.** Deep cavity with probable pulpal involvement. Pulp should not be probed. (Usually included with D3 in data analysis.)

DIAGNOSIS AT THE DENTINAL LESION STAGE ONLY (THE "DICHOTOMOUS" SCALE):

Pits and fissures on the occlusal, vestibular, and lingual surfaces are carious when the explorer "catches" after insertion with moderate to firm pressure *and* when the "catch" is accompanied by one or more of the following signs of decay:

1. Softness at the base of the area.
2. Opacity adjacent to the area* provides evidence of undermining or demineralization.
3. Softened enamel adjacent to the area that may be scraped away by the explorer.

*These areas should be diagnosed as sound when there is apparent evidence of demineralization but no evidence of softness.
From Pitts NB, Fyffe HE. The effect of varying diagnostic thresholds upon clinical caries data for a low prevalence group. J Dent Res 1988;67:592–6; Horowitz HS. Clinical trials of preventives for dental caries. J Public Health Dent 1972;32:229–33.

quantity of words on the subject. Different traditions about defining a lesion in the "gray area," where it is difficult to tell whether or not the disease is irreversibly established, have grown up and are still adhered to. Apart from the inherent problem of diagnosing a borderline lesion, the major philosophical issue is how to score the early carious lesion that has not yet become cavitated, whether diagnosed clinically or radiographically. These lesions appear as a discolored fissure without loss of substance, as a "white spot" on visible smooth surfaces, or radiographically as an early interproximal shadow. The issue is that not all noncavitated lesions progress to become dentinal lesions requiring restorative treatment; a good proportion of them remain static or even regress, especially smooth surface lesions.[39] These lesions are thus reversible, as opposed to a dentinal lesion, which is usually considered irreversible. Because there are usually more noncavitated than cavitated lesions at any one time in both high-caries and low-caries populations,[9, 21, 40] the decision of whether to include or exclude them can make a substantial difference in the oral health profiles obtained.

Examples of these two different approaches to diagnostic criteria for dental car-

ies are shown in Table 14–1. Traditionally, European investigators have recorded caries on a scale that extends through the full range of disease from the earliest detectable noncavitated lesion through to pulpal involvement.[3] The full-range criteria in Table 14–1 are based on those first published by WHO in 1979,[51] and are now referred to as the *D1-D3* scale. On the other hand, investigators in North America, Britain, and the other English-speaking countries have traditionally recorded caries as a dichotomous condition, meaning caries is diagnosed only as present or absent. (We will refer to this as the dichotomous scale.) In the dichotomous recording, caries is noted only when it has reached the level of dentinal involvement[18] (i.e., the D3 level). Use of the D1-D3 scale requires the teeth to be dried and a longer, more meticulous survey examination. Although there are more diagnostic decisions to make in the D1-D3 scale, adequate examiner reliability can be maintained when examiners have been trained in this system.[39]

The D1-D3 scale is of extreme value in research studies on dental caries, for it permits identification of lesion progression as well as initiation. Research questions on the conditions under which early lesions progress, regress, or remain static can thus be answered only with such a measurement scale. Its use demands meticulous examiner training, for if D1 lesions are capable of regressing back to sound enamel, it becomes difficult to differentiate examiner error from natural phenomena. There is less consensus on whether the D1-D3 scale should be used in large-scale surveys. Arguments can be made both ways, but on balance we believe that more benefit is gained from surveys continuing to diagnose caries at the D3 level only (i.e., using the dichotomous scale).[11]

Caries diagnosis by clinical means, irrespective of the criteria used, has traditionally used visual-tactile means (i.e., explorer as well as vision). Indeed, the criteria listed in the dichotomous scale in Table 14–1 explicitly require use of the explorer. With our current understanding of caries, however, routine use of the explorer this way is likely to damage the enamel matrix of noncavitated lesions where remineralization is taking place. As a result, European criteria for diagnosing caries in the 1990s have moved more toward exclusively visual criteria. Initial studies with a group of dentists using extracted teeth that later were sectioned and histologically examined found that the explorer did not add to the value of exclusively visual diagnosis.[32, 33] The series of surveys for monitoring caries in British children that is carried out by the British Association for the Study of Community Dentistry uses the exclusively visual approach in its protocol. Caries is recorded at the D3 level, and the criterion for caries is: ". . . if, in the opinion of a trained examiner, after visual inspection there is a carious lesion into dentine,"[39] then caries is recorded. This criterion requires extensive examiner training and meticulous drying of the teeth. The third National Health and Nutrition Examination Survey (NHANES III) in the United States, 1988–1994, retained the traditional dichotomous criteria shown in Table 14–1.[22]

Caries diagnosis is also complicated by *hidden* caries, the name given to dentinal caries found radiographically beneath an apparently sound occlusal surface.[27, 39, 48] This condition is poorly understood, although it is hardly rare. One study found hidden caries in 7.5% of a group of children.[49] Some see it as a by-product of the fluoride age, in which the original break in the enamel remineralizes before the dentinal lesion has reached the pulp, but its natural history is really unknown. Additional research on this condition

is clearly needed. Hidden caries has led to a further look at the use of radiographs for caries diagnosis at a time when they generally are not used in caries epidemiologic studies and clinical trials for ethical reasons (unnecessary exposure when not used in the course of treatment), costs, and the risk of bias, which comes from the refusal of some study participants to be radiographed.

Newer methods of caries diagnosis, such as fiberoptic transillumination (FOTi) and electrical conductance have shown promise[27, 34] and may find a role in epidemiologic study, as well as in patient care. These diagnostic aids do not change the philosophical approach to measuring caries; if reliable they permit noncavitated lesions to be detected at earlier stages of development. Whether this is always necessary depends on the aims of the study and the purposes for which the resulting data are used.

ROOT CARIES

The criteria most frequently used to diagnose root caries were first described in 1980.[7] The clinical examination was carried out after a thorough prophylaxis, after which root caries was diagnosed according to the criteria shown in Table 14–2. Although these criteria have proved to be versatile, there are several diagnostic conditions in root caries that have not yet been fully settled. These problems include the lack of a universally accepted case definition,[8] inability to detect active from nonactive lesions,[24] and uncertainties with diagnostic reliability.[6]

Root lesions are becoming increasingly difficult to detect because they are more commonly found as small, discrete lesions on a

Table 14–2. CRITERIA FOR DIAGNOSING ROOT SURFACE CARIES

1. There was a discrete, well-defined, and discolored soft area.
2. The explorer entered easily and displayed some resistance to withdrawal.
3. The lesion was located either at the cemento-enamel junction or wholly on the root surface.
4. Restored root lesions were counted only if it was obvious that the lesion originated at the cemento-enamel junction or was confined to the root surface completely.

From Banting DW, Ellen RP, Fillery ED. Prevalence of root surface caries among institutionalized older persons. Community Dent Oral Epidemiol 1980;8:84–8.

single root surface rather than circumscribing a root.[43] Although most lesions occur on exposed root surfaces, approximately 15% of all root lesions have been found on surfaces without gingival recession, although they have loss of periodontal attachment.[12, 30, 43] It is not yet clear whether these root lesions form in periodontal pockets, or whether an exposed root surface later becomes covered by the overgrowth of inflamed gingiva. Problems in locating the cementoenamel junction, because of obliteration by restorations or calculus, can add to the diagnostic difficulties.[24]

Root caries can be expressed by a simple prevalence figure, meaning the proportion of a defined population with at least one root lesion, and from the mean number of carious or restored root lesions per person (i.e., a DFS count). For the most complete profile of root caries activity, however, these values should be accompanied by the number of missing teeth and by Root Caries Index (RCI) scores.

The RCI, first described in 1980,[23] was intended to make the simple prevalence measures more specific by including the concept of teeth at risk (in contrast to the DMF). A tooth was considered to be at risk of root caries if enough gingival recession has occurred to expose part of the cemental surface to the oral environment. The RCI is computed by scoring root lesions and restorations and noting teeth with gingival recession, according to the following formula:

$$\frac{\text{Root surfaces: decayed } + \text{ filled}}{\begin{array}{c}\text{(Root surfaces with loss of}\\ \text{periodontal attachment:}\\ \text{Decayed } + \text{ Filled } + \text{ Sound)}\end{array}} \times 100$$

The index can be computed for an individual, particular tooth types, or for a population at large. An RCI of 7% means that of all teeth with gingival recession, 7% were decayed or filled on the root surfaces. As with any index scores, results are most useful if a distribution measure is also presented, as means can be unduly weighted by a small number of individuals with severe disease.

The original description of the RCI acknowledged the chance of underestimation brought on by exclusion of subgingival lesions,[23] but at the time these were considered unusual. As noted previously, however, approximately 15% or more of root lesions since recorded are subgingival. Accordingly, it is now recommended that the RCI be applied to both supragingival and subgingival le-

sions, but that the scores for each type of lesion be recorded separately.[25] This recommendation is made because we are not yet sure if the subgingival lesions are etiologically distinct from supragingival lesions and because of the likely difficulties in recording subgingival lesions (i.e., they can be underestimated because of the diagnostic problems in finding them).

CARIES TREATMENT NEEDS

Assessment of the caries treatment needs of a group, at first glance, appears to be nothing more than the D segment of a mean DMF score assessed from a survey. This approach, however, has been shown not to work for the following reasons:

- Criteria used to diagnose caries in a survey usually are not the same as those used by practitioners in forming a patient's treatment plan.
- A patient's own perceived needs, level of interest in his dental conditions, and ability or willingness to pay all influence the level of treatment carried out.
- A practitioner has to judge if a minor lesion will develop into a major lesion over time, and also if a lesion in a primary tooth can safely remain untreated for the life of the tooth. A survey scores a tooth by how it appears at the present time.
- Treatment philosophies change with expanding knowledge and technologic developments; a treatment that is standard today may not be so tomorrow.

Because surveys are usually conducted in less than ideal conditions, relative to the dental office, it would be expected that surveys detect fewer carious lesions than do practitioners. Although that has been shown to be true,[31, 38] it begs the question of which assessment is "correct." Field surveys can miss early lesions, but practitioners can also overtreat. In addition, treatment plans for the same patients vary drastically from dentist to dentist.[4, 15, 36]

Difficulties in determining treatment need by survey have been illustrated by an important series of reports from Scotland. They began with a 1978 national dental survey in Britain, in the course of which 720 dentate adults in Scotland agreed to permit their dental records to be followed over subsequent years. After 3 years, records showed that whereas 863 teeth in this group had been assessed as needing restorative care in the survey, 3108 actually had been restored. One might think that this finding could be explained by lesions missed under the poorer survey conditions, but if that explanation is accepted, then the next finding has no logic. Of the 863 teeth classified as needing restorative treatment in the survey, only 271 (31%) were in the 3108 restored.[35] This shows that the care, rather than being an extension of the survey results, in fact bore no relation to them. There were similar findings with prosthetic treatment.[14]

Dental needs in the United States were assessed by examiners in the first National Health and Examination Survey (NHANES I) of 1971–1974; 65% of the population was judged as being in need of care.[44] A similar assessment was made with the first national survey of schoolchildren in 1979–1980, when 37% of schoolchildren were judged to be in need of restorative care.[45] The validity of these figures is debatable, and they have received little use. In later national surveys,[46, 47] treatment needs assessments were not carried out.

The World Health Organization (WHO) includes a subjective treatment-need assessment by the examiner as part of its Pathfinder survey method,[50] although it has not been determined how well these estimates approximate treatment actually carried out. WHO also has developed a broad-based approach to determining needs in an economically undeveloped country through what it calls a *Situation Analysis*, an enhancement of Pathfinder survey data with information on population trends, school enrollment figures, per capita income, and health care resources.[52]

Public health directors in the United States are required to submit information on health needs, including dental care needs, to qualify for Maternal and Child Health Block Grant funds from the federal government (Chapter 8). From what has been said on the difficulty of gathering treatment need information from surveys, this would seem to present a problem. However, the American Association of State and Territorial Dental Directors has developed a detailed manual[2] to help public health personnel in collecting the necessary data. The approach is similar in spirit to WHO's Situation Analysis and relies on using existing data from national surveys to derive broad categories of need, such as proportions of children with caries, oral injuries, fluorosis, or baby bottle tooth decay, or

the extent of health risks such as tobacco use. When added to existing data from the census, and from routinely collected information (e.g., the extent of water fluoridation, fluoride mouthrinsing programs), a broad but not overly-detailed community profile can be constructed. This approach to estimating caries treatment needs, broad though it is, is probably as detailed as treatment need assessment ever needs to be.

REFERENCES

1. Ainsworth NJ. Mottled teeth. Br Dent J 1933;55:233–50, 274.
2. American Association of State and Territorial Dental Directors. Assessing oral health needs: ASTDD seven-step model. ASTDD, undated typescript.
3. Backer-Dirks O, Houwink B, Kwant GW. The results of $6\frac{1}{2}$ years of artificial drinking water in the Netherlands: The Tiel-Culemborg experiment. Arch Oral Biol 1961;5:284–300.
4. Bader JD, Shugars DA. Agreement among dentists' recommendations for restorative treatment. J Dent Res 1993;72:891–6.
5. Bader JD, Shugars DA, Rozier RG. Relationship between epidemiologic coronal caries assessments and practitioners' treatment recommendations in adults. Community Dent Oral Epidemiol 1993;21:96–101.
6. Banting DW. Diagnosis and prediction of root caries. Adv Dent Res 1993;7:80–6.
7. Banting DW, Ellen RP, Fillery ED. Prevalence of root surface caries among institutionalized older persons. Community Dent Oral Epidemiol 1980;8:84–8.
8. Billings RJ, Banting DW. Future directions for root caries research. Gerodontol 1993;10:114–9.
9. Bjarnason S, Kohler B, Ranggard L. Dental caries in a group of 15 to 16-year-olds from Göteborg. Part I. Swed Dent J 1992;16:143–9.
10. Bodecker CF, Bodecker HWC. A practical index of the varying susceptibility to dental caries in man. Dent Cosmos 1931;73:707–16.
11. Burt BA. How useful are cross-sectional data from surveys of dental caries? Community Dent Oral Epidemiol 1997;25:36–41.
12. Burt BA, Ismail AI, Eklund SA. Root caries in an optimally fluoridated and a high-fluoride community. J Dent Res 1986;65:1154–8.
13. Dean HT, Arnold FA, Jr, Elvove E. Domestic water and dental caries. V. Additional studies of the relation of fluoride domestic waters to dental caries experience in 4,425 white children aged 12–14 years of age in 13 cities in 4 states. Public Health Rep 1942;57:1155–79.
14. Eddie S, Elderton RJ. Comparison of dental status determined in an epidemiological survey with prosthetic treatment need. Community Dent Oral Epidemiol 1983;11:271–7.
15. Espelid I, Tveit AB, Haugejorden O, Riordan PJ. Variation in radiographic interpretation and restorative treatment decisions on approximal caries among dentists in Norway. Community Dent Oral Epidemiol 1985;13:26–9.
16. Grainger RM. Epidemiological data. In: Chilton NW. Design and analysis in dental and oral research. 1st ed. Philadelphia: JB Lippincott, 1967:311–53.

17. Gruebbel AO. A measure of dental caries prevalence and treatment service for deciduous teeth. J Dent Res 1944;23:163–8.

18. Horowitz HS. Clinical trials of preventives for dental caries. J Public Health Dent 1972;32:229–33.

19. Hyatt TP. Report of an examination made of two thousand one hundred and one high school pupils. Dent Cosmos 1920;52:507–11.

20. Hyatt TP. Prophylactic odontotomy. Dent Cosmos 1923;65:234–41.

21. Ismail AI, Brodeur JM, Gagnon P, et al. Prevalence of non-cavitated and cavitated carious lesions in a random sample of 7–9-year-old schoolchildren in Montreal, Quebec. Community Dent Oral Epidemiol 1992;20:250–5.

22. Kaste LM, Selwitz RH, Oldakowski RJ, et al. Coronal caries in the primary and permanent dentition of children and adolescents 1–17 years of age: United States, 1988–1991. J Dent Res 1996;75(Spec Issue):631–41.

23. Katz RV. Assessing root caries in populations: The evolution of the Root Caries Index. J Public Health Dent 1980;40:7–16.

24. Katz RV. The clinical diagnosis of root caries: Issues for the clinician and the researcher. Am J Dent 1995;8:335–41.

25. Katz RV. The RCI revisited after 15 years: Used, reinvented, modified, debated, and natural logged. J Public Health Dent 1996;56:28–34.

26. Katz RV, Meskin LH. Testing the internal and external validity of a simplified dental caries index on an adult population. Community Dent Oral Epidemiol 1976;4:227–31.

27. Kidd EA, Ricketts DNJ, Pitts NB. Occlusal caries diagnosis: A changing challenge for clinicians and epidemiologists. J Dent 1993;21:323–31.

28. Kingman A. A method of utilizing the subject's initial caries experience to increase efficiency in caries clinical trials. Community Dent Oral Epidemiol 1979;7:87–90.

29. Klein H, Palmer CE, Knutson JW. Studies on dental caries: I. Dental status and dental needs of elementary school children. Public Health Rep 1938;53:751–65.

30. Locker D, Slade GD, Leake JL. Prevalence of and factors associated with root decay in older adults in Canada. J Dent Res 1989;68:768–72.

31. Long LM Jr, Rozier RG, Bawden JW. Estimation of actual caries prevalence and treatment needs from field survey caries information on a child population in USA. Community Dent Oral Epidemiol 1979;7:322–9.

32. Lussi A. Validity of diagnostic and treatment decisions of fissure caries. Caries Res 1991;25:296–303.

33. Lussi A. Comparison of different methods for the diagnosis of fissure caries without cavitation. Caries Res 1993;27:409–16.

34. Lussi A, Firestone A, Schoenberg V, et al. In vivo diagnosis of fissure caries using a new electrical resistance monitor. Caries Res 1995;29:81–7.

35. Nuttall NM. Capability of a national epidemiological survey to predict General Dental Service treatment. Community Dent Oral Epidemiol 1983;11:296–301.

36. Nuttall NM, Pitts NB, Fyffe HE. Assessment of reports by dentists of their restorative treatment thresholds. Community Dent Oral Epidemiol 1993;21:273–8.

37. Pedersen PO. Dental disease in Europe and Greenland. J Royal Soc Health 1971;91:23–7.

38. Pickles TH. The relationship of caries prevalence data and diagnosed treatment needs in a child population. Med Care 1970;8:463–73.

39. Pitts NB. Current methods and criteria for caries diagnosis in Europe. J Dent Educ 1993;57:409–14.

40. Pitts NB, Fyffe HE. The effect of varying diagnostic thresholds upon clinical caries data for a low prevalence group. J Dent Res 1988;67:592–6.

41. Poulsen S, Horowitz H. An evaluation of a hierarchical method of describing the pattern of dental caries attack. Community Dent Oral Epidemiol 1974;2:7–11.

42. Sheiham A, Maizels J, Maizels A. New composite indicators of dental health. Community Dent Health 1987;4:407–14.

43. Stamm JW, Banting DW, Imrey PB. Adult root caries survey of two similar communities with contrasting natural water fluoride levels. J Am Dent Assoc 1990;120:143–9.

44. US Public Health Service, National Center for Health Statistics. Basic data on dental examination findings of persons aged 1–74 years; United States. DHEW Publication No. (PHS) 79–1662, Series 11 No 214. Washington DC: Government Printing Office, 1979.

45. US Public Health Service, National Institute of Dental Research. Dental treatment needs of United States children. NIH Publication No 83–2246. Washington DC: Government Printing Office, 1982.

46. US Public Health Service, National Institute of Dental Research. Oral health of United States adults; national findings. NIH Publication No 87–2868. Washington DC: Government Printing Office, 1987.

47. US Public Health Service, National Institute of Dental Research. Oral health of United States children. NIH Publication No 89–2247. Washington DC: Government Printing Office, 1989.

48. Weerheijm KL, Groen HJ, Bast AJ, et al. Clinically undetected occlusal dentine caries: a radiographic comparison. Caries Res 1992;26:305–9.

49. Weerheijm KL, Gruythuysen RJ, van Amerongen WE. Prevalence of hidden caries. J Dent Child 1992;59:408–12.

50. World Health Organization. Oral health surveys; basic methods. 4th ed. Geneva: WHO, 1997.

51. World Health Organization. A guide to oral health epidemiological investigations. Geneva: WHO, 1979.

52. World Health Organization. Planning oral health services. Geneva: WHO Offset Publication No 53, 1980.

15

Measuring Periodontal Diseases

Gingivitis ◆ Periodontitis ◆ Periodontal Treatment
Needs ◆ Plaque and Calculus ◆ Partial-Mouth
Periodontal Measurements

In contrast to the stability of the DMF index for caries over a 50-year period, the philosophical basis for measuring periodontal disease has changed several times over a shorter time. In the early days of modern periodontal research (i.e., the 1950–1960s), "periodontal disease" was seen as a single entity, which began with gingivitis and progressed to periodontitis and tooth loss. This view is now obsolete (Chapter 20), so that indexes based on it are considered invalid. The separate clinical measures now used for gingivitis and periodontitis were first described 40 years ago, although some measures based on molecular biology are emerging at the end of the 20th century.

GINGIVITIS

The oldest reversible index is the P-M-A (Papillary-Marginal-Attached), which dates from the immediate post-World War II period.[33] With better understanding of the inflammatory process, it gave way to the Gingival Index (GI) of Löe and Silness[30] in the early 1960s. The GI grades the gingiva on the mesial, distal, buccal, and lingual surfaces of the teeth. Each area is scored on a 0 to 3 ordinal scale according to the criteria shown in Table 15–1. The GI has been used on selected teeth in the mouth,[42] as well as on all erupted teeth.[29] The GI, an index of gingivitis that takes no account of deeper changes in the periodontium, is sufficiently sensitive to distinguish between groups with little and with severe gingivitis, although it may not discriminate as well between the middle ranges.

The use of gingival bleeding after gentle probing as a measure of gingivitis has become a standard measure in clinical trials. Although visual assessments of inflammation (color, swelling) are subjective, the appearance of spots of blood after gently running the probe around the gingival margin is more sensitive[20] and more objective in those sites that are difficult to view directly.[21] Validity against the GI has also been demonstrated.[35] The major subjective area with a gingival bleeding index is "gentle probing," which has been shown to vary between 3 and 130 grams with different examiners.[37] A further refinement of the bleeding indexes came with the Eastman Interdental Bleeding Index,[13] which may be more sensitive than other measures of papillary bleeding.[14]

Gingival bleeding indexes, as opposed to visually determined gingivitis, are not recommended in public health programs for three reasons:

• This degree of sensitivity is rarely required

Table 15–1. SCORES AND CRITERIA FOR THE GINGIVAL INDEX (GI)

0:	Normal gingiva.
1:	Mild inflammation—slight change in color, slight edema. No bleeding on probing.
2:	Moderate inflammation—redness, edema, and glazing. Bleeding on probing.
3:	Severe inflammation—marked redness and edema. Ulceration. Tendency to spontaneous bleeding.

From Löe H, Silness J. Periodontal disease in pregnancy. I. Prevalence and severity. Acta Odont Scand 1963;21:533–51.

in surveys or screening programs; it may be needed in cohort and case-control studies.

- They have uncertain discriminatory power in field conditions.[31]
- Concerns about infection control make the deliberate inducement of gingival bleeding in surveys or screening programs hard to justify.

The Modified Gingival Index (MGI) was developed to eliminate the use of bleeding on probing while still providing high visual sensitivity with incipient gingivitis.[28] Gingivitis is an area where valid nonclinical measures would be highly beneficial.

PERIODONTITIS

Many early epidemiologic studies of periodontal diseases were based on radiographic surveys of alveolar bone loss.[15, 40, 41] However, radiography, although a standard diagnostic procedure in periodontitis clinical trials, is impractical and probably unethical in field studies. The attempt was therefore made to develop reversible indexes, which were both sensitive and clinically manageable in field conditions. In this group, the most widely used periodontal index for many years was the Periodontal Index (PI), described by Russell in 1956.[39]

The PI was a composite index, meaning that it scored both gingivitis and periodontitis on the same scale. It represented the thinking of its time, but in light of modern concepts of periodontitis, the PI is invalid because it did not measure loss of attachment, graded all pockets of 3 mm or more equally, and scored gingivitis and periodontitis on the same weighted scale. Its compression of all information into a group mean also failed to illuminate the disease distribution, and a primary research interest today centers on people with either no disease or severe periodontitis. In the 1960s, however, the PI was seen as an ideal field index and was used in a series of epidemiologic studies that correlated disease scores with clinical and social determinants. These correlations (Chapter 20) soon became accepted as basic knowledge.[44]

The same fundamental problem of a composite index was evident in the Periodontal Disease Index (PDI), intended as a more sensitive version of the PI for use in clinical trials.[38] Although the PDI is also no longer used, the indirect method of measuring loss of periodontal attachment (LPA) that Ramfjord[38] described then is still used today. The PDI also gave us the "Ramfjord teeth," an examination of 6 teeth taken to represent the whole mouth. The "Ramfjord teeth" are the maxillary right first molar, left central incisor, left first bicuspid, the mandibular left first molar, right central incisor, and right first bicuspid. Ramfjord chose this group of teeth to save time in clinical examinations. (Partial-mouth recording is discussed later in this chapter.)

Periodontitis in field studies today is still usually measured by Ramfjord's technique for the indirect measurement of LPA.[38] The approach is shown graphically in Figure 15–1. First, the examiner measures from the gingival crest to the base of the pocket to record pocket depth. Second, the cementoenamel junction (CEJ) is located by touch and the depth from the CEJ to the gingival crest recorded. The difference between the two gives an indirect measure of LPA. These measurements are usually carried out at between 2 and 6 sites per tooth, depending on the purposes of the study, either for selected teeth or the whole dentition. Measuring 6 sites per tooth for an intact dentition can take 30 to 40 minutes per examination, even for an experienced examiner.

A more recent measure, the Extent and Severity Index (ESI), records the percent of sites with LPA greater than 1 mm, and the mean LPA for those affected sites.[12] When amended to make the cut-off at 2 mm, the ESI has yielded some useful summary information,[9] although its use is descriptive rather than analytic. Despite its name, the ESI is a method of summarizing data rather than a true index. Its measurements are made by the Ramfjord method.

Although the indirect method of scoring LPA is generally considered the best available measure of periodontitis in epidemiology, by itself it is far from ideal because LPA records the scars of past disease rather than present disease activity. More useful would be combining these clinical measures of past disease with some measure of current disease activity. Cytokines, inflammatory mediators found in gingival crevicular fluid, are showing promise as markers of active periodontitis.[24–26] If this research results in identification of valid, reliable, and practical tests for active periodontitis, both research and patient care will be greatly enhanced.

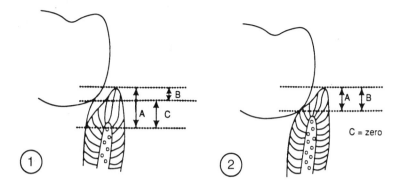

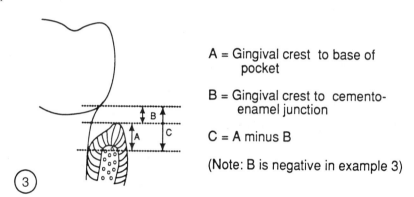

Figure 15–1. The indirect method of measuring loss of periodontal attachment and pocket depth. (From Ramfjord SP. Indices for prevalence and incidence of periodontal disease. J Periodontol 1959;30:51–59.)

A = Gingival crest to base of pocket

B = Gingival crest to cemento-enamel junction

C = A minus B

(Note: B is negative in example 3)

PERIODONTAL TREATMENT NEEDS

Any assessment of periodontal treatment needs has the same limitations seen with caries. Treatment plans are subjective, depending on some dentist-patient factors that are not part of a clinical examination, and standard treatment for a given condition can change as knowledge develops (e.g., treatment of periodontal pockets has shifted considerably from surgical removal of pockets to scaling and root planing). Despite these limitations, a number of methods for assessing periodontal treatment needs have been used.

The Periodontal Treatment Need System (PTNS), which categorized patients into levels of treatment need and assigned times for the type of treatment required, received some use in Norway.[10] In the 1977 edition of its survey procedures manual,[45] the World Health Organization (WHO) recommended something similar, although only a year later that evolved into what became known as the "621" method (from its WHO technical series publi-

cation number): examination of the Ramfjord teeth in 4 age-groups for calculus, depth of pocket, and presence or absence of bleeding.[47] Within a few years, the "621" method evolved into the Community Periodontal Index of Treatment Needs (CPITN).

The CPITN was first described in 1982[3] and with some promotion from WHO, it has received worldwide use.[2] It differs from earlier indexes in several ways. The most obvious to an examiner is that it requires its own periodontal probe, which has a 0.5 mm diameter ball at its tip, a black band for visibility between 3.5 and 5.5 mm, and circular markings at 8.5 and 11.5 mm. The purpose of the ball is to assist in feeling subgingival calculus and to help prevent the probe from being pushed through inflammatory tissue at the base of a pocket. Probing pressure is recommended to be no more than 20 grams (described as the pressure at which the probe can be inserted under a fingernail without discomfort). Another difference is that CPITN data are presented in categorical form rather than as mean values; members of an examined group are placed into treatment categories according to the most severe finding in the mouth.

For a treatment need survey, the mouth is divided into sextants. For adults aged 20 or more, the first and second molars are examined in the four posterior sextants, the upper right central incisor in the upper anterior sextant, and the lower left central incisor in the lower anterior sextant. For persons aged 19 or under, the second molars are not examined.[46] Codes 0 to 4 are ascribed to the teeth examined according to the clinical criteria (Table 15–2), and from those findings the patient is categorized into 1 of 4 treatment groups on the basis of the most severe condition found. CPITN used to assign the examined populations into 4 treatment categories, depending on these clinical findings. Because treatment philosophies have changed since the index was first described, these treatment categories are no longer used.[46]

Widespread use of the CPITN has produced substantial contributions to WHO's Global Oral Data Bank (Chapter 20), and a number of national dental associations have encouraged the use of CPITN by its practitioner members. In the United States, the Indian Health Service used CPITN in its treatment planning until the American Dental Association began to promote a slightly modified version as the PSR, or Periodontal Screening Record.[34] Another modification of CPITN appeared in Britain, where it was called the BPE, or British Periodontal Examination.[36]

The validity of the CPITN/PSR continues to be debated; it appears that the index underestimates in some areas and overestimates in others.[5–7] It must be remembered that CPITN/PSR is not a research tool, but rather a measure of treatment need; it should not be used as a measure of periodontitis in research studies.[8] Some periodontists have criticized its measurement of pockets rather than LPA, but others respond that pockets are what periodontists treat. Modifications to the index were suggested as a result of a workshop on the index in Manila in 1994.[2, 23, 36] These included a recommendation that CPITN remain the global standard for data on health planning but that the treatment need codes be eliminated, as they have become obsolete in view of the current model for periodontal diseases.[36] Some of these recommendations seem to have been accepted by WHO, for the fourth edition of its handbook on Pathfinder surveys includes an optional inclusion of LPA measurements, and the index itself is referred to as CPI (rather than CPITN) thoughout.[46]

PLAQUE AND CALCULUS

The OHI-S, the Simplified Oral Hygiene Index,[18, 19] has had wide use in surveys. It is quick and practical, although its lack of sensitivity makes it less useful in the individual patient than in a group. The OHI-S scores calculus and plaque together, both supragingivally and subgingivally. It has not been used much in recent years, especially with the current focus on subgingival plaque and calculus, rather than supragingival, as potential risk factors in periodontitis.

Silness and Löe[42] developed a Plaque Index (PlI) designed to be used along with their GI. The same surfaces of the same teeth are scored as in the GI and a 0-to-3 ordinal scale is again used. The principal difference between the PlI and the OHI-S approach is that the PlI scores plaque according to its thickness at the gingival margin rather than its coronal extent, a measure claimed to be more valid.[4] The PlI is still used in the 1990s; criteria for its use are shown in Table 15–3.

WHO, after several earlier efforts to develop a simple measure of oral hygiene status,[45] settled for its measure of subgingival calculus as part of CPITN.[46] Soft plaque deposits are ignored. Because calculus appears

Table 15–2. CODES AND CRITERIA USED IN THE CPITN (COMMUNITY PERIODONTAL INDEX OF TREATMENT NEEDS)

0: Healthy gingiva.
1: Bleeding observed, directly or by using the mouth mirror, after "sensing" (i.e., gentle probing).
2: Calculus felt during probing but all the black area of the probe visible (3.5–5.5 mm from ball tip).
3: Pocket 4 or 5 mm (gingival margin situated on black area of probe, i.e., 3.5–5.5 mm from probe tip).
4: Pocket > 6 mm (black area of probe not visible).
X: Excluded segment (fewer than two teeth present).
9: Not recorded.

From World Health Organization. Oral health surveys: Basic methods. 4th ed. Geneva: WHO, 1997.

Table 15–3. CRITERIA FOR USE OF THE PLAQUE INDEX

0:	No plaque in the gingival area.
1:	A film of plaque adhering to the free gingival margin and adjacent area of the tooth. The plaque may be recognized only by running a probe across the tooth surface.
2:	Moderate accumulation of soft deposits within the gingival pocket, on the gingival margin and/or adjacent tooth surface, which can be seen by the naked eye.
3:	Abundance of soft matter within the gingival pocket and/or on the gingival margin and adjacent tooth surface.

From Löe H. The Gingival Index, the Plaque Index, and the Retention Index Systems. J Periodontol, part II, 1967;38(Suppl):610–6.

to be the oral hygiene measure most closely associated with periodontitis,[32] a simple measure of its presence or absence, as WHO uses in CPITN, would be sufficient for many purposes. As always, however, the index chosen depends on the purpose of a survey and how the data are to be used.

The Volpe-Manhold Index (VMI),[43] has been widely used in the United States in trials to test agents for plaque control and calculus inhibition.[27] It is intended to score new deposits of supragingival calculus, following a prophylaxis to remove all calculus, in clinical trials. (The reasoning is that all new calculus over a 3-month period, the approximate length of a clinical trial to test calculus-inhibiting products, will be supragingival.) The VMI scores calculus deposits on 3 planes of each of the lower 6 anterior teeth: gingival, distal, and mesial. A probe is used to measure the linear extent of calculus in increments of 0.5 mm, from 0 to 5.0 mm. The tooth score is the sum of the scores in the 3 planes; patient total score is the sum of the tooth scores.

PARTIAL-MOUTH PERIODONTAL MEASUREMENTS

Because full-mouth examinations for gingival bleeding, LPA, plaque, and calculus can be time-consuming, investigators have tried using various indexes on a subset of teeth to save time. The expectation is that the subset of teeth will act as a "representative sample" of all teeth in the mouth, yielding information that can be applied to the whole mouth but taking much less time to do it. Partial-mouth

recording was pioneered by Ramfjord with his PDI in 1959,[38] and the CPITN uses it today.

There seems to be agreement that partial-mouth recording is valid for plaque and gingivitis,[1, 16, 17, 22] both of which are generalized conditions. Partial-mouth recording is less satisfactory for the site-specific conditions of LPA and pocketing, where systematic underreporting occurs.[1, 6, 16, 22] Partial-mouth recording is adequate for surveys where a degree of measurement bias is a trade-off for lower costs, but it is not recommended for clinical trials, or any other situation that demands a high degree of precision in the data.

The National Institute of Dental Research (NIDR) was criticized for the method it chose for measuring periodontitis in the National Survey of Employed Adults and Seniors in 1985–1986. Two randomly chosen quadrants were examined, one maxillary and one mandibular, and probing depth and LPA measured at two sites, the mesiobuccal and buccal. Critics thought this method would underestimate the true prevalence of periodontitis because:

- The site specificity of periodontitis meant that severity would be underestimated by measuring only 2 quadrants instead of the whole mouth.
- Severity would be further underestimated by measuring only 2 sites per tooth, neither of them a lingual site.

That underestimation may be real, but the same method was used for measuring periodontitis in the NHANES III national survey of 1988–94.[11] In fairness, the method may be sufficiently valid for the purposes of the survey, and it represents a great savings of time (and hence cost). It is a pragmatic measure, not recommended for analytic research but probably adequate for surveys.

REFERENCES

1. Ainamo J, Ainamo A. Partial indices as indicators of the severity and prevalence of periodontal disease. Int Dent J 1985;35:322–6.
2. Ainamo J, Ainamo A. Validity and relevance of the criteria of the CPITN. Int Dent J 1994;44(Suppl 1):527–32.
3. Ainamo J, Barmes D, Beagrie G, et al. Development of the World Health Organization (WHO) Community Periodontal Index of Treatment Needs (CPITN). Int Dent J 1982;32:281–91.
4. Ainamo J, Bay I. Problems and proposals for recording gingivitis and plaque. Int Dent J 1975;25:229–35.

5. Almas K, Bulman JS, Newman HN. Assessment of periodontal status with CPITN and conventional periodontal indices. J Clin Periodontol 1991;18:654–9.

6. Aucott DM, Ashley FP. Assessment of the WHO partial recording approach in identification of individuals highly susceptible to periodontitis. Community Dent Oral Epidemiol 1986;14:152–5.

7. Baelum V, Manji F, Wanzala P, Fejerskov O. Relationship between CPITN and periodontal attachment loss findings in an adult population. J Clin Periodontol 1995;22:146–52.

8. Baelum V, Papapanou PN. CPITN and the epidemiology of periodontal disease. Community Dent Oral Epidemiol 1996;24:367–8.

9. Beck JD, Koch GG, Rozier RG, Tudor GE. Prevalence and risk indicators for periodontal attachment loss in a population of older community-dwelling blacks and whites. J Periodontol 1990;61:521–8.

10. Bellini HT, Gjermo P. Application of the Periodontal Treatment Need System (PTNS) in a group of Norwegian industrial employees. Community Dent Oral Epidemiol 1973;1:22–9.

11. Brown LJ, Brunelle JA, Kingman A. Periodontal status, 1988–91: Prevalence, extent, and demographic variation. J Dent Res 1996;75(Spec Issue):672–83.

12. Carlos JP, Wolfe MD, Kingman A. The Extent and Severity Index: A simple method for use in epidemiological studies of periodontal disease. J Clin Periodontol 1986;13:500–5.

13. Caton J, Polson AM. The Interdental Bleeding Index: A simplified procedure for monitoring gingival health. Compend Contin Educ Dent 1985;6:88–92.

14. Caton J, Polson A, Bouwsma O, et al. Associations between bleeding and visual signs of interdental gingival inflammation. J Periodontol 1988;59:722–7.

15. Dunning JM, Leach LB. Gingival-bone count: A method for epidemiological study of periodontal disease. J Dent Res 1960;39:506–13.

16. Fleiss JL, Park MH, Chilton NW, et al. Representativeness of the "Ramfjord teeth" for epidemiologic studies of gingivitis and periodontitis. Community Dent Oral Epidemiol 1987;15:221–4.

17. Goldberg P, Matsson L, Anderson H. Partial recording of gingivitis and dental plaque in children of different ages and in young adults. Community Dent Oral Epidemiol 1985;13:44–6.

18. Greene JC, Vermillion JR. The oral hygiene index: A method for classifying oral hygiene status. J Am Dent Assoc 1960;61:172–9.

19. Greene JC, Vermillion JR. The simplified oral hygiene index. J Am Dent Assoc 1964;68:7–13.

20. Greenstein G. The role of bleeding upon probing in the diagnosis of periodontal disease. J Periodontol 1984;55:684–8.

21. Greenstein G, Caton J, Polson AM. Histologic characteristics associated with bleeding after probing and visual signs of inflammation. J Periodontol 1981;52:420–5.

22. Hunt RJ. Efficiency of half-mouth examinations in estimating the prevalence of periodontal disease. J Dent Res 1987;66:1044–8.

23. Khocht A, Zohn H, Deasy M, Chang KM. Assessment of periodontal status with PSR and traditional clinical periodontal examination. J Am Dent Assoc 1995;126:1658–65.

24. Kjeldsen M, Holmstrup P, Bendtzen K. Marginal periodontitis and cytokines: A review of the literature. J Periodontol 1993;64:1013–22.

25. Lamster IB. The host response in gingival crevicular fluid: Potential applications in periodontitis clinical trials. J Periodontol 1992;63(12 Suppl):1117–23.

26. Lee HJ, Kang IK, Chung CP, Choi SM. The subgingival microflora and gingival crevicular fluid cytokines in refractory periodontitis. J Clin Periodontol 1995;22:885–90.

27. Lobene RR. A clinical comparison of the anticalculus effect of two commercially available dentifrices. Clin Preven Dent 1987;9(4):3–8.

28. Lobene RR, Mankodi SM, Ciancio SG, et al. Correlation among gingival indices: A methodology study. J Periodontol 1989;60:159–62.

29. Löe H. The Gingival Index, the Plaque Index, and the Retention Index systems. J Periodontol, part II, 1967;38(Suppl):610–6.

30. Löe H, Silness J. Periodontol disease in pregnancy. I. Prevalence and severity. Acta Odont Scand 1963;21:533–51.

31. Macaulay WR, Taylor GO, Lennon MA, et al. The suitability of three periodontal indices for epidemiological studies conducted for planning purposes. Community Dent Health 1988;5:113–9.

32. Mandel ID, Gaffar A. Calculus revisited. J Clin Periodontol 1986;13:249–57.

33. Massler M, Schour I, Chopra B. Occurrence of gingivitis in suburban Chicago schoolchildren. J Periodontol 1950;21:146–64.

34. Nasi JH. Background to, and implementation of, the Periodontal Screening and Recording (PSR) procedure in the USA. Int Dent J 1994;44(Suppl 1):585–8.

35. Nowicki D, Vogel RI, Melcer S, Deasy MJ. The gingival bleeding time index. J Periodontol 1981;52:260–2.

36. Page RC, Morrison EC. Summary of outcomes and recommendations of the workshop on CPITN. Int Dent J 1994;44(Suppl 1):589–94.

37. Polson AM, Caton JG. Current status of bleeding in the diagnosis of periodontal diseases. J Periodontol 1985;56 (Spec Issue):1–3.

38. Ramfjord SP. Indices for prevalence and incidence of periodontal disease. J Periodontol 1959;30:51–9.

39. Russell AL. A system of scoring for prevalence surveys of periodontal disease. J Dent Res 1956;35:350–9.

40. Sandler HC, Stahl SS. Measurement of periodontal disease prevalence. J Am Dent Assoc 1959;58:93–7.

41. Schei O, Waerhaug J, Lovdal A, Arno A. Alveolar bone loss as related to oral hygiene and age. J Periodontol 1959;30:7–16.

42. Silness J, Löe H. Periodontal disease in pregnancy. II. Correlation between oral hygiene and periodontal condition. Acta Odontol Scand 1964;22:112–35.

43. Volpe AR, Kupczak LJ, King WJ. In vivo calculus assessment. Part III. Scoring techniques, rate of calculus formation, partial mouth exams vs. full mouth exams, and intra-examiner reproducibility. Periodontics 1967;5:184–93.

44. Waerhaug J. Epidemiology of periodontal disease—review of literature. In: Ramfjord SP, Kerr DA, Ash MM, eds. World workshop in periodontics. Ann Arbor, MI: University of Michigan Press, 1966:181–220.

45. World Health Organization. Oral health surveys: Basic methods. 2nd ed. Geneva: WHO, 1977.

46. World Health Organization. Oral health surveys: Basic methods. 4th ed. Geneva: WHO, 1997.

47. World Health Organization. Epidemiology, etiology, and prevention of periodontal diseases. Tech Rep Series No 621. Geneva: WHO, 1978.

16

Measuring
Dental Fluorosis

Dean's Fluorosis Index ◆ Tooth Surface Index of
Fluorosis (TSIF) ◆ The Thylstrup-Fejerskov Index (TF) ◆
Fluorosis Risk Index (FRI) ◆ Developmental Defects of
Dental Enamel Index (DDE)

This chapter describes methods for measuring dental fluorosis. Dental fluorosis is a hypomineralization of the dental enamel caused by excessive ingestion of fluoride during tooth development.[13] Depending on the quantity and timing of fluoride ingestion during this period, the clinical appearance of fluorosis can range from barely noticeable to a severe and ugly brown stain with pitting and flaking of friable enamel.

DEAN'S FLUOROSIS INDEX

The first index for fluorosis came from the initial investigations of fluorosis in the 1930s (Chapter 23). Dean's first Fluorosis Index set criteria for categorizing dental fluorosis on a 7-point ordinal scale: normal, questionable, very mild, mild, moderate, moderately severe, and severe. Dean used this 7-point scale for his Fluorosis Index for some time,[3, 8] but by 1939 his experience led him to combine the moderately severe and severe categories into a single "severe" category.[9] By 1942, Dean had revised his Fluorosis Index into the 6-point scale (including "normal") that is still used today.[4] Dean's criteria for his revised version of the Fluorosis Index are shown in Table 16–1.

A spin-off from the Fluorosis Index was the Community Fluorosis Index (CFI), which Dean arbitrarily defined in 1935[6] on a 7-point ordinal scale, again ranging from negative and borderline to marked and very marked. Figure 16–1 shows the distributional data from 10 communities[7] on which he based the CFI; he later added numerical weights to these categories to derive a numerical CFI.[4] Dean related this index to the concentration of fluoride in a water supply and was able to show a linear correlation, as one of his original charts demonstrates (Fig. 16–2). Dean also stated, although only in a footnote, that CFI scores below 0.4 were of no "public health significance."[5] With cosmetic awareness likely to be more sensitive now than it was in the 1930s, however, Dean's estimates on "public health significance" of fluorosis may be less relevant today.

TOOTH SURFACE INDEX OF FLUOROSIS (TSIF)

Fluorosis was the subject of surprisingly little study after the initial studies of controlled water fluoridation[20] until the 1980s, when research was spurred by suggestions that its prevalence might be increasing.[16] During the 1980s, the Tooth Surface Index of Fluorosis (TSIF) was developed and used by researchers in the National Institute of Dental Research.[10, 15] Criteria for the TSIF are shown in Table 16–2. The TSIF scale is probably more sensitive than Dean's index for the mildest forms of fluorosis. The TSIF ascribes a score, on a 0-to-7 scale, to each tooth surface in the mouth, whereas Dean's index applies only to the two worst teeth in the mouth. The World Health Organization (WHO), however, still recommends use of Dean's index in its basic survey manual.[24] TSIF results are given as an ordinal distribution rather than as mean scores.

Table 16–1. CRITERIA FOR DEAN'S FLUOROSIS INDEX

DIAGNOSIS	CRITERIA
Normal	The enamel represents the usual translucent semivitriform type of structure. The surface is smooth, glossy, and usually of a pale creamy white color.
Questionable	The enamel discloses slight aberrations from the translucency of normal enamel, ranging from a few white flecks to occasional white spots. This classification is utilized in those instances where a definite diagnosis of the mildest form of fluorosis is not warranted and a classification of "normal" not justified.
Very mild	Small, opaque, paper white area scattered irregularly over the tooth but not involving as much as approximately 25% of the tooth surface. Frequently included in this classification are teeth showing no more than about 1 to 2 mm of white opacity at the tip of the summit of the cusps of the bicuspids or second molars.
Mild	The white opaque areas in the enamel of the teeth are more extensive but do not involve as much as 50% of the tooth.
Moderate	All enamel surfaces of the teeth are affected, and surfaces subject to attrition show marked wear. Brown stain is frequently a disfiguring feature.
Severe	Includes teeth formerly classified as "moderately severe" and "severe." All enamel surfaces are affected, and hypoplasia is so marked that the general form of the tooth may be altered. The major diagnostic sign of this classification is the discrete or confluent pitting. Brown stains are widespread, and teeth often present a corroded appearance.

From Dean HT. The investigation of physiological effects by the epidemiological method. In: Moulton FR, ed: Fluorine and dental health. Washington DC: American Association for the Advancement of Science, 1942:23–71.

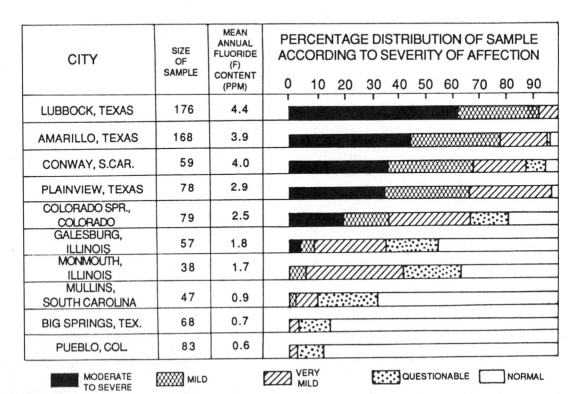

Figure 16–1. Data from Dean's studies to show the distribution of fluorosis severity related to fluoride concentration of the drinking water in 10 communities. (From Dean HT, Elvove E. Further studies on the minimal threshold of chronic endemic dental fluorosis. Public Health Rep 1937;52:1249–64.)

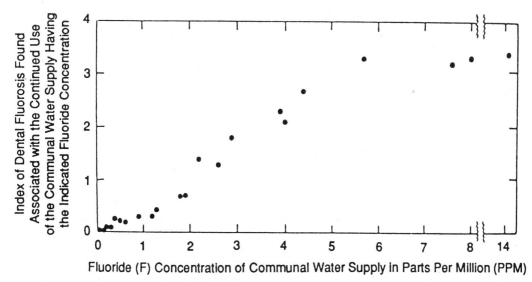

Figure 16–2. Data from Dean's studies to show the relation between mean Fluorosis Index scores and the fluoride concentration of the drinking water. (From Dean HT. The investigation of physiological effects by the epidemiological method. In: Moulton FR, ed: Fluorine and Dental Health. Washington DC: American Association for the Advancement of Science, 1942, pp 23–71.)

The TSIF is seen as a "public health" index rather than a research tool. It does not call for drying of the teeth before scoring, on the grounds that when the appearance of teeth is judged in everyday life, it is done so with the teeth wet. The very mildest forms of fluorosis are therefore likely to be missed with the TSIF.

THE THYLSTRUP-FEJERSKOV INDEX (TF)

With studies of fluorosis being carried out in many regions of the world, Dean's Fluorosis Index inevitably became modified to meet specific needs, such as increasing its sensitivity at the higher end of the scale for use where fluorosis was more severe than any Dean had to deal with.[23] This Thylstrup-Fejerskov (TF) index has a stronger biologic basis than Dean's more or less arbitrary index, because the index scores were developed by relating them to histologic features of affected enamel. The criteria for the TF index are shown in Table 16–3. Because its use calls for drying of the teeth, the TF is the most sensitive of existing indexes. At the same time, it requires assessment of only one sur-

Table 16–2. CLINICAL CRITERIA AND SCORING SYSTEM FOR THE TOOTH SURFACE INDEX OF FLUOROSIS

0:	Enamel shows no evidence of fluorosis.
1:	Enamel shows definite evidence of fluorosis, namely areas with parchment-white color that total less than one-third of the visible enamel surface. This category includes fluorosis confined only to incisal edges of anterior teeth and cusp tips of posterior teeth ("snowcapping").
2:	Parchment-white fluorosis totals at least one-third of the visible surface, but less than two-thirds.
3:	Parchment-white fluorosis totals at least two-thirds of the visible surface.
4:	Enamel shows staining in conjunction with any of the preceding levels of fluorosis. Staining is defined as an area of definite discoloration that may range from light to very dark brown.
5:	Discrete pitting of the enamel exists, unaccompanied by evidence of staining of intact enamel. A pit is defined as a definite physical defect in the enamel surface with a rough floor that is surrounded by a wall of intact enamel. The pitted area is usually stained or differs in color from the surrounding enamel.
6:	Both discrete pitting and staining of the intact enamel exist.
7:	Confluent pitting of the enamel surface exists. Large areas of enamel may be missing and the anatomy of the tooth may be altered. Dark-brown stain is usually present.

From Horowitz HS, Driscoll WS, Meyers RJ, et al. A new method for assessing the prevalence of dental fluorosis—the Tooth Surface Index of Fluorosis. J Am Dent Assoc 1984;109:37–41. Copyright © 1984 American Dental Association. Reprinted with permission of ADA Publishing Co., Inc.

Table 16–3. CLINICAL CRITERIA AND SCORING FOR THE THYLSTRUP-FEJERSKOV FLUOROSIS INDEX

0:   Normal translucency of enamel remains after prolonged air-drying.
1:   Narrow white lines located corresponding to the perikymata.
2:   *Smooth surfaces:*
     More pronounced lines of opacity which follow the perikymata. Occasionally confluence of adjacent lines.
     Occlusal surfaces:
     Scattered areas of opacity < 2 mm in diameter and pronounced opacity of cuspal ridges.
3:   *Smooth surfaces:*
     Merging and irregular cloudy areas of opacity. Accentuated drawing of perikymata often visible between opacities.
     Occlusal surfaces:
     Confluent areas of marked opacity. Worn areas appear almost normal but usually circumscribed by a rim of opaque enamel.
4:   *Smooth surfaces:*
     The entire surface exhibits marked opacity or appears chalky white. Parts of surface exposed to attrition appear less affected.
     Occlusal surfaces:
     Entire surface exhibits marked opacity. Attrition is often pronounced shortly after eruption.
5:   *Smooth and occlusal surfaces:*
     Entire surface displays marked opacity with focal loss of outermost enamel (pits) < 2 mm in diameter.
6:   *Smooth surfaces:*
     Pits are regularly arranged in horizontal bands < 2 mm in vertical extension.
     Occlusal surfaces
     Confluent areas < 3 mm in diameter exhibit loss of enamel. Marked attrition.
7:   *Smooth surfaces:*
     Loss of outermost enamel in irregular areas involving < 1/2 of entire surface.
     Occlusal surfaces
     Changes in the morphology caused by merging pits and marked attrition.
8:   *Smooth and occlusal surfaces:*
     Loss of outermost enamel involving > 1/2 of surface.
9:   *Smooth and occlusal surfaces:*
     Loss of main part of enamel with change in anatomic appearance of surface.
     Cervical rim of almost unaffected enamel is often noted.

From Thylstrup A, Fejerskov O. Clinical appearance of dental fluorosis in permanent teeth in relation to histologic changes. Community Dent Oral Epidemiol 1978;6:315–28.

face per tooth because fluorosis affects all tooth surfaces equally.[14] It can be used on selected teeth or the whole dentition, and results are expressed by distributions rather than by mean scores. An example of a TF distribution is shown in Figure 16–3.

FLUOROSIS RISK INDEX (FRI)

The Fluorosis Risk Index[18] is designed for analytic studies that seek to identify risk factors for fluorosis; it explicitly recognizes that the risk of fluorosis is related to fluoride exposure at particular stages of dentition development. It divides the buccal and occlusal surfaces of each permanent tooth into 4 zones based on the age at which calcification begins and selectively assigns each zone into one of 2 classifications.[17] When related to the history of fluoride exposure, fluorosis that develops during the maturation phase of enamel can be differentiated from that which develops

earlier. Wider use of this index is likely in studies on fluorosis risk factors.

DEVELOPMENTAL DEFECTS OF DENTAL ENAMEL INDEX (DDE)

The intent of the Developmental Defects of Dental Enamel (DDE) index was to avoid the necessity for diagnosing fluorosis before recording enamel opacities,[12] a requirement that some think may introduce measurement bias. The DDE has been used a number of times since its introduction,[2, 11, 21, 22] but the large amount of data generated has led to problems with presenting results in a meaningful fashion. Following a national survey of children in Ireland, modifications of the DDE were suggested[1] to make it simpler. On that same issue of distinguishing between milder forms of fluorosis and nonfluoride enamel opacities, Table 16–4 shows Russell's description[19] of differential diagnostic features of

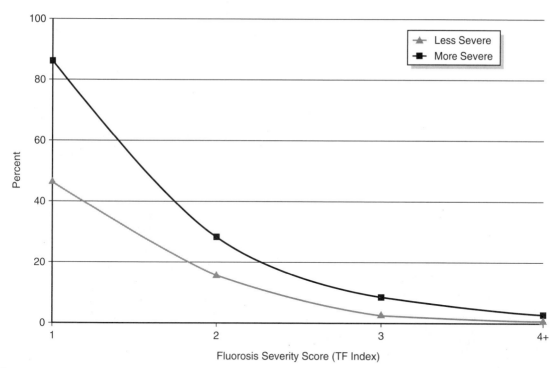

Figure 16–3. Unpublished data to show the distribution of fluorosis in two child populations, as measured by the TF index.

Table 16–4. DIFFERENTIAL DIAGNOSIS BETWEEN MILDER FORMS OF DENTAL FLUOROSIS (QUESTIONABLE, VERY MILD, AND MILD) AND NONFLUORIDE OPACITIES OF ENAMEL

CHARACTERISTIC ENAMEL OPACITIES	MILDER FORMS OF FLUOROSIS	NONFLUORIDE OPACITIES
Area Affected	Usually seen on or near tips of cusps or incisal edges.	Usually centered in smooth surface; may affect entire crown
Shape of Lesion	Resembles line shading in pencil sketch; lines follow incremental lines in enamel, form irregular caps on cusps.	Often round or oval.
Demarcation	Shades off imperceptibly into surrounding normal enamel.	Clearly differentiated from adjacent normal enamel.
Color	Slightly more opaque than normal enamel; "paper-white." Incisal edges, tips of cusps may have frosted appearance. Does not show stain at time of eruption (in these milder degrees, rarely at any time).	Usually pigmented at time of eruption; often creamy-yellow to dark reddish-orange.
Teeth Affected	Most frequent on teeth that calcify slowly (cuspids, bicuspids, second and third molars). Rare on lower incisors. Usually seen on six or eight homologous teeth. Extremely rare in deciduous teeth.	Any tooth may be affected. Frequent on labial surfaces of lower incisors. May occur singly. Usually one to three teeth affected. Common in deciduous teeth.
Gross Hypoplasia	None. Pitting of enamel does not occur in the milder forms. Enamel surface has glazed appearance, is smooth to point of explorer.	Absent to severe. Enamel surface may seem etched, be rough to explorer.
Detection	Often invisible under strong light; most easily detected by line of sight tangential to tooth crown.	Seen most easily under strong light on line of sight perpendicular to tooth surface.

From Russell AL. The differential diagnosis of fluoride and nonfluoride enamel opacities. J Public Health Dent 1961;21:143–6.

each. Although this guide dates from 1961, it is still relevant today in what can be a difficult diagnostic process. An accurate history of drinking water locations, as well as use of fluoride tablets, toothpaste, and rinses, should all be sought by practitioners as aids to diagnosing the nature of enamel disturbances in patients.

REFERENCES

1. Clarkson J, O'Mullane D. A modified DDE index for use in epidemiological studies of enamel defects. J Dent Res 1989;68:445–50.
2. Cutress TW, Suckling GW, Pearce EIF, Ball BE. Defects of tooth enamel in children in fluoridated and non-fluoridated water areas of Auckland. NZ Dent J 1985;81:12–9.
3. Dean HT. Chronic endemic dental fluorosis (mottled enamel). In: Gordon SM, ed: Dental science and dental art. Philadelphia: Lea and Febiger, 1938:387–414.
4. Dean HT. The investigation of physiological effects by the epidemiological method. In: Moulton FR, ed: Fluorine and Dental Health. Washington DC: American Association for the Advancement of Science, 1942:23–71.
5. Dean HT. Epidemiological studies in the United States. In: Moulton FR, ed: Dental caries and fluorine. Washington DC: American Association Advancement Science, 1946:5–31.
6. Dean HT, Dixon RM, Cohen C. Mottled enamel in Texas. Public Health Rep 1935;50:424–42.
7. Dean HT, Elvove E. Some epidemiological aspects of chronic endemic dental fluorosis. Am J Public Health 1936;26:567–75.
8. Dean HT, Elvove E. Further studies on the minimal threshold of chronic endemic dental fluorosis. Public Health Rep 1937;52:1249–64.
9. Dean HT, Elvove E, Poston RF. Mottled enamel in South Dakota. Public Health Rep 1939;54:212–28.
10. Driscoll WS, Horowitz HS, Meyers RJ, et al. Prevalence of dental caries and dental fluorosis in areas with negligible, optimal, and above-optimal fluoride concentrations in drinking water. J Am Dent Assoc 1986;113:29–33.
11. Dummer PM, Kingdon A, Kingdon R. Prevalence of enamel developmental defects in a group of 11- and 12-year-old children in South Wales. Community Dent Oral Epidemiol 1986;14:119–22.
12. Fédération Dentaire Internationale, Commission on Oral Research and Epidemiology. An epidemiological index of developmental defects of dental enamel (DDE index). Int Dent J 1982;32:159–67.
13. Fejerskov O, Manji F, Baelum V. The nature and mechanisms of dental fluorosis in man. J Dent Res 1990;69(Spec Issue):692–700.
14. Fejerskov O, Manji F, Baelum V, Møller IJ. Dental fluorosis: A handbook for health workers. Copenhagen: Munksgaard, 1988.
15. Horowitz HS, Driscoll WS, Meyers RJ, et al. A new method for assessing the prevalence of dental fluorosis—the Tooth Surface Index of Fluorosis. J Am Dent Assoc 1984;109:37–41.
16. Leverett DH. Fluorides and the changing prevalence of dental caries. Science 1982;217:26–30.
17. Pendrys DG. The Fluorosis Risk Index: A method for investigating risk factors. J Public Health Dent 1990;50:291–8.
18. Pendrys DG, Katz RV. Risk of enamel fluorosis associated with fluoride supplementation, infant formula, and fluoride dentifrice use. Am J Epidemiol 1989;130:1199–1208.
19. Russell AL. The differential diagnosis of fluoride and nonfluoride enamel opacities. Public Health Dent 1961;21:143–6.
20. Russell AL. Dental fluorosis in Grand Rapids during the seventeenth year of fluoridation. J Am Dent Assoc 1962;65:608–12.
21. Suckling GW, Brown RH, Herbison GP. The prevalence of defects of enamel in nine-year-old children in New Zealand in a health and development study. Community Dent Health 1985;2:303–13.
22. Suckling GW, Pearce EIF. Developmental defects of enamel in a group of New Zealand children. Community Dent Oral Epidemiol 1984;12:177–84.
23. Thylstrup A, Fejerskov O. Clinical appearance of dental fluorosis in permanent teeth in relation to histologic changes. Community Dent Oral Epidemiol 1978;6:315–28.
24. World Health Organization. Oral health surveys: Basic methods. 4th ed. Geneva: WHO, 1997.

17

Measuring Other Conditions in Oral Epidemiology

Malocclusions ◆ Oral Cancers ◆ Cleft Lip and
Palate ◆ Oral Health and the Quality of Life

There are other conditions which have been studied in oral epidemiology with varying degrees of success. Some, such as temporomandibular disorders, present so many inherent difficulties that they will probably always be extremely difficult to measure. Others, such as soft tissue lesions other than oral cancer and precancers (e.g., oral pemphigus, lichen planus) have not attracted much attention.

MALOCCLUSION

Malocclusion is a difficult entity to define because of wide variation in individual perceptions of what constitutes a malocclusion problem. Many malocclusion indexes have been devised, but probably because of this perceptual problem none has ever emerged as a standard. Thoughtful, still-valid commentaries on the problems of classifying and scoring malocclusions date from the 1970s.[9, 11]

Angle's classification, which dates from the 19th century,[1] may still be useful in treatment planning, but is of no use in epidemiologic surveys because it is a nominal categorization. Most other indexes are limited because they record specific conditions rather than the status of the whole occlusion. The Malalignment Index[23] assesses rotation and tooth displacement, whereas the Occlusal Feature Index[18] records crowding, cuspal interdigitation, and vertical and horizontal overbite. The HLD Index[7] received considerable public health use when it was used for assessing treatment needs in the 1960s and

1970s when a public orthodontic program was initiated in New York State. (HLD is said to stand for Handicapping Labio-lingual Deviations, though unkind critics have pointed out that it is also the initials of the developer of the index.) Grainger developed the Treatment Priority Index (TPI) for assessing treatment needs. This index was used once, but only once, in a national study of orthodontic needs of children.[22] None of these indexes has seen much use in the years beyond their introduction. The Occlusal Index (OI)[21] measures 9 characteristics: dental age, molar relation, overbite, overjet, posterior crossbite, posterior openbite, tooth displacement, midline relations, and missing permanent maxillary incisors. It demands a fair degree of examiner skill and training, but is probably closer to a complete malocclusion index than the others.

In Europe, the Index of Orthodontic Treatment Need (IOTN) has received some use since it was first introduced in 1989.[2] It was modified from an existing Swedish scale and combines both a functional and an aesthetic measure. Functional occlusion is categorized in 5 different grades, and the aesthetic measure is on a 10-point ordinal scale, which allows the individual to determine her own aesthetic perception of her dentition.

The very proliferation of these indexes, all developed around the same time, underlined the difficulties in measuring this complex issue. The World Dental Federation (FDI) jumped on the bandwagon with its attempt to develop an internationally accepted and simplified method of determining malocclusion.[8] It was not successful; the result was a carefully qualified method of measuring occlusal traits. It has been used,[6] but seems to be of no more value than the other indexes described.

The complexities of malocclusion and the frustrations that have grown up with the inadequacies of these indexes have led many researchers to believe that functional malocclusion is virtually unmeasurable for epidemiologic purposes. In terms of trying to interpret group data on overbites, crowding, and other clinical conditions, that may well be true. Orthodontic indexes developed in the late 1980s, however, take a different philosophical approach in that they assess aesthetics rather than clinical measures of function. One is the Dental Aesthetic Index (DAI), published in 1986 after years of testing.[5] The DAI starts from the premise that the impact of malocclusion on other oral pathology is doubtful, and the main benefit of orthodontic treatment is in the individual's social and psychological well-being. The DAI makes objective measurements of aesthetic acceptability according to social norms, for which it has been validated in a number of different countries.

The World Health Organization (WHO), for its Pathfinder survey protocol,[24] suggests using DAI criteria to record malocclusion in the following categories:

- Missing incisor, canine, and bicuspid teeth
- Incisal crowding in maxillary and mandibular anterior segments
- Spacing in the maxillary and mandibular anterior segments
- Diastema between the two maxillary central incisors
- Largest irregularity in the front four maxillary anterior incisors (rotations or displacement from normal alignment)
- Largest irregularity in the front four mandibular anterior incisors
- Anterior maxillary and mandibular overjet
- Vertical anterior open bite
- Anteroposterior molar relation

ORAL CANCERS

Like other cancers, oral cancer is usually expressed as a proportion or rate. The age-adjusted rate of years of life lost from oral cancer, for example, dropped from 23.1 per 100,000 population in 1970 to 19.9 per 100,000 in 1985.[15] Five-year survival rates are also use-

ful cancer measures; a 5-year survival rate of 67%, for example, means that 67% of persons who had the condition diagnosed 5 years ago are still alive.

Cancer data are maintained in registries in most (but not all) states; information is reported to the registry by physicians and hospitals. Eleven of these population-based registries in the United States participate in the SEER program (Surveillance, Epidemiology, and End Results), which is conducted by the National Cancer Institute. This program is the nation's principal source for national estimates of site-specific cancer incidence and trends, and it is the primary source of the research data used in analytic epidemiologic studies.

CLEFT LIP AND PALATE

The occurrence of cleft lip and palate is also usually expressed as a proportion; about 1 birth in 700 exhibits this condition.[10] Soft tissue abnormalities of various kinds, as well as the more rare types of oral pathoses, are also most suitably expressed as proportions or rates. Cleft lip and palate, as a congenital abnormality, is supposed to be recorded on birth certificates in the United States, although such recording is unfortunately far from universal.

ORAL HEALTH AND THE QUALITY OF LIFE

Although philosophically it is desirable to measure health rather than disease, in practice epidemiology concerns itself with measuring disease because health is so difficult to define in operational terms (Chapter 4). When definition of a concept is difficult to state, so is its measurement. Several extensive research efforts have been made to develop an index of oral health.[3, 4, 12, 14, 16, 17] These approaches have been largely empirical, meaning based on what dentists consider oral health to be, and they require some form of weighting about what conditions are more serious than others. They do not consider any subjective measures.

Given that health is more than the absence of disease, several commentators have argued that an individual's subjective assessment of her own oral health is at least as valid as a dentist's, and probably more so. This is a different philosophical approach to disease measurement, because subjective indicators and clinical indicators of oral health are poorly correlated.[13] One index that attempts to measure the social impact of oral conditions as perceived by the individual is The Oral Health Impact Profile, derived initially from statements given in interviews with dental patients and later refined and tested extensively for validity and reliability.[20] Because indexes such as this one have considerable potential for ranking oral disorders in terms of their impacts on peoples' daily lives, they are a boon to both clinical treatment planning and research.

Objective measures of caries or periodontitis are relatively simple when compared with assessing the subjective impacts of oral disease and disabilities on peoples' lives. A 1996 conference at Chapel Hill, North Carolina, explored the various measures for assessing quality-of-life.[19] This conference was exploratory in nature and came to no general conclusions. It is likely to be a baseline against which further development in this complex area is measured.

REFERENCES

1. Angle EH. Classification of malocclusion. Dent Cosmos 1899;41:248–64.
2. Brook PH, Shaw WC. The development of an index of orthodontic treatment priority. Eur J Orthodont 1989;11:309–20.
3. Bulman JS, Richards ND, Slack GL, Willcocks AJ. Demand and need for dental care: A socio-dental study. London: Oxford University Press, 1968.
4. Burke FJ, Wilson NH. Measuring oral health: an historical view and details of a contemporary oral health index (OHX). Int Dent J 1995;45:358–70.
5. Cons NC, Jenny J, Kohaut FJ. DAI: The Dental Aesthetic Index. Iowa City IA: University of Iowa, 1986.
6. Cons NC, Mruthyunjaya YC, Pollard ST. Distribution of occlusal traits in a sample of 1,337 children, ages 15–18, residing in upstate New York. Int Dent J 1978;28:154–64.
7. Draker HL. Handicapping labio-lingual deviations

8. Fédération Dentaire Internationale. Commission on Classification and Statistics for Oral Conditions. A method for measuring occlusal traits. Int Dent J 1973;23:530–7.
9. Foster TD. The public health interest in assessment for orthodontic treatment. J Public Health Dent 1979;39:137–42.
10. Greene JC. Epidemiology of congenital clefts of the lip and palate. Public Health Rep 1963;78:589–602.
11. Jago JD. The epidemiology of dental occlusion; a critical appraisal. J Public Health Dent 1974;34:80–93.
12. Koch AL, Gershen JA, Marcus M. A children's oral health status index based on dentists' judgment. J Am Dent Assoc 1985;110:36–42.
13. Locker D, Slade GD. Association between clinical and subjective indicators of oral health status in an older adult population. Gerodontol 1994;11:108–14.
14. Marcus M, Koch AL, Gershen JA. Construction of a population index of adult oral health status derived from dentists' preferences. J Public Health Dent 1983;43:284–94.
15. Myers MH, Glockler Ries LA. Cancer patient survival rates: SEER program results for 10 years of follow-up. CA 1989;39:21–32.
16. Nikias MK, Sollecito WA, Fink R. An empirical approach to developing multidimensional oral status profiles. J Public Health Dent 1978;38:148–58.
17. Nikias MK, Sollecito WA, Fink R. An oral health index based on ranking of oral status profiles by panels of dental professionals. J Public Health Dent 1979;39:16–26.
18. Poulton DR, Aaronson SA. The relationship between occlusion and periodontal status. Am J Orthodont 1961;47:690–9.
19. Slade GD, ed: Measuring oral health and quality of life. Chapel Hill, NC: University of North Carolina, 1997.
20. Slade GD, Spencer AJ. Development and evaluation of the Oral Health Impact Profile. Community Dent Health 1994;11:3–11.
21. Summers CJ. The Occlusal Index; a system for identifying and scoring occlusal disorders. Am J Orthodont 1971;59:552–67.
22. US Public Health Service, National Center for Health Statistics. Orthodontic treatment priority index. PHS Publ No 1000, Series 2 No 25. Washington DC: Government Printing Office, 1967.
23. Van Kirk LE Jr, Pennell EH. Assessment of malocclusion in population groups. Am J Orthodont 1959;45:752–8.
24. World Health Organization. Oral health surveys: Basic methods. 4th ed. Geneva: WHO, 1997.

proposed for public health purposes. Am J Orthodont 1960;46:295–305.

The Distribution of Oral Diseases and Conditions

18

Tooth Loss

The Historical Picture ◆ Edentulism ◆ Partial Tooth Loss ◆
Reasons for Tooth Loss ◆ Dental Care and Tooth Loss

Tooth loss, especially total tooth loss or edentulism, is the dental equivalent of death. Tooth loss diminishes the quality of life, often substantially.[53] If retaining teeth were just a matter of preventing disease conditions then the issue would be reasonably straightforward, but it is more complicated than that. Although loss of teeth is an end product of oral disease, it is also a reflection of patient and dentist attitudes, the dentist-patient relationship, the availability and accessibility of care, and the prevailing philosophies of care. This chapter reviews the issues and trends in tooth loss, and the reasons why people lose teeth.

THE HISTORICAL PICTURE

For centuries, tooth loss was considered an inevitable part of the human condition and was thus generally accepted with resignation. Long before dentistry emerged as a true profession (Chapter 1) the tooth-puller was a necessary part of most cultures, sometimes based in a village and sometimes plying an itinerant trade. As the profession of dentistry evolved during the 19th century, much of the work of dentists was still devoted to tooth extraction. Caries was rampant at this time (Chapter 19), restorative techniques crude and painful, prevention unknown. As a result, people expected to lose teeth and dentists expected to extract them.

Appalling oral health status marked by extensive loss of teeth extended well into the 20th century in the economically developed world. The oral condition of the millions drafted into the armies of many countries during World War I (1914–1918) was generally dreadful. The response of authorities was to extract more teeth, so that troops preparing to bayonet each other would not be bothered by toothache. Right after the war, surveys in New York found that schoolgirls aged 13–17 years had lost 13.5% of first molars and 2.5% of second molars, and adults of different ages had lost 22% to 47% of first molars.[31, 32] Things improved only slowly. In the Hagerstown studies of 1938, 15-year-old children averaged 1.1 lost permanent teeth per child, 94% of which were first molars.[37] Age-specific tooth loss among white-collar working adults in a large insurance office showed only mild improvement between 1927 and 1942,[21] and extensive tooth loss was still common among World War II (1939–1945) draftees in the United States.[48, 52]

Tooth retention in the 1990s is much improved in all the developed nations. Change came about with improvements in restorative dentistry (especially the development of the air-turbine dental engine in the late 1950s), increasing affluence and its accompanying more positive attitudes toward tooth retention, and significant research advances in preventing oral diseases. In that latter context, the advent of water fluoridation (Chapter 24) was probably the most profound influence, because it demonstrated to individuals and their families, in a way that dental treatment could not, that dental caries and subsequent tooth loss were not inevitable.

EDENTULISM

The sight of grandfather's false teeth in a glass of water was a familiar one to several generations of

203

Americans; the acquisition of false teeth was thought to go along with rheumatics, constipation, sensory diminution, and loss of memory as a normal part of growing old.[13]

That editorial comment from the mid-1980s conjured up an image that is fast becoming unknown to the present generation, for edentulism continues to decline steadily in the United States[12] and in other economically developed nations.[36, 49, 54] Figure 18–1 shows the proportion of adults edentulous, by age, in national surveys in the United States in 1957–1958, 1971, 1985–1986 and 1988–1994. It shows that edentulism has declined consistently in each age group with each succeeding survey. The relative decline in edentulism has been sharpest in the younger age groups, which suggests that the decline is going to become even more pronounced as today's younger cohorts grow older.

The third National Health and Nutrition Examination Survey (NHANES III) was conducted in two phases, one during 1988–1991 and the second during 1991–1994. A separate representative sample of the American population was drawn for each phase. Some data from NHANES III are given for the first phase, and some for the combined survey. In phase 1, 10.5% of Americans aged 18 or higher were found to be edentulous. There are sharply defined age-cohort differences; only some 1% of 25–34 year-olds were edentulous compared to 44% of those aged 75 or more.[43] One estimate of the decline in edentulism[64] suggested that by the year 2024, only 10% of Americans aged 65–74 would be edentulous, compared with the 28% edentulous in that age group in 1988–1991.[43] Many in the 65–74 age cohort for the year 2024 are the 25–34 year-old group from 1988–1991, a cohort benefiting from the caries decline (Chapter 19). This steady decline in edentulism among United States adults is expected to continue despite the aging of the population (Chapter 2).

This trend toward a continuing decline in edentulism is heartening. Many people, however, are puzzled by the apparently slow rate of progress when we constantly hear of rapid improvements in oral health status. The reason is in the nature of the condition. Looking at the data in Figure 18–1, the youngest person in the 75-and-over cohort for 1988–1994 was born in 1919, and most were born earlier. The early adult years for this group were in the Great Depression of the 1930s, and many of them then served in World War II. It is probable that a good proportion of this cohort first became edentulous during that

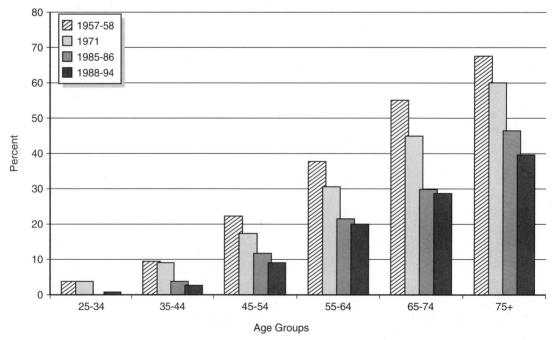

Figure 18–1. Proportion of the United States population edentulous in 1957–58; 1971; 1985–86; and 1988–94. By age. (From references 57–59, 61.)

war, and they have been influencing the statistics ever since. In time, these aging cohorts will be replaced by the "baby-boomers" who grew up in a totally different world of affluence and modern disease prevention, and with fundamentally more positive attitudes toward tooth retention. Already the emerging elderly cohorts, that is the 55–64 and 65–74 cohorts from the two most recent surveys in Figure 18–1, represent the "new elderly," a term coined to describe the post-World War II group who have experienced material affluence, higher education than their predecessors, and more of the benefits of modern preventive health care.[24] The level of total tooth loss among these age groups in 1985–1986 and 1988–1994 was already sharply lower than that in the 75-and-over groups in Figure 18–1. A survey of community-dwelling (rather than institutionalized), mostly healthy people aged 70 or more years in New England in the early 1990s found that only 37.6% were edentulous.[19]

The importance of nondisease factors in edentulism is shown in Table 18–1, which depicts the extent of total tooth loss among adults aged 35–44 in 8 economically developed countries in the 1970s. These data, most of them coming from the first International Collaborative Survey (ICS I) of the mid-1970s,[4] show a range in proportion of persons edentulous from one country to another that is too high to be explained solely in terms of dental disease. Health beliefs and societal attitudes affect the levels of edentulism. At the time the data in Table 18–1 were collected, there was still quite a high proportion of adults in New Zealand, for example, who attached no stigma to wearing full dentures.[18] In developing countries, where access to western-style dental care is limited, edentulism is uncommon.[5, 22, 41]

Historically, there has been a higher degree of edentulism among women than men, and women have tended to become edentulous at a younger age.[18, 26, 56, 59] These historical gender differences are not easy to explain; many think they reflected dentist-patient relationships more than disease occurrence. Data from the 1980s and later, however, suggest that the differences are fading, for there was no pattern of difference between men and women in the various age groups among the 4.2% of employed US adults who were edentulous in 1985–1986.[62] In the more representative sample seen in NHANES III (phase I) of 1988–1991, there was again no difference between men and women in the proportion edentulous.[43]

In the United States, there has been a greater degree of edentulism among whites than African-Americans,[59] perhaps because whites have traditionally had better access to dental care (see Chapter 2) and thus were at greater risk of having teeth extracted (see Dental Care and Tooth Loss later this chapter). Like gender differences, however, differences between the races have become less distinct since the 1980s, perhaps because edentulism overall is becoming so uncommon among younger cohorts. In both the national surveys of 1985–1986 and 1988–1991, only a slightly higher proportion of whites were edentulous compared to African-Americans.[44, 63] Figure 18–2 shows the proportions of people edentulous, by age, for the various racial and ethnic groups in the 1988–1994 national survey. It can be seen that only Mexican-Americans had notably less edentulism than the other groups.

Edentulism is considerably less prevalent in higher than in lower socioeconomic groups. These socioeconomic differences are found consistently in many societies and probably reflect expectations and health attitudes at least as much as oral diseases.[23, 25] Unpublished data from the 1985–1986 US survey show that the strongest risk indicator for edentulism in employed adults (other than

Table 18–1. PERCENTAGE OF PERSONS AGED 35–44 WHO WERE EDENTULOUS IN 8 COUNTRIES, 1968–1977

COMMUNITY	PERCENT EDENTULOUS
Yamanashi, Japan	0.0
Hannover, Germany	1.6
Trondelag, Norway	6.4
Ontario, Canada	8.7
Baltimore, USA	10.6
Sydney, Australia	13.2
England and Wales	22.0
Scotland	35.0
Canterbury, New Zealand	35.7

From Barmes DE. A progress report on adult data analysis in the WHO USPHS International Collaborative Study. Int Dent J 1978;28:348–60; Bonito AJ. The United States study of dental manpower systems in relation to oral health status: The private practice system. Final report for USPHS contract no NO1-DH-34051. Baltimore: University of Maryland Dental School, 1977; Gray PG, Todd JE, Slack GL, Bulman JS. Adult dental health in England and Wales 1968. London: Her Majesty's Stationery Office, 1970; Todd JE, Whitworth A. Adult dental health in Scotland, 1972, London: Her Majesty's Stationery Office, 1974.

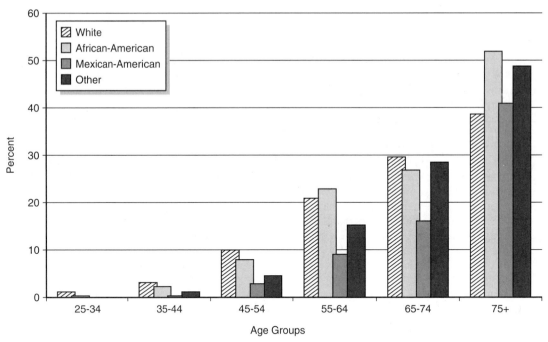

Figure 18–2. Proportion of the United States population edentulous, by age, racial and ethnic group, in the third National Health and Nutrition Examination Survey, 1988–94. (From US Department of Health and Human Services, National Center for Health Statistics. Third National Health and Nutrition Examination Survey, 1988–94. Public Use Data File No. 7–0627. Hyattsville MD: CDC, 1997.)

age) was socioeconomic status, with 10.2% of those with fewer than 8 years of education edentulous compared to 1.6% of those with 13 or more years. Figure 18–3 shows the proportions edentulous in three levels of income groupings, with clear and predictable differences between them. Similar socioeconomic differences have been demonstrated in regional studies in the United States[14, 29] and in Europe.[34] Edentulous people have also been found to have more risk factors for cardiovascular disease than dentate people,[33] and it should not be surprising that older people in good health enjoy greater tooth retention than do people of the same age in poor health.[40, 44]

PARTIAL TOOTH LOSS

As with edentulism, the extent of partial tooth loss has been diminishing in the United States as caries comes under control, more and better treatment is available, and attitudes toward tooth retention improve. In contrast to edentulism, where attitudes are a major factor in persons deciding to have all their teeth out, partial tooth loss appears to be more closely related to oral disease.[14]

For the same reasons as found with eden-

tulism, the sharpest improvement in reducing tooth loss is evident in younger age groups. To illustrate the extent of the improving trend, in the NHANES I survey of 1971–1974,[60] young people aged 12 to 17 on average had each lost 0.6 permanent teeth. Estimates from the 1986–1987 national survey of schoolchildren,[63] however, showed that average loss of permanant teeth in 12–17 year-olds had been reduced to 0.05, a remarkable 12-fold decrease over 14 years.

The change is naturally not as sharp among adults, because adults who lost first molars to caries in the "old days," while they were still young, will be influencing the data for a long time. However, comparison of data from the NHANES I survey of 1971–1974[60] with that from the 1985–1986 adult survey[62] showed a sharp improvement in tooth retention among dentate persons. In 1971–1974, 59.5% of adults aged 18 to 74 had lost 6 or fewer teeth, whereas in 1985–1986 80.6% of employed adults aged 18–64 had lost 6 or fewer. Figure 18–4 shows mean tooth loss among US adults in 1971–1974, 1985–1986, and in the NHANES III survey of 1988–1994. The likely higher socioeconomic status of the sample in the 1985–1986 survey underestimates the degree of tooth loss from that study

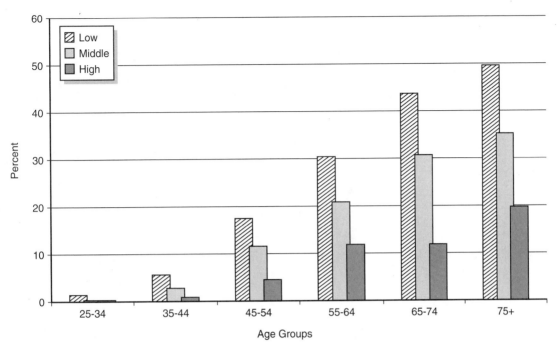

Figure 18–3. Proportion of the United States population edentulous, by age and poverty status, in the third National Health and Nutrition Examination Survey, 1988–94. (From US Department of Health and Human Services, National Center for Health Statistics. Third National Health and Nutrition Examination Survey, 1988–94. Public Use Data File No. 7–0627. Hyattsville MD: CDC, 1997.)

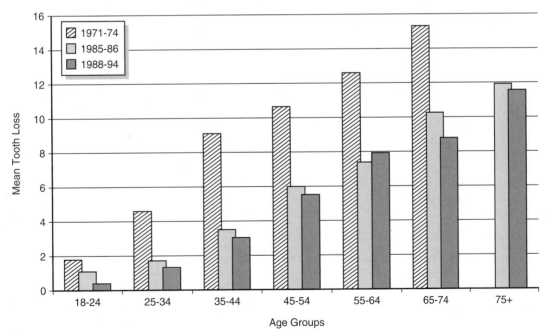

Figure 18–4. Mean number of missing teeth in dentate adults and seniors, by age, United States, 1971–74, 1985–86, and 1988–94. (From references 57, 59, 62.)

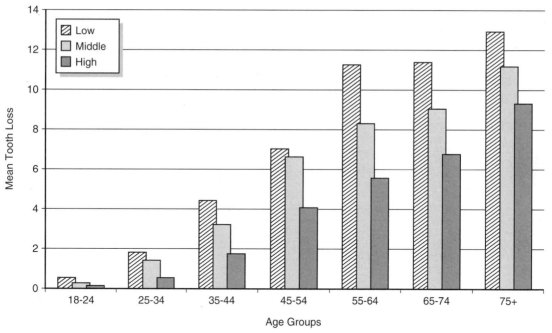

Figure 18–5. Mean number of missing teeth in dentate adults by income level and age, United States, 1988–94. (From US Department of Health and Human Services, National Center for Health Statistics. Third National Health and Nutrition Examination Survey, 1988–94. Public Use Data File No. 7–0627. Hyattsville MD: CDC, 1997.)

of employed persons; the true extent of the improvement in tooth retention can be seen when comparing the 1971–1974 data with that from 1988–1994. Tooth retention is improving at all ages.

Figure 18–5 shows the mean number of lost teeth according to income levels among dentate adults in 1988–1994. As was seen with edentulous persons, income (which reflects socioeconomic status) is an important risk indicator for tooth loss. Just as was seen with edentulousness, gender differences in partial tooth loss have diminished. Figure 18–6 shows the mean number of teeth remaining in dentate men and women in phase I of the NHANES III survey.

Longitudinal studies to identify risk factors that lead to tooth loss, either total or partial, have not been very successful.[27, 30] Smoking, not surprisingly, has been identified as a risk indicator,[23, 25, 28, 39] and early tooth loss was a strong predictor of subsequent edentulism.[23]

REASONS FOR TOOTH LOSS

Conventional wisdom for many years was that caries was the main reason for tooth loss before age 35, and periodontal disease was the main reason after age 35. This belief was based on some old and rather dubious data.[11, 50] The older of these reports stated that "periclasia" was the main reason for tooth loss "after maturity." Even as late as 1978 there was a report that 8%–10% of teeth are lost to periodontal disease by age 40, and that such loss increased rapidly after that age.[38]

This historical picture has changed considerably in recent years. Since the mid-1980s, studies from a number of countries and among different types of populations have consistently found that caries is the principal cause of tooth loss at most ages, with the possible exception of the oldest (i.e., those over 60 years). Data on which these conclusions were based came from surveys of practitioners[1, 2, 9, 10, 15, 17, 35] or reviews of dental records,[6, 16, 47, 55] or were asked for or diagnosed during survey examinations.[5, 21, 41, 42, 45] One exception to this trend came from Canada, where an Ontario survey found that periodontal diseases were the main reason given for extraction of most teeth in patients over 40 years of age, although multiple extractions in a relatively small number of patients can skew such data.[47] It is interesting to note that data were published as long ago as 1944[3] to show that most teeth were extracted for caries.

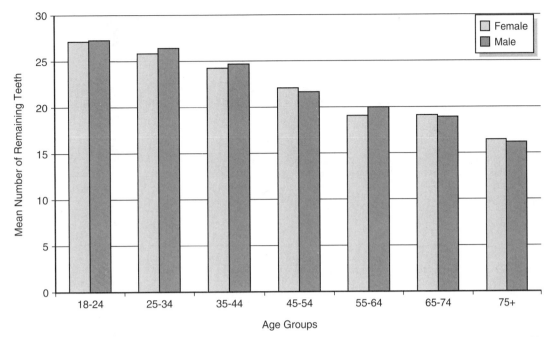

Figure 18–6. Mean number of teeth remaining in dentate men and women, by age. United States, 1988–91. (From Marcus SE, Drury TF, Brown LJ, Zion GR. Tooth retention and tooth loss in the permanent dentition of adults: United States, 1988–91. J Dent Res 1996; 75(special issue):684–95.)

A slight twist on this view came from a study of dental records of 1877 insured patients aged 40–69 years in the Kaiser Permanente system in the western United States. Of all teeth extracted in 1992, 51% were extracted for periodontal diseases and 35% for caries. When the patient was considered as the analytic unit, 58% of patients had an extraction for caries and 40% for periodontal diseases.[52] Caries tends to result in extraction of one aching tooth, whereas periodontal diseases (real or presumed) can lead to a treatment decision for a full clearance.

DENTAL CARE AND TOOTH LOSS

It is worth reminding ourselves that the main reason teeth are lost is that dentists extract them. To expand on that pearl of wisdom, "periodontal disease" may have been the chief reason for extraction in the era of "focal infection" (Chapter 1), because no doubt many teeth with no more than severe gingivitis were extracted in the name of periodontal disease. The reasons given for the extractions were honest enough; it just seems likely that the disease in many cases was probably not what today would be considered severe. With today's better understanding of periodontal diseases, most of these extractions have now ended. Probably the most important reason for improving tooth retention is the modern preventive philosophy governing dental treatment; most present-day dentists extract teeth only when there is no practical alternative.

In summary, tooth retention is improving because of better prevention and control of oral diseases, more positive attitudes toward tooth retention, and more conservative dental treatment philosophies. The result is that the proportion of people who are edentulous will continue to diminish until it levels off, probably at 3% to 4% of the population. Dentate persons will continue to maintain more teeth as extractions for all reasons become less common. The greater retention of teeth will continue despite the aging of society, so the older dentate patient will become more common in dental practice.

REFERENCES

1. Agerholm DM, Sidi AD. Reasons given for extraction of permanent teeth by general dental practitioners in England and Wales. Br Dent J 1988;164:345–8.
2. Ainamo J, Sarkki L, Kuhalampi ML, et al. The frequency of periodontal extractions in Finland. Community Dent Health 1984;1:165–72.

3. Allen EF. Statistical study of the primary causes of extractions. J Dent Res 1944;23:453–8.

4. Arnljot HA, Barmes DE, Cohen LK, et al. Oral health care systems: An international collaborative study. London: Quintessence/World Health Organization, 1985.

5. Baelum V, Fejerskov O. Tooth loss as related to dental caries and periodontal breakdown in adult Tanzanians. Community Dent Oral Epidemiol 1986;14:353–7.

6. Bailit HL, Braun R, Maryniuk GA, Camp P. Is periodontal disease the primary cause of tooth extraction in adults? J Am Dent Assoc 1987;114:40–5.

7. Barmes DE. A progress report on adult data analysis in the WHO/USPHS International Collaborative Study. Int Dent J 1978;28:348–60.

8. Bonito AJ. The United States study of dental manpower systems in relation to oral health status: the private practice system. Final report for USPHS contract no. NO1-DH-34051. Baltimore: University of Maryland Dental School, 1977.

9. Bouma J, Schaub RM, van de Poel F. Periodontal status and total tooth extraction in a medium-sized city in the Netherlands. Community Dent Oral Epidemiol 1985;13:323–7.

10. Bouma J, Schaub RM, van de Poel F. Relative importance of periodontal disease for full mouth extractions in the Netherlands. Community Dent Oral Epidemiol 1987;15:41–5.

11. Brekhus PJ. Dental disease and its relation to the loss of human teeth. J Am Dent Assoc 1929;16:2237–47.

12. Brown LJ. Trends in tooth loss among U.S. employed adults from 1971 to 1985. J Am Dent Assoc 1994;125:533–40.

13. Burt BA. The oral health of older Americans [editorial]. Am J Public Health 1985;75:1133–4.

14. Burt BA, Ismail AI, Morrison EC, Beltran ED. Risk factors for tooth loss over a 28-year period. J Dent Res 1990;69:1126–30.

15. Cahen PM, Frank RM, Turlot JC. A survey of the reasons for dental extractions in France. J Dent Res 1985;64:1087–93.

16. Chauncey HH, Glass RL, Alman JE. Dental caries. Principal cause of tooth extraction in a sample of US male adults. Caries Res 1989;23:200–5.

17. Corbet EF, Davies WIR. Reasons given for tooth extraction in Hong Kong. Community Dent Health 1991;8:121–30.

18. Cutress TW, Hunter PBV, Davis PB, et al. Adult oral health and attitudes to dentistry in New Zealand 1976. Wellington NZ: Medical Research Council, 1979.

19. Douglass CW, Jette AM, Fox CH, et al. Oral health status of the elderly in New England. J Gerontol 1993;48:M39–46.

20. Dunning JM, Klein H. Saving teeth among home office employees of the Metropolitan Life Insurance Company. J Am Dent Assoc 1944;31:1632–42.

21. Eckerbom M, Magnusson T, Martinsson T. Reasons for and incidence of tooth mortality in a Swedish population. Endod Dent Traumatol 1992;8:230–4.

22. Ekanayaka A. Tooth mortality in plantation workers and residents in Sri Lanka. Community Dent Oral Epidemiol 1984;12:128–35.

23. Eklund SA, Burt BA. Risk factors for total tooth loss in the United States: Longitudinal analysis of national data. J Public Health Dent 1994;54:5–14.

24. Ettinger RL, Beck JD. The new elderly: What can the dental profession expect? Special Care Dentistry 1982;2:62–9.

25. Gilbert GH, Duncan RP, Crandall LA, et al. Attitudinal and behavioral characteristics of older Floridians with tooth loss. Community Dent Oral Epidemiol 1993;21:384–9.

26. Gray PG, Todd JE, Slack GL, Bulman JS. Adult dental health in England and Wales 1968. London: Her Majesty's Stationery Office, 1970.

27. Hand JS, Hunt RJ, Kohout FJ. Five-year incidence of tooth loss in Iowans aged 65 and older. Community Dent Oral Epidemiol 1991;19:48–51.

28. Holm, G. Smoking as an additional risk for tooth loss. J Periodontol 1994;65:996–1001.

29. Hunt RJ, Beck DJ, Lemke JH, et al. Edentulism and oral health problems among elderly rural Iowans: The Iowa 65 + rural health study. Am J Public Health 1985;75:1177–81.

30. Hunt RJ, Drake CW, Beck JD. Eighteen-month incidence of tooth loss among older adults in North Carolina. Am J Public Health 1995;85:561–3.

31. Hyatt TP. Report of an examination made of two thousand one hundred and one high school girls. Dent Cosmos 1920;52:507–11.

32. Hyatt TP. Prophylactic odontotomy. Dent Cosmos 1923;65:234–41.

33. Johansson I, Tidehag P, Lundberg V, Hallmans G. Dental status, diet and cardiovascular risk factors in middle-aged people in northern Sweden. Community Dent Oral Epidemiol 1994;22:431–6.

34. Kalsbeek H, Truin GJ, Burgersdijk R, van't Hof M. Tooth loss and dental caries in Dutch adults. Community Dent Oral Epidemiol 1991;19:201–4.

35. Kay EJ, Blinkhorn AS. The reasons underlying the extraction of teeth in Scotland. Br Dent J 1986;160:287–90.

36. Klock KS, Haugejorden O. Primary reasons for extraction of permanent teeth in Norway: Changes from 1968 to 1988. Community Dent Oral Epidemiol 1991;19:336–41.

37. Knutson JW, Klein H. Studies on dental caries. IV. Tooth mortality in elementary school children. Public Health Rep 1938;53:1021–32.

38. Löe H, Ånerud A, Boysen H, Smith M. The natural history of periodontal disease in man. Tooth mortality rates before 40 years of age. J Periodont Res 1978;13:563–72.

39. Locker D. Smoking and oral health in older adults. Can J Public Health 1992;83:429–32.

40. Loesche WJ, Abrams J, Terpenning MS, et al. Dental findings in geriatric populations with diverse medical backgrounds. Oral Surg Oral Med Oral Pathol Oral Radiol Endod 1995;80:43–54.

41. Luan WM, Baelum V, Chen X, Fejerskov O. Tooth mortality and prosthetic treatment patterns in urban and rural Chinese aged 20–80 years. Community Dent Oral Epidemiol 1989;17:221–6.

42. Manji F, Baelum V, Fejerskov O. Tooth mortality in an adult rural population in Kenya. J Dent Res 1988;67:496–500.

43. Marcus SE, Drury TF, Brown LJ, Zion GR. Tooth retention and tooth loss in the permanent dentition of adults: United States, 1988–1991. J Dent Res 1996;75(Special Issue):684–95.

44. Miller Y, Locker D. Correlates of tooth loss in a Canadian adult population. J Can Dent Assoc 1994;60:549–55.

45. Mosha HJ, Lema PA. Reasons for tooth extraction among Tanzanians. East Afr Med J 1991;68:10–4.

46. Murray H, Locker D, Kay EJ. Patterns of and reasons for tooth extractions in general dental practice in

Ontario, Canada. Community Dent Oral Epidemiol 1996;24:196–200.

47. Niessen LC, Weyant RJ. Causes of tooth loss in a veteran population. J Public Health Dent 1989;49:19–23.

48. Nizel AE, Bibby BG. Geographic variations in caries prevalence in soldiers. J Am Dent Assoc 1944; 31:1619–26.

49. Osterberg T, Carlsson GE, Sundh W, Fyhrlund A. Prognosis of and factors associated with dental status in the adult Swedish population, 1975–1989. Community Dent Oral Epidemiol 1995;23:232–6.

50. Pelton WJ, Pennell EH, Druzina A. Tooth morbidity experience of adults. J Am Dent Assoc 1954;49:439–45.

51. Phipps KR, Stephens VJ. Relative contribution of caries and periodontal disease in adult tooth loss for an HMO dental population. J Public Health Dent 1995;55:250–2.

52. Schlack CA, Restarski JS, Dochterman EF. Dental status of 71,015 naval personnel at first examination in 1942. J Am Dent Assoc 1946;33:1141–6.

53. Slade GD, Spencer AJ. Social impact of oral conditions among older adults. Aust Dent J 1994;39:358–64.

54. Steele JG, Walls AW, Ayatollahi SM, Murray JJ. Major clinical findings from a dental survey of elderly people in three different English communities. Br Dent J 1996;180:17–23.

55. Stephens RG, Kogon SL, Jarvis AM. A study of the reasons for tooth extraction in a Canadian population sample. J Can Dent Assoc 1991;57:501–4.

56. Todd JE, Whitworth A. Adult dental health in Scotland, 1972. London: Her Majesty's Stationery Office, 1974.

57. US Department of Health and Human Services, National Center for Health Statistics. Third National Health and Nutrition Examination Survey, 1988–94. Public Use Data File No 7–0627. Hyattsville, MD: CDC, 1997.

58. US Public Health Service. Loss of teeth, United States June 1957–June 1958. PHS Publ No 584–B22, Series B No 22. Washington DC: Government Printing Office, 1960.

59. US Public Health Service, National Center for Health Statistics. Edentulous persons, United States 1971. DHEW Publ No (HRA) 74–1516, Series 10 No 89. Washington DC: Government Printing Office, 1974.

60. US Public Health Service, National Center for Health Statistics. Decayed, missing, and filled teeth among persons 1–74 years; United States. DHHS Publ No (PHS) 81–1673, Series 11 No 223. Washington DC: Government Printing Office, 1981.

61. US Public Health Service, National Center for Health Statistics. Use of dental services and dental health, United States 1986. DHHS Publ No (PHS) 88–1593, Series 10 No 165. Washington DC: Government Printing Office, 1988.

62. US Public Health Service, National Institute of Dental Research. Oral health of United States adults; national findings. NIH Publ No 87–2868. Washington DC: Government Printing Office, 1987.

63. US Public Health Service, National Institute of Dental Research. Oral health of United States children. NIH Publ No 89–2247. Washington DC: Government Printing Office, 1989.

64. Weintraub JA, Burt BA. Tooth loss in the United States. J Dent Educ 1985;49:368–76.

19

Dental Caries

Global Distribution ◆ Susceptibility of Different Teeth ◆ Regional Variations in the United States ◆ Secular Variations in Caries Experience ◆ Distribution in Caries Severity ◆ Caries Distribution: Demographic Risk Factors: Age, Gender, Race and Ethnicity, Socioeconomic Status, Familial and Genetic Patterns ◆ Caries Distribution: Risk Factors and Indicators, Bacterial Infection ◆ Nutrition ◆ Diet ◆ Early Theories on Diet and Caries ◆ Major Epidemiologic Studies on Diet and Caries ◆ Early Childhood Caries ◆ Root Caries

Dental caries is an ancient disease, dating back to at least the time that agriculture replaced hunting and gathering as the principal source of food. Examination of skulls in Britain suggests that caries experience changed little from the Anglo-Saxon period (5th–7th centuries) to the end of the Middle Ages, approximately the year 1500.[153, 154] Dental attrition was extensive and occurred early in life; some lesions in young persons seem to have begun in the occlusal fissures but developed no further because the rate of attrition was faster than the rate of caries progression. Most lesions found in human remains from this period were cervical or root caries; coronal caries was relatively uncommon. The modern pattern of caries in the industrialized nations, where a lesion usually begins in fissured surfaces and develops later on proximal surfaces, was not evident in Britain until the 16th century.[155]

Dietary changes during the 17th century, principally increased refinement of foods and greater availability of sugar, are considered chiefly responsible for the development of the modern pattern of caries. Later, import duties on sugar in Britain were relaxed in 1845 and completely removed by 1875,[155] a period during which the severity of caries greatly increased.[48, 118] By the end of the 19th century, dental caries was well established as an en-demic disease of massive proportions in most developed countries.[35]

This chapter examines the distribution of dental caries in populations, and the factors that influence that distribution. Although there is a rare disease of bone caries, we use the term *caries* in this chapter to refer to dental caries.

GLOBAL DISTRIBUTION

Although some of the ancient patterns of high attrition, little coronal caries, and moderate-to-high prevalence of root caries can still be found in remote places in the 20th century,[182–184] they are fast disappearing as once-isolated populations become infected with cariogenic bacteria and increasingly adopt the cariogenic diets and lifestyles of the developed world.

For most of the 20th century, caries was seen as a disease of the economically developed countries, with low prevalence in the developing world. There are several interrelated reasons why this historical pattern developed. The most obvious reason is diet; the high level of consumption of refined carbohydrates in the wealthier countries led to selective proliferation of cariogenic bacteria.[49] Poorer societies, on the other hand, survived on hunting and on subsistence farming, both of which provided diets low in fermentable carbohydrates.

Table 19-1. INCREASE IN CARIES EXPERIENCE NOTED AMONG CHILDREN AGED 10–14 IN SELECTED DEVELOPING COUNTRIES

COUNTRY	INCREASE IN DMFT		WITHIN NUMBER OF YEARS
	FROM	*TO*	
Ethiopia	0.2	1.6	17
Kenya	0.1	1.7	21
Iraq	0.7	3.5	9
Thailand	0.7	4.5	15
Vietnam	2.0	6.3	11
French Polynesia	negligible	7.5	50
Greenland	1.5	10.4	20

From Møller JJ. Impact of oral diseases across cultures. Int Dent J 1978;28:376–80.

By the late 20th century, however, this traditional pattern was changing in two ways. First, there was evidence that caries experience in some developing countries was rising sharply (Table 19–1). These data, taken from the Global Oral Data Bank of the World Health Organization (WHO) and published in 1978, show that caries in some countries had become a public health problem. However, the "developing world" is not a single entity, and caries levels in many such countries, especially those in Africa, still remain relatively low.[12, 46, 156, 157] Studies through the early 1990s show that dental caries is a major public health problem in the formerly socialist countries of eastern Europe,[23] which can be considered developing nations in the economic sense.

The second change is the marked reduction in caries experience among children and young adults in developed countries, a trend that first became evident in the late 1970s. This change, which has already had a marked impact on dental practice, will affect the oral conditions of the whole population in due course as today's younger cohorts progress through the life span.

In both the developed and the developing countries, there are distinct differences in caries experience from one country to another, and from region to region within a country. Intercountry differences are illustrated by the results of the first International Collaborative Study (ICS I), promoted by WHO with funding and cooperation from the US Public Health Service and the participating countries. These data were collected during the mid-1970s,[9] and the mean DMFT (see Chapter 14 for explanation of DMFT index) values for children aged 13–14 in the first seven participating countries are shown in Figure 19–1. These data were not from nationally representative population samples, but rather from selected communities. The data

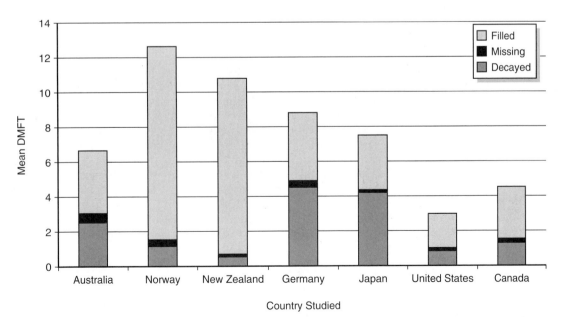

Figure 19–1. Decayed, missing, and filled permanent teeth in children aged 13–14 in seven countries. Data from the ICS I study, 1973–75. (From references 15, 26, and 66.)

from the United States, for instance, came from the metropolitan area of Baltimore, a city fluoridated since 1952. The areas chosen for examination in Australia and Canada also had been fluoridated for some years.

The data in Figure 19–1 provide some food for thought on caries treatment and its measurement. The two highest mean DMFT values are found in Norway (Trondelag) and New Zealand (Canterbury), both countries with extensive school dental services. The same two, it will be noticed, have the lowest mean D values, virtually no tooth loss, and by far the highest mean F values. With reference to the discussion of the DMF index in Chapter 14, the data in Figure 19–1 reflect dental treatment as much as disease.

SUSCEPTIBILITY OF DIFFERENT TEETH

When caries was more prevalent and severe than it is at present, it was found that teeth attacked by caries were affected within 2 to 4 years of eruption.[42] Although that can no longer be considered a rule, some teeth are still more susceptible to caries than others. In the pioneering studies of dental caries in Hagerstown, Maryland, carried out in 1937, the rank order of susceptibility of teeth to caries was listed as follows[107]:

- Mandibular first and second molars
- Maxillary first and second molars
- Mandibular second bicuspids, maxillary first and second bicuspids, maxillary central and lateral incisors
- Maxillary canines and mandibular first bicuspids
- Mandibular central and lateral incisors, mandibular canines (third molars had not erupted in the children studied)

Although overall caries experience is substantially less since the Hagerstown studies, it is not certain that this rank order of tooth vulnerability has changed. When caries first occurs today in the permanent dentition of young people, it does so predominantly in the first and second molars; it is now uncommon in all anterior teeth.

REGIONAL VARIATIONS IN THE UNITED STATES

Regional variations in caries experience in the United States were first documented

with the examination of young men in the Armed Forces during World War II.[101, 164, 186, 188] It is of interest to note that regional differences in caries prevalence among different tribes of Native Americans were demonstrated in the early 1930s,[103] with more severe disease among tribes in the Northwest than among those in the Southwest. This regional pattern is still seen today in the rest of the American population.[218]

The World War II surveys were in general agreement that the most severe caries experience was seen in recruits from New England, the Pacific Northwest, and the Great Lakes area, with distinctly less caries in young men from the South, the Southwest, and the Mountain States. In the years since World War II, some of these differences have been obscured by the spread of water fluoridation, but they were still apparent in the late 1960s.[128] The regional differences in a representative sample of youths aged 12–17 years from a national survey conducted in 1966–1970 are illustrated for whites and African-Americans in Figure 19–2.

Regional differences in caries experience are not unique to the United States, for just about every country exhibits similar variations. In Britain, for example, oral health is still poorer in Scotland and northern England than in southern England,[53, 54] despite an overall reduction in caries experience among children and improving tooth retention in adults.

SECULAR VARIATIONS IN CARIES EXPERIENCE

By the early 1980s, reports from local surveys suggested that the average prevalence and severity of caries among children in the United States were declining from their previously high levels.[34, 70, 84, 197] Similar information from other developed countries around the same time[7, 85, 86, 139, 180] indicated that this reduction in caries experience was widespread.

The decline in caries experience among children was confirmed for the United States by results from the National Dental Caries Prevalence Survey in US School Children of 1979–1980.[216] This survey showed that mean DMFS scores among children aged 5–17 years were 32% lower than those found in the first National Health and Nutrition Examination Survey (NHANES I) of 1971–1974.[214] The next national survey of US schoolchildren in 1986–

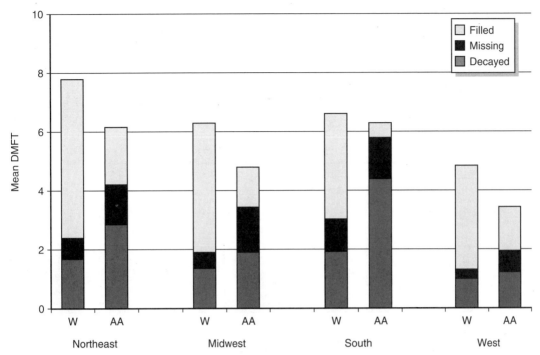

Figure 19–2. Decayed, missing, and filled permanent teeth in whites (W) and African-Americans (AA), aged 12–17, in four geographic areas of the United States, 1966–70. (From US Public Health Service, National Center for Health Statistics. Decayed, missing, and filled teeth among youths 12–17 years. United States. DHEW Pub. No. (HRA) 75–1626, Series 11 No. 144. Washington DC: Government Printing Office, 1974.)

1987 found that the decline was continuing,[219] with mean DMFS scores for 5–17 year-olds 36% lower than those from 7 years earlier; the decline was still continuing in the NHANES III survey of 1988–94.[210] Mean DMFS scores for schoolchildren in 1979–1980 and 1988–1994 are shown in Figure 19–3, and the reduction in caries experience is obvious. In the 1988–1994 data, there were few missing teeth, and the highest mean value for decayed surfaces was 1.14 for the 17-year-olds. This means that the index bars for 1988–1994 data in Figure 19–3 are made up predominantly of the F component. The decline has also been documented in primary teeth: mean df values (see Chapter 14 for explanation of df index) for 6-year-olds in the 1979–1980 survey was 4.76[216]; this was down to 3.73 in 1986–1987.[219]

The seemingly sudden caries decline among children in the economically developed nations was documented at a conference in Boston in 1982, the proceedings of which were published in a special issue of the *Journal of Dental Research* in November 1982. The caries decline in the permanent dentition among children of the developed nations has continued since then,[10, 24, 37, 55, 114, 136, 192] although caries experience in the primary den-

tition may have leveled out by the late 1980s.[37, 76, 95] Although the downward trend in caries experience (permanent teeth) among American and Canadian children was continuing through the 1990s, the rate of decrease must slow as overall caries experience approaches an irreducible minimum level. The main caries problem in the United States and some other countries today is the disparities in disease experience and treatment between different socioeconomic and racial/ethnic groups.

The reduction in caries has not occurred evenly across all kinds of tooth surfaces; it has been proportionately greater in free smooth surfaces and proximal surfaces than in pit-and-fissure surfaces.[25, 194] In a 3-year longitudinal study in Michigan in the early 1980s, 81% of all new lesions were on occlusal surfaces and in the pits and fissures of buccal and lingual molar surfaces, with no lesions on free smooth surfaces.[38] "As caries prevalence falls, the least susceptible sites (proximal and smooth surfaces) reduce by the greatest proportion, while the most susceptible sites (occlusal) reduce by the smallest proportion."[138] The net result is that while the total *number* of new carious lesions has been dropping, an

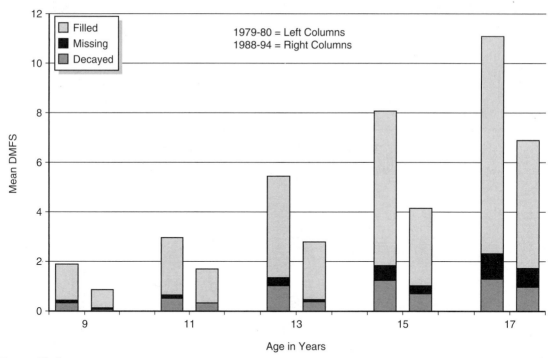

Figure 19–3. DMFS values for United States children, aged 5–17, in 1979–80 and in 1988–94. (From US Public Health Service, National Institute of Dental Research. The prevalence of dental caries in United States children, 1979–80. NIH Pub No 82–2245. Washington DC: Government Printing Office, 1981; US Department of Health and Human Services, National Center for Health Statistics. Third National Health and Nutrition Examination Survey, 1988–94. Public Use Data File No. 7–0627. Hyattsville MD: CDC, 1997.)

increasing *proportion* of them is made up of pit-and-fissure lesions. This trend has enhanced the attractiveness of fissure sealants as a preventive measure (see Chapter 26).

History has many examples of diseases that have waxed and waned without precise knowledge of why, and the caries decline is one of these. No clear reasons for the caries decline have been identified, although most researchers see the various uses of fluoride as the main reason.[31] Sugar consumption in the United States has increased (see Chapter 27) rather than diminished, and it is difficult to ascribe the decline to better oral hygiene, or to changes in the bacterial ecology of the oral cavity, whereas an influential role for fluoride is hard to reject.[36] The possible influence of widespread pediatric antibiotics on oral bacteria has been suggested as a contributory factor.[126] As with the cyclical nature of other diseases over time, however, it is quite likely that unidentified factors play a role.

DISTRIBUTION IN CARIES SEVERITY

For many years, the results of surveys and even research studies were presented only as mean DMFT values, usually with only a standard deviation to indicate the distribution. Although means are useful, they "compress" extreme values, meaning those with no caries and those with many teeth affected, into an average figure that sometimes can give a misleading profile. A landmark break from this convention came with the results of the National Preventive Dentistry Demonstration Program (NPDDP) in the mid-1980s. The NPDDP studied the effects of a series of preventive procedures among children in grades 1, 2, and 5 in 5 fluoridated and 5 nonfluoridated cities. One of the published reports from the NPDDP noted that although average caries experience in children was lower than the researchers had originally expected, there was still a significant minority with severe caries.[71] This type of distribution is illustrated in Figure 19–4, which shows data from the national surveys of schoolchildren in 1979–1980 and 1988–1994. Figure 19–3 illustrates the decline in mean DMFS scores between the two surveys; Figure 19–4 looks at the distributional changes. In the more recent survey, the proportion of caries-free children had increased, whereas the proportion with severe

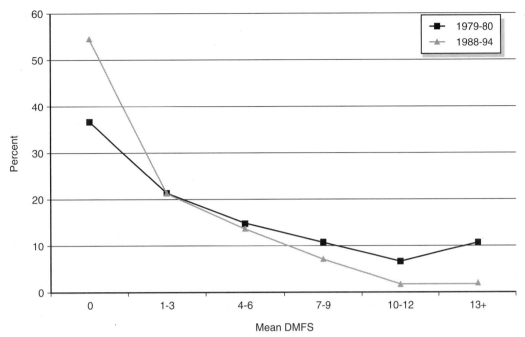

Figure 19–4. Distribution of mean DMFS values in schoolchildren aged 5–17, United States 1979–80 and 1988–94. (From US Public Health Service, National Institute of Dental Research. The prevalence of dental caries in United States children in 1979–80. NIH Pub No 82–2245. Washington DC: Government Printing Office, 1981; US Department of Health and Human Services, National Center for Health Statistics. Third National Health and Nutrition Examination Survey, 1988–94. Public Use Data File No. 7–0627. Hyattsville MD: CDC, 1997.)

caries had decreased. It must be noted, however, that the shape of the distribution remained much the same: highly skewed toward zero or few DMFS teeth, but with persistent "tails," meaning children at the severe end of the scale.

Although there is no generally accepted definition of *severe* caries, DMFS values of 7.0 or higher today can be considered severe in children up to age 17. In 1979–1980, 27.3% of all US children aged 5–17 were in this category; this percentage dropped to 17.3% by 1986–1987 and to 10.4% by 1988–1994. By this measure, 10% to 15% is a fair estimate of the proportion of US children who suffer from severe caries in the permanent dentition in the late 1990s.

Figure 19–5 is a cumulative frequency curve demonstrating that most caries occurs in a relatively small number of children. This figure is restricted to children of the same age (in this case, 15 years) so that the curve is not affected by age differences. According to the figure, 60% of all affected teeth are found in about 20% of children, and three-fourths of all affected teeth are in about one-fourth of the children. This concentration of disease in relatively few children has led to the concept

of targeting public health prevention programs toward that highly-affected minority, and has stimulated research into methods of predicting which children are likely to be found in that 10%–15% most affected (see Chapter 13).

CARIES DISTRIBUTION: DEMOGRAPHIC RISK FACTORS

Age

Mean DMF scores increase with age, as shown in Figure 19–3 for schoolchildren and Figure 19–6 for adults. The components of the DMF index are included in both figures. The increase with age for the childrens' cohorts comes largely from an increase in numbers of restored teeth, whereas for the adults (Fig. 19–6), most of the increase with age comes from missing teeth. Both figures are of cross-sectional data, so as younger cohorts in time replace today's older people the M component will drop (see Chapter 18). With fewer restorations being placed in younger people, the overall DMF values in older people are also likely to decline with time. The impact of the caries decline naturally takes longer to

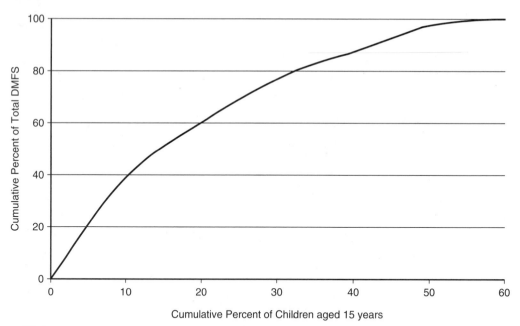

Figure 19–5. Cumulative frequency curve of the proportion of total DMFS teeth in schoolchildren aged 15 years, United States 1988–94. (From US Department of Health and Human Services National Center For Health Statistics. Third National Health and Nutrition Examination Survey, 1988–94. Public Use Data File No. 7–0627. Hyattsville MD: CDC, 1997.)

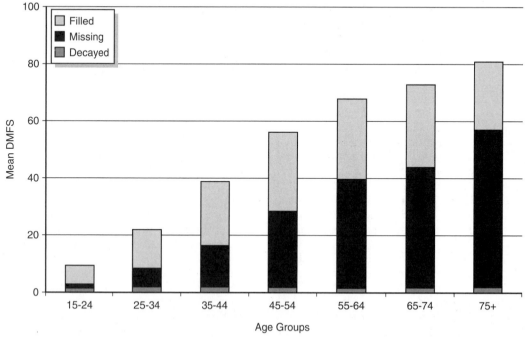

Figure 19–6. Mean DMFT values by age for adults, United States 1988–94. (From US Department of Health and Human Services, National Center for Health Statistics. Third National Health and Nutrition Examination Survey, 1988–94. Public Use Data File No. 7–0627. Hyattsville MD: CDC, 1997.)

become evident in adults than in children, because many adults depicted in Figure 19–6 had already experienced much of their DMF scores before the modern age of prevention.

Caries used to be considered a childhood disease, a perception that arose in days of greater caries severity when most susceptible surfaces were usually affected by the time a child reached adulthood. With younger people now reaching adulthood with many surfaces free of caries, the carious attack is spread out more throughout life. Adults of all ages can develop new coronal lesions,[56, 74] and caries has to be viewed as a lifetime disease.[61, 80] Even the disease distribution seen in youth (i.e., most disease being clustered in a relatively small number of people, as shown in Figure 19–5), is seen in the elderly.[141] In populations where caries experience is severe, the disease starts early in life and is common in the young. A more even occurrence of new lesions throughout life is characteristic of a lower community attack rate.

Gender

Females have usually demonstrated higher DMF scores than males of the same age,[212, 217, 219] although this finding is not universal. When observed in children, the difference has been attributed to the earlier eruption of teeth in females,[105, 205] but this explanation is hard to support when the differences are seen in older age groups. A treatment factor is more likely to be affecting the differences. In national survey data, males usually have more untreated decayed surfaces than females, and females have more restored teeth. Females visit the dentist more frequently (Chapter 2), so this observation is perhaps to be expected. In the NHANES III survey (phase I) of 1988–1991, females aged 12–17 years had the same mean number of decayed and missing surfaces as their male counterparts, but 25% more filled surfaces.[95] We cannot conclude from these figures that females are more susceptible to caries than are males; a combination of earlier tooth eruption plus a treatment factor is a more likely explanation for the observed differences.

Race and Ethnicity

Long-held contentions that certain races enjoy a high degree of resistance to dental caries probably came with early observations that some non-European races, such as those in Africa and India, enjoyed a greater freedom from caries than did Europeans. Today, however, we accept that global variations in caries experience result more from environment than from inherent racial attributes. For example, there is evidence that certain racial groups, once thought to be resistant to caries, quickly developed the disease when they migrated to areas with different cultural and dietary patterns.[17, 152, 176] In the United States, most surveys before the 1970s found that whites had higher DMF scores than African-Americans, although the latter usually had more decayed teeth as a result of lack of access to care. The National Health Examination Survey of 1960–1962 showed a marked difference in DMF scores between white and African-American adults of the same age group: a difference that remained even when the groups were standardized for income and education.[211] Figure 19–2, included to demonstrate regional differences in caries severity, also illustrates the differences in DMFT status between whites and African-Americans in the 1960s. It can be easily seen in Figure 19–2 that overall DMFT scores are higher among whites, although big differences in dental treatment are obvious. This difference was still evident in the NHANES I survey of 1971–1974,[214] although other studies from around that time were finding little difference in DMF scores between whites and African-Americans of the same age.[13, 81, 87]

By the time of the 1988–1994 NHANES III survey, however, there was little difference in total DMFS scores between whites and African-Americans, although whites still had a higher filled component and lower scores for decayed and missing surfaces (Figure 19–7 used the ages of 13, 15, and 17 for illustration). DMFS values for Mexican-Americans were between the two, and the "Other" racial-ethnic category had the highest overall DMFS scores of all (though this could have been influenced by small numbers in the "Other" category). Regional studies agree with these national findings.[52] This turnaround could reflect improving access to care for African-Americans, although it most likely reflects socioeconomic differences: the caries decline, as previously noted, is sharpest in the higher socioeconomic groups. The summary of relative DMFT scores for 12–15 year-old white and African-American children in 5 national surveys shown in Figure 19–8 illustrates the relative changes down the

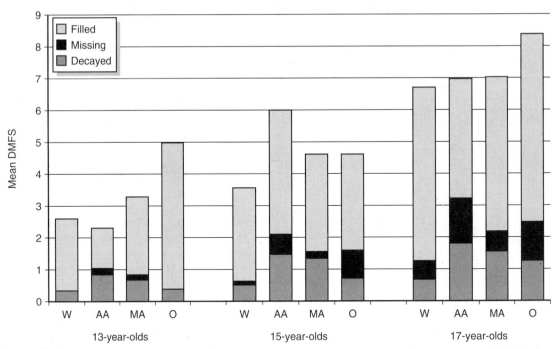

Figure 19–7. Mean DMFS values for 13-, 15-, and 17-year-old children in white (W), African-American (AA), Mexican-American (MA), and other (O) racial and ethnic groups, United States, 1988–94. (From US Department of Health and Human Services, National Center for Health Statistics. Third National Health and Nutrition Examination Survey, 1988–94. Public Use Data File No. 7–0627. Hyattsville MD: CDC, 1997.)

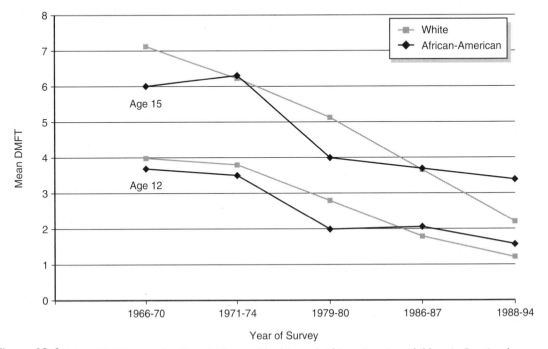

Figure 19–8. Mean DMFT scores for 12- and 15-year-old white and African-American children in 5 national surveys. United States, 1966–70 to 1988–94. (From references 210, 213, 214, 216, 219.)

years. (A word of caution when interpreting these data is that race-specific numbers in several of the national surveys are rather small.)

The caries status of Hispanic-Americans has not been as well studied, although valuable information came from the Hispanic Health and Nutrition Examination Survey (HHANES) of 1982–1983. Data from HHANES showed that DMF scores of Mexican-American adults were lower than the national average, but the D component was higher,[88] and a similar picture emerged from children in the Mexican-Americans of the Southwest, Cuban communities of Miami, and the Puerto Rican groups in New York.[89]

The overall pattern that emerges from these data is that there is little basis for believing in inherent differences in susceptibility to dental caries between African-Americans, people of Hispanic origin, and non-Hispanic whites. Socioeconomic differences (i.e., differences in education, self-care practices, attitudes, values, available income, and access to health care) appear to be far more important.

Socioeconomic Status

Socioeconomic status (SES) is a broad measure of an individual's background in terms of such factors as education, income, occupation, and attitudes and values. SES, which is referred to as social class in Britain, is a vital measure in many health studies because it is so closely correlated with many health-related characteristics. Attitudes toward health are often part of the set of values that follow from an individual's prestige in society and may explain some of the observed differences in health between SES groups. Obtaining a valid measure of SES, however, is always a problem because of its complexity. In the United States, it is usually measured by annual income or years of education, despite acknowledged shortcomings with that latter measure.[73]

SES is inversely related to the status of many diseases and to characteristics thought to affect health. The reasons in many cases seem obvious, but not always.[121] For example, differences in infant mortality by SES can be explained partly by differences in access to prenatal care, the ability to afford such care, the time to get to the care, probably less fatalistic attitudes, and perhaps some other factors.[67] Even after all these likely variables

have been factored into explaining the differences, however, there is still a considerable gap that defies explanation. In dental health, a similar finding came from Finland,[147] where differences in caries experience between children in the higher and lower social classes still remained after accounting for age, sex, reported frequency of toothbrushing, consumption of sugars, and ingestion of fluoride tablets. Children in Finland also have virtually equal access to publicly funded dental care, regardless of SES, which is not the case in the United States. Measurements used in science cannot always pick up all the subtleties embedded in SES.

As part of some landmark research in caries epidemiology during the 1930s–1940s, Klein and Palmer[106] observed that overall DMF values were not different between the SES groups, but aspects of treatment were. Lower SES groups had higher values for D and M, lower for F. In the first national survey of US children in 1963–1965, white children in the higher SES strata actually had higher DMF scores than did white children in the lower strata, but African-American children showed the opposite trend.[212] In both white and African-American children, the mean number of D teeth diminished with increasing SES, and M showed little change. In white children, the F component ballooned so much with increasing SES that it lifted the whole DMF index. By contrast, the F component in the African-American children did not change, with the net result that DMF diminished with increasing SES. As mentioned earlier, these results from 1963–1965 showed that a "treatment effect" (Chapter 14) was artificially inflating the DMF data in the white children, and the values for the African-American children were likely to be more valid.

In today's lower overall caries experience, however, the position has been reversed. The NPDDP showed that the higher SES groups have enjoyed the sharpest decline in caries experience,[71] so that the DMF values of children in the higher SES strata are now considerably below those of children in the lower SES strata. This is illustrated in Figure 19–9, which shows the components of the DMFS index for 15-year-old children in low, medium, and high SES groups from the NHANES III national survey of 1988–1994. Figure 19–10 shows the same distribution for adults in 3 age groups, and the same patterns can be seen relative to SES. Among the older

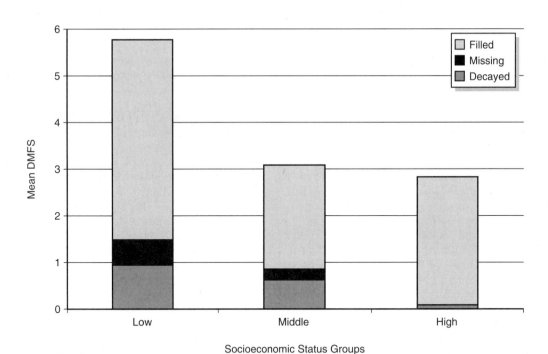

Figure 19–9. Mean DMFS scores for 15-year-old children in three socioeconomic levels, United States, 1988–94. (From US Department of Health and Human Services, National Center for Health Statistics. Third National Health and Nutrition Examination Survey, 1988–94. Public Use Data File No. 7–0627. Hyattsville MD: CDC, 1997.)

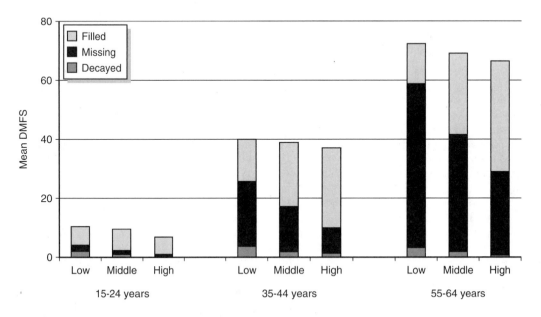

Figure 19–10. Mean DMFS scores in adults aged 15–24 years, 35–44 years, and 55–64 years in three socioeconomic levels. United States, 1988–94. (From US Department of Health and Human Services, National Center for Health Statistics. Third National Health and Nutrition Examination Survey, 1988–94. Public Use Data File No. 7–0627. Hyattsville MD: CDC, 1997.)

adults, adults in the higher SES groups had fewer missing and more filled surfaces. In the younger group, however, both total DMFS and all of its components were lower in the higher SES groups. The data in Figure 19–10 suggest that there may be a treatment effect in older age groups who grew up before the caries decline, but among the 15–24 year-olds, the higher SES groups clearly have lower caries experience.

The demonstrated relationships between caries status and SES in the United States have also been reported from Britain[43–45, 166] and from elsewhere in Europe.[79, 137] Using appropriate measures of social status in a nonindustrialized society, they have also been observed in Africa.[142] The British studies noted that although fluoridation of water supplies (Chapter 24) reduces the difference between the social classes, it does not entirely remove it.

These studies collectively demonstrate that dental caries in the United States today can be looked on as a disease of poverty. The greatest reductions in caries experience have been enjoyed by the upper social groups, whereas reductions in the lower social groups have been more modest. When planning treatment programs, caries experience can be expected to be more extensive and severe among lower SES populations.

Familial and Genetic Patterns

Familial tendencies ("bad teeth run in families") are seen by many dentists and have been demonstrated by research.[69, 104, 108, 171] However, these studies do not pin down whether such tendencies have a genetic basis or whether they stem from bacterial transmission or continuing familial dietary or behavioral traits. Husband-wife similarities clearly have no genetic origin, and intrafamilial transmission of cariogenic flora, especially from mother to infant, is accepted as a primary way for cariogenic bacteria to become established in children.[110, 111, 172] The lack of a genetic influence by race weakens the case for genetic inheritance of a susceptibility or resistance to caries, although Klein[102] concluded that the similarities within families involved "strong familial vectors which very likely have a genetic basis, perhaps sex-linked." Studies with identical twins concluded that whereas genetic factors could affect caries experience to some extent, the

influence of environmental variables was stronger.[133]

With the explosion of research discoveries of genetic influences in many diseases in the late 1990s, dental caries is being looked at in a different light. It is likely that some attributes that affect an individual's caries experience, such as salivary flow and composition, are genetically determined, and the genetics of the cariogenic bacteria must also be a factor. The rapid growth of research technology and interest in genetics holds promise for a new view of caries emerging in the future.

CARIES DISTRIBUTION: RISK FACTORS AND INDICATORS

Many factors are considered part of the causal web in dental caries: bacteria, diet, plaque deposits, saliva quantity and quality, enamel quality, and tooth morphology have all been so considered. We do not attempt to detail the role of each of these factors in caries development; instead the reader is referred to texts such as *Textbook of Clinical Cariology*[204] or *Cariology.*[162] The role of bacteria and diet as risk factors (according to the definition given in Chapter 12) for caries, however, is worth considering here.

Bacterial Infection

Dental caries is a bacterial disease. Bacteria are a necessary condition for its occurrence, and regardless of any other factor, it cannot occur in the absence of bacteria.[60, 125] The bacteria principally involved, the mutans streptococci and lactobacilli, are normal constituents of the flora in most mouths, so in that sense caries can be seen as an ecologic imbalance rather than an exogenous infection. It has been described as a carbohydrate-modified bacterial infectious disease, in which a cariogenic diet selectively favors cariogenic bacteria.[220] It is a transmissible disease, usually passed along from mother to child.[111, 113, 172]

When studied in groups, caries experience usually is inversely related to counts of mutans streptococci in saliva or plaque,[19, 27, 109] although this relationship is not always strong. At the individual level, however, bacterial counts by themselves are a poor predictor of future caries.[3, 190] Whereas negative predictive values can be high (i.e., low bacterial counts predict the nondevelopment of caries fairly well), positive predictive values are not (i.e., high bacterial counts do not predict the development of future caries).[98]

The evidence is not yet clear enough to permit quantification of the risk attributable to specific bacteria, which in any case may vary in different populations. However, because infection with cariogenic bacteria is a necessary condition for caries to occur, it is obviously a risk factor for caries.

Nutrition and Caries

The term *diet* refers to the total oral intake of substances that provide nourishment and energy, whereas *nutrition* refers to the absorption of nutrients. In view of nutrition's fundamental role in human health, it is natural that its etiologic function in caries should have received a lot of attention. The suggestion that a deficiency of vitamin D was a causative factor in subsequent hypoplasia and development of dental caries dates from 1934,[143] and was most likely influenced by contemporary findings on the importance of vitamins in human health. Subsequent research with animals suggested that nutritional imbalances may affect postdevelopmental resistance to caries, a hypothesis supported by one series of animal studies[144–146, 159] and questioned by others.[30] Among humans, there is evidence from studies of children in Peru that chronic and severe malnutrition during the first year of life is associated with increased caries years later, although this association is difficult to demonstrate because malnutrition delays eruption and exfoliation of the primary teeth.[5] Chronic malnutrition among children in India has been shown to reduce salivary flow, which could be one reason for a causative link.[91]

The epidemiologic evidence shows that before modern preventive methods, the prevalence of caries was lowest in countries where living standards were also lowest: even where generalized malnutrition was the norm, dental caries was uncommon.[1, 57, 132, 134, 175–178, 203] This pattern is unlikely to have arisen because of "protective" factors in the unprocessed diet in poor societies because it is hard to identify how such factors actually function in humans.[28] It is far more likely that the observed pattern came from nonexposure to the cariogenic diets more commonly found in developed countries. Even in those developing countries where caries prevalence is increasing, this increase is largely confined to urban populations in which both dietary and cultural changes are occurring rapidly. Traditional village populations in Africa still show little sign of dental caries, although many of them suffer from some degree of malnutrition.[2, 12, 46, 150, 156–158, 165, 180] In the United States, no relation between nutritional adequacy and DMF scores could be found in the NHANES I survey of 1971–1974.[215]

The limited epidemiologic evidence thus favors the conclusion that severe, chronic malnutrition during infancy can predispose people to later dental caries. This situation is found in countries where malnourishment during early childhood is common but where there is later exposure to cariogenic foods; the malnutrition itself does not produce caries without the later cariogenic challenge. In the developed nations, this degree of severe malnutrition is seen only in unusual circumstances.

Diet and Caries

In contrast to nutrition, dietary factors have a clear influence on caries development. In particular, the relation between the intake of refined carbohydrates, especially sugars, and the prevalence and severity of caries is so strong that sugars are clearly a major etiologic factor in the causation of caries. This link has been recognized for many years,[22, 29, 63, 129, 130, 135, 160, 161, 173, 189, 193] and more recent evidence has confirmed the relationship.[39, 47, 83, 93, 221] Added sugars are not the only dietary factor involved in the etiology of caries, because a limited degree of caries occurs in populations who consume only naturally occurring sugars.[181]

Although the evidence that consumption of sugars is a major risk factor for caries can be described as overwhelming, sugars are not the only food sources likely to be involved in the carious process. Cooked or milled starches can be broken down to low molecular weight carbohydrates by the salivary enzyme amylase and thus act as a substrate for cariogenic bacteria. It has been asserted that sugar-starch mixtures are more cariogenic than sugars alone,[21] and there is some animal evidence to support that view.[64] The issue may never be totally clarified in the human condition, but it is reasonable and prudent to view all foods containing sugars and cooked or milled starches as potentially cariogenic. By contrast, the large molecular weight carbohydrates in uncooked or lightly cooked vegetables are considered virtually noncariogenic

because little breakdown of these foods occurs in the mouth.[112, 163]

Early Theories on Diet and Caries

The great exploratory voyages of the 17th
and 18th centuries led to the discovery of
peoples previously unknown to Europeans,
such as the islanders of the South Pacific, who
appeared to live an idyllic life free of the
diseases that afflicted Europe at the time. It is
not surprising that the concept of the "noble
savage"[58] developed during the latter part of
the 18th century. An understandable offshoot
from this ideal was the belief that the apparent freedom from caries enjoyed by so-called
primitive races could be attributed to the
"natural" diet on which they existed. Eating
hard, fibrous, and unprocessed food, so the
theory went, led to better development of the
jaws and teeth and helped to clear food debris
from the teeth. By contrast, Europeans were
even then eating a lot of processed food, high
in fermentable carbohydrates, which was
thought to exercise the masticatory apparatus
insufficiently and lead eventually to tooth decay. It was against the background of these
beliefs that Miller, in the late 19th century,
put forward his chemoparasitic theory of the
development of dental caries. Miller's theory,
developed during the "golden age of bacteri-
ology," was based on the action of microorganisms on fermentable carbohydrates that
adhered to the tooth's surface.[148]

Theories about the preventive value of
hard and fibrous foods became more widespread in the early 20th century and became
established dogma in many places. One article of faith stated that accumulations of fermentable carbohydrates could be removed by
eating hard and fibrous foods,[227] the so-called
cleansing or detersive foods. Another view
was that if a meal was finished with a salivary stimulant such as an apple, the mouth
would be kept free of fermentation both by
the physical cleansing effect of the fibrous
food and also because of the salivary flow
induced by it.[169]

As stated previously, "protective" factors
in an unrefined diet have proven hard to
identify. High-fiber diets with a good proportion of unprocessed vegetables are today recommended by all health authorities. The reduced cariogenicity of these diets, however,
is attributable not to the presence of hard and
fibrous foods but to the relative absence of
fermentable carbohydrates.[151]

Major Epidemiologic Studies on Diet and Caries

World War II Studies. Strict food rationing
in Japan made sugar virtually unobtainable
during World War II. After the war, the mean
DMFT for 10-year-old children in 1950 was
considerably below values recorded in 1940.
By 1957, however, DMFT values had returned
to just higher than 1940 levels.[202]

Norway was occupied by German forces
for much of World War II, a 5–6 year period
during which strict food rationing was enforced. Among children 8–14 years old, average height and weight were reduced, indicating nutritional inadequacies. Dental effects
during the occupation included delayed eruption of teeth, which began to be seen a year
or two after rationing began and reached a
peak after the war, returning to normal only
in the 1950s.[206] Caries in the permanent dentition was drastically reduced, even after
allowing for the effects of delayed eruption,
with the number of caries-free children aged
7 to 8 increasing 3 to 4 times between 1941
and 1946.[207] Caries prevalence returned to
1941 levels by 1949, after rationing had
ended.[208] Perhaps the most fascinating part of
Toverud's Norwegian studies is that they
were done at all, given the conditions of the
occupation.

Tristan da Cunha. The people on this remote island in the South Atlantic are mostly
of European descent. The island's limited
contacts with the outside world were gradually increasing when a volcanic eruption in
the early 1960s led to the temporary evacua-
tion of the entire community to England.
They returned when the island was habitable
again, after which the establishment of some
industry created an economy and a demand
for consumer goods. Much of the diet now
consists of processed food. The Tristan da
Cunhans were dentally examined on the island in 1932, 1937, and 1953; in England in
1962; and again on the island in 1966. The
results show that the prevalence of caries in
the first permanent molars of 6- to 19-year-
olds was 0% in 1932 and 1937, but increased
to 50% in 1962 and to 80% in 1966.[65] It would
be intriguing to have more recent data to find
out if Tristan da Cunha has shared in the
caries decline of more recent years.

Hopewood House. This institution in Australia provided an opportunity for a 15-year
study of a group of children living on a basically vegetarian diet with severely restricted

sucrose intake. The study began with 81 children, aged 4 to 9 years, of whom 63 (77.8%) were caries-free.[120] At age 13, 53% of the children were still caries-free, compared with 0.4% of the local noninstitutionalized population of the same age.[198] Over the years some of the dietary restrictions in the institution were relaxed, but at the conclusion of the study 34.7% of 13-year-olds were still caries-free.[77] Although this study used small numbers and lacked a rigid research design, the differences between the Hopewood House children and the nearby population were so profound that the dental effects of dietary control were difficult to question.

Anthropologic Studies. There are numerous reports of the disastrously rapid increase in caries that occurs when a previously remote society comes in contact with the diet and lifestyle of the developed world. Although the changes in such people's lives are often so profound and abrupt that it is difficult to be sure that all changes in caries prevalence are due to diet, there is little question that the dietary factors are important. Examples of such instances have been reported from Polynesia,[16] Ghana,[140] Greenland,[90, 152, 168] among the Inuit people of Canada's Northwest,[50] among Australian aborigines,[183, 184] and among children in a remote Scottish island where a 20th-century lifestyle has replaced traditional ways.[75]

Heredity Fructose Intolerance. The rare disease of hereditary fructose intolerance (HFI) requires that people who have it minimize their sugar intake on a lifelong basis. Studies of persons with HFI, hard to conduct because of the rarity of the condition, show that they experience virtually no caries compared with normal subjects without HFI.[163] Although the numbers of people studied are necessarily small, the differences in the intake of sugars and in caries experience are extreme and obvious.

Vipeholm. Probably the best-known attempt to conduct an experimental study on the effect of diet on dental decay in humans was the Vipeholm study, conducted in Sweden between 1945 and 1952.[72] The study was conducted in a mental institution, and by today's standards is considered unethical because it gave high quantities of sugars to people unable to give their consent to this regimen. Its conclusions have profoundly influenced the way we view the role of sugars in dental decay. The study design was complicated and not free of flaws. Briefly, inmates

Table 19–2. CONCLUSIONS FROM THE VIPEHÖLM STUDY, 1946–1952

1. Sugar consumption increases caries activity.
2. The risk of increased caries activity is greater if the sugar is in sticky form.
3. The risk is greatest if the sugar is taken between meals and in a sticky form.
4. The increase in caries under uniform conditions shows great individual variation.
5. The increase in caries disappears upon withdrawal of sticky foodstuffs from the diet.
6. Caries can still occur in the absence of refined sugar, natural sugars, and total dietary carbohydrates.

From Gustafsson BE, Quensel C-E, Swenander Lanke L, et al. The Vipehölm dental caries study. The effect of different levels of carbohydrate intake on caries activity in 436 individuals observed for five years. Acta Odont Scand 1954;11:232–364.

of the institution were divided into groups with controlled consumption of refined sugars that varied in amount, frequency, physical form, and whether they were taken with or between meals. The extremes of intake were from (a) no added sugars at all in one group to (b) daily between-meal consumption of 24 sticky toffees, each of which was too large to be swallowed and so had to be sucked and chewed, in another. The differences in caries incidence between the groups were pronounced. Some of the conclusions from Vipehölm can be challenged in light of more recent research, but they are listed in Table 19–2 because of the historical importance of the study.

Sugars-Caries Relationships in Today's Low Caries Environment

The major studies were conducted at a time when caries was widespread and severe in the industrialized world. In light of modern research protocols, design and analysis can be criticized in virtually all of them. All studies except the Vipehölm study were cross-sectional, and analysis considered only sugar intake (measured in various ways) and caries status. Factors such as exposure to fluoride, which obviously would also influence caries development, were not considered. Since the caries decline was recognized, however, we have to think that the "Vipehölm rules" have changed. Are all the caries-free children we see today not consuming sugar, or do other factors have a major influence? Studies such as those suggesting that oral hygiene is an important co-variable in the sugar-caries relationship,[78, 100, 200] have served to question the validity of the Vipehölm findings.

Two prospective studies reported in the 1980s, one in Britain and one in the United States, measured diet and caries incidence concurrently and included more analytic detail than did any previous research. The British study followed 405 children with an average initial age of 11.5 years for 2 years.[174] The children, all from a low-fluoride area near Newcastle, completed 5 food diaries, each for a 3-day period, for a total of 15 days of recorded diet over the 2 years. Interviews with a dietitian followed each 3-day period to clarify uncertainties and to quantify amounts. The mean DMFS incidence of the group was 3.63 over the 2 years, with 57% of new lesions in pits and fissures, a lower caries increment than the authors had expected. Average consumption of all sugars was 118 grams per day, providing 21% of energy intake. The results showed that caries increment was significantly but weakly correlated with total intake of sugars, but poorly correlated with frequency of intake. The authors stated that because of the lower-than-expected caries increment, more clear-cut results would have been likely if the study had been extended for another year.

The second study was based in the low-fluoride area of Coldwater, Michigan. It followed 499 children, initially aged 11 to 15, for 3 years.[38] The majority completed 4 24-hour dietary recall interviews with a dietitian, although 27% completed more. The boys in the study averaged 156 grams of sugar intake per day, the girls 127 grams, and sugars accounted for 26% of energy intake. Both of these measures are higher than was found in the British group. Caries incidence, however, was lower than in the British group, averaging 2.9 DMF surfaces over the 3 years, of which 81% were pit-and-fissure lesions (buccal pits and lingual extensions as well as occlusal lesions). Nearly 30% of the group developed no caries at all over the 3 years, and only 51 children (10.2%) developed 2 or more proximal lesions during the study. Only among this latter "high-caries" group was caries experience weakly related to total intake of sugars, and no relationships between caries experience and frequency of consumption could be discerned. The risk of caries from high sugar consumption relative to low sugar consumption was low[41]; each additional 5 grams of sugars ingested daily was associ-

ated with a 1% increase in the probability of developing caries.[201]

These 2 independent studies are among the few prospective studies of sugar intake and caries experience. Despite some differences in study protocols, findings were generally similar. Between them, the studies indicated that consumption of sugars is not a major risk factor for many children (i.e., those who were caries-free, who still ate a lot of sugar), but it is for those who are still clearly susceptible to caries (broadly defined here as those getting proximal-surface caries). These studies remind us that caries is a multifactorial disease, and that caries risk is not always related directly to sugar consumption.[115, 226] The relationship between consumption of sugars and caries experience is by no means linear.

The much-stressed role of frequency of consumption of sugars ("it's not how much you eat, it's how often you eat it") is clearly questioned from the studies in Newcastle and Michigan, as it has been from others in Sweden.[20, 196, 199] The importance of frequency of consumption was a major finding of the Vipehölm study, and it has dominated dental health education ever since. However, the importance of frequency in Vipehölm was principally based on the caries experience of the group that consumed 24 large toffees between meals each day, a frequency of consumption not approached in either the British or the Michigan study. The British children averaged 6.8 food or drink intakes per day (an intake being food or drink at least 15 minutes after the last one), the Michigan children 4.3 (with at least 20 minutes between intakes). The results from the highly artificial circumstances of the Vipehölm study may be misleading when applied to the general population. (The implications of these findings for dental health education are discussed in Chapter 27).

EARLY CHILDHOOD CARIES

Early childhood caries, also known as nursing caries and as baby bottle tooth decay, is a distressing syndrome. This condition is diagnosed by caries in the primary maxillary incisors of infants, typically 1 to 3 years old. Tooth crowns can be totally destroyed in severe cases, and it is difficult and expensive to treat. Uncertainty over the name of the condition has resulted because it was originally thought to be attributable solely to prolonged infant feeding by either bottle or breast. The holding of these sweetened liquids in contact with the teeth for hours at a time, often while the child was sleeping, was assumed to be the prime causative factor. That etiology is clear in some instances, although it is now understood that broader use of cariogenic diets can also be involved.[209]

Prevalence in the developed countries is estimated at between 1% and 12% of the infant populations, but in highly affected groups it can be as high as 70%.[149] A cursory visual inspection of children aged 12 to 23 months in the NHANES III (phase I) survey of 1988–1991 found a 2% prevalence, with most cases in children of Mexican-American heritage.[95] It is prevalent among immigrants to the United States and among Native Americans,[32, 228] as well as among indigenous peoples elsewhere.[4, 6] It is more prevalent in low-SES populations, or where infants are being cared for by persons with little education.[149] It has been associated with lower-than-average growth among affected infants,[11] and children with the condition seem to be at greater risk for caries in the permanent dentition later in life.[94] These latter observations may reflect chronically poor and cariogenic diets rather than direct cause and effect.

Research into the condition has been hampered by absence of a clear case definition. Caries of the primary maxillary incisors, often with little if any caries of primary molars, is the most common case definition, but some investigators have used generalized rampant caries or the presence of caries on the buccal and lingual surfaces of the incisors. It is possible that these different clinical manifestations come from different dietary practices. Prevention has been based largely on education, but it is clear that simply pointing out to parents the dangers of excessive feeding with sugary liquids is by itself ineffective.[228]

The proceedings of a conference at the National Institutes of Health on early childhood caries were published in *Community Dentistry and Oral Epidemiology* in 1998. The conference confirmed that a better understanding of the social and cultural factors involved among the population groups most affected is clearly needed if the prevalence of early childhood caries is to be seriously reduced.

ROOT CARIES

Root caries is defined as caries that begins on cemental root surfaces below the cementoenamel margin. It thus is found only where loss of periodontal attachment has led to exposure of the roots to the oral environment, and hence to the accumulation of bacterial plaque around these exposed roots. Root caries appears to be polymicrobial,[187, 221] with the bacterial composition of dental plaque in root lesions apparently little different from that found in coronal lesions.[33, 59, 68] As with coronal caries, sugars are an etiologic factor.[167]

Root caries has been with humankind since our earliest days; indeed most of the caries found in skulls dating from the Stone Age or earlier is root caries.[96, 97, 153] A similar pattern can be found today in some developing countries.[127, 131, 185] In the developed countries, general awareness of root caries grew only in the early 1980s, when it became clear that older adults were keeping more teeth than they used to. Subsequent studies have confirmed that root caries is highly prevalent among older persons in developed countries.[14, 18, 117, 122, 124, 179, 224, 225]

In the NHANES III survey (phase I, 1988–1991), the prevalence of root caries among American adults aged 18 or more was 25.1%.[230] Prevalence rose to more than 50% in men aged 65 or more, and in women aged 75 or more. Prevalence varies in more localized surveys according to the age and nature of the population seen. It was 71% in a group of adults aged 50 and higher in Ontario, Canada,[123] while in an Australian population aged 60 or more it was 27%.[191] In New England, prevalence among community-dwelling adults aged 70 or more was 52%, with 22% of lesions being untreated.[92] Prevalence in Scandinavia was estimated to be almost 100% among dentate adults aged 60 or more.[62] Other localized surveys in parts of the United States and Canada have found that incidence can range from 0.3 to 0.6 surfaces per person per year,[74, 116, 119] depending on the population seen.

Figure 19–11 shows the prevalence of root caries by age among dentate adults in the NHANES III survey of 1988–1994. Males appear to be more affected than females. Although the condition is more prevalent in older age groups it is also quite common among younger people. It is not yet clear whether these data are a cohort pattern, or whether the younger age groups will look

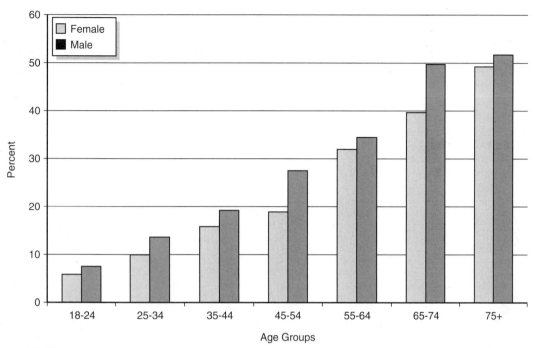

Figure 19–11. Prevalence of root caries in adults and seniors, by gender, United States 1988–94. (From US Department of Health and Human Services, National Center for Health Statistics. Third National Health and Nutrition Examination Survey, 1988–94. Public Use Data File No. 7–0627. Hyattsville MD: CDC, 1997.)

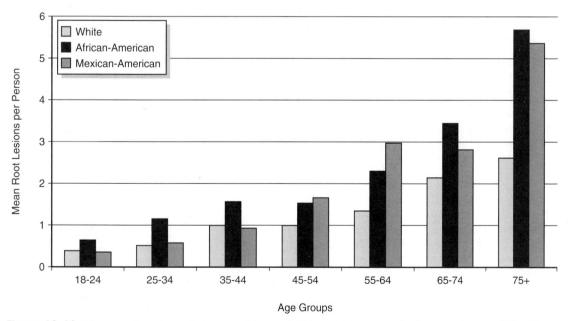

Figure 19–12. Mean number of root lesions in whites and African-Americans and other races by age, United States 1988–94. (From US Department of Health and Human Services, National Center for Health Statistics. Third National Health and Nutrition Examination Survey, 1988–94. Public Use Data File No. 7–0627. Hyattsville MD: CDC, 1997.)

like the current older cohorts in the future. One argument is that as more teeth are retained, the number of surfaces at risk of root caries will increase. But if gingival recession becomes less common, then the overall prevalence and severity may not change much.

Root caries, by definition, is strongly associated with the loss of periodontal attachment.[116, 123, 170, 191, 229] Other correlates that have been found associated with root caries are primarily socioeconomic, such as years of education, number of remaining teeth, use of dental services, oral hygiene levels, and preventive behavior.[18, 51, 82, 99, 223] An important risk factor is also the use of multiple medications among the elderly,[99] a common practice in nursing homes that can promote xerostomia. Xerostomia (salivary diminution) has long been known as a major risk factor for caries among people of any age and is particularly prevalent among those who have received radiation treatment for oral cancers.[8] People who suffer from coronal caries also seem likely to be at risk of root caries when gingival recession occurs,[222] and root caries is not nearly as common in high-fluoride areas as it is in low-fluoride communities.[40, 195] Smokers exhibit more root caries than nonsmokers, and prevalence tends to be inversely related to the number of teeth remaining.[18, 123]

In terms of racial distribution, Figure 19–12 shows the average number of root lesions in whites, African-Americans, and Mexican-Americans from the NHANES III survey. This graphic suggests that African-Americans of all ages average more root lesions per person than do whites.

Root caries seems to be a particular problem among older people of lower socioeconomic status, who have lost some teeth, do not maintain good oral hygiene, and do not visit the dentist regularly. Because of the aging population and increasing retention of teeth, the dimensions of the problem are likely to continue growing, even if the number of lesions per person shows little change. Dental practitioners should increasingly try to treat and prevent root caries in adults, as less time is needed to deal with coronal caries in children.

REFERENCES

1. Afonsky D. Some observations on dental caries in central China. J Dent Res 1951;30:53–61.
2. Akpata ES. Pattern of dental caries in urban Nigerians. Caries Res 1979;13:242–9.
3. Alaluusua S, Kleemola-Kujala E, Gronroos L, Evalahti M. Salivary caries-related tests as predictors of future caries increment in teenagers. A three-year longitudinal study. Oral Microbiol Immunol 1990;5:77–81.
4. Albert RJ, Cantin RY, Cross HG, Castaldi CR. Nursing caries in the Inuit children of the Keewatin. J Can Dent Assoc 1988;54:751–8.
5. Alvarez JO. Nutrition, tooth development, and dental caries. Am J Clin Nutr 1995;61:410S–6S.
6. Amaratunge A. Rampant dental caries in Papua New Guinean children. Odontostomatol Trop 1989;12:14–6.
7. Anderson RJ, Bradnock G, James PMC. The changes in the dental health of 12-year-old school children in Shropshire. Br Dent J 1981;150:278–81.
8. Anneroth G, Holm LE, Karlsson G. The effect of radiation on teeth. A clinical, histologic and microradiographic study. Int J Oral Surg 1985;14:269–74.
9. Arnjlot HA, Barmes DE, Cohen LK, et al. Oral health care systems: An international collaborative study. London: Quintessence/World Health Organization, 1985.
10. Athanassouli I, Mamai-Homata E, Panagopoulos H, et al. Dental caries changes between 1982 and 1991 in children aged 6–12 in Athens, Greece. Caries Res 1994;28:378–82.
11. Ayhan H, Suskan E, Yildirim S. The effect of nursing or rampant caries on height, body weight and head circumference. J Clin Pediatr Dent 1996;20:209–12.
12. Baelum V, Fejerskov O, Manji F. The "natural history" of dental caries and periodontal diseases in developing countries: some consequences for health care planning. Tandlaegebladet 1991;95:139–48.
13. Bagramian RA, Russell AL. Epidemiologic study of dental caries experience and between-meal eating patterns. J Dent Res 1973;52:342–7.
14. Banting DW. Epidemiology of root caries. Gerodontol 1986;5:5–11.
15. Barmes DE. Features of oral health care across cultures. Int Dent J 1976;26:353–68.
16. Baume LJ. Caries prevalence and caries intensity among 12,344 schoolchildren of French Polynesia. Arch Oral Biol 1969;14:181–205.
17. Beal JF. The dental health of five-year-old children of different ethnic origins resident in an inner Birmingham area and a nearby borough. Arch Oral Biol 1973;18:305–12.
18. Beck JD. The epidemiology of root surface caries: North American studies. Adv Dent Res 1993;7:42–51.
19. Beighton D, Manji F, Baelum V, et al. Associations between salivary levels of Streptococcus mutans, Streptococcus sobrinus, lactobacilli, and caries experience in Kenyan adolescents. J Dent Res 1989; 68:1242–6.
20. Bergendal B, Hamp SE. Dietary pattern and dental caries in 19-year-old adolescents subjected to preventive measures focused on oral hygiene and/or fluorides. Swed Dent J 1985;9:1–7.
21. Bibby BG. The cariogenicity of snack foods and confections. J Am Dent Assoc 1975;90:121–32.
22. Bibby BG. Dental caries. Caries Res 1978; 12(Suppl):3–6.
23. Bjarnason S, Berzina S, Care R, et al. Oral health in Latvian 15-year-olds. Euro J Oral Sci 1995;103:274–9.
24. Bjarnason S, Finnbogason SY, Holbrook P, Kohler B. Caries experience in Icelandic 12-year-old urban children between 1984 and 1991. Community Dent Oral Epidemiol 1993;21:195–7.

25. Bohannan HM. Caries distribution and the case for sealants. J Public Health Dent 1983;43:200–4.

26. Bonito AJ. The United States study of dental manpower systems in relation to oral health status: The private practice system. Final report for USPHS contract NO1–DH–34051. Baltimore: University of Maryland, 1977.

27. Bowden GH. Mutans streptococci caries and chlorhexidine. J Can Dent Assoc 1996;62:700, 703–7.

28. Bowen WH. Food components and caries. Adv Dent Res 1994;8:215–20.

29. Bowen WH. Role of carbohydrates in dental caries. In Shaw JH, Roussos GG, eds. Sweeteners and dental caries. Washington DC: IRL Press, 1978, pp 147–52.

30. Bowen WH, Amsbaugh SM, Monell-Torrens S, Brunelle J. Effect of varying intervals between meals on dental caries in rats. Caries Res 1983;17:466–71.

31. Bratthall D, Hänsel Petersson G, Sundberg H. Reasons for the caries decline: What do the experts believe? Euro J Oral Sci 1996;104:416–22.

32. Broderick E, Mabry J, Robertson D, Thompson J. Baby bottle tooth decay in Native American children in Head Start centers. Public Health Rep 1989;104:50–54.

33. Brown LR, Billings RJ, Kaster AG. Quantitative comparisons of potentially cariogenic microorganisms cultured from noncarious and carious root and coronal tooth surfaces. Infect Immun 1986;51:765–70.

34. Bryan ET, Collier DR, Vancleave ML. Dental health status of children in Tennessee: A 25-year comparison. J Tenn Dent Assoc 1982;62:31–3.

35. Burt BA. Influences for change in the dental health status of populations: An historical perspective. J Public Health Dent 1978;38:272–88.

36. Burt BA. The future of the caries decline. J Public Health Dent 1985;45:261–9.

37. Burt BA. Trends in caries prevalence in North American children. Int Dent J 1994;44(Suppl 1):403–13.

38. Burt BA, Eklund SA, Morgan KJ, et al. The effects of sugars intake and frequency of ingestion on dental caries increment in a three-year longitudinal study. J Dent Res 1988;67:1422–9.

39. Burt BA, Ismail AI. Diet, nutrition, and food cariogenicity. J Dent Res 1986;65(Special Issue):1475–84.

40. Burt BA, Ismail AI, Eklund SA. Root caries in an optimally fluoridated and a high-fluoride community. J Dent Res 1986;65:1154–58.

41. Burt BA, Szpunar SM. The Michigan Study: The relationship between sugars intake and dental caries over three years. Int Dent J 1994;44:230–40.

42. Carlos JP, Gittelsohn AM. Longitudinal studies of the natural history of caries. II. A life-table study of caries incidence in the permanent teeth. Arch Oral Biol 1965;10:739–51.

43. Carmichael CL, French AD, Rugg-Gunn AJ, Furness JA. The relationship between social class and caries experience in five-year-old children in Newcastle and Northumberland after twelve years' fluoridation. Community Dent Health 1984;1:47–54.

44. Carmichael CL, Rugg-Gunn AJ, Ferrell RS. The relationship between fluoridation, social class and caries experience in 5-year-old children in Newcastle and Northumberland in 1987. Br Dent J 1989;167:57–61.

45. Carmichael CL, Rugg-Gunn AJ, French AD, Cranage JD. The effect of fluoridation upon the relationship between caries experience and social class in 5-year-old children in Newcastle and Northumberland. Br Dent J 1980;149:163–7.

46. Chironga L, Manji F. Dental caries in 12-year-old urban and rural children in Zimbabwe. Community Dent Oral Epidemiol 1989;17:31–3.

47. Committee on Medical Aspects of Food Policy. Dietary sugars and human disease. Report on Health and Social Subjects no 37. London: HMSO, 1989.

48. Corbett ME, Moore WJ. Distribution of dental caries in ancient British populations. IV: The 19th century. Caries Res 1976;10:401–14.

49. Coykendall AL. On the evaluation of *Streptococcus mutans* and dental caries. In: Stiles HM, Loesche WJ, O'Brien TC, eds: Proceedings of microbial aspects of dental caries. Microbial Abstr 1976;3(Special Suppl):703–12.

50. Curzon ME, Curzon JA. Dental caries in Eskimo children of the Keewatin District in the Northwest Territories. J Canad Dent Assoc 1970;36:342–4.

51. DePaola PF, Soparkar PM, Tavares M, Kent RL Jr. The clinical profiles of individuals with and without root caries. Gerodontol 1989;8:9–16.

52. Disney JA, Graves RC, Stamm JW, et al. The University of North Carolina Caries Risk Assessment Study. II. Baseline caries prevalence. J Public Health Dent 1990;50:178–85.

53. Dowell TB, Evans DJ. The dental caries experience of 5 year old children in Great Britain. A survey coordinated by the British Association for the Study of Community Dentistry in 1987–88. Community Dent Health 1989;6:271–9.

54. Downer MC. The improving dental health of United Kingdom adults and prospects for the future. Br Dent J 1991;170:154–8.

55. Downer MC. Caries prevalence in the United Kingdom. Int Dent J 1994;44(Suppl 1):365–70.

56. Drake CW, Hunt RJ, Beck JD, Koch GG. Eighteen-month coronal caries incidence in North Carolina older adults. J Public Health Dent 1994;54:24–30.

57. Dreizen S, Mann AW, Spies TD, Hunt FM. Prevalence of dental caries in malnourished children. Am J Dis Child 1947;74:265–7.

58. Dubos R. The mirage of health. New York: Doubleday, 1959.

59. Ellen RP, Banting DW, Fillery ED. *Streptococcus mutans* and *Lactobacillus* detection in the assessment of dental root surface caries risk. J Dent Res 1985;64:1245–9.

60. Emilson CG, Krasse B. Support for and implications of the specific plaque hypothesis. Scand J Dent Res 1985;93:96–104.

61. Fejerskov O, Baelum V, Luan WM, Manji F. Caries prevalence in Africa and the Peoples' Republic of China. Int Dent J 1994;44(Suppl 1):425–33.

62. Fejerskov O, Baelum V, Ostergaard ES. Root caries in Scandinavia in the 1980's and future trends to be expected in dental caries experience in adults. Adv Dent Res 1993;7:4–14.

63. Finn SB, Glass RB. Sugar and dental decay. World Rev Nutr Dietet 1975;22:304–26.

64. Firestone AR, Schmid R, Mühlemann HR. Effect on the length and number of intervals between meals on caries in rats. Caries Res 1984;18:128–33.

65. Fisher FJ. A field survey of dental caries, periodontal disease and enamel defects in Tristan da Cunha. Br Dent J 1968;125:447–53.

66. Foster MK, Hunt AM. A study of dental manpower systems in relation to oral health status. Part 1: Ontario. Final report for Health and Welfare grant 606–1334–43. Toronto: University of Toronto, 1978.

67. Fuchs V. Who shall live? Health, economics, and social choice. New York: Basic Books, 1974.

68. Fure S, Romaniec M, Emilson CG, Krasse B. Proportions of *Streptococcus mutans*, lactobacilli and *Actinomyces* spp in root surface plaque. Scand J Dent Res 1987;95:119–23.

69. Garn SM, Rowe NH, Cole PE. Husband-wife similarities in dental caries experience. J Dent Res 1977;56:186.

70. Glass RL. Secular changes in caries prevalence in two Massachusetts towns. Caries Res 1981;15:445–50.

71. Graves RC, Bohannan HM, Disney JA, et al. Recent dental caries and treatment patterns in US children. J Public Health Dent 1986;46:23–9.

72. Gustafsson BE, Quensel C-E, Swenander Lanke L, et al. The Vipeholm dental caries study. The effect of different levels of carbohydrate intake on caries activity in 436 individuals observed for five years. Acta Odont Scand 1954;11:232–364.

73. Hadden WC. The use of educational attainment as an indicator of socioeconomic position. Am J Public Health 1996;86:1525–6.

74. Hand JS, Hunt RJ, Beck JD. Incidence of coronal and root caries in an older adult population. J Public Health Dent 1988;48:14–9.

75. Hargreaves JA. Changes in diet and dental health of children living in the Scottish Island of Lewis. Caries Res 1972;6:355–76.

76. Hargreaves JA, Wagg BJ, Thompson GW. Changes in caries prevalence of Isle of Lewis children, a historical comparison from 1937 to 1984. Caries Res 1987;21:277–84.

77. Harris R. Biology of the children of Hopewood House, Bowral, Australia. 4. Observations on dental caries experience extending over five years (1957–1961). J Dent Res 1963;42:1387–99.

78. Hausen H, Heinonen OP, Paunio I. Modification of occurrence of caries in children by toothbrushing and sugar exposure in fluoridated and nonfluoridated areas. Community Dent Oral Epidemiol 1981;9:103–7.

79. Hausen H, Milen A, Heinonen OP, Paunio I. Caries in primary dentition and social class in high and low fluoride areas. Community Dent Oral Epidemiol 1982;10:33–6.

80. Heft MW, Gilbert GH. Tooth loss and caries prevalence in older Floridians attending senior activity centers. Community Dent Oral Epidemiol 1991;19:228–32.

81. Heifetz SB, Horowitz HS, Korts DC. Prevalence of dental caries in white and black children in Nelson County, Virginia, a rural southern community. J Public Health Dent 1976;36:79–87.

82. Hix JO, O'Leary TJ. The relationship between cemental caries, oral hygiene status and fermentable carbohydrate intake. J Periodontol 1976;47:398–404.

83. Holbrook WP. Dental caries and cariogenic factors in preschool urban Icelandic children. Caries Res 1993;27:431–7.

84. Hughes JT, Rozier RG. The survey of dental health in the North Carolina population: Selected findings. In: Bawden JW, De Friese GH, eds. Planning for dental care on a statewide basis: The North Carolina dental manpower project. Chapel Hill, NC: Dental Foundation of North Carolina, 1981:21–37.

85. Hugoson A, Koch G, Hallonsten A-L, et al. Dental health 1973 and 1978 in individuals aged 3–20 years in the community of Jonkopping, Sweden. Swed Dent J 1980;150:217–29.

86. Hunter PBV. The prevalence of dental caries in 5-year-old New Zealand children. NZ Dent J 1979;75:154–7.

87. Infante PF, Russell AL. An epidemiologic study of dental caries in preschool children in the United States by race and socioeconomic level. J Dent Res 1974;53:393–6.

88. Ismail AI, Burt BA, Brunelle JA. Prevalence of total tooth loss, dental caries, and periodontal disease in Mexican-American adults: Results from the Southwestern HHANES. J Dent Res 1987;66:1183–8.

89. Ismail AI, Szpunar SM. The prevalence of dental caries and periodontal disease among Mexican-Americans, Cubans, and Puerto Ricans. Findings from HHANES, 1982–84. Am J Public Health 1990;80(Suppl):66–70.

90. Jakobsen J. Recent reorganization of the Public Dental Health Service in Greenland in favor of caries prevention. Community Dent Oral Epidemiol 1979;7:75–81.

91. Johansson I, Saellstrom AK, Rajan BP, Parameswaran A. Salivary flow and dental caries in Indian children suffering from chronic malnutrition. Caries Res 1992;26:38–43.

92. Joshi A, Douglass CW, Jette A, Feldman H. The distribution of root caries in community-dwelling elders in New England. J Public Health Dent 1994;54:15–23.

93. Kalsbeek H, Virrips GH. Consumption of sweet snacks and caries experience of primary school children. Caries Res 1994;28:477–83.

94. Kaste LM, Marianos D, Chang R, Phipps KR. The assessment of nursing caries and its relationship to high caries in the permanent dentition. J Public Health Dent 1992;52:64–8.

95. Kaste LM, Selwitz RH, Oldakowski RJ, et al. Coronal caries in the primary and permanent dentition of children and adolescents 1–17 years of age: United States, 1988–1991. J Dent Res 1996;75(Special Issue):631–41.

96. Keene HJ. Dental caries prevalence in early Polynesians from the Hawaiian Islands. J Dent Res 1986;65:935–8.

97. Kerr NW. The prevalence and pattern of distribution of root caries in a Scottish medieval population. J Dent Res 1990;69:857–60.

98. Kingman A, Little W, Gomez I, et al. Salivary levels of *Streptococcus mutans* and lactobacilli and dental caries experiences in a US adolescent population. Community Dent Oral Epidemiol 1988;16:98–103.

99. Kitamura M, Kiyak HA, Mulligan K. Predictors of root caries in the elderly. Community Dent Oral Epidemiol 1986;14:34–8.

100. Kleemola-Kujala E, Rasanen L. Relationship of oral hygiene and sugar consumption to risk of caries in children. Community Dent Oral Epidemiol 1982;10:224–33.

101. Klein H. The dental status and dental needs of young adult males, rejectable or acceptable for military service, according to Selective Service dental requirements. Public Health Rep 1941;56:1369–87.

102. Klein H. The family and dental disease. IV. Dental disease (DMF) experience in parents and offspring. J Am Dent Assoc 1946;33:735–43.

103. Klein H, Palmer CE. Dental caries in American Indian children. Public Health Bull No 239. Washington DC: Government Printing Office, 1937.

104. Klein H, Palmer CE. Studies on dental caries. V. Familial resemblance in the caries experience of siblings. Public Health Rep 1938;53:1353–64.

105. Klein H, Palmer CE. Studies on dental caries. VII. Sex differences in dental caries experience of elementary school children. Public Health Rep 1938; 53:1685–90.

106. Klein H, Palmer CE. Community economic status and the dental problem of school children. Public Health Rep 1940;55:187–205.

107. Klein H, Palmer CE. Studies on dental caries. XII. Comparison of the caries susceptibility of the various morphological types of permanent teeth. J Dent Res 1941;20:203–16.

108. Klein H, Shimizu T. The family and dental disease. I. DMF experience among husbands and wives. J Am Dent Assoc 1945;32:945–55.

109. Kohler B, Bjarnason S, Finnbogason SY, Holbrook WP. Mutans streptococci, lactobacilli and caries experience in 12-year-old Icelandic urban children, 1984 and 1991. Community Dent Oral Epidemiol 1995;23:65–8.

110. Kohler B, Bratthall D. Intrafamilial levels of *Streptococcus mutans* and some aspects of the bacterial transmission. Scand J Dent Res 1978;86:35–42.

111. Kohler B, Bratthall D, Krasse B. Preventive measures in mothers influence the establishment of the bacterium *Streptococcus mutans* in their infants. Arch Oral Biol 1983;28:225–31.

112. Krasse B. Oral effects of other carbohydrates. Int Dent J 1982;32:24–32.

113. Krasse B. Biological factors as indicators of future caries. Int Dent J 1988;38:219–25.

114. Kumar J. Green E, Wallace W, Bustard R. Changes in dental caries prevalence in upstate New York schoolchildren. J Public Health Dent 1991;51:158–63.

115. Larsson B, Johansson I, Ericson T. Prevalence of caries in adolescents in relation to diet. Community Dent Oral Epidemiol 1992;20:133–7.

116. Lawrence HP, Hunt RJ, Beck JD. Three-year root caries incidence and risk modeling in older adults in North Carolina. J Public Health Dent 1995;55:69–78.

117. Leake JL. A review of regional studies on the dental health of older Canadians. Gerodontology 1988; 7:7–11.

118. Lennon MA, Davies RM, Downer MC, Hull PS. Tooth loss in a 19th century British population. Arch Oral Biol 1974;19:511–6.

119. Leske GS, Ripa LW. Three-year root caries increments: an analysis of teeth and surfaces at risk. Gerodontol 1989;8:17–22.

120. Lilienthal B, Goldsworthy NE, Sullivan HR, Cameron DA. The biology of the children of Hopewood House, Bowral, NSW. I. Observations on dental caries extending over five years (1947–1952). Med J Aust 1953;1:878–81.

121. Link BG, Phelan JC. Understanding sociodemographic differences in health: The role of fundamental social causes [editorial]. Am J Public Health 1996;86:471–3.

122. Lo EC, Schwarz E. Tooth and root conditions in the middle-aged and the elderly in Hong Kong. Community Dent Oral Epidemiol 1994;22:381–5.

123. Locker D, Leake JL. Coronal and root decay experience in older adults in Ontario, Canada. J Public Health Dent 1993;53:158–64.

124. Locker D, Slade GD, Leake JL. Prevalence of and factors associated with root decay in older adults in Canada. J Dent Res 1989;68:768–72.

125. Loesche WJ. Dental caries: A treatable infection. 2nd ed. Grand Haven MI: ADQ Publications, 1993.

126. Loesche WJ, Eklund SA, Mehlisch D, Burt BA. Possible effect of medically administered antibiotics on the mutans streptococci: Implications for reductions in decay. Oral Microbiiol Immunol 1989;4:77–81.

127. Luan WM, Baelum V, Chen X, Fejerskov O. Dental caries in adult and elderly Chinese. J Dent Res 1989;68:1771–6.

128. Ludwig TG, Bibby BG. Geographic variations in the prevalence of dental caries in the United States of America. Caries Res 1969;3:32–43.

129. Makinen KK. The role of sucrose and other sugars in the development of dental caries: A review. Int Dent J 1972;22:363–86.

130. Mandel ID. Dental caries. Am Sci 1979;67:680–8.

131. Manji F, Fejerskov O, Baelum V. Pattern of dental caries in an adult rural population. Caries Res 1989;23:55–62.

132. Mann AW, Dreizen S, Spies TD, Hunt FM. A comparison of dental caries activity in malnourished and well nourished patients. J Am Dent Assoc 1947;34:244–52.

133. Mansbridge JN. Heredity and dental caries. J Dent Res 1959;38:337–47.

134. Marshall Day CD. Nutritional deficiencies and dental caries in Northern India. Br Dent J 1944;76:115–22.

135. Marthaler TM. Epidemiological and clinical dental findings in relation to intake of carbohydrates. Caries Res 1967;1:22–38.

136. Marthaler TM, Steiner M, Menghini G, Bandi A. Caries prevalence in Switzerland. Int Dent J 1994;44(Suppl 1):393–401.

137. Martinsson T. Socio-economic investigation of school children with high and low caries frequency. III. A dietary study based on information given by the children. Odont Revy 1972;23:93–113.

138. McDonald SP, Sheiham A. The distribution of caries on different tooth surfaces at varying levels of caries—a compilation of data from 18 previous studies. Community Dent Health 1992;9:39–48.

139. McEniery TM, Davies GN. Brisbane dental survey 1977. A comparative study of caries experience of children in Brisbane, Australia, over a 20-year period. Community Dent Oral Epidemiol 1979;7:42–50.

140. McGregor AB. Changing diet and its effect on caries prevalence in Ghana [abstract]. J Dent Res 1963;42:1086–7.

141. McGuire SM, Fox CH, Douglass CW, et al. Beneath the surface of coronal caries: Primary decay, recurrent decay, and failed restorations in a population-based survey of New England elders. J Public Health Dent 1993;53:76–82.

142. McNulty JA, Fos PJ. The study of caries prevalence in children in a developing country. J Dent Child 1989;56:129–36.

143. Mellanby M. Diet and the teeth. Part III. The effect of diet on dental structure and disease in man. London: His Majesty's Stationery Office, 1934.

144. Menaker L, Navia JM. Effect of undernutrition during the perinatal period on caries development in the rat. II. Caries susceptibility in underfed rats supplemented with protein or caloric additions during the suckling period. J Dent Res 1973;52:680–7.

145. Menaker L, Navia JM. Effect of undernutrition during the perinatal period on caries development in the rat. III. Effect of undernutrition on biochemical parameters in the developing submandibular salivary glands. J Dent Res 1973;52:688–91.

146. Menaker L, Navia JM. Effect of undernutrition during the perinatal period on caries development in

the rat. IV. Effects of differential tooth eruption and exposure to a cariogenic diet on subsequent dental caries incidence. J Dent Res 1973;52:692–7.

147. Milen A. Role of social class in caries occurrence in primary teeth. Int J Epidemiol 1987;16:252–6.

148. Miller WD. Agency of micro-organisms in decay of human teeth. Dent Cosmos 1883;25:1–12.

149. Milnes AR. Description and epidemiology of nursing caries. J Public Health Dent 1996;56:38–50.

150. Møller IJ. Impact of oral diseases across cultures. Int Dent J 1978;28:376–80.

151. Møller IJ, Pindborg JJ, Roed-Petersen B. The prevalence of dental caries, enamel opacities and enamel hypoplasia in Ugandans. Arch Oral Biol 1972;17:9–22.

152. Møller IJ, Poulsen S, Nielsen VO. The prevalence of dental caries in Godhavn and Scoresbysund districts, Greenland. Scand J Dent Res 1972;80:169–80.

153. Moore WJ, Corbett ME. The distribution of dental caries in ancient British populations. I. Anglo-Saxon period. Caries Res 1971;5:151–68.

154. Moore WJ, Corbett ME. The distribution of dental caries in ancient British populations. II. Iron Age, Romano-British and Mediaeval periods. Caries Res 1973;7:139–53.

155. Moore WJ, Corbett ME. The distribution of dental caries in ancient British populations. III. The 17th century. Caries Res 1975;9:163–75.

156. Mosha HJ, Ngilisho LA, Nkwera H, et al. Oral health status and treatment needs in different age groups in two regions of Tanzania. Community Dent Oral Epidemiol 1994;22:307–10.

157. Mosha HJ, Robison VA. Caries experience of the primary dentition among groups of Tanzanian urban preschoolchildren. Community Dent Oral Epidemiol 1989;17:34–7.

158. Mosha HJ, Scheutz F. Dental caries in the permanent dentition of schoolchildren in Dar es Salaam in 1979, 1983 and 1989. Community Dent Oral Epidemiol 1992;20:381–2.

159. Navia JM. Nutrition in oral health and disease. In: Stallard RE, ed. A textbook of preventive dentistry. Philadelphia: WB Saunders, 1982:90–146.

160. Newbrun E. Dietary carbohydrates: their role in cariogenicity. Med Clin North Am 1979;63:1069–86.

161. Newbrun E. Sugar and dental caries: A review of human studies. Science 1982;217:418–23.

162. Newbrun E. Cariology. 3rd ed. Chicago: Quintessence, 1989.

163. Newbrun E, Hoover C, Mettraux G, Graf H. Comparison of dietary habits and dental health of subjects with hereditary fructose intolerance and control subjects. J Am Dent Assoc 1980;101:619–26.

164. Nizel AE, Bibby BG. Geographic variations in caries prevalence in soldiers. J Am Dent Assoc 1944; 31:1619–26.

165. Ojofeitimi EO, Hollist NO, Banjo T, Adu TA. Effect of cariogenic food exposure of prevalence of dental caries and fee and non-fee-paying Nigerian schoolchildren. Community Dent Oral Epidemiol 1984; 12:274–77.

166. Palmer JD, Pitter AFV. Differences in dental caries levels between 8-year-old children in Bath from different socio-economic groups. Community Dent Health 1988;5:363–7.

167. Papas AS, Joshi A, Palmer CA, et al. Relationship of diet to root caries. Am J Clin Nutr 1995;61:423S–9S.

168. Pedersen PO. Dental disease in Europe and Greenland. J R Soc Health 1971;91:88–91.

169. Pickerill HP. The prevention of dental caries and oral sepsis. 3rd ed. London: Bailliere, Tindall and Cox, 1923.

170. Ringelberg ML, Gilbert GH, Antonson DE, et al. Root caries and root defects in urban and rural adults: The Florida Dental Care Study. J Am Dent Assoc 1996;127:885–91.

171. Ringelberg ML, Matonski GM, Kimball AW. Dental caries-experience in three generations of families. J Public Health Dent 1974;34:174–80.

172. Rogers AH. Evidence for the transmissibility of dental caries. Austr Dent J 1977;22:53–6.

173. Rugg-Gunn AJ, Edgar WM. Sugar and dental caries; a review of the evidence. Community Dent Health 1984;1:85–92.

174. Rugg-Gunn AJ, Hackett AF, Appleton DR, et al. Relationship between dietary habits and caries increment assessed over two years in 405 English adolescent school children. Arch Oral Biol 1984;29:983–92.

175. Russell AL. International nutrition surveys: A summary of preliminary dental findings. J Dent Res 1963;42:233–44.

176. Russell AL. World epidemiology and oral health. In: Kreshover SJ, McClure FJ, eds. Environmental variables in oral disease. Washington DC: American Association Advancement Science Publ No 81, 1966:21–39.

177. Russell AL. Dental caries and nutrition in Lebanon. J Dent Res 1966;45:957–63.

178. Russell AL, Leatherwood EC, Le Van Hien, Van Reen R. Dental caries and nutrition in South Vietnam. J Dent Res 1965;44:102–11.

179. Salonen L, Allander L, Bratthall D, et al. Oral health status in an adult Swedish population. Prevalence of caries. A cross-sectional epidemiological study in the Northern Alvsborg county. Swed Dent J 1989;13:111–23.

180. Sardo Infirri J, Barmes DE. Epidemiology of oral diseases: Differences in national problems. Int Dent J 1979;29:183–90.

181. Schamschula RG, Adkins BL, Barmes DE, et al. WHO study of dental caries etiology in Papua New Guinea. WHO Offset Publ No 40. Geneva: WHO, 1978.

182. Schamschula RG, Barmes DE, Keyes PH, Gulbinat W. Prevalence and interrelationships of root surface caries in Lufa, Papua New Guinea. Community Dent Oral Epidemiol 1974;2:295–304.

183. Schamshula RG, Cooper MH, Adkins BL, et al. Oral conditions in Australian children of Aboriginal and Caucasian descent. Community Dent Oral Epidemiol 1980;8:365–9.

184. Schamshula RG, Cooper MH, Wright MC, Agus HM, Un PSH. Oral health of adolescent and adult Australian Aborigines. Community Dent Oral Epidemiol 1980;8:370–4.

185. Schamschula RG, Keyes PH, Hornabrook KRW. Root surface caries in Lufa, New Guinea. I. Clinical observations. J Am Dent Assoc 1972;85:603–8.

186. Schlack CA, Restarske JS, Dochterman EF. Dental status of 71,015 naval personnel at first examination in 1942. J Am Dent Assoc 1946;33:1141–6.

187. Schupbach P, Osterwalder V, Guggenheim B. Human root caries: Microbiota in plaque covering sound, carious and arrested carious root surfaces. Caries Res 1995;29:382–95.

188. Senn WW. Incidence of dental caries among aviation cadets. Mil Surg 1943;93:461–4.

189. Shaw JH. Nutrition and dental caries. In: National Research Council, Committee on Dental Health. Survey of the literature on dental caries. Nat Res Council Publ No 225. Washington DC: Nat Acad Sciences, 1952:415–567.

190. Sigurjons H, Magnusdottir MO, Holbrook WP. Cariogenic bacteria in a longitudinal study of approximal caries. Caries Res 1995;29:42–5.

191. Slade GD, Spencer AJ, Gorkic E, Andrews G. Oral health status and treatment needs of non-institutionalized persons aged 60+ in Adelaide, South Australia. Aust Dent J 1993;38:373–80.

192. Spencer AJ, Davies M, Slade G, Brennan D. Caries prevalence in Australia. Int Dent J 1994;44(Suppl 1):415–23.

193. Sreebny LM. Sugar and human dental caries. World Rev Nutr Diet 1982;40:19–65.

194. Stamm JW. Is there a need for dental sealants? Epidemiological indications in the 1980s. J Dent Educ 1984;48:9–17.

195. Stamm JW, Banting DW, Imrey PB. Adult root caries survey of two similar communities with contrasting natural water fluoride levels. J Am Dent Assoc 1990;120:143–9.

196. Stecksen-Blicks C, Arvidsson S, Holm A-K. Dental health, dental care, and dietary habits in children in different parts of Sweden. Acta Odontol Scand 1985;43:59–67.

197. Stookey GK, Sergeant JW, Park KK, et al. Prevalence of dental caries in Indiana school children: results of a 1982 survey. Pediatr Dent 1985;7:8–13.

198. Sullivan HR, Harris R. The biology of the children of Hopewood House, Bowral, NSW. II. Observations extending over five years (1952–1956). 2. Observations on oral conditions. Aust Dent J 1958;3:311–7.

199. Sundin B, Birkhed D, Granath L. Is there not a strong relationship nowadays between caries and consumption of sweets? Swed Dent J 1983;7:103–8.

200. Sundin B, Granath L, Birkhed D. Variation of posterior approximal caries incidence with consumption of sweets with regard to other caries-related factors in 15–18 year-olds. Community Dent Oral Epidemiol 1992;20:76–80.

201. Szpunar SM, Eklund SA, Burt BA. Sugar consumption and caries risk in schoolchildren with low caries experience. Community Dent Oral Epidemiol 1995;23:142–6.

202. Takeuchi M. Epidemiological study on dental caries in Japanese children before, during, and after World War II. Int Dent J 1961;11:443–57.

203. Taylor GF, Marshall Day CD. Osteomalacia and dental caries. Br Dent J 1940;69:316–8.

204. Thylstrup A, Fejerskov O, eds. Textbook of clinical cariology. 2nd ed. Copenhagen: Munksgaard, 1994.

205. Todd JE. Children's dental health in England and Wales, 1973. London: Her Majesty's Stationery Office, 1975.

206. Toverud G. The influence of war and post-war conditions on the teeth of Norwegian school children. I. Eruption of permanent teeth and status of deciduous dentition. Milbank Mem Fund Quart 1956;34:354–430.

207. Toverud G. The influence of war and post-war conditions on the teeth of Norwegian school children. II. Caries in the permanent teeth of children aged 7–8 and 12–13 years. Milbank Mem Fund Quart 1957;35:127–96.

208. Toverud G. The influence of war and post-war conditions on the teeth of Norwegian school children. III. Discussion of food supply and dental condition in Norway and other European countries. Milbank Mem Fund Quart 1957;35:373–459.

209. Tsubouchi J, Tsubouchi M, Maynard RJ, et al. A study of dental caries and risk factors among Native American infants. J Dent Child 1995;62:283–7.

210. US Department of Health and Human Services, National Center for Health Statistics. Third National Health and Nutrition Examination Survey, 1988–94. Public Use Data File No. 7–0627. Hyattsville MD: CDC, 1997.

211. US Public Health Service, National Center for Health Statistics. Decayed, missing, and filled teeth in adults, United States, 1960–1962. PHS Publ No 1000, Series 11 No 23. Washington DC: Government Printing Office, 1967.

212. US Public Health Service, National Center for Health Statistics. Decayed, missing, and filled teeth among children; United States. DHEW Publ No (HSM) 72–1003, Series 11 No 106. Washington DC: Government Printing Office, 1971.

213. US Public Health Service, National Center for Health Statistics. Decayed, missing, and filled teeth among youths 12–17 years, United States. DHEW Publ No (HRA) 75–1626, Series 11 No 144. Washington DC: Government Printing Office, 1974.

214. US Public Health Service, National Center for Health Statistics. Decayed, missing, and filled teeth among persons 1–74 years, United States 1971–1974. DHHS Publ No (PHS) 81–1678, Series 11 No 223. Washington DC: Government Printing Office, 1981.

215. US Public Health Service, National Center for Health Statistics. Diet and dental health; a study of relationships. DHHS Publ No (PHS) 82–1675, Series 11 No 225. Washington DC: Government Printing Office, 1982.

216. US Public Health Service, National Institute of Dental Research. The prevalence of dental caries in United States children, 1979–80. NIH Publ No 82–2245. Washington DC: Government Printing Office, 1981.

217. US Public Health Service, National Institute of Dental Research. Oral health of United States adults; national findings. NIH Publ No 87–2868. Washington DC: Government Printing Office, 1987.

218. US Public Health Service, National Institute of Dental Research. Oral health of United States adults; regional findings. NIH Publ No 88–2869. Washington DC: Government Printing Office, 1988.

219. US Public Health Service, National Institute of Dental Research. Oral health of United States children. NIH Publ No 89–2247. Washington DC: Government Printing Office, 1989.

220. van Houte J. Role of micro-organisms in caries etiology. J Dent Res 1994;73:672–81.

221. van Houte J, Lopman J, Kent R. The predominant cultivable flora of sound and carious human root surfaces. J Dent Res 1994;73:1727–34.

222. Vehkalahti MM. Relationship between root caries and coronal decay. J Dent Res 1987;66:1608–10.

223. Vehkalahti MM, Paunio IK. Occurrence of root caries in relation to dental health behavior. J Dent Res 1988;67:911–14.

224. Vehkalahti M, Rajala M, Tuominen R, Paunio I. Prevalence of root caries in the adult Finnish population. Community Dent Oral Epidemiol 1983; 11:188–90.

225. Wagg BJ. Root surface caries: A review. Community Dent Health 1984;1:11–20.

226. Walker AR, Walker BF, Glatthaar II. Perplexing fea-

tures in the occurrence of dental caries and its relationship to sugar intake. J R Soc Health 1992; 112:74–7.

227. Wallace JS. The cause and prevention of decay in teeth. 2nd ed. London: Churchill, 1902.

228. Weinstein P. Research recommendations: Pleas for enhanced research efforts to impact the epidemic of dental disease in infants. J Public Health Dent 1996;56:55–60.

229. Whelton HP, Holland TJ, O'Mullane DM. The prevalence of root surface caries amongst Irish adults. Gerodontol 1993;10:72–5.

230. Winn DM, Brunelle JA, Selwitz RH, et al. Coronal and root caries in the dentition of adults in the United States, 1988–1991. J Dent Res 1996;75(Spec No):642–51.

20

Periodontal Diseases

Periodontal Infections and Host Response ◆ Current
Models of Periodontal Diseases ◆ Distribution of
Periodontal Diseases ◆ Geographic Distribution ◆
Gingivitis ◆ Periodontitis: Prevalence and Incidence ◆
Demographic Risk Factors: Gender and Race,
Age, Socioeconomic Status ◆ Risk Factors for
Periodontitis: Oral Hygiene, Plaque, Microbiota ◆
Local Factors ◆ Nutrition ◆ Tobacco Use ◆
Periodontitis and Systemic Conditions: Diabetes,
HIV Infection, Cardiovascular Diseases ◆
Predicting Periodontitis

Periodontal diseases have been prevalent throughout human history, although without the obvious secular variations that characterize dental caries. Human remains from the early Christian era show clear evidence of periodontal bone loss.[108, 109]

The term *periodontal disease* has been recognized for some time as a generic term used to describe a group of diseases,[137] so it should more correctly be used in the plural form. The singular term is as imprecise and nonspecific as is the term *fever* is in the medical context. It is generally more useful to refer specifically to gingivitis and periodontitis; the term *periodontal disease* should be reserved only for those situations in which the generic term is specifically intended.

This chapter describes the epidemiology of gingivitis and adult periodontitis, their distribution, and the risk factors and background characteristics associated with them.

PERIODONTAL INFECTIONS AND HOST RESPONSE

Like caries, both gingivitis and periodontitis result from bacterial infections. The causative bacteria are found in dental plaque. *Gingivitis* is defined as an inflammatory process

of the gingiva in which the junctional epithelium, although altered by the disease, remains attached to the tooth at its original level.[53] Most forms of gingivitis are plaque-induced; nonspecific bacterial deposits in the supragingival plaque are associated with early lesions, although up to one-fourth of plaque bacteria in chronic gingivitis can be made up of gram-negative species.[35] There are initial, early, and established gingivitis lesions; and a sequential microbial colonization leads to bacteriologically more complex plaque as the lesions progress.[124]

Periodontitis is also an inflammatory condition of the gingival tissues, characterized by loss of attachment of the periodontal ligament and the bony support of the tooth.[53] Periodontitis is thought to develop as an extension of gingivitis, although only a few gingivitis sites make this transition, and the mechanisms by which they do so are not well understood.[124] Inflammatory mediators play an important role in the progression of periodontitis.[117, 125] A large number of microbial species have been associated with destructive periodontitis. Most of them are spirochetes and gram-negative rods,[98] but it is unlikely that all of these bacteria are essential players in the disease.[127] The bacteria associated with periodontitis can vary with the rate of tissue destruction, disease activity, and host resistance. Some of these species have been implicated in a number of serious systemic diseases.[49, 162]

The other side of periodontal infections is the nature and extent of the host response to these infections. Only a small proportion of virtually any population is susceptible to severe, generalized periodontitis, even though most people have these infections to some degree,[54] which shows that the host response to these infections is crucial to whether or not clinical disease is manifested. This has led to the hypothesis that there are two distinct models of periodontitis. One is the *plaque and local factor* model, in which specific pathogens dominate the host response in controlling disease expression. The second is the *compromised host* model, in which severity and rate of progression are often rapid and not well correlated with local factors such as plaque.[117] The compromised host model is less common, responds much less favorably to standard treatments, and is thought to be the type of disease found in early-onset, refractory, and diabetes-associated periodontitis. Neutrophil abnormalities have been associated with these forms of the disease,[126] and at least for early-onset periodontitis, the compromised host response is thought to be of genetic origin.[42] Genetic influences have also been proposed as an etiologic factor in adult periodontitis.[107]

There is an extensive classification of these and related conditions for diagnostic and treatment purposes,[53] and the evolution of these disease classifications is well documented in the various World Workshops held through the years. These workshops are international gatherings of experts to review the state of knowledge in the periodontal field, and have been held in 1966,[134] 1977,[78] 1989,[116] and 1996 (reported in the first issue of *Annals of Periodontology*). Disease classifications have traditionally been based on clinical manifestations rather than etiologic factors, and at least four types of periodontitis have become generally recognized: adult, rapidly progressive, juvenile, and prepubertal.[128] These classifications were expanded at the 1989 World Workshop to include early-onset periodontitis and other conditions listed in Table 20–1. It is becoming increasingly accepted that the periodontal diseases are a family of more-or-less related conditions, and advances in molecular biology may provide a new basis for classifying them in the future.

Although different categories of peri-

Table 20–1. SUGGESTED CLASSIFICATION OF PERIODONTITIS CONDITIONS BY THE 1989 WORLD WORKSHOP IN CLINICAL PERIODONTICS

I. Adult Periodontitis
II. Early-Onset Periodontitis
   A. Prepubertal Periodontitis
      1. Generalized
      2. Localized
   B. Juvenile Periodontitis
      1. Generalized
      2. Localized
   C. Rapidly Progressive Periodontitis
III. Periodontitis Associated with Systemic Disease
IV. Necrotizing Ulcerative Periodontitis
V. Refractory Periodontitis

From Consensus report, discussion session 1. In: Nevins M, Becker W, Kornman K (eds): Proceedings of the World Workshop on Clinical Periodontics. Chicago: American Academy of Periodontology, 1990:123–31.

odontitis are recognized, there are no generally accepted definitions of *serious* or *moderate* periodontitis, terms used in clinical practice, epidemiology, and public health. Several definitions of serious periodontitis used in epidemiologic studies are shown in Table 20–2. Two of these definitions use similar combinations of loss of periodontal attachment (LPA) sites added to the presence of pockets; the third uses a cut-point on a statistical distribution. As used in this chapter, the term *serious periodontitis* refers to a degree of periodontitis severe enough to cause or threaten the loss of teeth. There is moderate agreement in the literature that LPA of 6 mm

Table 20–2. SOME SUGGESTED MEASURES OF "SERIOUS" PERIODONTITIS

4 or more sites with loss of periodontal attachment (LPA) $\geq$ 5 mm, with 1 or more of those sites with pocket depth $\geq$ 4 mm*

2 or more teeth with LPA $\geq$ 6 mm, plus 1 or more sites with pocket depth $\geq$ 5 mm†

Mean LPA in the top 20th percentile of the distribution‡

From *Beck JD, Koch GG, Kozier RG, Tudor GE. Prevalence and risk indicators for periodontal attachment loss in a population of older community-dwelling blacks and whites. J Periodontol 1990;61:521–8; †Machtei EE, Christenson LA, Grossi SG, et al. Clinical criteria for the definition of "established periodontitis." J Periodontol 1992;63:206–14; ‡Locker D, Leake JL. Risk indicators and risk markers for periodontal disease experience in older adults living independently in Ontario, Canada. J Dent Res 1993;72:9–17.

or more is a reasonable cut-off point between serious and moderate periodontitis; the latter term is usually applied to LPA of 4 to 5 mm or less. *Moderate periodontitis* is used in this chapter when pocketing, LPA, or even some bone loss can be clinically or radiographically demonstrated; but the condition is not severe enough to threaten the loss of teeth.

CURRENT MODELS OF PERIODONTAL DISEASES

As mentioned in Chapter 15, perceptions of the nature of periodontal diseases changed radically as a result of research during the 1980s. Before then the "old" view of periodontal disease is summarized in this statement from a 1961 report by an Expert Committee of the World Health Organization (WHO):

> *Periodontal disease is one of the most widespread diseases of mankind. No nation and no area of the world is free from it and in most it has a high prevalence, affecting in some degree approximately half the child population and almost the entire adult population. Research and clinical evidence indicate that the damage caused to the supporting structures of the teeth by periodontal disease in early adult life is irreparable, whilst in the middle adult life it destroys a large part of the natural dentition and deprives many people of all their teeth long before old age. The total effects of periodontal disease on the general health of the populations is unassessable.*[179]

Note that the disease is referred to in the singular, and the whole passage conjures up the vision of helpless peoples, all equally susceptible and suffering en masse. It was also accepted that gingivitis invariably progressed to periodontitis, a view that has now changed to recognize that few gingivitis lesions actually make the transition into periodontitis.

Challenges to the concept of universal susceptibility came as studies were conducted in developing countries, places from which little data had previously been available. The results of these surveys were broadly similar in that they found massive deposits of plaque and calculus, and thus high levels of prevalence and severity of gingivitis.[16] Contrary to expectations, however, they also found that the prevalence of serious, generalized periodontitis in the developing world was little different from that in the highly treated populations of western countries.[10, 11, 13, 83, 93, 119] Further substantial modification to the traditional

perception of periodontitis came with the demonstration, in the early 1980s, that the periodontal tissues apparently had some capacity to repair themselves.[57] This finding was incorporated into what became known as the *burst theory* of periodontitis.[157] This theory states that periodontitis progresses in a series of relatively short, acute "bursts" of rapid tissue destruction, followed by some tissue repair and with long periods of remission.[86] This view was the converse of the "linear" type of progression, which had been assumed until that time, and resulted from analyzing measurements from individual sites rather than using pooled, mean data as had generally been the method used. The burst theory of periodontal destruction has been accepted by most researchers, and there is now good epidemiologic evidence to support it.[24]

Basic, clinical, and epidemiologic research from the late 1970s onward (about the same time that the caries decline was recognized) therefore have led to a perception of the periodontal diseases, by the 1990s, that can be summarized as shown in Table 20–3.

As described in Chapter 15, much of the confusion surrounding periodontal diseases came from the difficulties in measuring the conditions. Although the diseases are constantly becoming better understood, the measurement problems have not disappeared.

Table 20–3. A CURRENT MODEL OF PERIODONTAL DISEASES

- Only a small proportion of persons (7%–15%) exhibit severe periodontitis, "severe" meaning that tooth loss occurs or is threatened. Mild gingivitis is common, as is mild-to-moderate periodontitis: Most adults exhibit some loss of bony support and loss of probing attachment while still maintaining a functioning dentition.
- Gingivitis and periodontitis are associated with bacterial flora that have some similarities but also some differences. Gingivitis precedes periodontitis, but only a fraction of sites with gingivitis later develop periodontitis.
- Although usually related to age in cross-sectional surveys, periodontitis is not a natural consequence of aging.
- Periodontitis is not the major cause of tooth loss in adults, except perhaps in the oldest age groups in some populations.
- Periodontitis is usually a site-specific condition, only occasionally seen in generalized forms. Generalized periodontitis is usually severe, and of the early-onset type.
- Periodontitis is usually thought to proceed in bursts of destructive activity with quiescent periods between the bursts.

Until research finds a suitable way of measuring active disease, we are left with LPA, pocket depth, radiographic bone loss, and gingival bleeding to serve as clinical and epidemiologic measures of periodontal diseases, cumbersome and inappropriate for some purposes though they are.

DISTRIBUTION OF PERIODONTAL DISEASES

Geographic Distribution

More than 70% of adults in all parts of the world have some degree of gingivitis or periodontitis.[15] Under the old perception of periodontal disease, prevalence and severity were considered greater in developing countries and more moderate in the developed world.[142] However, data collected since 1980 in WHO's Global Oral Data Bank,[130, 131] when added to the results of other epidemiologic studies,[9] suggest that although gingivitis and calculus are more prevalent and severe in developing nations, there are fewer global differences in the prevalence of severe periodontitis. Gingivitis and calculus are controlled by personal oral hygiene and professional dental care, so it is to be expected that they are less severe in economically developed nations. If severe periodontitis is the result of the host response interacting with periodontal infections, then that process is less amenable to control by oral hygiene and professional care. This profile is consistent with the compromised host model of periodontitis described previously.

Gingivitis

At the population level, gingivitis is found in early childhood, is more prevalent and severe in adolescence, and tends to level off after adolescence. The prevalence of gingivitis among schoolchildren in the United States has ranged from 40% to 60% in various national surveys.[29, 168] In the national survey of employed adults in 1985–1986, 47% of males and 39% of females aged 18–64 exhibited at least one site that bled on probing.[170] The mean number of bleeding sites per person was higher in the older age groups in males, but not in females. In the first national survey of adults that measured gingivitis, conducted in 1960–1962, 85% of men and 79% of women were affected.[167] Even allowing for

the differences in measurement techniques between the two surveys, there appears to have been an improvement in gingival health over that period.

Gingivitis is closely correlated with plaque deposits, a relationship long considered one of cause and effect. Studies on the natural history of periodontal diseases in Norway and Sri Lanka found no increase in prevalence and severity of gingivitis between the late teen years and age 40 in the Norwegian professionals and students, among whom oral hygiene was excellent.[6] Among the Sri Lankan tea workers, both the gingival condition and oral hygiene was poorer at all ages. Surveys among other developing nations show that gingivitis, associated with extensive plaque and calculus deposits, is the norm among adults.[9]

It is generally believed that gingivitis has declined over recent years in the United States because of greater attention to oral hygiene as a part of personal grooming. The main research interest in gingivitis today is why some lesions progress to periodontitis and some do not, as well as the factors that may predict these outcomes.

Prevalence of Periodontitis

Interpretation of epidemiologic data from before 1980 is extremely difficult because the indexes used to measure the conditions then are no longer considered valid (Chapter 15). The impression created by these data was summed up in the WHO quote cited earlier: "periodontal disease" was extensive and serious in most populations. Later research, however, in which the use of disaggregated indexes in epidemiology played a prominent part, has led to an almost total reversal of that concept. Data from many parts of the world, collected during the 1980s and 1990s, have shown that the prevalence of generalized, severe periodontitis is in the range of 7% to 15% in almost all populations, regardless of their state of economic development, oral hygiene, or availability of dental care.[43, 59] This relatively low proportion is a fundamental shift away from the old view of universal susceptibility, even though it still represents many people with serious periodontitis.

Any assessment of the prevalence of a condition, and the form of its distribution in a population, must begin with a case definition of the disease. Here is the first difficulty, for as described previously, there is no clear agreement with regard to defining moderate and serious levels of periodontitis. We stated earlier that 6 mm LPA is generally considered serious and 4 to 5 mm moderate, but to many it seems reasonable to say that *any* LPA should be considered disease. Philosophically that might be true, but in practical terms, the consideration of all LPA as disease is not helpful. Figure 20–1 shows the proportion of adults in the United States with at least one site showing 2 mm LPA. A high proportion of even the younger age groups are affected, and this condition soon becomes almost universal. LPA of at least 2 mm is so common, and is so often found in persons with functional dentitions, that one has to question whether philosophically it should be thought of as disease in a clinical sense. Certainly any measure that is so common is not appropriate in epidemiologic research, where risk factors are being sought. Treatment for this level of LPA is also very conservative.[53]

The ideal would be some measure of current disease activity added to a record of LPA, which is a "scar" from past disease. However, a measure of current disease activity does not yet exist; only after-the-fact measures of attachment levels can disclose it. Pocket depth added to clinical signs of inflammation serves as a surrogate for disease activity, but a more valid measure may be developed from detection of inflammatory mediators at a suspected active site. In the meantime, researchers and clinicians use radiographs of bone loss, plus clinical measures of LPA, pocket depth, gingival bleeding, and presence of plaque and calculus (Chapter 15).

Attachment loss is considered to be the most valid measure of periodontitis,[56] although it measures past disease rather than present activity. If 2 mm LPA is too common to discriminate between people who are susceptible or nonsusceptible to serious periodontitis, where should the cut-off be? Figure 20–2 shows the proportion of adults with at least one site with LPA of 2 mm, 4 mm, and 6 mm. If the use of a 2 mm measure is not sensitive enough (i.e., includes too many false-negative results), a 6 mm cut-off may be not specific enough (i.e., it could exclude too many true-positive results). We stated earlier that 4 to 5 mm LPA has generally been considered moderate periodontitis in the literature, so LPA of at least 3 mm at the upper level of mild periodontitis seems a reasonable basis for a case definition of periodontitis. In incidence studies, 3 mm LPA is taken as the

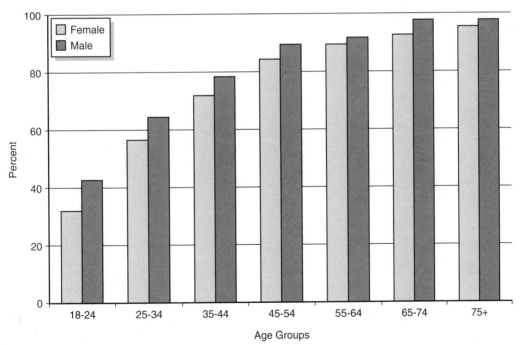

Figure 20–1. Percent of adults with at least one site with loss of periodontal attachment (LPA) of 2 mm or more. By age and gender, United States, 1985–94. (From US Department of Health and Human Services, National Center for Health Statistics. Third National Health and Nutrition Examination Survey, 1988–94. Public Use Data File No. 7–0627. Hyattsville MD: CDC, 1997.)

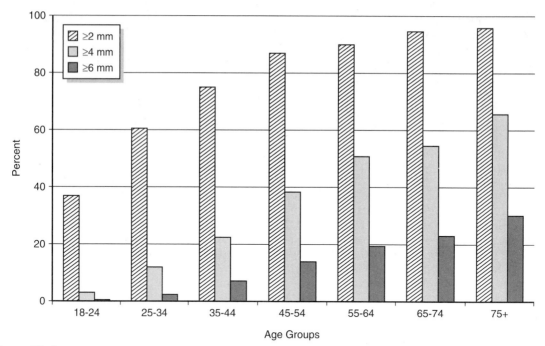

Figure 20–2. Proportion of adults with at least one site with loss of periodontal attachment (LPA) of 2 mm or more, 4 mm or more, and 6 mm or more. By age, United States, 1988–94. (From US Department of Health and Human Services, National Center for Health Statistics. Third National Health and Nutrition Examination Survey, 1988–94. Public Use Data File No. 7–0627. Hyattsville MD: CDC, 1997.)

criterion for a case of incident periodontitis because this level is outside the change that could reasonably be attributed to error by a trained, experienced examiner.[21]

Incidence of Periodontitis

Longitudinal studies of periodontitis onset and progression in community-dwelling populations are inherently expensive and difficult, so it is not surprising that only a few have been conducted. One important study is the Piedmont project in North Carolina, so named for the 5-county geographic region in which a community-dwelling sample (i.e., neither institutionalized nor taken from patient lists at a dental school) aged 65 to 80 years, mostly rural and of low income, received a series of periodontal examinations in their own homes over a 3-year period. Periodontal conditions in this group were generally not good. Although the mean number of affected sites at baseline was only a little more than that found in younger age groups, the severity of disease in those sites was considerably greater.[22] Tobacco use and the presence of specific bacteria were risk indicators for severe disease in both African-

Americans and whites. When disease incidence (defined as an increase in LPA of at least 3 mm) was assessed for the first 18 months and for the second 18 months separately, LPA during the first period was positively related to LPA in the second period at the person level, but not at the site level.[20] This finding supports the episodic, randomized model of periodontitis in susceptible persons. At the mesiobuccal sites examined, most disease incidence came from increased pocket depth rather than from gingival recession, whereas for buccal sites, most incidence came from gingival recession.[19] Also, over the 3 years of observation, 41% of the participants had no change in baseline attachment levels, 27% recorded only new lesions (i.e., lesions in sites that were scored as healthy at baseline), 11% only had progression in existing lesions, and 20% had both. The research team found that risk factors (related to new disease) were not the same as the *prognostic factors* (their term for risk factors related to the progression of existing disease). However, factors common to both groups were low income, tobacco use, and taking medications likely to result in soft tissue reactions.[19] The authors suggest that different disease processes may be at work here.

A longitudinal project of major importance was the 15-year study of periodontitis among 480 tea workers in Sri Lanka.[93] The group studied had virtually no dental treatment of the type found in developed countries, so the data reflected the natural history of periodontitis. Based on tooth loss and interproximal attachment levels, it was concluded that some 8% demonstrated rapid progression, 81% moderate progression, and 11% no progression beyond gingivitis. This study provided important evidence for demonstrating the range of susceptibility to periodontitis. Subsequent findings on disease incidence in this group were that gingival recession over time progressed on virtually all surfaces, whereas in a comparison group of upper-socioeconomic status (SES) Norwegians, it was largely confined to the buccal surfaces. The buccal-only recession was thought to come from toothbrush abrasion, whereas the all-surfaces recession among the Sri Lankans was seen as plaque-related.[92]

Clinical studies that have followed groups of patients over time have contributed valuable information toward our understanding of periodontitis.[55, 63, 89] These should not be called epidemiologic studies, for when only a group of patients is followed then all participants, by definition, are susceptible to the disease. Whereas epidemiology is better at defining risk factors, clinical studies are valuable for studying disease progression in susceptible subjects.

DEMOGRAPHIC RISK FACTORS IN PERIODONTITIS

Gender and Race

Surveys of periodontal conditions usually show that men have poorer periodontal health than women. This has long been observed, and is still the case in the most recent national survey in the United States. Figure 20–1 (and later in Figures 20–7 and 20–9) shows that in measures of LPA and the presence of pockets and subgingival calculus, women consistently look better than men. In older surveys[167, 169] this finding was obscured by the greater extent of tooth loss among women, tooth loss assumed to reflect the ravages of periodontal disease. The differences in tooth loss between the sexes are no longer evident (Chapter 18). Women usually exhibit better oral hygiene than do men,[170] which

would explain the differences seen with gingivitis. Current knowledge of the pathogenesis of periodontitis, when added to the epidemiologic evidence, is that there are no inherent differences between men and women in susceptibility to periodontitis.

There is little evidence to suggest different susceptibility to periodontitis among different races, although the emergence of genetic research is likely to provide conclusive answers to this issue. Early epidemiologic studies showed considerable differences between nations,[133, 143] but no consistent relationships with race or ethnicity when persons of the same age and oral hygiene status were compared. Reviews presented at World Workshops on Periodontics in 1966[173] and 1977[37] also found no differences in disease prevalence that could be attributed to race or ethnicity, and that view essentially still prevails.[9] On the other hand, an analysis of data from the 1986–1987 national survey of schoolchildren found the prevalence of early-onset periodontitis in 13–17 year-olds to be 10.0% among African-Americans, 5.0% among Hispanics, and only 1.3% among whites.[3] Early-onset periodontitis was defined as at least one site with LPA of at least 3 mm.

Figure 20–6 shows the prevalence of severe periodontitis among four racial/ethnic groups in the United States in the NHANES III survey of 1988–1994. Data are not consistent from one age group to another, except that prevalence is higher at all ages among African-Americans, and these are likely to be associated with SES differences rather than true racial differences. The WHO Global Oral Data Bank, which maintains data from many nations collected by the Community Periodontal Index of Treatment Needs (CPITN) index, suggests a rather remarkable uniformity of conditions around the world.[130, 131] Overall, the evidence suggests that race and ethnicity in themselves cannot be considered demographic risk factors for periodontitis.

Age

The relationship between age and periodontitis is not always easy to understand. Much of the problem dates back to the older perception of the disease, in which the interpretation of cross-sectional survey data was generally that the severity of the disease increased with advancing age. However, today we consider that periodontitis is not a disease of aging. The greater prevalence and severity of LPA in older people in cross-sectional surveys do not come from greater susceptibility of older people but to the cumulative progression of lesions over time.[31]

Figure 20–2 shows the distribution of sites by degree of LPA among adults in the NHANES III survey in United States during 1988–1994. These cross-sectional data show that there is a linear relationship between age and the proportion of people with at least one site with 4 or 6 mm LPA. By contrast, the proportion of people with at least one site with 2 mm LPA rises rapidly with age and then tends to flatten out at a high level. This suggests that people who get only this low level of periodontitis get it early in life, and as discussed previously, it is too common to be of value in discriminating between disease and nondisease.

Figure 20–7 shows that the relationship between age and the presence of at least one pocket of 4 mm or more is not as direct as that found with LPA. If pockets are taken to reflect active disease (as opposed to LPA being a "scar" of past disease), this weak relationship with age is not surprising.

Age-related findings were a feature of the Sri Lankan studies described previously.[93] Earlier reports from these researchers compared the Sri Lankans with a group of college students and professors in Oslo, Norway, a high-SES, dentally aware group with high utilization of dental care.[6, 94, 95] The oral hygiene status of the Oslo group was excellent, with no increase in the prevalence and severity of gingivitis from the late teenage years to approximately 40 years of age. Mean annual LPA in the Oslo group was 0.07 to 0.13 mm.

The Sri Lankan group was followed for 15 years. As described earlier, the members were categorized into 3 groups in terms of rate of disease progression: rapid, moderate, and little-to-none. In the first 2 groups, periodontitis progressed with age, although naturally much more rapidly in the first group, virtually all of whom had become edentulous by 40 to 45 years of age. In the moderate progression group, the annual mean rate of LPA increased from 0.3 mm, when the members were in their 20s, to 0.5 mm 15 years later. By contrast, annual LPA in the rapidly progressing group averaged 1.04 mm when they were aged 25 to 29. In the nonprogressing group, average annual LPA was approximately 0.05 mm and did not change with age.

Rather than an increased susceptibility to

periodontitis with increasing age, post-1980 epidemiology supports the view that those who retain their teeth into old age are likely to be the less susceptible. When periodontitis occurs in susceptible individuals, it is evident when they are young.[4, 7, 10, 11, 13, 34, 39, 40, 65, 67, 81, 93, 103, 178] Although none of these studies demonstrating moderate LPA in young people followed their subjects into later life, it is likely that at least some of this disease is early-onset periodontitis, and that these persons may be in that minority with severe, generalized periodontitis later in life. (Early-onset periodontitis cannot be separated from adult periodontitis in a survey examination.) They may also fit the compromised host disease model,[117] although without case-control studies or additional longitudinal data, this cannot be stated unequivocally. It would fit with the pattern of many diseases, however, if the persons most susceptible to severe periodontitis were those who exhibit the disease in their youth. (We are referring here to adult and early-onset periodontitis, not to the specific condition of localized juvenile periodontitis, which is thought to affect 0.1% to 0.2% of the adolescent population.)[172]

The likelihood that older, dentate people may be the less susceptible members of the population is strengthened by the findings that serious disease is not as common among such groups as once thought.[69] As shown in Figure 20–3, the distribution of people by their most severe LPA is skewed, and this skewed distribution is largely independent of age.[67] Other analyses of cross-sectional national survey data have challenged the view that age is a major determinant of periodontitis.[1, 32]

Even though there are indications from clinical studies that the aging periodontium does not tolerate plaque as well as it used to, that the nature of the plaque itself might change with age, and that the aging periodontium recovers from injury more slowly, these potential problems are overshadowed by the patient's susceptibility to disease.[171] This information further supports the idea that when a patient is susceptible to periodontitis, the tendency is seen early. Adult periodontitis in the elderly is characterized by infrequent and slow progression[122] and does not usually lead to tooth loss. Even where periodontitis is reported as a leading cause of tooth loss in the elderly (Chapter 18), it is likely that many of the teeth extracted then have been seri-

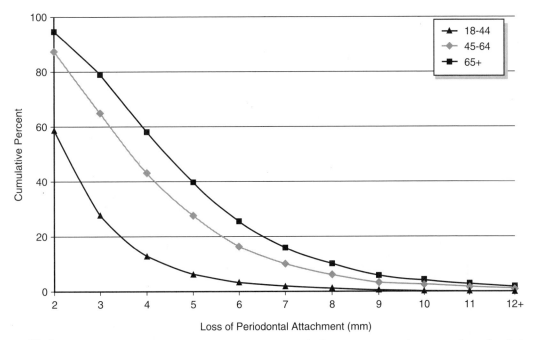

Figure 20–3. Proportion of adults, in age-groups 18–44, 45–64, and 65 or more years, whose worst loss of periodontal attachment site is stated level or greater. United States, 1988–94. (From US Department of Health and Human Services, National Center for Health Statistics. Third National Health and Nutrition Examination Survey, 1988–94. Public Use Data File No. 7–0627. Hyattsville MD: CDC, 1997.)

ously diseased for years rather than becoming that way in old age.

To summarize the data on age and periodontitis, cross-sectional survey data invariably show, on average, a greater extent of LPA among older than younger persons. Pockets and subgingival calculus have a less direct relationship with age in cross-sectional data, indicating that the apparent increase of LPA with age is more a lifetime accumulation of effects rather than greater susceptibility in the older years. Limited longitudinal data suggest that LPA increases rapidly with age among the 7% to 15% of any population susceptible to serious disease, and to a lesser extent among the majority that exhibits moderate disease. Those susceptible to serious disease exhibit LPA and bone loss when young, often in the teenage years.

Socioeconomic Status

Levels of periodontal disease, when recorded by composite indexes, have historically been related to lower SES.[167, 169] Gingivitis and poorer oral hygiene are clearly related to lower SES, but the relationship between periodontitis and SES is less direct. Figure 20–4 shows that there are obvious SES differences only among younger people when LPA

is 2 mm or more, but this is not a sensitive measure. When SES groups are compared by LPA of at least 6 mm (Fig. 20–5), a more consistent difference is seen, especially at younger ages. When the measure is the prevalence of pockets of at least 4 mm, Figure 20–8 also shows SES differences that are most pronounced among the young. Subgingival calculus is more prevalent among lower SES groups (Fig. 20–10).

The widely observed relation between SES levels and gingival health is a function of better oral hygiene among the more educated, and a greater frequency of dental visits among the more dentally aware and those with dental insurance (who are more likely to be white-collar employees, that is, those with more education). SES is a complex and multifaceted variable that can include a variety of cultural factors, and it is virtually impossible to remove the effect of SES as a confounder in the race/ethnicity relationships seen in Figure 20–6.

RISK FACTORS FOR PERIODONTITIS

Oral Hygiene, Plaque, and Microbiota

Like some other long-term beliefs in periodontal disease, the relationship between oral

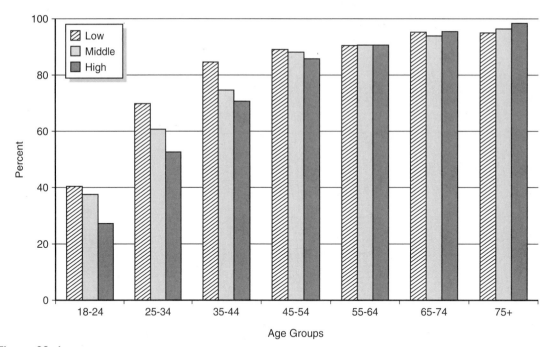

Figure 20–4. Proportion of adults with at least one site with loss of periodontal attachment (LPA) of 2 mm or more. By age and socioeconomic status, United States, 1988–94. (From US Department of Health and Human Services, National Center for Health Statistics. Third National Health and Nutrition Examination Survey, 1988–94. Public Use Data File No. 7–0627. Hyattsville MD: CDC, 1997.)

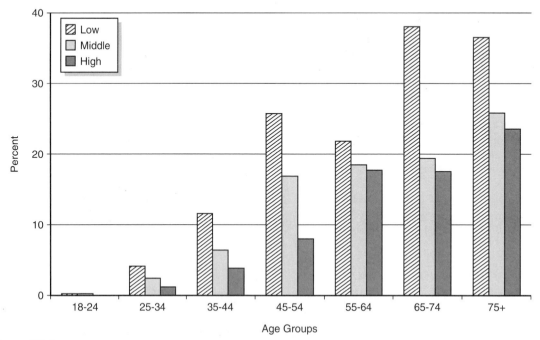

Figure 20–5. Proportion of adults with at least one site with loss of periodontal attachment (LPA) of 6 mm or more. By age and socioeconomic status, United States, 1988–94. (From US Department of Health and Human Services, National Center for Health Statistics. Third National Health and Nutrition Examination Survey, 1988–94. Public Use Data File No. 7–0627. Hyattsville MD: CDC, 1997.)

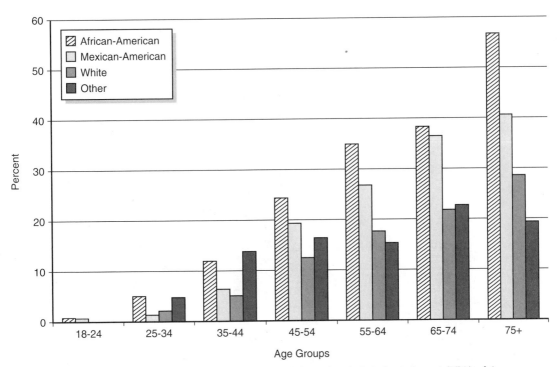

Figure 20–6. Proportion of adults with at least one site with loss of periodontal attachment (LPA) of 6 mm or more. By age and race/ethnicity, United States, 1988–94. (From US Department of Health and Human Services, National Center for Health Statistics. Third National Health and Nutrition Examination Survey, 1988–94. Public Use Data File No. 7–0627. Hyattsville MD: CDC, 1997.)

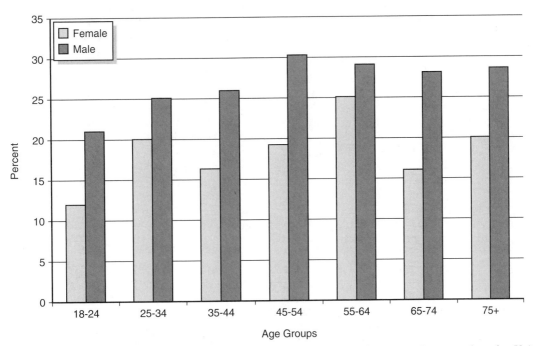

Figure 20–7. Proportion of adults with at least one periodontal pocket of 4 mm or more. By age and gender, United States, 1988–94. (From US Department of Health and Human Services, National Center for Health Statistics. Third National Health and Nutrition Examination Survey, 1988–94. Public Use Data File No. 7–0627. Hyattsville MD: CDC, 1997.)

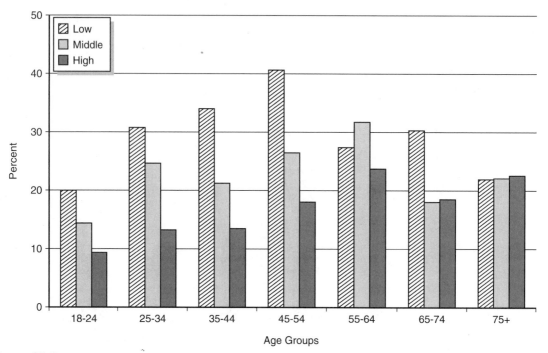

Figure 20–8. Proportion of adults with at least one periodontal pocket of 4 mm or more. By age and socioeconomic status, United States, 1988–94. (From US Department of Health and Human Services, National Center for Health Statistics. Third National Health and Nutrition Examination Survey, 1988–94. Public Use Data File No. 7–0627. Hyattsville MD: CDC, 1997.)

hygiene status and various manisfestations of periodontal diseases is not as straightforward as it once appeared to be. Periodontal conditions measured by the composite indexes in use before the 1980s invariably were more severe when accompanied by poor oral hygiene.[58, 99, 144, 148, 152, 153, 167, 169] However, we can now see that much of this association was dominated by the link between plaque deposits and gingivitis; the relationship between plaque deposits and periodontitis is less clear.

The classic studies in experimental human gingivitis, conducted in the mid-1960s,[96] showed the relation between plaque deposits and gingivitis to be one of cause and effect. Gingivitis is a nonspecific infection caused by bacteria found in supragingival plaque.[124] In the economically developed countries where oral hygiene is of high cultural value, there is less gingivitis than in poorer societies where oral hygiene practices are not a normal part of the daily routine. There is also less calculus, both supragingival and subgingival, as a result of better oral hygiene and more professional dental care. As well as the intercountry differences,[130, 131] these patterns are also evident between the genders and socioeconomic strata within the United States, as seen in

Figures 20–9 and 20–10, although it can be seen that subgingival calculus is quite prevalent even among higher-SES American adults.

In view of our current knowledge of the infections that characterize periodontitis, subgingival plaque may be a necessary cause of periodontitis.[35] However, plaque and calculus deposits correlate poorly with severe periodontitis in population studies.[10, 11, 13, 45, 71, 83, 92, 93, 105, 119] It is also possible that subgingival calculus is a result of periodontitis rather than a cause, which would make it a marker for periodontitis.[12] These studies in populations with poor oral hygiene and little dental treatment suggest that, although gingivitis and calculus are more severe,[5] the prevalence and severity of periodontitis are not that different from conditions in developed nations.[9, 59, 130, 131]

Quantity of plaque accumulation has also been shown to be only weakly correlated with periodontitis.[8, 60, 61, 63, 85, 102, 129] This does not mean that oral hygiene is not an important factor in periodontitis, for periodontal infections are clearly part of the disease etiology. Cross-sectional associations between putative periodontopathogens and clinical periodontitis have been reported,[23, 158] although

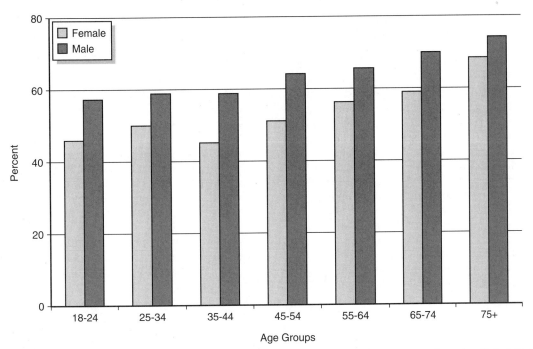

Figure 20–9. Proportion of adults with at least one site with subgingival calculus. By age and gender, United States, 1988–94. (From US Department of Health and Human Services, National Center for Health Statistics. Third National Health and Nutrition Examination Survey, 1988–94. Public Use Data File No. 7–0627. Hyattsville MD: CDC, 1997.)

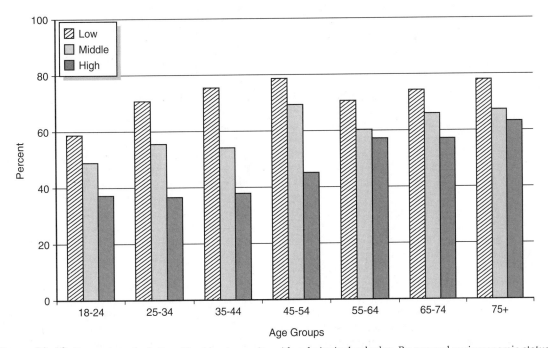

Figure 20–10. Proportion of adults with at least one site with subgingival calculus. By age and socioeconomic status, United States, 1988–94. (From US Department of Health and Human Services, National Center for Health Statistics. Third National Health and Nutrition Examination Survey, 1988–94. Public Use Data File No. 7–0627. Hyattsville MD: CDC, 1997.)

the ability of microbial counts to predict future attachment loss has been limited.[87, 89, 174] However, these findings do suggest that for those who are not susceptible to severe disease, the deposits of plaque and calculus will not by themselves induce severe disease.

Among patients who are being maintained after receiving treatment for periodontitis, some clinicians see the role of plaque control as vital to the maintenance of periodontal health.[25, 140] Although other authorities are less stringent on the importance of oral hygiene at this time,[135] and some data to support the contention are inconsistent,[25] no one suggests that periodontitis patients should not do all they reasonably can to maintain excellent oral hygiene. This line of thinking is not inconsistent with the epidemiologic data, because periodontal patients, by definition, are disease-susceptible individuals. The etiologic role of oral hygiene in periodontitis might be similar to that of sugar in dental caries (Chapter 19): a sensitive etiologic factor among susceptible persons, less so among the less susceptible.

Local Factors

Gingival overhangs make the maintenance of periodontal health difficult because cleaning under them is difficult, and the growth of pathogenic flora can therefore be encouraged.[80] Although gingival overhangs are common,[30] they are not associated with serious periodontitis, at least in young people.[84] Local factors of this nature are generally considered to be of minor importance in the etiology of periodontitis when compared to the nature of the infection and the host response.[123]

Nutrition

Despite the centuries-old observation that sailors suffering from scurvy (severe deficiency of ascorbic acid, or vitamin C) had bleeding gums, no nutritional or dietary factors have been shown to be directly related to the prevalence or intensity of periodontitis. The possibility that generalized malnutrition may influence its severity, however, cannot be ignored.[33, 145] In the well-fed societies of the developed world, generalized malnutrition is not a public health problem, although it can be found in some individuals with eating disorders. Ascorbic acid is probably the nutrient most often thought to be a factor, but has

been shown to be associated with periodontitis only at the lowest levels of intake, 25% or less of the Recommended Dietary Allowance for the United States.[73]

A series of worldwide epidemiologic studies in the 1960s found only thin evidence for a relationship between periodontal disease and poor nutrition, although they used the PI index and lacked rigor in their measurement of nutritional deficiencies.[141] These studies were important at the time, but their relevance today is questionable. Subsequent studies suggest that there may be a relationship between more extensive gingival bleeding and ascorbic acid deficiency,[74, 82] but whether such a mechanism relates to bone loss or LPA is not known. Nutritional adequacy is of course a precondition for successful treatment of virtually any disease, but there is no evidence to support the use of ascorbic acid, or any other nutrient, in the treatment of periodontitis.

Tobacco Use

An analysis of data from the 1971–1975 National Health and Nutrition Examination Survey in the United States (NHANES I) showed a clear association between smoking and periodontal diseases, independent of oral hygiene, age, or any other factor.[72] The evidence to identify smoking as a risk factor for periodontitis has continued to mount since then,[26, 60, 61, 90] and assessments of randomly-chosen patient groupings invariably show a higher prevalence of periodontitis among smokers.[62, 66, 76]

Experimental studies have shown no difference between smokers and nonsmokers in amounts of plaque accumulation,[47, 62] or prevalence of the principal bacteria considered pathogenic for periodontitis.[132, 160] Rather than affecting the expression of periodontitis through oral hygiene or microbiota, smoking is thought to suppress the vascular reaction that follows gingivitis. In experimental plaque-induced gingivitis, despite the rate of plaque accumulation being equal in smokers and nonsmokers, the increase in gingival vascularity in smokers was only half that seen in the nonsmokers.[27] In effect, this is a masking effect on the signs of inflammation.[28] This finding might explain the results of the one epidemiologic study in which smoking was not associated with periodontal diseases.[104] In this study of a representative sample of the Finnish population, the periodontal assessment was through the Periodontal Treatment Need System (PTNS) index (Chapter 15), which weights gingival inflammation and plaque deposits. The effect of smoking in suppressing the signs of gingival inflammation could have led to the negative findings.

There is also some evidence that smoking is associated with osteoporosis; its role in alveolar bone loss is still being investigated.[75] A study of denture requirements among postmenopausal women found that twice as many smokers as nonsmokers required dentures after age 50, and that the lowest need was among nonosteoporotic nonsmokers.[46] Smoking may also be a factor in the association between refractory periodontitis and a polymorphonuclear (PMN) leukocyte defect in the peripheral blood.[100] The risk of periodontitis attributable to tobacco, compared to its nonuse, is in the order of 2.5 to 6.0 or even higher.[28] The collective evidence clearly shows that smoking is a major risk factor for periodontitis.

PERIODONTITIS AND SYSTEMIC CONDITIONS

Systemic predisposition to periodontitis is associated with unusual syndromes associated with PMN defects (e.g., Chediak-Higashi syndrome), Down syndrome, Papillon-Lefévre syndrome, and the rare condition of Ehlers-Danlos syndrome.[35, 175] Adverse pregnancy outcomes have been associated with periodontitis,[118] and so has bacterial pneumonia.[149] The principal conditions associated with periodontitis, however, are diabetes, human immunodeficiency virus (HIV) infection, and cardiovascular diseases.

Diabetes

Both type 1 (insulin-dependent diabetes mellitus, or IDDM, formerly referred to as early-onset diabetes) and type 2 diabetes (non-insulin-dependent diabetes mellitus, NIDDM, formerly referred to as adult-onset diabetes) are risk factors for periodontitis. Younger adult patients with IDDM, especially those in whom the disease is of long duration, have more gingivitis and more deep pockets than nondiabetics.[48, 52, 68, 147] Among patients of similar age with long-duration IDDM and similar plaque levels, those with poorer metabolic control had greater LPA and alveolar bone loss than did those with better con-

trol.[146, 150, 151] Periodontitis also progresses more rapidly in poorly controlled diabetics,[151] and early age of onset of diabetes is a risk factor for more severe disease.[164] Poorly controlled diabetics also exhibit higher levels of the enzyme β-glucuronidase in their gingival crevicular fluid than do well-controlled patients.[121]

The most extensive periodontitis studies among NIDDM patients have been with the Gila River community in Arizona, a group among whom NIDDM prevalence is unusually high. NIDDM patients had substantially greater LPA, loss of alveolar bone, and tooth loss.[114, 154] When age, sex, and oral hygiene are statistically accounted for, the increased risk of developing destructive periodontitis as a result of NIDDM was 2.81 for LPA and 3.43 for bone loss.[51] These degrees of risk are similar to the odds ratio of 2.32 for severe LPA in diabetics (variety not specified) compared to nondiabetics in an adult population in upstate New York.[61] Metabolic control is a prime factor in maintaining periodontal health among NIDDM patients,[2, 36, 121] and there is evidence for the converse, namely that severe periodontitis may adversely affect medical treatment aimed at diabetic control.[162]

A study of quantitative and qualitative aspects of microflora in both type 1 and type 2 diabetics revealed no notable differences between diabetics and nondiabetics.[163] Tests of subgingival plaque samples from participants in the Gila River studies suggest that diabetics react differently to the putative pathogens than do nondiabetics, although the significance of these findings is uncertain.[182] Other suggested mechanisms by which diabetes may contribute to periodontitis include vascular changes, PMN dysfunction, abnormal collagen synthesis, and genetic predisposition.[44, 77, 120] Although the mechanism by which diabetes exacerbates periodontal destruction is still not fully understood, diabetes is clearly a risk factor for periodontitis. Poor diabetic control exacerbates the risk even further.

HIV Infection

Many studies on HIV infection and periodontitis have not been rigorously designed,[139] and as a result the role of HIV infection as a risk factor for periodontitis is not clear. Initial research was limited to cross-sectional studies of convenience samples of homosexual men.[176, 177] The microbiology of periodontitis in HIV-infected persons, relative to those not infected, is not clear, for both little difference[112, 113, 136] and significant differences[110] have been reported. Reports on the occurrence of yeasts in subgingival flora of HIV-positive patients are inconsistent.[110, 183]

Some clinical studies of the periodontal conditions of persons with HIV infection are only descriptive studies of groups of patients without controls.[79, 138] Several studies have examined the periodontal condition of patients taking part in clinical trials for the drug zidovudine (AZT). One found the periodontal health of patients in the early stages of HIV disease to be generally good,[50] but a longitudinal study of 30 HIV-infected patients found a greater progression of periodontitis over 18 months in this group in comparison to 10 HIV-negative controls.[180] In neither study, however, was there analysis of periodontal diseases in the AZT patients compared to the others.

In a follow-up of 114 homosexual or bisexual men conducted over 20 months, periodontal changes were related to HIV-1 serostatus, immune status, age, and plaque deposits. The risk of LPA of 3 mm or more over the 20 months was 6.16 times higher in the more immunosuppressed patients (CD4 + counts <200) than in the less immunosuppressed patients, and this finding was more pronounced in older subjects.[17] Seropositive patients showed a more sensitive reaction to plaque than did the seronegative patients. This well-conducted study concluded that immunosuppression, especially in combination with older age, was a risk factor for progression of LPA, and that seropositivity, independent of immune status, was a risk factor for gingivitis.

In a cross-sectional study of 230 HIV-infected military personnel, however, the relation between periodontal health and immune status was less clear.[161] A detailed follow-up on 474 patients from the same population, aged 18 to 49 and 85% male, found LPA of 5 mm or more in 20% of the patients. In this group, neither the clinical stage of the disease nor the CD4 + counts were good independent predictors of severe LPA when other significantly associated variables (e.g., tobacco use) were accounted for.[165]

The overall picture of periodontal conditions in HIV + persons is thus best described as unclear. With improved treatment for HIV, and with the HIV + population continuing to expand, further well-controlled research in this group is sorely needed.

Cardiovascular Diseases

The possibility that periodontal infections could be a risk factor for cardiovascular diseases is intriguing.[18, 24] One study analyzed clinical periodontal data from the NHANES I survey of 1971–1975 and matched it with cardiovascular data obtained from death certificates, personal interviews, and records from hospitals and nursing homes. The report concluded that persons with periodontitis at baseline had 1.25 times the risk of subsequent coronary heart disease than did those without periodontitis.[49] The relative risk was strongest (1.72) for men under age 50 at baseline. While thought-provoking, this evidence by itself is not conclusive because periodontal conditions were measured by the now-defunct Periodontal Index, and periodontal conditions were measured only once (at baseline). This analysis also found that periodontitis and poor oral hygiene were more strongly associated with total mortality than with coronary heart disease, which could indicate that neglect of oral health is more an indicator of poor health practices in general than a causal factor.

Associations of varying strength between cardiovascular disease and periodontitis have been reported from different populations.[97, 115, 156, 159] Evidence for a causal link, however, can be found in an animal study in which rats with both catheter-induced aortic valve vegetations and periodontitis were subjected to tooth extractions. A subsequent bacteremia was observed, and 3 days later 90% of the rats had endocarditis.[111]

Infections that characterize periodontitis have been associated with a variety of systemic conditions;[106] *Actinobacillus actinomycetemcomitans* in particular has been involved with endocarditis and brain abscesses.[181] It has been suggested that specific properties of bacteria, such as ability to adhere to damaged heart valves, might be more important than simply the numbers that enter the bloodstream in a bacterial shower.[14]

It is interesting to reflect that what is being discussed here is essentially the "focal infection" issue, first raised in 1911,[70] which subsequently became the underlying rationale for mass extractions over subsequent decades. The focal infection theory faded in the 1950s, and now may be reemerging. Research with regard to the link between periodontitis and heart disease continues.

PREDICTING PERIODONTITIS

When everyone was thought to be equally susceptible to periodontitis, there was little need for methods of predicting the circumstances under which future disease would occur. The realization that periodontitis is found in a skewed distribution and that only 7% to 15% of the population is affected by serious periodontitis led to different imperatives. How can we identify this susceptible minority? What characterizes these people relative to those who have moderate or no periodontitis? What tests can a practitioner carry out that will allow these individuals to be identified before the disease has progressed? The situation is not all that different from that described for caries (Chapter 19), where the caries decline prompted research to permit identification of susceptible individuals.

Research on predictive methods has often been mixed with attempts to discern markers of active disease. Clinical parameters such as plaque, calculus, and gingival bleeding have proved to be poor predictors of disease activity in longitudinal clinical studies,[38, 64] and research into markers of disease activity now is focusing on inflammatory mediators.[117] It is not surprising, in view of the pathogenesis of periodontitis, that gingivitis failed to predict periodontitis in another 3-year clinical study.[88] Increase in probing pocket depth, over a period of years, has predicted LPA better than other clinical parameters,[8, 38] and LPA of 4 mm or more is highly predictive of subsequent bone loss.[55]

Microbiologic research has sought to identify infections that might predict the subsequent development of clinical periodontitis, although with only modest success.[87, 89, 174] Within the general profile of gram-negative anerobes and spirochetes being the principal periodontopathogens, however, the research is complicated because of the long list of bacteria associated with periodontitis.[123] Presumptive evidence is mounting, however, that three organisms in particular are likely to be major pathogens: *Actinobacillus acetomycetemcomitans*, *Porphyromonas gingivalis*, and *Prevotella intermedia*. In a series of studies of 196 adults with advanced disease in 405 sites, only one lesion failed to show the presence of at least one of these three.[155] In another study of LPA in adolescents, the greatest odds for the presence of LPA was associated with the presence of *P. intermedia* together with subgingival calculus and gingival bleeding.[34] However, these organisms are not the only periodontal pathogens. The presence of specific organisms has not been shown to predict the subsequent development of disease with any high probability, although it seems likely that infection with one or more of these bacteria is a necessary condition for the development of periodontitis.

REFERENCES

1. Abdellatif HM, Burt BA. An epidemiological investigation into the relative importance of age and oral hygiene status as determinants of periodontitis. J Dent Res 1987;66:13–8.
2. Ainamo J, Lahtinen A, Uitto VJ. Rapid periodontal destruction in adult humans with poorly controlled diabetes. A report of 2 cases. J Clin Periodontol 1990;17:22–8.
3. Albandar JM, Brown LJ, Löe H. Clinical features of early-onset periodontitis. J Am Dent Assoc 1997;128:1393–9.
4. Al-Kufaishi KA, Hirschmann PN, Lennon MA. The radiographic assessment of early periodontal bone loss in adolescents. Br Dent J 1984;157:91–3.
5. Ånerud A, Löe H, Boysen H. The natural history and clinical course of calculus formation in man. J Clin Periodontol 1991;18:160–70.
6. Ånerud A, Löe H, Boysen H, Smith M. The natural history of periodontal disease in man: Changes in gingival health and oral hygiene before 40 years of age. J Periodont Res 1979;14:526–40.
7. Ånerud KE, Robertson PB, Löe H, et al. Periodontal disease in three young adult populations. J Periodont Res 1983;18:655–68.
8. Badersten A, Nilveus R, Egelberg J. Scores of plaque, bleeding, suppuration and probing depth to predict probing attachment loss. Five years of observation following nonsurgical periodontal therapy. J Clin Periodontol 1990;17:102–7.
9. Baelum V, Chen X, Manji F, et al. Profiles of destructive periodontal disease in different populations. J Perio Res 1996;31:17–26.
10. Baelum V, Fejerskov O, Karring T. Oral hygiene, gingivitis, and periodontal breakdown in adult Tanzanians. J Periodont Res 1986;21:221–32.
11. Baelum V, Fejerskov O, Manji F. Periodontal diseases in adult Kenyans. J Clin Periodontol 1988;15:445–52.
12. Baelum V, Luan W-M, Chen X, Fejerskov O. Predictors of destructive periodontal disease incidence and progression in adult and elderly Chinese. Community Dent Oral Epidemiol 1997;25:265–72.
13. Baelum V, Luan W-M, Fejerskov O, Xia C. Tooth mortality and periodontal conditions in 60–80-year-old Chinese. Scand J Dent Res 1988;96:99–107.
14. Barco CT. Prevention of infectious endocarditis: A review of the medical and dental literature. J Periodontol 1991;62:510–23.

15. Barmes DE. Epidemiology of dental disease. J Clin Periodontol 1977;4:80–93.

16. Barmes DE, Leous PA. Assessment of periodontal status by CPITN and its applicability to the development of long-term goals on periodontal health of the population. Int Dent J 1986;36:177–81.

17. Barr C, Lopez MR, Rua-Dobles A. Periodontal changes by HIV serostatus in a cohort of homosexual and bisexual men. J Clin Periodontol 1992;19:794–801.

18. Beck JD, Garcia R, Heiss G, et al. Periodontal disease and cardiovascular disease. J Periodontol 1996;67(Suppl):1123–37.

19. Beck JD, Koch GG. Characteristics of older adults experiencing periodontal attachment loss as gingival recession or probing depth. J Periodontol Res 1994;29:290–8.

20. Beck JD, Koch GG, Offenbacher S. Attachment loss trends over 3 years in community-dwelling older adults. J Periodontol 1994;65:737–43.

21. Beck JD, Koch GG, Offenbacher S. Incidence of attachment loss over 3 years in older adults—new and progressing lesions. Community Dent Oral Epidemiol 1995;23:291–6.

22. Beck JD, Koch GG, Rozier RG, Tudor GE. Prevalence and risk indicators for periodontal attachment loss in a population of older community-dwelling blacks and whites. J Periodontol 1990;61:521–8.

23. Beck JD, Koch GG, Zambon JJ, Tudor GE. Evaluation of oral bacteria as risk indicators for periodontitis in older adults. J Periodontol 1992;63:93–9.

24. Beck JD, Slade GD. Epidemiology of periodontal diseases. Curr Opin Periodontol 1996;3:3–9.

25. Becker W, Berg L, Becker BE. The long-term evaluation of periodontal treatment and maintenance in 95 patients. Int J Periodont Restor Dent 1984;4:54–71.

26. Bergstrom J, Floderus-Myrhed B. Co-twin control study of the relationship between smoking and some periodontal disease factors. Community Dent Oral Epidemiol 1983;11:113–6.

27. Bergstrom J, Persson L, Preber H. Influence of cigarette smoking on vascular reaction during experimental gingivitis. Scand J Dent Res 1988;96:34–9.

28. Bergstrom J, Preber H. Tobacco use as a risk factor. J Periodontol 1994;65:545–50.

29. Bhat M. Periodontal health of 14–17 year-old US schoolchildren. J Public Health Dent 1991;51:5–11.

30. Brunsvold MA, Lane JJ. The prevalence of overhanging dental restorations and their relationship to periodontal disease. J Clin Periodontol 1990; 17:67–72.

31. Burt BA. Periodontitis and aging: Reviewing recent evidence. J Am Dent Assoc 1994;125:273–9.

32. Burt BA, Ismail AI, Eklund SA. Periodontal disease, tooth loss, and oral hygiene among older Americans. Community Dent Oral Epidemiol 1985;13:93–6.

33. Carlos JP, Wolfe MD. Methodological and nutritional issues in assessing the oral health of aged subjects. Am J Clin Nutr 1989;50:1210–8.

34. Carlos JP, Wolfe MD, Zambon JJ, Kingman A. Periodontal disease in adolescents: Some clinical and microbiologic correlates of attachment loss. J Dent Res 1988;67:1510–4.

35. Caton J. Periodontal diagnosis and diagnostic aids. In: Nevins M, Becker W, Kornman K, eds: Proceedings of the World Workshop in Clinical Periodontics. Chicago: American Academy of Periodontology, 1990:11–21.

36. Cherry-Peppers G, Ship JA. Oral health in patients with type II diabetes and impaired glucose tolerance. Diabetes Care 1993;16:638–41.

37. Chilton NW, Miller MF. Epidemiology. In: International Conference on Research in the Biology of Periodontal Disease. Chicago: University of Illinois School of Dentistry, 1977:119–43.

38. Claffey N, Nylund K, Kiger R, et al. Diagnostic predictability of scores of plaque, bleeding, suppuration and probing depth for probing attachment loss. 3½ years of observation following initial periodontal therapy. J Clin Periodontol 1990;17:108–14.

39. Clerehugh V, Lennon MA. The radiographic measurement of early periodontal bone loss and its relationship with loss of attachment. Br Dent J 1986;161:141–4.

40. Clerehugh V, Lennon MA. A two-year longitudinal study of early periodontitis in 14- to 16-year-old schoolchildren. Community Dent Health 1986;3:135–41.

41. Consensus report, discussion session 1. In: Nevins M, Becker W, Kornman K, eds: Proceedings of the World Workshop in Clinical Periodontics. Chicago: American Academy of Periodontology, 1990:123–31.

42. Consensus report. Periodontal diseases: Pathogenesis and microbial factors. Ann Periodontol 1996;1:926–32.

43. Consensus report. Periodontal diseases: Epidemiology and diagnosis. Ann Periodontol 1996;1:216–22.

44. Cutler CW, Eke P, Arnold RR, Van Dyke TE. Defective neutrophil function in an insulin dependent diabetes mellitus patient. A case report. J Periodontol 1991;62:394–401.

45. Cutress TW, Powell RN, Ball ME. Differing profiles of periodontal disease in two similar South Pacific island populations. Community Dent Oral Epidemiol 1982;10:193–203.

46. Daniell HW. Postmenopausal tooth loss. Contributions to edentulism by osteoporosis and cigarette smoking. Arch Intern Med 1983;143:1678–82.

47. Danielsen B, Manji F, Nagelkerke N, et al. Effect of cigarette smoking on the transition dynamics in experimental gingivitis. J Clin Periodontol 1990;17:159–64.

48. de Pommereau V, Dargent-Pare C, Robert JJ, Brion M. Periodontal status in insulin-dependent diabetic adolescents. J Clin Periodontol 1992;19:628–32.

49. DeStefano F, Anda RF, Kahn HS, et al. Dental disease and risk of coronary heart disease and mortality. Br Med J 1993;306:688–91.

50. Drinkard CR, Decher L, Little JW, et al. Periodontal status of individuals in early stages of human immunodeficiency virus infection. Community Dent Oral Epidemiol 1991;19:281–5.

51. Emrich LJ, Shlossman M, Genco RJ. Periodontal disease in non-insulin-dependent diabetes mellitus. J Periodontol 1991;62:123–31.

52. Galea H, Aganovic I, Aganovic M. The dental caries and periodontal disease experience of patients with early onset insulin dependent diabetes. Int Dent J 1986;36:219–24.

53. Genco RJ. Classification and clinical and radiographic features of periodontal disease. In: Genco RJ, Goldman HM, Cohen DW, eds: Contemporary periodontics. St. Louis: Mosby, 1990:63–81.

54. Genco RJ, Slots J. Host responses in periodontal diseases. J Dent Res 1984;63:441–51.

55. Goodson JM, Haffajee AD, Socransky SS. The relationship between attachment level loss and alveolar bone loss. J Clin Periodontol 1984;11:348–59.

56. Goodson JM. Selection of suitable indicators of periodontitis. In: Bader JD, ed: Risk assessment in dentistry. Chapel Hill: University of North Carolina, 1990:69–74.

57. Goodson JM, Tanner ACM, Haffajee AD, et al. Patterns of progression and regression of advanced destructive periodontal disease. J Clin Periodontol 1982;9:472–81.

58. Greene JC. Oral hygiene and periodontal disease. Am J Public Health 1963;53:913–22.

59. Griffiths GS, Wilton JM, Curtis MA, et al. Detection of high-risk groups and individuals for periodontal diseases. Clinical assessment of the periodontium. J Clin Periodontol 1988;15:403–10.

60. Grossi SG, Genco RJ, Machtei EE, et al. Assessment of risk for periodontal disease. II. Risk indicators for alveolar bone loss. J Periodontol 1995;66:23–9.

61. Grossi SG, Zambon JJ, Ho AW, et al. Assessment of risk for periodontal disease. I. Risk indicators for attachment loss. J Periodontol 1994;65:260–7.

62. Haber J, Wattles J, Crowley M, et al. Evidence for cigarette smoking as a major risk factor for periodontitis. J Periodontol 1993;64:16–23.

63. Haffajee AD, Socransky SS, Dzink JL, et al. Clinical, microbiological and immunological features of subjects with destructive periodontal diseases. J Clin Periodontol 1988;15:240–6.

64. Haffajee AD, Socransky SS, Goodson JM. Clinical parameters as predictors of destructive disease activity. J Clin Periodontol 1983;10:257–65.

65. Hoover JN, Ellegaard B, Attstrom R. Radiographic and clinical examination of periodontal status of first molars in 15–16 year-old Danish schoolchildren. Scand J Dent Res 1981;89:260–3.

66. Horning GM, Hatch CL, Cohen ME. Risk indicators for periodontitis in a military treatment population. J Periodontol 1992;63:297–302.

67. Hugoson A, Jordan T. Frequency distribution of individuals aged 20–70 years according to severity of periodontal disease. Community Dent Oral Epidemiol 1982;10:187–92.

68. Hugoson A, Thorstensson H, Falk H, Kuylenstierna J. Periodontal conditions in insulin-dependent diabetics. J Clin Periodontol 1989;16:215–23.

69. Hunt RJ, Levy SM, Beck JD. The prevalence of periodontal attachment loss in an Iowa population aged 70 and older. J Public Health Dent 1990;50:251–6.

70. Hunter W. The role of sepsis and antisepsis in medicine. Lancet 1911 Jan 14;79–86.

71. Ismail AI, Burt BA, Brunelle JA. Prevalence of total tooth loss, dental caries, and periodontal disease in Mexican-American adults: results from the Southwestern HHANES. J Dent Res 1987;66:1183–8.

72. Ismail AI, Burt BA, Eklund SA. Epidemiologic patterns of smoking and periodontal disease in the United States. J Am Dent Assoc 1983;106:617–21.

73. Ismail AI, Burt BA, Eklund SA. Relation between ascorbic acid intake and periodontal disease in the United States. J Am Dent Assoc 1983;107:927–31.

74. Jacob RA, Omaye ST, Skala JH, et al. Experimental vitamin C depletion and supplementation in young men. Nutrient interactions and dental health effects. Ann NY Acad Sci 1987;498:333–46.

75. Jeffcoat MK, Chesnut CH III. Systemic osteoporosis and oral bone loss: Evidence shows increased risk factors. J Am Dent Assoc 1993;124:49–56.

76. Jette AM, Feldman HA, Tennstedt SL. Tobacco use: A modifiable risk factor for dental disease among the elderly. Am J Public Health 1993;83:1271–6.

77. Katz PP, Wirthlin MR Jr, Szpunar SM, et al. Epidemiology and prevention of periodontal disease in individuals with diabetes. Diabetes Care 1991;14:375–85.

78. Klavan B, Genco R, Löe H, et al., eds: International conference on research in the biology of periodontal disease. Chicago: University of Illinois, 1977.

79. Klein RS, Quart AM, Small CB. Periodontal disease in heterosexuals with acquired immunodeficiency syndrome. J Periodontol 1991;62:535–40.

80. Lang NP, Kiel RA, Anderhalden A. Clinical and microbiological effects of subgingival restorations with overhanging or clinically perfect margins. J Clin Periodontol 1983;10:563–78.

81. Latcham NL, Powell RN, Jago JD, et al. A radiographic study of chronic periodontitis in 15-year-old Queensland children. J Clin Periodontol 1983;10:37–45.

82. Leggott PJ, Robertson PB, Rothman DL, et al. The effect of controlled ascorbic acid depletion and supplementation on periodontal health. J Periodontol 1986;57:480–5.

83. Lembariti BS, Frencken JE, Pilot T. Prevalence and severity of periodontal conditions among adults in urban and rural Morogoro, Tanzania. Community Dent Oral Epidemiol 1988;16:240–3.

84. Lervik T, Riordan PJ, Haugejorden O. Periodontal disease and approximal overhangs on amalgam restorations in Norwegian 21-year-olds. Community Dent Oral Epidemiol 1984;12:264–8.

85. Lindhe J, Okamoto H, Yoneyama T, et al. Longitudinal changes in periodontal disease in untreated subjects. J Clin Periodontol 1989;16:662–70.

86. Listgarten MA. Pathogenesis of periodontitis. J Clin Periodontol 1986;13:418–30.

87. Microbiological testing in the diagnosis of periodontal disease. J Periodontol 1992;63:332–7.

88. Listgarten MA, Schifter CC, Laster L. Three-year longitudinal study of the periodontal status of an adult population with gingivitis. J Clin Periodontol 1985;12:225–38.

89. Listgarten MA, Slots J, Nowotny AH, et al. Incidence of periodontitis recurrence in treated patients with and without cultivable *Actinobacillus actinomycetemcomitans*, *Prevotella intermedia*, and *Porphyromonas gingivalis*: A prospective study. J Periodontol 1991;62:377–86.

90. Locker D. Smoking and oral health in older adults. Can J Public Health 1992;83:429–32.

91. Locker D, Leake JL. Risk indicators and risk markers for periodontal disease experience in older adults living independently in Ontario, Canada. J Dent Res 1993;72:9–17.

92. Löe H, Ånerud A, Boysen H. The natural history of periodontal disease in man: prevalence, severity, and extent of gingival recession. J Periodontol 1992;63:489–95.

93. Löe H, Ånerud A, Boysen H, Morrison E. Natural history of periodontal disease in man: Rapid, moderate, and no loss of attachment in Sri Lankan laborers 14 to 46 years of age. J Clin Periodontol 1986;13:431–40.

94. Löe H, Ånerud A, Boysen H, Smith M. The natural history of periodontal disease in man. Study design and baseline data. J Periodont Res 1978;13:550–62.

95. Löe H, Ånerud A, Boysen H, Smith M. The natural history of periodontal disease in man: The rate of periodontal destruction before 40 years of age. J Periodontol 1978;49:607–20.

96. Löe H, Theilade E, Jensen SB. Experimental gingivitis in man. J Periodontol 1965;36:177–87.

97. Loesche WJ. Periodontal disease as a risk factor for heart disease. Compend Cont Educ 1994;25:976, 978–82, 985–6.

98. Loesche WJ, Syed SA, Schmidt E, Morrison EC. Bacterial profiles of subgingival plaques in periodontitis. J Periodontol 1985;56:447–56.

99. Lovdal A, Arno A, Waerhaug J. Incidence of clinical manifestation of periodontal disease in light of oral hygiene and calculus formation. J Am Dent Assoc 1958;56:21–33.

100. MacFarlane GD, Herzberg MC, Wolff LF, Hardie NA. Refractory periodontitis associated with abnormal polymorphonuclear leukocyte phagocytosis and cigarette smoking. J Periodontol 1992;63:908–13.

101. Machtei EE, Christenson LA, Grossi SG, et al. Clinical criteria for the definition of "established periodontitis." J Periodontol 1992;63:206–14.

102. Machtei EE, Christersson LA, Zambon JJ, et al. Alternative methods for screening periodontal disease in adults. J Clin Periodontol 1993;20:81–7.

103. Mann J, Cormier PP, Green P, et al. Loss of periodontal attachment in adolescents. Community Dent Oral Epidemiol 1981;9:135–41.

104. Markkanen H, Paunio I, Tuominen R, Rajala M. Smoking and periodontal disease in the Finnish population aged 30 years and over. J Dent Res 1985;64:932–5.

105. Matthesen M, Baelum V, Aarslev I, Fejerskov O. Dental health of children and adults in Guinea-Bissau, West Africa, in 1986. Community Dent Health 1990;7:123–33.

106. Mendieta C, Reeve CM. Periodontal manifestations of systemic disease and management of patients with systemic disease. Curr Opin Periodontol 1993;18–27.

107. Michalowicz BS, Aeppli DM, Virag JG, et al. Periodontal findings in adult twins. J Periodontol 1991;62:293–9.

108. Moore WJ, Corbett ME. The distribution of dental caries in ancient British populations. I. Anglo-Saxon period. Caries Res 1971;5:151–68.

109. Moore WJ, Corbett ME. The distribution of dental caries in ancient British populations. II. Iron Age, Romano-British and Mediaeval periods. Caries Res 1973;7:139–53.

110. Moore LV, Moore WE, Riley C, et al. Periodontal microflora of HIV-positive subjects with gingivitis or adult periodontitis. J Periodontol 1993;64:48–56.

111. Moreillon P, Overholser CD, Malinverni R, et al. Predictors of endocarditis in isolates from cultures of blood following dental extractions in rats with periodontal disease. J Infect Dis 1988;157:990–5.

112. Murray PA, Grassi M, Winkler JR. The microbiology of HIV-associated periodontal lesions. J Clin Periodontol 1989;16:636–42.

113. Murray PA, Winkler JR, Peros WJ, et al. DNA probe detection of periodontal pathogens in HIV-associated periodontal lesions. Oral Microbiol Immunol 1991;6:34–40.

114. Nelson RG, Shlossman M, Budding LM, et al. Periodontal disease and NIDDM in Pima Indians. Diabetes Care 1990;13:836–40.

115. Nery EB, Meister FJ, Ellinger RF, et al. Prevalence of medical problems in periodontal patients obtained from three different populations. J Periodontol 1987;58:564–8.

116. Nevins M, Becker W, Kornman K, eds: Proceedings of the World Workshop in Clinical Periodontics. Chicago: American Academy of Periodontology, 1990.

117. Offenbacher S, Collins JG, Yalda B, Haradon G. Role of prostaglandins in high-risk periodontitis patients. In: Genco RJ, Hamada S, Lehner T, et al., eds: Molecular pathogenesis of periodontal disease. Washington DC: American Society for Microbiology, 1994.

118. Offenbacher S, Katz V, Fertik G, et al. Periodontal infection as a possible risk factor for preterm low birth weight. J Periodontol 1996;67(Suppl):1103–13.

119. Okamoto H, Yoneyama T, Lindhe J, et al. Methods of evaluating periodontal disease data in epidemiological research. J Clin Periodontol 1988;15:430–9.

120. Oliver RC, Tervonen T. Diabetes—a risk factor for periodontitis in adults? J Periodontol 1994;65:530–8.

121. Oliver RC, Tervonen T, Flynn DG, Keenan KM. Enzyme activity in crevicular fluid in relation to metabolic control of diabetes and other periodontal risk factors. J Periodontol 1993;64:358–62.

122. Page RC. Periodontal diseases in the elderly: A critical evaluation of current information. Gerodontol 1984;3:63–70.

123. Page RC. Current understanding of the aetiology and progression of periodontal disease. Int Dent J 1986;36:153–61.

124. Page RC. Gingivitis. J Clin Periodontol 1986;13:345–59.

125. Page RC. The role of inflammatory mediators in the pathogenesis of periodontal disease. J Periodontol Res 1991;26(3 Pt 2):230–42.

126. Page RC. Host response tests for diagnosing periodontal diseases. J Periodontol 1992;63(Suppl 4):356–66.

127. Page RC. Critical issues in periodontal research. J Dent Res 1995;74:1118–28.

128. Page RC, Schroeder HE. Periodontitis in man and other animals: A comparative review. New York: Karger, 1982.

129. Peretz B, Machtei EE, Bimstein E. Changes in periodontal status of children and young adolescents: A one year longitudinal study. J Clin Pediatr Dent 1993;18:3–6.

130. Pilot T, Barmes DE, Leclercq MH, et al. Periodontal conditions in adults, 35–44 years of age: An overview of CPITN data in the WHO Global Oral Data Bank. Community Dent Oral Epidemiol 1986;14:310–2.

131. Pilot T, Barmes DE, Leclercq MH, et al. Periodontal conditions in adolescents, 15–19 years of age: An overview of CPITN data in the WHO Global Oral Data Bank. Community Dent Oral Epidemiol 1987;15:336–8.

132. Preber H, Bergstrom J, Linder LE. Occurrence of periodontopathogens in smoker and nonsmoker patients. J Clin Periodontol 1992;19:667–71.

133. Ramfjord SP, Emslie RD, Greene JC, et al. Epidemiological studies of periodontal disease. Am J Public Health 1968;58:1713–22.

134. Ramfjord SP, Kerr DA, Ash MM, eds. World workshop in periodontics. Ann Arbor: University of Michigan Press, 1966.

135. Ramfjord SP, Morrison EC, Burgett FG, et al. Oral hygiene and maintenance of periodontal support. J Periodontol 1982;53:26–30.

136. Rams TE, Andriolo M Jr, Feik D, et al. Microbiological study of HIV-related periodontitis. J Periodontol 1991;62:74–81.

137. Ranney RR. Pathogenesis of periodontal disease. In: International Conference on Research in the Biology of Periodontal Disease. Chicago: University of Illinois School of Dentistry, 1977:223–300.

138. Riley C, London JP, Burmeister JA. Periodontal health in 200 HIV-positive patients. J Oral Pathol Med 1992;21:124–7.

139. Robinson P. Periodontal diseases and HIV infection. A review of the literature. J Clin Periodontol 1992;19:609–14.

140. Rosling B, Nyman S, Lindhe J. The effect of systematic plaque control on bone regeneration in infrabony pockets. J Clin Periodontol 1976;3:38–53.

141. Russell AL. International nutrition surveys: A summary of preliminary dental findings. J Dent Res 1963;42:233–44.

142. Russell AL. World epidemiology and oral health. In: Kreshover SJ, McClure FJ, eds: Environmental variables in oral disease. AAAS Publ No 81. Washington DC: American Association Advancement Science, 1966:21–39.

143. Russell AL. Epidemiology of periodontal disease. Int Dent J 1967;17:282–96.

144. Russell AL, Ayers P. Periodontal disease and socioeconomic status in Birmingham, Alabama. Am J Public Health 1960;50:206–14.

145. Russell AL, Leatherwood EC, Consolazio CF, Van Reen R. Periodontal disease and nutrition in South Vietnam. J Dent Res 1965;44:775–82.

146. Safkan-Seppala B, Ainamo J. Periodontal conditions in insulin-dependent diabetes mellitus. J Clin Periodontol 1992;19:24–9.

147. Sandholm L, Swanjung O, Rytomaa I, et al. Periodontal status of Finnish adolescents with insulin-dependent diabetes mellitus. J Clin Periodontol 1989;16:617–20.

148. Schei O, Waerhaug J, Lovdal A, Arno A. Alveolar bone loss as related to oral hygiene and age. J Periodontol 1959;30:7–16.

149. Scannopieco FA, Mylotte JM. Relationships between periodontal disease and bacterial pneumonia. J Periodontol 1996;67(Suppl):1114–22.

150. Seppala B, Ainamo J. A site-by-site follow-up study on the effect of controlled versus poorly controlled insulin-dependent diabetes mellitus. J Clin Periodontol 1994;21:161–5.

151. Seppala B, Seppala M, Ainamo J. A longitudinal study on insulin-dependent diabetes mellitus and periodontal disease. J Clin Periodontol 1993; 20:161–5.

152. Sheiham A. The epidemiology of chronic periodontal disease in Western Nigerian schoolchildren. J Periodont Res 1968;3:257–67.

153. Sheiham A. Dental cleanliness and chronic periodontal disease: studies on populations in Britain. Br Dent J 1970;120:413–8.

154. Shlossman M, Knowler WC, Pettitt DJ, Genco RJ. Type 2 diabetes mellitus and periodontal disease. J Am Dent Assoc 1990;121:532–6.

155. Slots J. Bacterial specificity in adult periodontitis: A summary of recent work. J Clin Periodontol 1986;13:912–7.

156. Smith AJ, Adams D. The dental status and attitudes of patients at risk from infective endocarditis. Br Dent J 1993;174:59–64.

157. Socransky SS, Haffajee AD, Goodson JM, Lindhe J. New concepts of destructive periodontal disease. J Clin Periodontol 1984;11:21–32.

158. Socransky SS, Haffajee AD, Smith C, Dibart S. Relation of counts of microbial species to clinical status at the sampled site. J Clin Periodontol 1991;18:766–75.

159. Stansby G, Byrne MT, Hamilton G. Dental infection in vascular surgical patients. Br J Surg 1994;81:1119–20.

160. Stoltenberg JL, Osborn JB, Pihlstrom BL, et al. Association between cigarette smoking, bacterial pathogens, and periodontal status. J Periodontol 1993; 64:1225–30.

161. Swango PA, Kleinman DV, Konzelman JL. HIV and periodontal health. A study of military personnel with HIV. J Am Dent Assoc 1991;12:49–54.

162. Taylor GW, Burt BA, Becker MP, et al. Severe periodontitis and risk for poor glycemic control in patients with non-insulin dependent diabetes mellitus. J Periodontol 1996;67(Suppl):1085–93.

163. Tervonen T, Oliver RC, Wolff LF, et al. Prevalence of periodontal pathogens with varying metabolic control of diabetes mellitus. J Clin Periodontol 1994;21:375–9.

164. Thorstensson H, Hugoson A. Periodontal disease experience in adult long-duration insulin-dependent diabetics. J Clin Periodontol 1993;20:352–8.

165. Tomar SL, Swango PA, Kleinman DV, Burt BA. Loss of periodontal attachment in HIV-seropositive military personnel. J Periodontol 1995;66:421–8.

166. US Department of Health and Human Services, National Center for Health Statistics. Third National Health and Nutrition Examination Survey, 1988–94. Public Use Data File No. 7–0627. Hyattsville MD: CDC, 1997.

167. US Public Health Service, National Center for Health Statistics. Periodontal disease in adults, United States, 1960–62. PHS Publ No 1000, Series 11 No 12. Washington DC: Government Printing Office, 1965.

168. US Public Health Service, National Center for Health Statistics. Periodontal disease and oral hygiene among children, United States. DHEW Publ No (HSM) 72–1060, Series 11 No 117. Washington DC: Government Printing Office, 1972.

169. US Public Health Service, National Center for Health Statistics. Basic data on dental examination findings of persons 1–74 years, United States, 1971–1974. DHEW Publ No (PHS) 79–1662, Series 11 No 214. Washington DC: Government Printing Office, 1979.

170. US Public Health Service, National Institute of Dental Research. Oral health survey of United States adults; national findings. NIH Publ No 87–2868. Washington DC: Government Printing Office, 1987.

171. Van der Velden U. Effect of age on the periodontium. J Clin Periodontol 1984;11:281–94.

172. Van der Velden U, Abbas F, Van Steenbergen TJ, et al. Prevalence of periodontal breakdown in adolescents and presence of *Actinobacillus actinomycetemcomitans* in subjects with attachment loss. J Periodontol 1989;60:604–10.

173. Waerhaug J. Epidemiology of periodontal disease: A review of literature. In: Ramfjord SP, Kerr DA, Ash MM, eds: World Workshop in Periodontics. Ann Arbor MI: University of Michigan, 1966:181–271.

174. Wennstrom J, Dahlen G, Svensson J, Nyman S. *Actinobacillus actinomycetemcomitans, Bacteroides gingivalis,* and *Bacteroides intermedius*: Predictors of attachment loss? Oral Microbiol Immunol 1987;2:158–63.

175. Wilton JM, Griffiths GS, Curtis MA, et al. Detection of high-risk groups and individuals for periodontal diseases. Systemic predisposition and markers of general health. J Clin Periodontol 1988;15:339–46.

176. Winkler JR, Grassi M, Murray PA. Clinical description and etiology of HIV-associated periodontal diseases. In: Robertson PB, Greenspan JS, eds: Perspectives on oral manifestations of AIDS. Littleton MA: PSG Publishing, 1988:49–70.

177. Winkler JR, Robertson PB. Periodontal disease associated with HIV infection. Oral Surg Oral Med Oral Pathol 1992;73:145–50.

178. Wolfson SM, Lewis MH. A survey of periodontal conditions in Saskatchewan adolescents. J Can Dent Assoc 1985;51:486–9.

179. World Health Organization. Periodontal disease. Tech Report Series No 207. Geneva: WHO, 1961.

180. Yeung SC, Stewart GJ, Cooper DA, Sindhusake D. Progression of periodontal disease in HIV seropositive patients. J Periodontol 1993;64:651–7.

181. Zambon JJ. *Actinobacillus actinomycetemcomitans* in human periodontal disease. J Clin Periodontol 1985;12:1–20.

182. Zambon JJ, Reynolds H, Fisher JG, et al. Microbiological and immunological studies of adult periodontitis in patients with noninsulin-dependent diabetes mellitus. J Periodontol 1988;59:23–31.

183. Zambon JJ, Reynolds HS, Genco RJ. Studies of the subgingival microflora in patients with acquired immunodeficiency syndrome. J Periodontol 1990;61:699–704.

21

Dental Fluorosis

Definition ◆ Prevalence of Fluorosis in the United
States ◆ Risk Factors ◆ Dental Fluorosis and
Caries ◆ Dental Fluorosis as a Public Health Problem

DEFINITION

Dental fluorosis is defined as a permanent hypomineralization of enamel, characterized by greater surface and subsurface porosity than in normal enamel, that results from excess fluoride (F) reaching the developing tooth during developmental stages.[22] Pre-eruptive enamel maturation consists of an increase in mineralization within the developing tooth and a concurrent loss of early-secreted matrix proteins. Excess F available to the enamel during maturation disrupts mineralization and results in excessive retention of enamel proteins.[5, 15] Although sufficiently high F concentrations might affect enamel at all developmental stages,[16, 60] early pre-eruptive maturation appears to be the time when enamel is most sensitive to the effects of F, both in animals[17, 54] and in humans.[20] Elegantly-designed human studies have shown that this "critical period" for the development of fluorosis in the human maxillary central incisor begins around the age of 22 months and extends for periods of up to several years after that for later-developing teeth.[20]

In its mildest forms, fluorosis appears as barely-discernible fine, lacy markings that follow the perikymata across the width of the enamel surface. At this level, an experienced dental examiner is required to detect it. At the opposite extreme, the most severe forms of fluorosis manifest as heavily stained, pitted, and friable enamel that can result in loss of dental function. Fluorosis is a dose-response condition; gradations between these two extremes appear as more obvious white lacy markings through to a nontranslucent white coloration of the whole enamel surface. The brown stain that often accompanies moderate fluorosis is a posteruptive feature that comes from certain dietary ingredients being picked up by proteins in the porous outer enamel[23]; it is only seen when porous enamel has formed before eruption.

Fluorosed surface enamel contains higher F concentrations than does unaffected enamel, and the enamel F content increases with the severity of the condition.[53] Teeth that mineralize later in life generally show more severe fluorotic disturbances than do those that mineralize earlier.[3, 36-38] On that theme, fluorosis is less common in the primary than in the permanent dentition, although it has been reported in both a fluoridated and a nonfluoridated area in Britain,[66] and is common in the primary dentition in high-fluoride areas of the world.[37, 41, 45, 46, 63]

Because dental fluorosis is a dose-response condition, the higher the intakes during the crucial period of tooth development, the more severe the fluorosis.[14, 18, 22] It was previously believed that fluorosis would be probable following intakes of 0.1 mg F/kg body weight or more during infancy.[25] More recent evidence, however, has lowered that threshold: 0.03 to 0.1 mg F/kg body weight has been suggested as the borderline zone,[24] at least for European children. Studies in Kenya have found fluorosis with average intakes as low as 0.04 mg F/kg body weight.[3] Because this range encompasses the range of 0.05 to 0.07 mg F/kg body weight/day, the so-called "optimum intake" range (Chapter 23), it is not clear whether other factors (e.g., nutrition) lead to these different estimates or

whether they merely reflect biological variation. Certainly a range of fluorosis severity is
seen among individuals who appear to have
similar exposures to F.

PREVALENCE OF FLUOROSIS IN THE UNITED STATES

Fluorosis in the United States was first
mapped out by Dean during his classic studies of the 1930s and early 1940s. These studies
are discussed in Chapter 23; they are an integral part of the story of how fluorosis and
caries experience were first associated with F
concentrations in drinking water.

One part of the United States that received a lot of attention from Dean was northern Illinois, where there is an extensive belt
of naturally fluoridated drinking water. Seven
of these communities, naturally fluoridated to
varying degrees, were revisited by researchers from the National Institute of Dental and
Craniofacial Research (NIDCR) in 1980 and
1985.[30] Relating age to fluorosis and tooth calcification, the authors concluded that F intake
had increased during the 1970–1977 period,
but had not increased subsequently. A follow-
up study in 1990 found that age-standardized
fluorosis prevalence and severity had
changed little since 1980 at all levels of water F.[57]

Although there are difficulties in comparing data from 60 years apart, it is clear that
the prevalence of dental fluorosis in the
United States has increased since the time
of Dean.[11, 61] Prevalence among children was
reported as 22.3% in the 1986–1987 National
Survey of Dental Caries in US School Children, ranging by age from 18.5% of 17-year-
olds to 25.8% of 9-year-olds.[7] This higher
prevalence in the younger children hints that
prevalence might still be increasing, and more
recent data do not refute that possibility.[11]
Almost all of the fluorosis recorded in the
1986–1987 survey was of the mild/very mild
variety. Although there is little firm evidence,
it is possible that a slight increase in fluorosis
severity has accompanied the large increase
in prevalence.[64]

Fluorosis prevalence has increased considerably since Dean's time, and the fact that
the biggest relative increase has been seen in
nonfluoridated areas (Fig. 21–1) suggests that

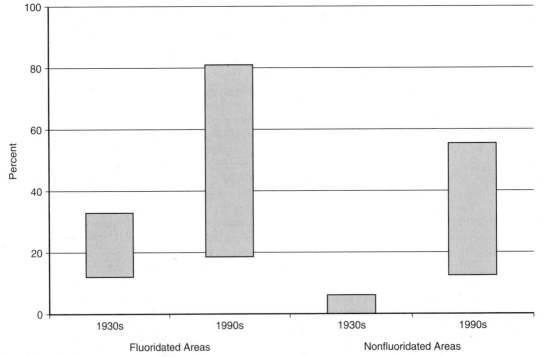

Figure 21–1. Increase in dental fluorosis prevalence in North America since initial studies in the 1930s. The bars
represent the prevalence range reported from Dean's studies compared to those from the late 1980s and early 1990s.
(From Clark DC. Trends in the prevalence of dental fluorosis in North America. Community Dent Oral Epidemiol
1994;22:148–52; Dean HT. The investigation of physiological effects by the epidemiological. In: Moulton FR [ed]: Fluorine
and dental health. Washington DC: American Association for the Advancement of Science 1942:23–31.)

the risk of fluorosis from fluoridated water may be coming from its use in processed foods and drinks, as well as from direct consumption.

RISK FACTORS FOR DENTAL FLUOROSIS

Because fluorosis is a disturbance of enamel resulting from excessive F intake during the developmental period, risk factors are related to the intake of F at the crucial periods of pre-eruptive tooth development. Fluoridated water is a risk factor; it was documented long ago that even around 1.0 ppm F in the United States, 7% to 16% of children born and reared in the area exhibit mild or very mild dental fluorosis in the permanent dentition.[1, 14, 56] This degree of prevalence was recorded at a time when drinking water was virtually the only source of exposure to F. Even small changes in F concentrations in drinking water can lead to considerable change in fluorosis prevalence and severity.[21, 62]

F dietary supplements, in the form of tablets, drops, or F-vitamin combinations, have been used for years in nonfluoridated areas to prevent caries (Chapter 25). Regardless of F supplements' role in preventing caries, there is now strong evidence that supplements are a risk factor for mild-to-moderate fluorosis. Case-control studies in nonfluoridated areas of New England have found that exposure to F supplements during the first 6 years of life, together with higher socioeconomic status, significantly increased the risk of developing fluorosis.[49, 51] Later research found the risk to be extremely high when supplements were used in fluoridated areas, a clearly inappropriate procedure.[50] Other studies during the 1990s have demonstrated the link between supplements and fluorosis risk.[2, 32, 35, 52] It was this evidence that led the American Dental Association (ADA), in 1994, to reduce the recommended F supplement dosage for caries prevention in children (Chapter 25).

Young children, in whom the swallowing reflex is not yet fully developed, can ingest up to 0.3 to 0.5 g of toothpaste (0.3 to 0.5 mg F) at each brushing.[4, 6, 28] These findings naturally raise the issue of whether overenthusiastic use of F toothpaste in young children is a risk factor for fluorosis. One study in the fluoridated Toronto area found that early use of F toothpaste (before 2 years of age) and prolonged use of infant formula made up with fluoridated water were strong risk factors for the later development of fluorosis.[47] Although most of the fluorosis seen in that Toronto study was very mild, later studies were able to confirm a clear risk of fluorosis with early use of F toothpaste.[35, 43, 50, 55, 58] The extent of the risk from early use of F toothpaste, however, was usually not as high as that seen with F supplements.

Infant formula has been recognized as a risk factor for fluorosis, both for its own F content and especially when mixed with fluoridated water.[47, 50] Soy-based formulas contain higher F concentrations than do milk-based formulas.[33, 42]

There is no reason to believe that F mouthrinses and professionally applied gels and varnishes are risk factors for fluorosis. Obviously, the protocols for use of these products must be designed to minimize ingestion.

DENTAL FLUOROSIS AND CARIES

Dean's studies showed that caries experience dropped sharply as the F concentration of drinking water rose from negligible to 1.0 ppm, and that it tended to level off after that (Chapter 23). When F concentration reaches a point where severe fluorosis is common and the enamel of affected individuals becomes friable and liable to fracture, caries experience has been observed to increase.[26] This phenomenon has been demonstrated in the United States, from the NIDCR studies in the 7 communities in northern Illinois described previously, in 1980, 1985, and again in 1990.[57] The results of the caries examinations, related to F concentrations in drinking water, are shown in Figure 21–2. Data for each year describes a J-shaped curve: with increasing F levels, caries experience diminishes to a certain point and then starts to rise again. Dean showed that caries experience in the 1930s continued to drop at least as far as a water F level of 2.6 ppm[13]; unfortunately he did not publish caries data from the higher F communities that he studied earlier in his career.

These data suggest that the true relationship between water F levels and caries is the J-shaped curve, with the turning point in the J being something between 3 and 4 times the optimum level. However, this hypothesis is not supported by the data in Figure 24–1, where caries experience of adults in a community with 5 times the optimum fluoride

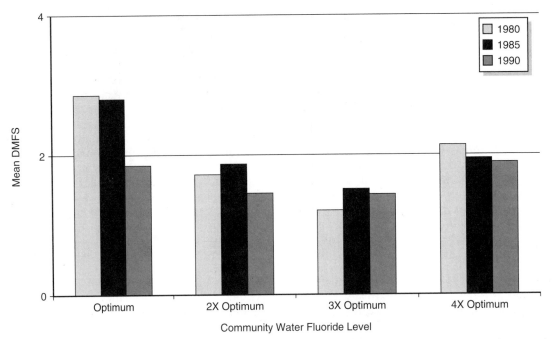

Figure 21–2. Caries experience of children, age-adjusted for comparability, in 7 Illinois communities, relative to the degree of fluoride in the drinking water: 1980, 1985, and 1990. (From Selwitz RH, Nowjack-Raymer RE, Kingman A, Driscoll WS. Prevalence of dental caries and dental fluorosis in areas with optimal and above-optimal water fluoride concentrations: A 10-year follow-up survey. J Public Health Dent 1995;55:85–93.)

level in drinking water was below that found in a neighboring community with optimum level. An earlier Texas study also found that caries experience in 12–15 year olds continued to diminish even when community F levels reached 6 to 8 times optimum.[19]

Figure 21–3 shows the relation between caries experience and water F levels, age-standardized and restricted to permanent residents, among participants in the 1986–1987 National Survey of Caries in United States Schoolchildren. It makes an interesting comparison with the comparable data from Dean's studies (see Fig. 23–1), for although absolute caries levels are much lower, there is a much less pronounced relationship between caries and water F levels in Figure 21–3. These 2 factors together indicate the importance of F from sources other than drinking water that has arisen since Dean's time. The J-shaped relationship between caries and F level of drinking water (see Fig. 21–2) is still evident. Figure 21–4 shows fluorosis prevalence data from the same national survey, and here fluorosis seems to fall into 3 stages: the lowest prevalence from zero to 0.5 ppm F, a plateau from 0.6 to 1.2 ppm F, and the highest prevalence at 1.3 ppm F and above.

Caries could increase with higher F levels

in drinking water because restorative treatment is sought for fluorosed enamel, or because pitted and friable enamel is diagnosed as carious. Although friable enamel can certainly lead to loss of function and require dental restoration, it is not necessarily carious. It is possible, however, that broken enamel makes a tooth more vulnerable to caries. Whatever the link, severe fluorosis is obviously a condition to be avoided as far as possible.

DENTAL FLUOROSIS AS A PUBLIC HEALTH PROBLEM

At what point does dental fluorosis become a public health problem? There is no reason to call it such in a community where it is found only in its mildest forms, even those in the United States where prevalence is around 50% in children. On the other hand, its high prevalence and severity make it a public health problem in some countries of East Africa [9, 27, 39, 40, 44, 46, 65, 67] and in parts of India.[8, 34, 59] It is an urgent problem in those regions of Ethiopia and India where skeletal fluorosis is found.[27, 34]

The relatively greater increase in fluoro-

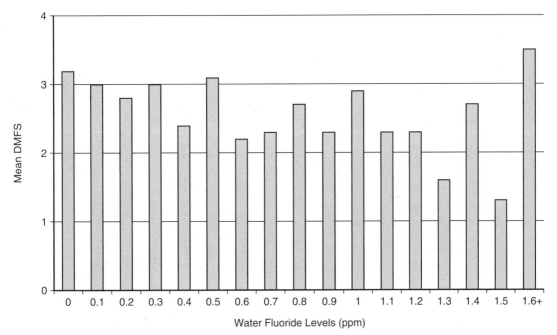

Figure 21-3. Caries experience of children aged 5–17 years by fluoride level of drinking water. Age-adjusted and restricted to permanent residents in the 1986–87 National Survey of Caries in US Schoolchildren. (From Heller KE, Eklund SA, Burt BA. Dental caries and dental fluorosis at varying water fluoride concentrations. J Public Health Dent 1997;57:136–43.)

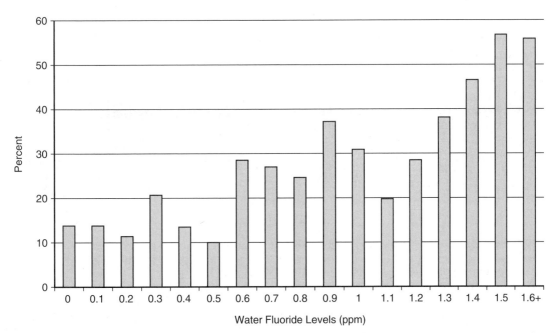

Figure 21-4. Fluorosis prevalence of children aged 7–17 years by fluoride level of drinking water. Age-adjusted and restricted to permanent residents in the 1986–87 National Survey of Caries in US Schoolchildren. (From Heller KE, Eklund SA, Burt BA. Dental caries and dental fluorosis at varying water fluoride concentrations. J Public Health Dent 1997;57:136–43.)

sis prevalence in nonfluoridated communities, relative to fluoridated areas (see Fig. 21–1), must be largely attributable to an increase in F ingestion from sources other than drinking water. The risk of fluorosis from dental products, notably toothpaste and F supplements, was described previously. Estimates of F intake from dietary sources were given previously; F ingestion can be high from soft drinks and fruit juices processed with fluoridated water.[12, 48] For most people, drinking water is now just one of numerous exposures to F.

Dental fluorosis cannot be classed as a public health problem in the United States and other countries where controlled water fluoridation is extensive. It would be a mistake, however, to assume that it could not become so. There is evidence that members of the public are quite aware of the presence of even the milder forms of fluorosis on their teeth.[10, 29, 55] If high-F toothpastes become widely marketed, and if the aesthetic perceptions of the public regarding fluorosis become more stringent, dentistry could be faced with that problem. Increased public pressure to restrict F is best avoided by prudent use of F now, especially for children during the formative years of the permanent dentition.

Public policy on any issue usually has to be established without complete information, and water fluoridation is no exception. Bearing in mind that adults, on average, ingest 1 to 3 mg F per day in their normal diets, that 9 to 10 million Americans (and many other people around the world) have been drinking naturally fluoridated water for a long time, and that more than 100 million Americans have been drinking F-supplemented water for generations, there is a lot of empirical evidence to say that fluoridation at 1.0 ppm is not harmful. Certainly there is no credible evidence that F in these amounts leads to serious ill health. The scientific method cannot "prove a negative"; we take inability to reject the null hypothesis for specific conditions (Chapter 12) as evidence of safety. The occasional allegation of a sensitivity reaction should be investigated seriously, but with the passage of time the probability becomes greater that fluoridation at 1.0 ppm produces no undesirable side effects. Although some aspects of F in human health are still not fully understood, we support the policy of the US Public Health Service that F be added to drinking water at the recommended concentrations.

REFERENCES

1. Ast DB, Smith DJ, Wachs B, Cantwell KT. The Newburgh-Kingston caries-fluorine study. XIV. Combined clinical and roentgenographic dental findings after ten years of fluoride experience. J Am Dent Assoc 1956;52:314-25.
2. Awad MA, Hargreaves JA, Thompson GW. Dental caries and fluorosis in 7–9 and 11–14 year old children who received fluoride supplements from birth. J Can Dent Assoc 1994;60:318-22.
3. Baelum V, Fejerskov O, Manji F, Larsen MJ. Daily dose of fluoride and dental fluorosis. Tandlaegebladet 1987;91:452-6.
4. Barnhart WE, Hiller LK, Leonard GJ, Michaels SE. Dentifrice usage and ingestion among four age groups. J Dent Res 1974;53:1317-22.
5. Bawden JW, Crenshaw MA, Wright JT, LeGeros RZ. Concise review: Consideration of possible biologic mechanisms of fluorosis. J Dent Res 1995;74:1349-52.
6. Baxter PM. Toothpaste ingestion during toothbrushing by school children. Br Dent J 1980;148:125-8.
7. Brunelle JA. The prevalence of dental fluorosis in U.S. children, 1987 [abstract]. J Dent Res 1989;68(Spec Issue):995.
8. Chandra S, Sharma R, Thergaonkar VP, Chaturvedi SK. Determination of optimal fluoride concentration in drinking water in an area in India with dental fluorosis. Community Dent Oral Epidemiol 1980;8:92-6.
9. Chibole O. Epidemiology of dental fluorosis in Kenya. J R Soc Health 1987;107:242-3.
10. Clark DC. Evaluation of aesthetics for the different classifications of the Tooth Surface Index of Fluorosis. Community Dent Oral Epidemiol 1995;23:80-3.
11. Clark DC. Trends in the prevalence of dental fluorosis in North America. Community Dent Oral Epidemiol 1994;22:148-52.
12. Clovis J, Hargreaves JA. Fluoride intake from beverage consumption. Community Dent Oral Epidemiol 1988;16:11-5.
13. Dean HT. Endemic fluorosis and its relation to dental caries. Public Health Rep 1938;53:1443-52.
14. Dean HT. The investigation of physiological effects by the epidemiological method. In: Moulton FR, ed: Fluorine and dental health. Washington DC: American Association for the Advancement of Science, 1942:23-31.
15. Den Besten PK. Effects of fluoride on protein secretion and removal during enamel development in the rat. J Dent Res 1986;65:1272-7.
16. Den Besten PK, Crenshaw MA. Studies on the changes in developing enamel caused by ingestion of high levels of fluoride in the rat. Adv Dent Res 1987;1:176-80.
17. Den Besten PK, Thariani H. Biological mechanisms of fluorosis and level and timing of systemic exposure to fluoride with respect to fluorosis. J Dent Res 1992;71:1238-43.
18. Eklund SA, Burt BA, Ismail AI, Calderone JJ. High-fluoride drinking water, fluorosis, and dental caries in adults. J Am Dent Assoc 1987;114:324-8.
19. Englander HR, DePaola PF. Enhanced anticaries action from drinking water containing 5 ppm fluoride. J Am Dent Assoc 1979;98:35-9.
20. Evans RW, Stamm JW. An epidemiologic estimate of the critical period during which maxillary central incisors are most susceptible to fluorosis. J Public Health Dent 1991;51:251-9.

21. Evans RW, Stamm JW. Dental fluorosis following downward adjustment of drinking water. J Public Health Dent 1991;51:91-8.

22. Fejerskov O, Manji F, Baelum V. The nature and mechanisms of dental fluorosis in man. J Dent Res 1990;69(Spec Issue):692-700.

23. Fejerskov O, Manji F, Baelum V, Møller IJ. Dental fluorosis—a handbook for health workers. Copenhagen: Munksgaard, 1988.

24. Fejerskov O, Stephen KW, Richards A, Speirs R. Combined effect of systemic and topical fluoride treatments on human deciduous teeth—case studies. Caries Res 1987;21:452-9.

25. Forsman B. Early supply of fluoride and enamel fluorosis. Scand J Dent Res 1977;85:22-30.

26. Grobler SR, van Wyk CW, Kotze D. Relationship between enamel fluoride levels, degree of fluorosis and caries experience in communities with a nearly optimal and a high fluoride level in the drinking water. Caries Res 1986;20:284-8.

27. Haimanot RT, Fekadu A, Bushra B. Endemic fluorosis in the Ethiopian Rift Valley. Trop Geog Med 1987;39:209-17.

28. Hargreaves JA, Ingram GS, Wagg BJ. A gravimetric study of the ingestion of toothpaste by children. Caries Res 1972;6:236-43.

29. Hawley GM, Ellwood RP, Davies RM. Dental caries, fluorosis and the cosmetic implications of different TF scores in 14-year-old adolescents. Community Dent Health 1996;13:189-92.

30. Heifetz SB, Driscoll WS, Horowitz HS, Kingman A. Prevalence of dental caries and dental fluorosis in areas with optimal and above-optimal water-fluoride concentrations: A 5-year follow-up survey. J Am Dent Assoc 1988;116:490-5.

31. Heller KE, Eklund SA, Burt BA. Dental caries and dental fluorosis at varying water fluoride concentrations. J Public Health Dent 1997;57:136-43.

32. Ismail AI, Brodeur J-M, Kavanagh M, et al. Prevalence of dental caries and dental fluorosis in students, 11–17 years of age, in fluoridated and nonfluoridated cities in Quebec. Caries Res 1990;24:290-7.

33. Johnson J Jr, Bawden JW. The fluoride content of infant formulas available in 1985. Pediatr Dent 1987;9:33-7.

34. Jolly SS, Singh BM, Mathur OC, Malhotra KC. Epidemiological, clinical, and biochemical study of endemic dental and skeletal fluorosis in Punjab. Br Med J 1968;4:427-9.

35. Lalumandier JA, Rozier RG. The prevalence and risk factors of fluorosis among patients in a pediatric dental practice. Pediatr Dent 1995;17:19-25.

36. Larsen MJ, Kirkegaard E, Poulsen S. Patterns of dental fluorosis in a European country in relation to the fluoride concentration of drinking water. J Dent Res 1987;66:10-2.

37. Larsen MJ, Richards A, Fejerskov O. Development of dental fluorosis according to age at start of fluoride administration. Caries Res 1985;19:519-27.

38. Larsen MJ, Senderovitz F, Kirkegaard E, et al. Dental fluorosis in the primary and the permanent dentition in fluoridated areas with consumption of either powdered milk or natural cow's milk. J Dent Res 1988;67:822-5.

39. Manji F, Baelum V, Fejerskov O. Dental fluorosis in an area of Kenya with 2 ppm fluoride in the drinking water. J Dent Res 1986;65:659-62.

40. Manji F, Kapila S. Fluorides and fluorosis in Kenya. Part III: Fluorides, fluorosis and dental caries. Odont-Stomatol Trop 1986;9:135-39.

41. McInnes PM, Richardson BD, Cleaton-Jones PE. Comparison of dental fluorosis and caries in primary teeth of preschool-children living in arid high and low fluoride villages. Community Dent Oral Epidemiol 1982;10:182-6.

42. McKnight-Hanes MC, Leverett DH, Adair SM, Shields CP. Fluoride content of infant formulas: Soy-based formulas as a potential factor in dental fluorosis. Pediatr Dent 1988;10:189-94.

43. Milsom K, Mitropolous CM. Enamel defects in 8-year-old children in fluoridated and nonfluoridated parts of Cheshire. Caries Res 1990;24:286-9.

44. Møller IJ, Pindborg JJ, Gedalia I, Roed-Petersen B. The prevalence of dental fluorosis in the people of Uganda. Arch Oral Biol 1970;15:213-25.

45. Nair KR, Manji F. Endemic fluorosis in deciduous dentition. A study of 1276 children in typically high fluoride area (Kiambu) in Kenya. Odont-Stomatol Trop 1982;5:177-84.

46. Olsson B. Dental findings in high-fluoride areas in Ethiopia. Community Dent Oral Epidemiol 1979;7:51-6.

47. Osuji OO, Leake JL, Chipman ML, et al. Risk factors for dental fluorosis in a fluoridated community. J Dent Res 1988;67:1488-92.

48. Pang DTY, Phillips CL, Bawden JW. Fluoride intake from beverage consumption in a sample of North Carolina children. J Dent Res 1992;71:1382-8.

49. Pendrys DG, Katz RV. Risk of enamel fluorosis associated with fluoride supplementation, infant formula, and fluoride dentifrice use. Am J Epidemiol 1989;130:1199-208.

50. Pendrys DG, Katz RV, Morse DE. Risk factors for enamel fluorosis in a fluoridated population. Am J Epidemiol 1994;140:461-71.

51. Pendrys DG, Katz RV, Morse DE. Risk factors for enamel fluorosis in a nonfluoridated population. Am J Epidemiol 1996;143:808-15.

52. Pendrys DG, Stamm JW. Relationship of total fluoride intake to beneficial effects and enamel fluorosis. J Dent Res 1990;69(Spec Issue):529-38.

53. Richards A, Fejerskov O, Baelum V. Enamel fluoride in relation to severity of human dental fluorosis. Adv Dent Res 1989;3:147-53.

54. Richards A, Kragstrup J, Josephsen K, Fejerskov O. Dental fluorosis developed in post-secretory enamel. J Dent Res 1986;65:1406-9.

55. Riordan PJ. Perceptions of dental fluorosis. J Dent Res 1993;72:1268-74.

56. Russell AL. Dental fluorosis in Grand Rapids during the seventeenth year of fluoridation. J Am Dent Assoc 1962;65:608-12.

57. Selwitz RH, Nowjack-Raymer RE, Kingman A, Driscoll WS. Prevalence of dental caries and dental fluorosis in areas with optimal and above-optimal water fluoride concentrations: A 10-year follow-up survey. J Public Health Dent 1995;55:85-93.

58. Skotowski MC, Hunt RJ, Levy SM. Risk factors for dental fluorosis in pediatric dental patients. J Public Health Dent 1995;55:154-9.

59. Subbareddy VV, Tewari A. Enamel mottling at different levels of fluoride in drinking water in an endemic area. J Ind Dent Assoc 1985;57:205-12.

60. Suckling G, Thurley DC, Nelson DGA. The macroscopic and scanning electron-microscopic appearance and microhardness of the enamel, and the related histological changes in the enamel organ of erupting sheep incisors resulting from a prolonged low daily dose of fluoride. Arch Oral Biol 1988;33:361-73.

61. Szpunar SM, Burt BA. Trends in the prevalence of dental fluorosis in the United States: A review. J Public Health Dent 1987;47:71-9.

62. Szpunar SM, Burt BA. Dental caries, fluorosis, and fluoride exposure in Michigan schoolchildren. J Dent Res 1988;67:802-6.

63. Thylstrup A. Distribution of dental fluorosis in the primary dentition. Community Dent Oral Epidemiol 1978;6:329-37.

64. US Public Health Service, Ad Hoc Subcommittee on Fluoride. Review of fluoride benefits and risks. Washington DC: Government Printing Office, 1991.

65. Walvekar SV, Qureshi BA. Endemic fluorosis and partial defluoridation of water supplies: A public health concern in Kenya. Community Dent Oral Epidemiol 1982;10:156-60.

66. Weeks KJ, Milsom KM, Lennon MA. Enamel defects in 4- to 5-year old children in fluoridated and non-fluoridated parts of Cheshire, UK. Caries Res 1993;27:317-20.

67. Wenzel A, Thylstrup A, Melsen B, Fejerskov O. The relationship between water-borne fluoride, dental fluorosis and skeletal development in 11-15 year old Tanzanian girls. Arch Oral Biol 1982;27:1007-11.

22

Oral Cancer and Other Oral Conditions

Oral Cancer ◆ Other Soft-Tissue Lesions ◆ Cleft Lip and Palate ◆ Malocclusion ◆ Temporomandibular Joint Disorders

With the decline in dental caries among children, and the realization that periodontal disease may not be the monster it was once thought to be, dental professionals are in a position to spend more time on the diagnosis and treatment of conditions that traditionally have not occupied much time in the dental office. This chapter looks at the distribution of some of these conditions and at the risk factors and risk indicators associated with them.

ORAL CANCER

Of all conditions that dental professionals see and treat, oral cancer is the one that literally has life-and-death implications. It is sobering to note that age-adjusted mortality rates from oral cancer in the United States showed only slight improvement from 1960 to the mid-1980s; and only since the late 1980s has a modest trend toward improvement in mortality among males become evident (Fig. 22–1). Although mortality rates among American females have always been low, they have not changed over the 30-year period depicted in Figure 22–1.

The term oral cancer includes disease category numbers 140–149 of the International Classification of Diseases, known as ICD-9.[34] Oral cancers are also listed as classifications C00 to C14 of the Application of the International Classification of Diseases to Dentistry and Stomatology, known as ICD-DA.[90] This range includes cancers of the lip, tongue, buccal mucosa, floor of the mouth, salivary glands, and pharynx. It does not include

throat cancer. The occurrence of oral cancer and its site distribution within the mouth vary widely in different parts of the world,[58, 62, 76] presumably because of the environmental factors with which they are associated. Squamous cell carcinomas of the oral mucosa, tongue, and lip comprise 80% of all oral cancers on a global basis.[35] The risk factor most consistently identified on a global basis is the use of tobacco in its various forms.[62] In India, for example, 30% to 40% of all reported cancers are oral cancers,[2, 14] a remarkably high prevalence that is closely associated with several forms of tobacco smoking and chewing in that country.

Table 22–1 shows the extent of the oral cancer problem within the United States and compares data for 1997 with that from 1988. There were more cancers of all kinds in 1997 than in 1988, but the number of new oral cancers had grown only slightly. This means that cancers of the oral cavity constituted 2.2% of all new cases reported in 1997, down from 3.1% in 1988. Mortality from oral cancers has also declined, both in absolute numbers and proportionately, and was 1.5% of all cancer deaths in 1997. The proportionate decline in mortality rates is attributable both to the slight drop in absolute numbers of oral cancers and to the absolute increase in mortality from other types of cancers.

Although these overall trends in the United States seem to be moving in the right direction, oral cancer remains twice as prevalent in males as in females (Table 22–1), and annual incidence among males in the 1988–92 period remained more than twice the rate seen in females (Fig. 22–2), and nearly twice

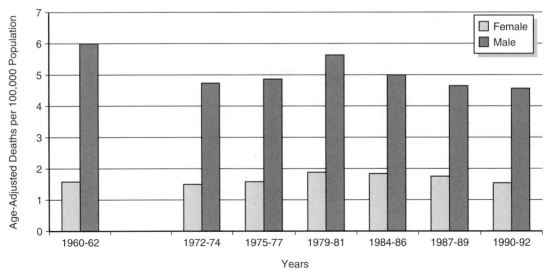

Figure 22–1. Age-adjusted mortality rates, per 100,000 population, from oral cancer for males and females. United States, selected years 1960–92. (Data from American Cancer Society. Cancer facts and figures, 1997. Atlanta: ACS, 1997.)

as many deaths occur in males as in females. There is considerable difference between males and females in the specific sites within the oral cavity in which oral cancer is found (Table 22–2), and there are no obvious explanations for these differences.

Oral cancer is closely related to increasing age, as shown by the fact that over 83% of the 8278 deaths from oral cancer registered in 1991 were for persons 55 years or older.[86] This age-related mortality proportion has remained consistent over the years.

Mortality also varies considerably by race and ethnicity in the United States. Overall annual mortality among African-Americans from 1988 to 1992 was 5.2 per 100,000, nearly double the rate of 2.7 in whites.[81] Not only was the overall mortality higher, but as shown in Figure 22–3, the mortality among younger people was much higher in African-Americans. The peak mortality age is seen in African-Americans 20 years before the peak occurs in whites (Fig. 22–3). The occurrence of oral cancer is most likely related to low socioeconomic status in the United States, as it has been shown to be in Britain.[60]

Table 22–1. NEW CANCER CASES AND DEATHS, BY SEX, FOR ALL CANCERS AND FOR ORAL CANCERS. UNITED STATES, 1988 AND ESTIMATED FOR 1997

SITE	YEAR	.TOTAL	MEN	WOMEN
NEW CASES				
All cancers (in thousands)	1988	985	495	490
	1997	1382	786	596
Oral cancers (thousands)	1988	30.2	20.5	9.7
	1997	30.8	20.9	9.9
Oral cancer as percent of	1988	3.1	4.1	2.0
all cancers	1997	2.2	2.7	1.7
DEATHS				
All cancers (thousands)	1988	494	263	231
	1997	560	294	266
Oral cancers (thousands)	1988	9.1	6.0	3.1
	1997	8.4	5.6	2.8
Oral cancer as percent of	1988	1.8	2.3	1.3
all cancer deaths	1997	1.5	1.9	1.1

From Parker SL, Tong T, Bolden S, Wingo PA. Cancer statistics, 1997. CA 1997;47:5–27; Silverberg E, Lubera JA. Cancer statistics, 1988. CA 1988;38:5–22.

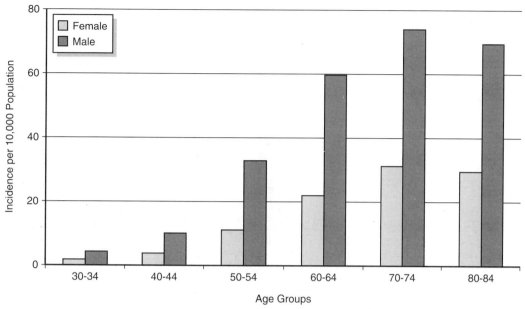

Figure 22–2. Annual incidence rates, per 10,000 population, of oral cancer by age and gender. United States, 1988–92. (From Parker SL, Tong T, Bolden S, Wingo PA. Cancer Statistics, 1997. CA 1997;47:5–27.)

A standard measure of cancer severity is the 5-year relative survival rate, which is the proportion of people still alive 5 years after diagnosis, adjusted for those who died for some other reason during the 5 years. Figure 22–4 shows these rates for men and women since 1974. It is evident that they have not changed much. Although survival seems to have improved slightly for women, it has deteriorated for men, for reasons that are unknown. Survival is also much more favorable for whites than for African-Americans since 1974, and the survival gap between the races has clearly not improved over that time (Fig. 22–5). Survival rates have also diminished in parts of Europe over recent years, a finding attributed to increasing alcohol consumption[3] and to social deprivation.[45]

The prospects for survival are considerably higher when the cancer is confined to a local lesion, as opposed to regional or distant spread having already occurred when the diagnosis is made.[1] Five-year survival is 4 times greater when tumors are diagnosed at localized stages rather than after metastasis has occurred.[81] It follows that cancers and precancerous lesions should be diagnosed as early as possible if treatment is to have a good prognosis, but there is nothing in the data to suggest that the proportion of oral cancers diagnosed at earlier, more localized stages has improved since 1973.[81]

Table 22–2. SITE OCCURRENCE OF ORAL CANCER, FOR ESTIMATED NEW CASES AND FOR DEATHS, FOR MEN AND WOMEN, SHOWN AS PERCENT OF ALL ORAL CANCERS. UNITED STATES, 1997

SITE	NEW CASES			DEATHS		
	TOTAL	MEN	WOMEN	TOTAL	MEN	WOMEN
Tongue	20.8	20.1	22.3	21.6	21.4	21.8
Mouth*	37.5	32.1	43.7	29.6	25.0	38.7
Pharynx	28.6	30.6	24.4	24.1	26.8	18.7
Other sites†	14.9	17.2	9.6	24.7	26.8	20.8

*Floor of the mouth, buccal mucosa, gingiva, palate, salivary glands.
†Lip, both internal and external.
From Parker SL, Tong T, Bolden S, Wingo PA. Cancer statistics, 1997. CA 1997;47:5–27.

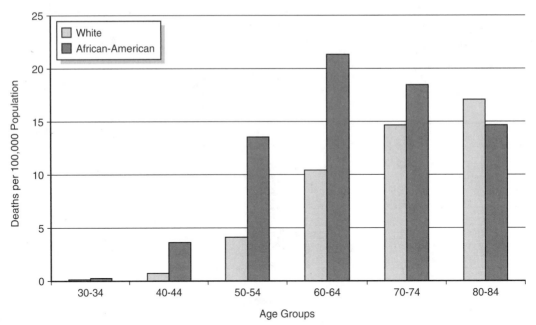

Figure 22–3. Mortality rates, per 100,000 population, from oral cancer, by age and race. United States, 1988–92. (From Parker SL, Tong T, Bolden S, Wingo PA. Cancer Statistics, 1997. CA 1997;47:5–27.)

Studies of oral cancer have shown that smoking and other uses of tobacco are the most consistently identified risk factors. High relative risks, in the range of 6:1 to 14:1, for the development of oral cancers in smokers compared with nonsmokers, continue to be reported from a number of countries.[21, 22, 36, 44,] [49, 51, 57, 79] The risk of developing oral cancer from smoking is just as high for women as for men,[37] and risk diminishes with elapsed time since quitting.[22, 51] The risk of oral cancer in association with smoking is greatest for phanyngeal cancers and lowest for lip cancer.[44, 49]

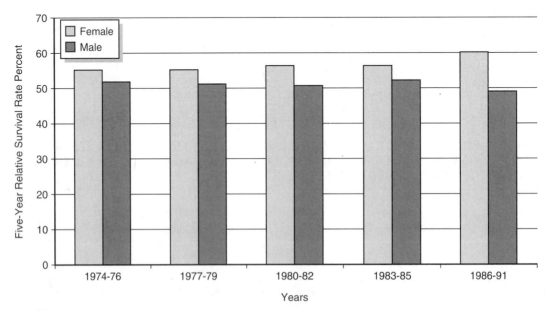

Figure 22–4. Five-year relative survival rates for males and females diagnosed with oral cancer. United States, 1974–91. (Data from American Cancer Society. Cancer facts and figures, 1997. Atlanta: ACS, 1997.)

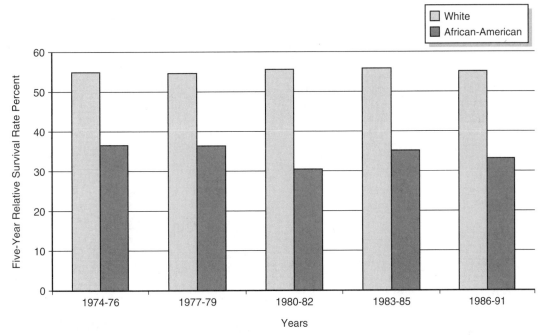

Figure 22–5. Five-year relative survival rates for persons diagnosed with oral cancer. For whites and African-Americans, United States, 1974–91. (Data from American Cancer Society. Cancer facts and figures, 1997. Atlanta: ACS, 1997.)

Research into the extraordinarily high prevalence of oral cancer in India has focused on the widespread habits of chewing the areca nut (betel) in that country. Betel is usually chewed in a mix with tobacco, with lime and other ingredients sometimes added to the betel-tobacco mix. Some studies concluded that the cancer risk came largely from the tobacco, with little role for betel.[29] More recently, however, betel has been identified as a major etiologic factor in the development of oral submucous fibrosis, a precancerous condition that has a high rate of malignant transformation.[55, 56, 75] Nodular leukoplakia, a precancerous condition that may be associated with oral submucous fibrosis, also shows a high rate of malignant transformation. Tobacco users with nodular leukoplakia are at especially high risk of oral cancer.[27] Intervention studies to curtail tobacco and betel chewing have had moderate success in reducing leukoplakia formation in India and confirm that chewing tobacco and betel are major risk factors for oral cancer.[28]

Over recent years, the resurgence of smokeless tobacco[8] has presented the United States with a relatively new risk factor for oral cancer. Because its recent use is predominantly by young people,[9] it has so far made little impact on incidence and mortality data, although if its widespread use continues, it could lead to a sharp increase in the incidence of oral cancer in the years ahead. The dimensions of smokeless tobacco use, its effects on human health, and what dental professionals can do about it are discussed in Chapter 29.

Alcohol consumption is also identified as a risk factor, especially with heavier consumption, although not all studies have identified it as a risk factor independent of tobacco use.[44, 51, 79] There is frequently some degree of confounding between smoking and heavy use of alcohol since the two habits are often found together.

Other risk factors have been identified, although the evidence is less consistent than it is for smoking and alcohol. Painful and ill-fitting dentures are still often listed as a risk factor,[92] although supportive evidence is lacking. Long-term exposure to strong sunlight is seen as a risk factor in lip cancer, although evidence for that contention is not easy to find other than a higher prevalence in sunnier climates.[77] Chronic inflammation, such as that found with lichen planus, has also been suggested as a possible risk factor.[12]

In terms of diagnosis, concern has been expressed that survival rates of oral cancer are unnecessarily low because of delays by patients in seeking attention for lesions and because of delays in diagnosis by health professionals.[26] Dentists and hygienists must be sensitive to the presence of leukoplakia and other precancerous conditions, especially in patients who present with known risk factors in their history. Leukoplakia has long been known as a precancerous condition; that is, it has been documented to precede the development of cancer.[27] It has also been pointed out that mucosal erythroplasia, rather than leukoplakia, is often the first sign of cancerous change in a lesion.[49] A related issue is the unusually high rate of second primary cancers among patients who have previously had oral cancer, a finding that is also correlated with higher tobacco and alcohol consumption.[10]

The genetic role in oral cancers is likely to be strong, although it requires further definition at present. Although mutation of the p53 cancer-suppression gene has long been recognized as an etiologic factor in many forms of cancer, its role in oral cancer has not been well defined.[41] Further research in oral cancer is likely to focus on the genetic influences and molecular risk markers, but the importance of reducing the most common risk factors still remains.

OTHER SOFT-TISSUE LESIONS

As a general statement, the epidemiology of soft-tissue lesions other than cancer has not been well studied. Precancerous conditions are obviously the lesions of most concern. A precancerous lesion is defined as morphologically altered tissue in which cancer is more likely to occur than in its apparently normal counterpart.[91] The principal precancerous conditions for oral cancer are generally recognized as leukoplakia and erythroplakia.[20]

Leukoplakia, already mentioned in reference to use of tobacco, is usually defined as a white patch or plaque that cannot be characterized clinically or by pathologic examination as anything else[42, 87]; this is a definition-by-default that is not very satisfactory. There is no general figure for the prevalence of leukoplakia in the population; it seems to have been studied only in connection with known cancer risk factors such as smoking. The rate of transformation of leukoplakia lesions to oral cancer varies in different parts of the world, but is generally about 6%.[80] Erythroplakia is a bright red or velvety plaque that cannot be characterized clinically or pathologically as being due to anything else,[91] another definition-by-default. When these le-

sions are found, or even suspected, immediate biopsy is indicated.

In general, little is known about the distribution of other soft tissue conditions, including papillary hyperplasia, candidiasis, pemphigus and pemphigoid, lichen planus, and the prevalence of herpes infections.[20] Not surprisingly, risk factors have not been defined for these conditions (except that papillary hyperplasia is associated with ill-fitting dentures). There is a clear need for some basic epidemiologic research on all of these poorly understood conditions.

CLEFT LIP AND PALATE

Clefts are predominantly of genetic origin, and there is evidence of genetic-environmental interactions in their etiology.[6, 33, 73] The occurrence of cleft lip, cleft palate, or both in the United States each year was estimated years ago at 1 in 700 live births.[24] There is nothing to suggest that the rate has changed since then.

Attempts to isolate some of the environmental variables that are potential risk factors have proved difficult for several reasons. One is that the relatively low occurrence of clefts means that a large number of birth records need to be examined to establish statistical correlations. Second, although cleft lip and palate as a congenital malformation is supposedly recorded on birth certificates in the United States, this requirement is sometimes neglected.[46]

While the problems with these studies are recognized, epidemiologic correlations reported from several studies[25, 66, 69] are as follows:

- More facial clefts occur in boys, but more isolated cleft palates occur in girls.
- Cleft lip and palate appear more frequently in plural births than in single births.
- Babies with clefts generally are of lower birth weight, and a relation has been found between clefts and prematurity. There is a higher infant mortality rate among children born with clefts,[32] and 35% of those born with clefts have associated malformations. The higher mortality rate is attributed more to these associated malformations; clefts without associated malformations do not present an increased risk of infant mortality.[18]

The occurrence of clefts is also associated with:

- Threatened spontaneous abortion during the first and second trimesters of pregnancy
- Influenza and fever in the first trimester
- Maternal drug consumption during the first trimester

It has also been shown that among various ethnic groups in the United States, the lowest reported prevalence was among African-Americans and the highest among persons of Japanese ancestry.[25] It is not clear whether advancing age of parents is a risk factor, and no correlation has been reported between birth order and clefts. Research on the risk of clefts after maternal smoking during pregnancy has shown a weak role for tobacco exposure alone,[39, 89] although there is some evidence for a gene-environment interaction between maternal smoking during pregnancy and the infant genotype.[33, 73]

The small number of studies on clefts means that the probability of chance correlations being reported is moderately high. As a result, more study is needed to confirm the associations described.

MALOCCLUSION

The difficulties of quantifying malocclusion were described in Chapter 6. Differing cultural perceptions of what constitutes a malocclusion, differing perceptions of malocclusion between orthodontic specialists and general dentists, and difficulties in achieving a sufficient degree of examiner consistency in use of malocclusion indexes all make summary statements difficult.

Since the 1980s, no attempts have been made to measure malocclusions in national surveys because of the problems just mentioned, so existing national data are now old enough to be of questionable value. Malocclusion was last measured in the 1966–1970 National Health Examination survey of youths aged 12 to 17 in the United States.[85] This survey of a nationally representative sample of youths used the TPI (Treatment Priority Index), and results showed that a higher proportion of African-American than white youths seem to have either normal occlusion or minor malocclusion. There appeared to be little difference in malocclusions between young white males and females; however, a notably higher proportion of African-American females seem to have very severe malocclusion relative to African-American males.

A 1985 review of the prevalence of malocclusion in the United States[50] concluded that there was good epidemiologic evidence for significant departures from "normal occlusion" in American children, and that a majority of American children "would benefit from orthodontic treatment." Unfortunately that conclusion remains as problematic as it always was, because normal occlusion was not defined; in fact, the authors seemed to be referring to ideal occlusion. Whether these children would really benefit, or whether orthodontic treatment would make no difference to their oral status, is a matter of conjecture.

TEMPOROMANDIBULAR JOINT DISORDERS

Disturbances of the temporomandibular joint, usually referred to as TMD or TMPDS (temporomandibular pain and dysfunction sydrome), are a group of extremely painful and distressing conditions. There are 3 times as many women patients as men, although no one knows why.[30] Diagnosis is not easy because TMD is often accompanied by generalized pain in the head and neck region. There is no agreement on what constitutes standard treatment procedures, and treatment outcomes are mixed.[16] It is hardly surprising that the epidemiology of these conditions is poorly understood.[7, 11, 82, 83]

The difficulty in defining risk factors in TMD stems from the absence of a suitable case definition of TMD. To put the problem in perspective, disagreements on criteria for diagnosing caries (Chapter 14) exist only over a narrow range of clinical detection of an agreed-upon pathology. TMD conditions, however, go far beyond these relatively restricted definitional problems; they are more akin to the problems with measuring malocclusion. Where a condition cannot be defined, valid measurement is virtually impossible. Definitions of TMD exist,[64] but they tend to be all-encompassing and nonspecific, and hence of not much operational value for research purposes. Conferences on TMD have generally agreed that a case definition should include elements of pain and dysfunction, but agreement on specifics beyond that is hard to find.

Epidemiologic studies of TMD have measured various signs and symptoms in different population groups, so summation of the state of knowledge is difficult. Commonly measured signs and symptoms include pain in the joint or masseter muscles with joint movement, limitations in mandibular movement, mandibular deviations on opening, and joint clicking or crepitus. Studies have used both self-reported questionnaires and clinical examinations to obtain information. Many of what are referred to as epidemiologic studies in fact are clinical studies of patients receiving treatment, and so have to be interpreted cautiously.

There is agreement that the prevalence of the commonly measured conditions just listed is quite high, even among people who do not perceive that they have a problem that requires treatment.[13, 17, 19, 30, 52, 59, 63, 70, 78, 84, 88] One study of a representative population in Toronto found that 49% of adults responded positively to one or more of 9 questions regarding symptoms, although need for treatment was found in only 3% to 10%, depending on the case definition used.[43] It is far more difficult, however, to interpret what these data mean, for it is common to find prevalent symptoms having no clinical significance.[52, 65] Is a clicking joint, for example, a sign of impending trouble, or is it of no consequence? One longitudinal study found that a majority of patients with a painless click did develop joint pain in time,[4] although it should be noted that the group studied were already TMD patients for other reasons. Other longitudinal studies, however, have shown that many of these measured signs and symptoms are unstable over time, meaning that they come and go.[15, 47] It has been noted that signs and symptoms are as common in children and adolescents as they are in adults,[52, 82] although again the interpretation of these findings is unclear. Clicking joints in adolescents have been related to growth stages that come and go in response to "natural longitudinal fluctuations."[88] Cross-sectional studies therefore can yield misleading data with regard to prevalence and correlations.[40]

Although a great deal of TMD seems to have been treated by appliance therapy, the current view is that occlusal discrepancies such as attrition and premature contacts are not a factor in TMD[7, 31, 38, 72] and that TMD should be treated as a medical orthopedic problem rather than a purely dental one.[11, 23]

The need for a multidisciplinary approach to treatment is given weight by psychological studies of TMD patients. These studies are essential in dealing with the question of whether TMD is a discrete entity or whether it is part of broader psychological disturbances. Profiles of TMD patients have found that they tend to be of lower socioeconomic status,[5] that they tend to report their general health as being poorer than do nonpatients,[5, 30, 48] and that emotional distress and feelings of lack of control over their lives were common.[5, 71] (The cause-and-effect relationship is not necessarily defined as emotional stress leading to TMD. It could be the other way around, for continuing TMD, with no relief from pain despite treatment, could lead to emotional distress in otherwise normal persons.) Patients with complex orofacial pain conditions often do not respond as expected to treatment.[67] The state-of-the-art in terms of psychological correlates of TMD is confused, with contradictory findings in a number of studies.[53, 54, 68]

Research into this highly distressing condition has a long way to go before treatments with a firm scientific base can be formulated, let alone prevention strategies. The condition is highly complex and will require multidisciplinary effort for its better comprehension.

REFERENCES

1. American Cancer Society. Cancer facts and figures, 1997. Atlanta: ACS, 1997.
2. Binnie WH. Oral cancer. In: Dolby AE, ed: Oral mucosa in health and disease. Oxford, England: Blackwell, 1975:301-23.
3. Blot WJ, Devesa SS, McLaughlin JK, Fraumeni JF. Oral and pharyngeal cancers. Cancer Surv 1994; 19–20:23-42.
4. Brooke RI, Grainger RM. Long-term prognosis for the clicking jaw. Oral Surg Oral Med Oral Path 1988;65:668-70.
5. Carlsson GE, Kopp S, Wedel A. Analysis of background variables in 350 patients with TMJ disorders as reported in self-administered questionnaire. Community Dent Oral Epidemiol 1982;10:47-51.
6. Christensen K, Fogh-Andersen P. Cleft lip (+/- cleft palate) in Danish twins, 1970-1990. Am J Med Genet 1993;47:910-6.
7. Clark GT. Etiologic theory and the prevention of temporomandibular disorders. Adv Dent Res 1991; 5:60-6.
8. Connolly GN, Winn DM, Hecht SS, et al. The reemergence of smokeless tobacco. N Engl J Med 1986;314:1020-7.
9. Cullen JW, Blot W, Henningfield J, et al. Health consequences of using smokeless tobacco: Summary of the Advisory Committee's report to the Surgeon General. Public Health Rep 1986;101:355-73.
10. Day GL, Blot WJ, Shore RE, et al. Second cancers following oral and pharyngeal cancers: Role of tobacco and alcohol. J Natl Cancer Inst 1994;86:131-7.

11. de Bont LG, Dijkgraaf LC, Stegenga B. Epidemiology and natural progression of articular temporomandibular disorders. Oral Surg Oral Med Oral Pathol Oral Radiol Endod 1997;83:72-6.

12. Deeb ZE, Fox LA, deFries HO. The association of chronic inflammatory disease in lichen planus with cancer of the oral cavity. Am J Otolaryngol 1989;10:314-6.

13. Deng YM, Fu MK, Hagg U. Prevalence of temporomandibular joint dysfunction (TMJD) in Chinese children and adolescents. A cross-sectional epidemiological study. Eur J Orthodont 1995;17:305-9.

14. Dharkar D. Oral cancer in India: Need for fresh approaches. Cancer Detect Prev 1988;11:267-70.

15. Dibbets JM, van der Weele LT. Prevalence of TMJ symptoms and X-ray findings. Eur J Orthodont 1989;11:31-6.

16. Dolwick MF, Dimitroulis G. Is there a role for temporomandibular joint surgery? Br J Oral Maxillofac Surg 1994;32:307-13.

17. Droukas B, Lindee C, Carlsson GE. Relationship between occlusal factors and signs and symptoms of mandibular dysfunction. A clinical study of 48 dental students. Acta Odont Scand 1984;42:277-83.

18. Druschel CM, Hughes JP, Olsen CL. First year-of-life mortality among infants with oral clefts: New York State, 1983-1990. Cleft Palate Craniofac J 1996;33:400-5.

19. Ettala-Ylitalo UM, Syrjanen S, Halonen P. Functional disturbances of the masticatory system related to temporomandibular joint involvement by rheumatoid arthritis. J Oral Rehabil 1987;14:415-27.

20. Fischman SL. Oral health status in the United States: oral cancer and soft tissue lesions. J Dent Educ 1985;49:379-84.

21. Franceschi S, Talamini R, Barra S, et al. Smoking and drinking in relation to cancers of the oral cavity, pharynx, larynx, and esophagus in northern Italy. Cancer Res 1990;50:6502-7.

22. Franco EL, Kowalski LP, Oliveira BV, et al. Risk factors for oral cancer in Brazil: A case-control study. Int J Cancer 1989;43:992-1000.

23. Greene CS. Orthodontics and temporomandibular disorders. Dent Clin North Am 1988;32:529-38.

24. Greene JC. Epidemiology of congenital clefts of the lip and palate. Public Health Rep 1963;78:589-602.

25. Greene JC, Vermillion JR, Hay S, et al. Epidemiologic study of cleft lip and cleft palate in four states. J Am Dent Assoc 1964;68:387-404.

26. Guggenheimer J, Verbin RS, Johnson JT, et al. Factors delaying the diagnosis of oral and oropharyngeal carcinomas. Cancer 1989;64:932-5.

27. Gupta PC, Bhonsle RB, Murti PR, et al. An epidemiologic assessment of cancer risk in oral precancerous lesions in India with special reference to nodular leukoplakia. Cancer 1989;63:2247-52.

28. Gupta PC, Mehta FS, Pindborg JJ, et al. Primary intervention trial of oral cancer in India: A 10-year follow-up study. J Oral Pathol Med 1992;21:433-9.

29. Gupta PC, Pindborg JJ, Mehta FS. Comparison of carcinogenicity of betel quid with and without tobacco: An epidemiological review. Ecol Dis 1982;1:213-9.

30. Helkimo M. Epidemiological surveys of dysfunction of the masticatory system. Oral Science Rev 1976;7:54-69.

31. Houston F, Hanamura H, Carlsson GE, et al. Mandibular dysfunction and periodontitis. A comparative study of patients with periodontal disease and occlusal parafunctions. Acta Odont Scand 1987;45:239-46.

32. Hujoel PP, Bollen AM, Mueller BA. First-year mortality among infants with facial clefts. Cleft Palate Craniofac J 1992;29:451-5.

33. Hwang SJ, Beaty TH, Panny SR, et al. Association study of transforming growth factor alpha (TGF alpha) TaqI polymorphism and oral clefts: Indication of gene-environment interaction in a population-based sample of infants with birth defects. Am J Epidemiol 1995;141:629-36.

34. International Classification of Diseases, 9th revision, Clinical Modification, 4th ed. Los Angeles: Practice Management Information Corporation, 1994.

35. Johnson NW. Orofacial neoplasms: Global epidemiology, risk factors and recommendations for research. Int Dent J 1991;41:365-75.

36. Jones JB, Lampe HB, Cheung HW. Carcinoma of the tongue in young patients. J Otolaryngol 1989;18:105-8.

37. Kabat GC, Hebert JR, Wynder EL. Risk factors for oral cancer in women. Cancer Res 1989;49:2803-6.

38. Kampe T, Carlsson GE, Hannerz H, Haraldson T. Three-year longitudinal study of mandibular dysfunction in young adults with intact and restored dentitions. Acta Odont Scand 1987;45:25-30.

39. Khoury MJ, Gomez-Farias M, Mulinare J. Does maternal cigarette smoking during pregnancy cause cleft lip and palate in offspring? Am J Dis Child 1989;143:333-7.

40. Kirveskari P, Alanen P, Jamsa T. Association between craniomandibular disorders and occlusal interferences. J Prosth Dent 1989;62:66-9.

41. Koch WM, Boyle JO, Mao L, et al. p53 gene mutations as markers of tumor spread in synchronous oral cancers. Arch Otolaryngol Head Neck Surg 1994;120:943-7.

42. Kramer I, El-Labban N, Lee K. The clinical features and risk of malignant transformation in sublingual keratosis. Br Dent J 1978;144:171-80.

43. Locker D, Slade G. Prevalence of symptoms associated with temporomandibular disorders in a Canadian population. Community Dent Oral Epidemiol 1988;16:310-13.

44. Luce D, Guenel P, Leclerc A, et al. Alcohol and tobacco consumption in cancer of the mouth, pharynx, and larynx: A study of 316 female patients. Laryngoscope 1988;98:313-6.

45. Macfarlane GJ, Sharp L, Porter S, Francheschi S. Trends in survival from cancers of the oral cavity and pharynx in Scotland: A clue as to why the disease is becoming more common? Br J Cancer 1996;73:805-8.

46. Mackeprang M, Hay S, Lunde AS. Completeness and accuracy of reporting of malformations on birth certificates. HSMHA Health Rep 1972;87:43-9.

47. Magnusson T, Egermark-Eriksson I, Carlsson GE. Four-year longitudinal study of mandibular dysfunction in children. Community Dent Oral Epidemiol 1985;13:117-20.

48. Marbach JJ, Lennon MC, Dohrenwend BP. Candidate risk factors for temporomandibular pain and dysfunction syndrome: Psychosocial, health behavior, physical illness and injury. Pain 1988;34:139-51.

49. Mashberg A, Samit AM. Early detection, diagnosis, and management of oral and oropharyngeal cancer. CA 1989;39:67-88.

50. McLain JB, Proffitt WR. Oral health status in the United States: Prevalence of malocclusion. J Dent Educ 1985;49:386-96.

51. Merletti F, Boffetta P, Ciccone G, et al. Role of tobacco and alcoholic beverages in the etiology of cancer of

the oral cavity/oropharynx in Torino, Italy. Cancer Res 1989;49:4919-24.

52. Mintz SS. Craniomandibular dysfunction in children and adolescents: A review. Cranio 1993;11:224-31.

53. Moss RA, Adams HE. The assessment of personality, anxiety and depression in mandibular pain dysfunction subjects. J Oral Rehabil 1984;11:233-5.

54. Moss RA, Garrett JC. Temporomandibular joint disfunction syndrome and myofascial pain dysfunction syndrome: A critical review. J Oral Rehabil 1984;11:3-28.

55. Murti PR, Bhonsle RB, Gupta PC, et al. Etiology of submucous fibrosis with special reference to the role of areca nut chewing. J Oral Pathol Med 1995;24:145-52.

56. Murti PR, Gupta PC, Bhonsle RB, et al. Effect on the incidence of oral submucous fibrosis of intervention in the areca nut chewing habit. J Oral Pathol Med 1990;19:99-100.

57. Nandakumar A, Thimmasetty KT, Sreeramareddy NM, et al. A population-based case-control investigation on cancers of the oral cavity in Bangalore, India. Br J Cancer 1990;62:847-51.

58. Negri E, La Vecchia C, Levi F, et al. Comparative descriptive epidemiology of oral and oesophageal cancers in Europe. Eur J Cancer Prev 1996;5:267-79.

59. Nielsen L, Melsen B, Terp S. Prevalence, interrelation, and severity of signs of dysfunction from masticatory system in 14-16-year-old Danish children. Community Dent Oral Epidemiol 1989;17:91-6.

60. O'Hanlon S, Forster DP, Lowry RJ. Oral cancer in the North-East of England: Incidence, mortality trends and the link with material deprivation. Community Dent Oral Epidemiol 1997;25:371-6.

61. Parker SL, Tong T, Bolden S, Wingo PA. Cancer statistics, 1997. CA 1997;47:5-27.

62. Pindborg JJ. Epidemiological studies of oral cancer. Int Dent J 1977;27:172-8.

63. Pullinger AG, Seligman DA, Solberg WK. Temporomandibular disorders. Part I: Functional status, dentomorphologic features, and sex differences in a nonpatient population. J Prosthet Dent 1988;59:228-35.

64. Ramfjord SP, Ash MM, Jr. Occlusion. 3rd ed. Philadelphia: W.B. Saunders, 1983:175.

65. Riolo ML, TenHave TR, Brandt D. Clinical validity of the relationship between TMJ signs and symptoms in children and youth. J Dent Child 1988;55:110-3.

66. Robert E, Kallen B, Harris J. The epidemiology of orofacial clefts. I. Some general epidemiological characteristics. J Craniofac Genet Dev Biol 1996;16:234-41.

67. Rugh JD. Psychological components of pain. Dent Clin North Am 1987;31:579-94.

68. Rugh JD, Solberg WK. Psychological implications in temporomandibular pain and dysfunction. Oral Sci Rev 1976;7:3-30.

69. Saxen I. Epidemiology of cleft lip and palate; an attempt to rule out chance correlations. Br J Prevent Social Med 1975;29:103-10.

70. Schiffman EL, Fricton JR, Haley DP, Shapiro BL. The prevalence and treatment needs of subjects with temporomandibular disorders. J Am Dent Assoc 1990;120:295-303.

71. Schwartz RA, Greene CS, Laskin DM. Personality characteristics of patients with myofascial pain-dysfunction (MPD) syndrome unresponsive to conventional therapy. J Dent Res 1979;58:1435-9.

72. Seligman DA, Pullinger AG, Solberg WK. The prevalence of dental attrition and its association with fac-tors of age, gender, occlusion, and TMJ symptomatology. J Dent Res 1988;67:1323-33.

73. Shaw GM, Wasserman CR, Lammer EJ, et al. Orofacial clefts, parental cigarette smoking, and transforming growth factor-alpha gene variants. Am J Hum Genet 1996;58:551-61.

74. Silverberg E, Lubera JA. Cancer statistics, 1988. CA 1988;38:5-22.

75. Sinor PN, Gupta PC, Murti PR, et al. A case-control study of oral submucous fibrosis with special reference to the etiologic role of areca nut. J Oral Pathol Med 1990;19:94-8.

76. Smith CJ. Global epidemiology and aetiology of oral cancer. Int Dent J 1973;23:82-93.

77. Smith CJ, Pindborg JJ, Binnie WH, eds: Oral cancer; epidemiology, etiology, and pathology. New York: Hemisphere, 1990.

78. Solberg WK, Woo MW, Houston JB. Prevalence of mandibular dysfunction in young adults. J Am Dent Assoc 1979;98:25-34.

79. Spitz MR, Fueger JJ, Goepfert H, et al. Squamous cell carcinoma of the upper aerodigestive tract. A case comparison analysis. Cancer 1988;61:203-8.

80. Squier CA. Smokeless tobacco and oral cancer: A cause for concern? CA 1984;34:242-7.

81. Swango PA. Cancers of the oral cavity and pharynx in the United States: An epidemiologic overview. J Public Health Dent 1996;56:309-18.

82. Tallents RH. Etiologic theory and prevention of temporomandibular joint disorders: Reaction paper. Adv Dent Res 1991;5:67-8.

83. Tallents RH, Catania J, Sommers E. Temporomandibular joint findings in pediatric populations and young adults: A critical review. Angle Orthod 1991;61:7-16.

84. Tervonen T, Knuuttila M. Prevalence of signs and symptoms of mandibular dysfunction among adults aged 25, 35, 50 and 65 years in Ostrobothnia, Finland. J Oral Rehabil 1988;15:455-63.

85. US Public Health Service, National Center for Health Statistics. An assessment of the occlusion of the teeth of youths 12-17 years, United States. DHEW Publ No (HRA) 77-1644, Series 11 No 162. Washington DC: Government Printing Office, 1977.

86. US Public Health Service, National Center for Health Statistics. Vital statistics of the United States 1991. Vol 11: Mortality, part B. DHSS Publ No (PHS) 95-1102. Washington DC: Government Printing Office, 1995.

87. Waldron C, Shafer W. Leukoplakia revisited. A clinico-pathologic study of 3,256 oral leukoplakias. Cancer 1975;36:1386-92.

88. Wanman A, Agerberg G. Temporomandibular joint sounds in adolescents: A longitudinal study. Oral Surg Oral Med Oral Pathol 1990;69:2-9.

89. Werler MM, Lammer EJ, Rosenberg L, Mitchell AA. Maternal cigarette smoking during pregnancy in relation to oral clefts. Am J Epidemiol 1990;132:926-32.

90. World Health Organization. Application of the International Classification of Diseases to dentistry and stomatology. 3rd ed. Geneva: WHO, 1995.

91. World Health Organization, Collaborating Reference Centre for Oral Precancerous Lesions. Definition of leukoplakia and related lesions: An aid to studies on oral precancer. Oral Surg 1978;46:517-39.

92. Young TB, Ford CN, Brandenburg JH. An epidemiologic study of oral cancer in a statewide network. Am J Otolaryngol 1986;7:200-8.

section V

Prevention of Oral Diseases in Public Health

23

Fluoride: Human Health and Caries Prevention

A Classic Epidemiologic Study ◆ Environmental Fluoride ◆ Sources and Amounts of Fluoride Intake ◆ Fluoride Physiology ◆ Absorption, Retention, and Excretion ◆ ``Optimum Fluoride Intake'' ◆ Fluoride and Human Health: Early Studies, Mortality, Cancer, Down Syndrome, Bone Strength, Child Development ◆ Fluoride Toxicity ◆ Fluoride and Caries Control, Mechanisms of Action: Fluoride and Plaque, Enamel, Saliva ◆ Effects on Different Tooth Surfaces ◆ Effective Use of Fluoride

It is hard to describe adequately what caries used to look like in prefluoride days. Dentists commonly saw periapical abscesses and gaping anterior lesions. Extractions of first molars in young children were routine, and full extractions and complete dentures were virtually the norm for older people. Although higher educational levels, better technology, and the spread of middle-class standards have improved this situation, fluoride ranks as a primary influence in better oral health because its impact changed the way people thought about dental health. It demonstrated to patients and nonpatients alike that caries and subsequent tooth loss were not inevitable. Just as important, it helped dentists to reshape their attitudes toward tooth conservation and retention.

This chapter describes how fluoride's caries-inhibitory potential was first discovered, how the human physiology deals with fluoride when the material is ingested, fluoride's effect on our health, and how it works to prevent caries. The story begins with one of the great epidemiologic studies in health research.

A CLASSIC EPIDEMIOLOGIC STUDY

Dr. Frederick McKay, a new dental graduate in the early 1900s, headed west and opened a practice in Colorado Springs, Colorado. He soon noticed that many of his patients had a curious blotching of the enamel that he had not encountered before. People in the area called it "Colorado brown stain," and to them it was just a local oddity. It seemed harmless enough, although it was disfiguring in some cases. McKay was clearly a born scientist; he had an inquiring mind and fine powers of observation, and the condition piqued his curiosity. In 1908, he began to investigate the extent of Colorado brown stain in the surrounding area.

In his travels over the next few years, McKay found that the condition was highly prevalent in the Colorado Springs area. It was found only in long-term residents, individuals who had been born there or who had come to the area as babies. Since the stain was intrinsic, McKay reasoned that it must be caused by an environmental agent that was active during the period of enamel formation. To ensure that his findings attracted some attention, McKay was shrewd enough to enlist the collaboration of G.V. Black, a major figure in dental history, in writing the first description of what then came to be called *mottled enamel*.[13] This detailed report, in the elegant prose of the time, is a tribute to McKay's investigative thoroughness.

McKay found that mottled enamel was

endemic in many other communities along the Continental Divide and the plains to the east. It was most prevalent where deep artesian wells were the source of drinking water, and within any community the persons affected had almost invariably been users of the same water supply. By the 1920s, McKay had reached the conclusion that the etiologic agent had to be a constituent of some community water supplies, although chemical analyses all failed to identify likely constituents. In communities such as Andover and Britton, South Dakota, where he found severe mottling, he advised mothers to obtain their children's drinking water from sources other than the community supply. In Oakley, Idaho, McKay found that children living on the outskirts of the city, using water from a private spring, were free of mottling. He advised the citizens of Oakley to abandon their old supply and tap this spring for a new source, which the community did in 1925. McKay was right, for children born in Oakley subsequent to the change were free of mottled enamel.[125]

By 1930, new methods of spectrographic analysis of water had been developed. In 1931, McKay sent several samples of suspected waters to an Alcoa Company chemist named Churchill, who was using these new methods. Churchill identified fluoride (F) in each of the samples, in amounts ranging up to 14 parts per million (ppm).[23] Around the same time similar findings were reported from the University of Arizona[162] and from Morocco, still a French colony at the time, by a veterinary group studying *le darmous*, the local name given to an extreme degree of mottled enamel found in Moroccan sheep.[179]

The immediate reaction of the scientific community to the identification of F in drinking waters was one of concern, because F in high concentrations was known to be a protoplasmic poison. The discovery led to the appointment, in 1931, of the first dentist in the newly established National Institute of Health. This was H. Trendley Dean, who was transferred from elsewhere in the US Public Health Service to become the one-person Dental Hygiene Unit,[155] an odd name for a unit formed to investigate mottled enamel (although it subsequently became the National Institute of Dental Research [NIDR] in 1948).*

Amidst this flurry of concern, McKay

had also noted some benefits that seemed to accompany mottled enamel. In 1928, 3 years before F was identified in drinking waters, he was confident enough to publish his view that caries experience was reduced by the same waters that produced mottled enamel.[124] A similar observation was made shortly afterward in England by Ainsworth,[2] who, like McKay, was an observant dentist with an inquiring mind. While McKay was not the first to make this suggestion,[163] none of the earlier observers took the idea any further. McKay, and Dean too, are good examples of history putting the right people in the right place at the right time.

The task of defining the F-mottled enamel relationship now passed to Dean. His first task was to try to map out the prevalence of mottled enamel in the United States. Dean began like an investigative reporter, writing extensively to dental societies around the country to ask for their experiences. He received a good response, and published his first map on the distribution of mottled enamel in 1933.[30] His next step was to develop a 7-point, ordinal scale to classify the full range of mottled enamel, from the finest of lacy markings to the corroded, stained, and highly friable enamel seen with extreme hypomineralization.[31]

Dean began using the term *fluorosis* to replace mottled enamel in the mid-1930s.[37] He patiently surveyed children in many parts of the country, using his original fluorosis index, and built up a substantial body of information (what today would be called a database) for analysis. He devised a community index of fluorosis based on his original 7 grades of severity.[36] Studies through the mid-1930s analyzed many drinking water samples for minerals and other chemical constituents, but none apart from F could be related to fluorosis.[37, 39] Dean chose his words carefully to define a desirable fluoride concentration as follows:

> For public health purposes, we have arbitrarily defined the minimal threshold of fluoride concentration in a domestic water supply as the highest concentration of fluoride incapable of producing a definite degree of mottled enamel in as much as 10 percent of the group examined.[37]

By the mid-1930s, Dean had concluded that this "minimal threshold" level was 1.0 ppm F,[32] and that fluorosis below 1.0 ppm F was "of no public health significance."[38] Soon afterwards he called 1.0 ppm F "the permissible maximum."[43] Later in that decade of the

---

*NIDR became NIDCR, the National Institute of Dental and Craniofacial Research, in 1998.

Great Depression, Dean condensed his original 1934 fluorosis index to one using a 6-point ordinal scale (Chapter 16) by combining the moderately severe and severe categories.[40] He then added numerical values to the categories to permit quantitative comparisons among populations. By 1942, Dean had documented the prevalence of fluorosis for most of the United States.[34]

Although still documenting fluorosis in his studies, the main theme of Dean's research from now on was the F-caries relationship. In the mid-1930s, Dean matched his fluorosis data from children in parts of South Dakota, Colorado, and Wisconsin with the caries data from an earlier 26-state survey, in what today would be called an ecologic study (Chapter 12). Although he could hardly have failed to notice the low caries experience in communities with F-bearing waters during his early surveys, this was his first report in which he commented on the inverse relationship between fluorosis and caries.[33]

Encouraged by these preliminary data, Dean chose 4 cities in central Illinois as a study site in which to test the hypothesis that consumption of F-containing waters was associated with a reduced prevalence of caries. Galesburg and Monmouth, where Dean had already studied fluorosis,[38] used waters from deep wells that averaged 1.8 and 1.7 ppm F. Macomb and Quincy used surface waters averaging 0.2 ppm F. Clinical examinations of children aged 12 to 14 years, all with lifetime residence in their respective cities, showed that there were more than twice as many caries-free children in Galesburg and Monmouth than in the two low-F cities, and the mean number of permanent teeth affected by caries in Galesburg and Monmouth was half of that in the 2 low-F cities.[42] The evidence to support an F-caries hypothesis was now stronger.

Although caries prevalence and severity were low in Galesburg and Monmouth, fluorosis was an obvious problem in both communities. In the words of the investigators:

[It is] obvious that whatever effect the waters with relatively high fluoride content (over 2.0 ppm of F) have on dental caries is largely one of academic interest; the resultant permanent disfigurement of many of the users far outweighs any advantage that might accrue from the standpoint of partial control of dental caries. On the other hand, the demonstration of such marked dental caries differences as were observed at Galesburg and Quincy made advisable a quantitative study of the influ-ence on dental caries of waters with lower ranges of fluoride concentration. If marked inhibitory influences were operative at concentration levels as low as the minimal threshold of endemic fluorosis (1.0 ppm), the findings would be of considerable import.[41]

The next logical step was to define the lowest F level at which caries was clearly inhibited. This was done through a series of investigations that have become known collectively as the 21 Cities Study and that is rightly considered a landmark in dental research. The first part consisted of the results of clinical examinations of children aged 12 to 14 years who were lifetime residents in 8 suburban Chicago communities with various but stable mean F levels in their domestic waters.[41] The project was later expanded by adding data from 13 additional cities in Illinois, Colorado, Ohio, and Indiana.[35] The collective findings from the 21 Cities Study are shown graphically in Figures 23–1 and 23–2. Figure 23–1 shows that dental caries experience in different communities dropped sharply as F concentration rose toward 1.0 ppm, then leveled off. Figure 23–2 shows the dental fluorosis experience that Dean found among the 12 to 14 year-olds in the 21 cities. Dean's practice was to show questionable fluorosis separately in his reports, as we have done in Figure 23–2. The data in Figure 23–2 suggest that if questionable fluorosis had been included in the prevalence figures, then "acceptable fluorosis" may have been set at concentrations lower than 1.0 ppm F.

The results of the 21 Cities Study, being cross-sectional in design, confirmed the association but could not by themselves establish the cause-and-effect relationship between fluoridated water and reduced caries prevalence. The data in Figures 23–1 and 23–2, however, did lead to the adoption of 1.0 to 1.2 ppm as the appropriate concentration of F in drinking water for temperate climates, a standard that remains in place today. It also set the stage for a prospective test of the F-caries hypothesis. The years of study among people using waters with F levels much higher than the proposed 1.0 ppm (see later) was sufficient to convince public authorities that the prospective tests could be carried out in safety. These first prospective studies are described in Chapter 24.

Trendley Dean died in 1962. Those who knew him said that he could be autocratic, and the reverence he inspired in his colleagues may too often have been expressed

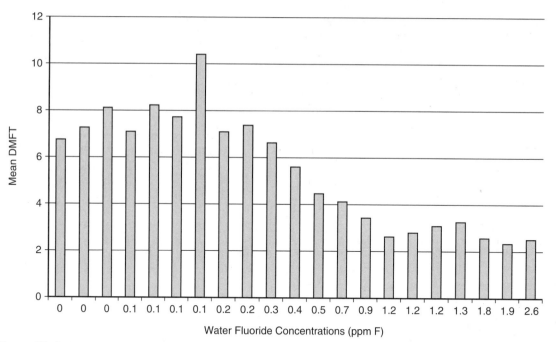

Figure 23–1. Caries experience of children aged 12–14 in 21 cities in the late 1930s, related to fluoride concentration of drinking water. (From Dean HT, Arnold FA Jr, Elvove E. Domestic water and caries. V. Additional studies of the relation of fluoride domestic waters to dental caries experience in 4,425 white children aged 2–14 years, of 13 cities in 4 states. Public Health Rep 1942; 57:1155–79; Dean HT, Jay P, Arnold FA Jr, Elvove E. Domestic water and dental caries. II. A study of 2,832 white children aged 12–14 years, of eight suburban Chicago communities, including *L. acidophilus* studies of 1,761 children. Public Health Rep 1941;56:761–92.)

as uncritical acceptance of all he did. Nevertheless, Dean had the researcher's virtues of dogged perseverance and remorseless logic as he progressed from one stage to the next. His grasp of the concept of "databasing" and his analytical mind make us wonder what he could have done with modern computer technology. Knowledge of F's effects has advanced considerably since those days, but we enjoy the benefits of F today because of the pioneering research of Dean and his colleagues. In time, it led to a substantial decline in dental caries in the economically developed nations, one of history's major public health success stories.

ENVIRONMENTAL FLUORIDE

Fluorine is one of the most reactive elements and therefore is never found naturally in its elemental form. The F ion, however, is abundant in nature and occurs almost universally in soils and waters in varying, but generally low, concentrations.[187] Seawater contains 1.2 to 1.4 ppm F.[186] Fresh surface waters generally have very low concentrations, 0.2

ppm F or less, whereas concentrations of up to 29.5 ppm F have been recorded in deep well waters in Arizona[117] and over 40 ppm in boreholes in Kenya.[110] F's ubiquity in soil and water means that all plants and animals contain F to some extent. Given this environmental ubiquity, it seems likely that all forms of life must have evolved to thrive with continuous exposure to small amounts of F.

SOURCES AND AMOUNTS OF FLUORIDE INTAKE

Humans absorb F from air, food, and water. Air intake is usually negligible, around 0.04 mg F/day.[185] Exceptions can occur around some industrial plants that work with F-rich material, such as aluminum smelters without safeguards to prevent the escape of F-containing compounds.[73] Such environmental hazards should be controlled to the extent possible, an issue that has nothing to do with the use of F to control caries.

F's abundance in soils and plants means that everyone consumes some F. Studies to estimate the average daily intake of F from

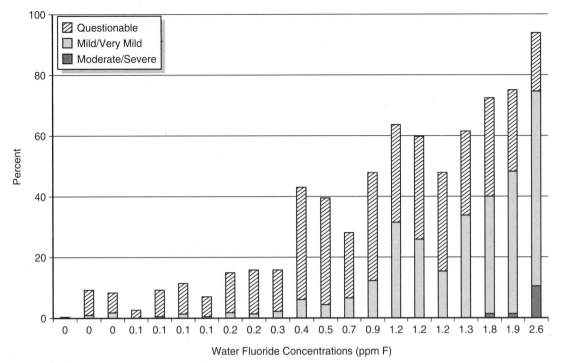

Figure 23–2. Fluorosis experience of children aged 12–14 in 21 cities in the late 1930s, related to the fluoride concentration of drinking water. (From Dean HT, Arnold FA Jr, Elvove E. Domestic water and caries. V. Additional studies of the relation of fluoride domestic waters to dental caries experience in 4,425 white children aged 2–14 years, of 13 cities in 4 states. Public Health Rep 1942; 57:1155–79; Dean HT, Jay P, Arnold FA Jr, Elvove E. Domestic water and dental caries. II. A study of 2,832 white children aged 12–14 years, of eight suburban Chicago communities, including *L. acidophilus* studies of 1,761 children. Public Health Rep 1941;56:761–92.)

all sources have provided fairly consistent results, despite both the variability of the human diet and methodologic difficulties inherent in analyzing such minute amounts.[172] Estimates for an adult North American male in a fluoridated area fall within the range of 1 to 3 mg F per day from food and beverages,[28, 60, 99, 138, 158, 159, 167, 173] decreasing to 1.0 mg F per day or less in a nonfluoridated area.[28, 99, 138, 158, 159] Estimates from "market basket" analyses are that 6-month-old infants ingest 0.21 to 0.54 mg F/day in 4 American cities with different F concentrations in the drinking water. For 2-year-olds in the same cities, the range was 0.41 to 0.61 mg F/day.[136, 137]

More refined estimates of F intake by infants came from a series of studies in Iowa during the 1990s, which recognized that F exposure was much more extensive than it used to be.[105] Infant formulas and baby foods contained variable amounts of F, fluoridated water was of course often used in their preparation, and some infants were exposed to F toothpaste and F supplements. The Iowa studies documented the F exposures of newborn infants at periodic intervals through ex-

tensive interviews about all likely sources of F exposure. Total F intakes from drinking water alone during the first 9 months of life, either consumed directly or when added to formula and juice, averaged 0.29 to 0.38 mg F/day, although in some infants was as high as 1.73 mg F/day.[106] Although mean intakes were similar to those estimated from the earlier market basket surveys, there was considerable range of intake. Approximately 25% of 9-month-old children, for example, were ingesting 0.49 mg F/day or more. Even without swallowing F toothpaste or taking F supplements, the risk of dental fluorosis is likely to be increased in these children because the upper limit of intake for 12-month-old children, beyond which the risk of detectable fluorosis is increased, has been estimated at 0.43 mg F/day.[18]

For most people, water and other beverages provide 75% of F intake, whether or not the drinking water is fluoridated.[159] This can occur because many soft drinks and fruit juices are processed in fluoridated cities, or it may reflect variable F content of the ingredients. One brand of grape juice in North Caro-

Table 23–1. THE FLUORIDE CONCENTRATION (PPM) OF VARIOUS BEVERAGES AVAILABLE IN A NONFLUORIDATED AND A FLUORIDATED COMMUNITY IN ALBERTA, CANADA, AND FROM VARIOUS COMMUNITIES IN NORTH CAROLINA

BEVERAGE	NONFLUORIDATED, CANADA	FLUORIDATED, CANADA	NORTH CAROLINA*
Drinking water	0.23	1.08	
Milk†	0.03	0.03	
Juice (commercially prepared)‡	0.80	0.80	0.36
Juice (home reconstituted)	0.21	1.06	
Carbonated drinks‡	0.80	0.80	0.74
Soup	0.21	1.06	
Tea	1.33	2.18	2.56
Coffee	0.23	1.08	
Gatorade			0.85

*Means of samples from six cities.
†Available fluoride.
‡Commercially available prepared juice and the carbonated drinks in Canada both came from a fluoridated large city.
Data from Clovis J, Hargreaves JA. Fluoride intake from beverage consumption. Community Dent Oral Epidemiol 1988;16:11–15; Pang DTY, Phillips CL, Bawden JW. Fluoride intake from beverage consumption in a sample of North Carolina children. J Dent Res 1992;71:1382–8.

lina, for example, was found to contain more than 1.6 ppm F, even when reconstituted with deionized water.[140] The F content of some tested beverages is shown in Table 23–1.

FLUORIDE PHYSIOLOGY

Although the use of F is a contribution to the public's health of which dentistry can be proud, F compounds must be handled responsibly and with respect. Everyone in dentistry should understand how the human body handles ingested F so that the material can be used safely and efficiently.

Absorption, Retention, and Excretion

Ingested F is absorbed mainly from the upper gastrointestinal tract. About 80% of F in food is absorbed, as is 85% to 97% of F in water.[27] Absorbed F is transported in the plasma, and is either excreted or deposited in the calcified tissues. Most absorbed F is excreted in the urine[88]; a single ingestion of 5.0 mg F is absorbed and cleared from the blood in 8 to 9 hours.[185] F ingested on an empty stomach produces a peak plasma level within 30 minutes. The time of the plasma peak is extended, and the level of the peak reduced, if F is taken with food. This is probably because of the binding of some F with calcium and other divalent and trivalent cations. When F absorption is inhibited this way, fecal excretion of F increases.[48]

Studies on what is called the *body burden* of F, meaning how much can be safely absorbed and at what point F absorption becomes a health concern, have mostly relied on urinary volumes and plasma concentrations as the primary measures. Samples of both are relatively simple to obtain, although both measures record only recent F intake (i.e., the previous 3 to 4 weeks) rather than lifetime intakes. Urinary concentrations can vary considerably with fluid intake during the period of F exposure[46] and require a 24-hour sample to be accurate. Accurate monitoring of plasma levels in individuals also requires frequent measures because of normal hour-to-hour fluctuations.[4, 47] Plasma F concentrations are more closely correlated with urinary flow rates than with urinary F concentrations.[49] Although there is no absolute measure of lifetime F intake, even theoretically, the nearest measure of long-term F intake would come from bone F content. For research purposes, however, this is a theoretical concept only; people don't volunteer to give a bone sample!

Fluoride balance is the net result from the accumulated effects of F ingestion, degree of F deposition in bones and teeth, mobilization rate of F from bone, and the efficiency of the kidneys in clearing absorbed F.[48]

Plasma F is found in ionic and nonionic forms. The biologic significance of the nonionic form has not yet been determined, and it seems to be independent of F intake.[71] Absorbed F is transported by plasma as ionic F; it is the level of this ionic F that rises temporarily after F ingestion and then drops rapidly; ionic F levels are not homeostatically regulated. In a healthy male living in a fluoridated area, plasma F levels are around 0.019 ppm (1 μmol/L), although this level fluctuates throughout the day.[48] Plasma levels are generally higher in persons living in fluoridated communities than in those living in nonfluoridated communities. Plasma F levels in persons with chronic kidney failure can rise to 0.05 to 0.09 ppm F (2.6 to 4.7 μmol/L)[88] without affecting health. Nephrotoxic plasma F values in healthy individuals have been estimated at 0.95 ppm F (50 μmol/L), although it is not clear whether it is this peak value itself, or the time for which it is maintained, that leads to kidney damage.[50]

F has an affinity for calcified tissues (i.e., bone and developing teeth). F that is not excreted is deposited in these hard tissues, although storage is dynamic rather than inert. Bone F levels (from postmortem assays) range from 800 to 10,000 ppm, depending on many factors, including age and F intake.[183] F levels in the outer few microns of dental enamel range from 400 to 3000 ppm and decrease rapidly with greater enamel depth. F concentrations in soft tissue rise or fall parallel to plasma F levels, but because healthy excretion and deposition mechanisms operate so rapidly there are negligible concentrations of F in the fluids of soft tissues other than the kidney.[186] Some F has been found in the aorta, associated with calcification of that blood vessel,[160] and deposition in the placenta is also associated with islets of calcified tissue.[55] A greater proportion of ingested F is excreted in older persons than in the young. It had been suggested that this was because children had lower renal clearance rates than adults,[166] but is now attributed to greater adsorption of F by the young skeleton.[186]

Because of the importance of the kidneys in maintaining F balance, the only disease condition which requires medical consideration in regard to more-or-less normal F ingestion is chronic kidney failure. Patients who receive renal dialysis for long periods with F-free water have maintained plasma levels of 0.06 ppm F, whereas some mistakenly dialyzed with fluoridated water (definitely not a recommended procedure) have recorded levels as high as 0.24 ppm F. Although plasma levels of around 0.09 ppm F had been suggested as the upper limit after which a patient on dialysis should reduce F intake, evidence for this recommendation has come only from a few case studies.[88] With today's standards for dialysate fluid, current medical opinion is that even persons with severe renal impairment can consume fluoridated water without ill effects as long as they are receiving regular dialysis treatment.

Aluminum, iron, and other minerals create greater technical problems for the renal dialysis process than does F. The standard for dialysate water set by the Association for Advancement of Medical Instrumentation is that the F content should not exceed 0.2 ppm.[92] Water used in renal dialysis should first be treated by reverse osmosis, which is superior to the older process of deionization in that it removes F and the other minerals almost entirely.[168]

"Optimum Fluoride Intake"

Frank McClure, a biochemist with the US Public Health Service, estimated in 1943 that the "average daily diet" contained 1.0 to 1.5 mg F, or about 0.05 mg F/kg body weight/day in children up to 12 years of age.[115] McClure's estimate somehow came to be interpreted as the lower limit of the range of "optimum" F intake. A widely quoted 1974 report[56] suggested 0.06 mg F/kg body weight/day as "optimum," although this estimate was based only on a number of personal opinions. The range of 0.05 to 0.07 mg F/kg body weight/day was suggested as "optimum" in 1980,[136] and has even been accepted by opponents of water fluoridation.[161] The estimate of 0.05 to 0.07 mg F/kg/day converts to 3.5 to 4.9 mg F per day for a man weighing 70 kg (154 lb). For a 10-kg infant (22 lb), that is a 12- to 18-month-old child, this "optimum" intake converts to 0.45 to 0.64 mg F/day. (As noted previously, the Iowa studies found that 25% of 9-month-old children were ingesting 0.49 mg F or more from water alone.)

The National Research Council, the body that establishes recommended dietary allowances for the United States, considers F to be a "beneficial element for humans" because of its positive impact on dental health.[132] The council at one time considered F an essential nutrient,[131] but has since backed away from that position because an essential role for F in human growth studies could not be confirmed, and because the physiologic mechanism by which F would influence growth was unknown. Available evidence did not justify classifying F as an essential element by accepted standards.[132]

The discussions about "optimum intake" are vague about what this intake is "optimum" for. The implication is that this degree of ingestion is "optimum" for caries resistance, but as will be described later in this chapter, little of F's action in caries control can be attributed to ingested F. It is also worth noting that McClure's 1943 comment was observational, although it somehow became a recommendation over time. Empiric evidence suggests that F intake of 0.05 to 0.07 mg/F/kg/day in childhood is a broad upper limit if unaesthetic fluorosis is to be avoided.[18] There is no evidence to link this range of F ingestion with caries inhibition, so we suggest that the term "optimum intake" be dropped from common usage.

FLUORIDE AND HUMAN HEALTH

Early Studies

Much was known about F at the time of Dean's appointment in the US Public Health Service in 1933,[114] but details of a safe range of F intake for humans were sketchy. The first study relating bone fracture experience to the F concentration in home water supplies, a subject revisited in the 1990s, concluded that there was no relationship.[116] McClure then demonstrated the close relationship between urinary F and the F levels of domestic water.[118] His balance studies during World War II, in which young men lived in rooms controlled for varying temperatures and humidity and received varying amounts of F in food and water, led to the conclusion that the elimination of absorbed F via urine and perspiration is almost complete when the quantity absorbed does not exceed 4 to 5 mg daily.[122] McClure suggested that this may be the F limit that could be ingested without "appreciable hazard" of excessive F storage in the body.

Higher F intakes were likely in such communities as Bartlett, Texas, where community water carried about 8.0 ppm F. A long-term study of the residents of Bartlett, conducted by a US Public Health Service team, began in 1943. Apart from severe dental fluorosis, the study found no adverse effects of long-term ingestion of this high-F water,[102] although postmortem bone F concentrations were high. Numerous animal studies in the early years of water fluoridation[101, 107, 113, 119, 121, 189-191] supported the results from studies with human populations.

Although not every possible hypothesis regarding F and human health was tested before beginning controlled fluoridation, there was sufficient research evidence to provide reasonable assurance that controlled fluoridation, with up to 1.2 ppm F in the drinking water, could be instituted in North America without any public health hazard.

Mortality

For the United States as a whole, no differences could be found in 1949–1950 death rates between 32 cities with 0.7 ppm F or more and 32 randomly selected nearby cities with 0.25 ppm F or less in the drinking water. Mortality rates were similar for cancer, heart disease, intracranial lesions, nephritis, and cirrhosis of the liver.[72] In 1979, mortality rates for 478 cities with populations of 25,000 or more were examined for the periods 1949–1950, 1959–1961, and 1969–1971. Data were collected on total deaths, as well as those attributed to cardiovascular disease, renal conditions, and cancer. No differences between fluoridated and nonfluoridated communities were found.[154]

Cancer

This 1979 mortality study[154] was produced as a response to 1975 testimony before a Congressional Committee, by Burk and Yiamouyiannis,[17] that fluoridation led to an increase in cancer deaths. Their argument was based on mortality data from the 10 largest fluoridated American cities between 1950 and 1970 compared with 10 selected nonfluoridated cities over the same period. The crude mortality data, unadjusted for age, sex, or race, showed a greater increase in cancer deaths in the fluoridated cities over the 20-year period. Criticism of this analysis was based on the inappropriateness of the crude mortality data, because the populations of the big cities during that 20-year period had become older and poorer and had changed in ethnic composition. Yiamouyiannis and Burk[188] repeated their work in 1977, this time with some age adjustment, and claimed that their data still showed an excess of cancer deaths in the fluoridated cities. A number of independent analyses of the same data, in both Britain and the United States, however, used more detailed age-sex-race adjustments; none could find a link between cancer incidence and consumption of fluoridated wa-ter.[44, 51, 81, 134, 145, 169]

One result of the Burk-Yiamouyiannis testimony was that a Congressional Committee directed the National Cancer Institute to carry out animal studies on the potential carcinogenicity of F. The National Toxicology Program (NTP) was responsible for the conduct of these studies, which were conducted in several animal species and used 4 levels of F concentration in the drinking water: 0, 11, 45, and 79 ppm F. (Use of extremely high levels of the test material is standard practice in toxicology studies to avoid having to use huge populations of animals.) The studies, which tested the effects of the water on the animals over 2 years, took longer than expected, but the NTP finally issued an extensive draft report in early 1990. Although a number of different cancers occurred in both test and control animals, the report found "equivocal evidence" of excess incidence of osteosarcoma, a rare form of bone cancer, in male rats of a particular strain.[176] Subsequent review of the data by statisticians, as well as a public hearing and considerable media attention, did not change this gray-zone conclusion.

In response, the Assistant Secretary for Health incorporated the NTP findings into a broader review of F and the environment, conducted by a special committee appointed by the US Public Health Service. The committee, in a thorough report, reached the following conclusion on cancer risk:

> *Optimal fluoridation of drinking water does not pose a detectable cancer risk to humans as evidenced by extensive human epidemiological data available to date, including the new studies prepared for this report. While the presence of fluoride in sources other than drinking water reduces the ability to discriminate between exposure in fluoridated as compared to non-fluoridated communities, no trends in cancer risk, including the risk of osteosarcoma, were attributed to the introduction of fluoride into drinking water in these new studies. During two time periods, 1973-1980 and 1981-1987, there was an unexplained increase of osteosarcoma in males under age 20. The reason for this increase remains to be clarified, but an extensive analysis reveals that it is unrelated to the introduction and duration of fluoridation.[177]*

The NTP report raised some interesting issues about risk assessment in the modern environment. Of the 538,000 estimated cancer deaths in the United States in 1994, 1075 (0.19%) were bone cancers of all kinds.[14] Case-control studies present the difficulty of documenting precisely all F exposure during a person's lifetime, which biases such studies toward the null (i.e., imprecise data make it more likely that the null hypothesis cannot be rejected). Risk assessment studies can be conducted with animals, but the question always remains as to what is the relevance of health effects in rats drinking water at 79 ppm F to humans drinking water at 1 to 4 ppm F. The inconclusive nature of the findings makes answering the question even more difficult. In addition, a large number of tests were conducted in the NTP studies, and statistical logic tells us that false results will occur about 5 times in each 100 tests (Chapter 12). In epidemiologic research with humans, neither ecologic[63, 127] nor case-control studies[64, 123] have found any association between osteosarcoma and previous F exposure.

Down Syndrome

A claim that water fluoridation caused an increase in the congenital malformation known as Down syndrome came with a series of papers in the mid-1950s.[141-143] The studies claimed to show from birth records in Wisconsin and Illinois that the incidence of Down syndrome was higher in fluoridated than in nonfluoridated areas, but there were errors in the research design.[149] The most serious error was to assume that the city of birth was the place of residence of the mother, which is clearly not the case for hospitals serving a large rural population. More rigorous independent studies in the United States and Britain have subsequently failed to show any correlation between fluoridation and Down syndrome.[12, 52, 53, 133]

Bone Density, Fracture Experience, and Osteoporosis

Bone fragility conditions (e.g., spontaneous vertebral fracture in the elderly as a result of osteoporosis) have been treated for years with high does of F combined with calcium, estrogen, and vitamin D. Controlled clinical trials have shown that high doses of F (30 to 60 mg/day), administered under medical supervision, can increase vertebral bone mass and reduce the vertebral fracture rate.[139] These favorable changes do not come without problems, however, for the new bone can be imperfectly mineralized and a good proportion of patients do not respond to treatment.[75]

Treatment also seems ineffective in preventing further fractures in patients who already have a fracture at first presentation.[95] The main concern is that the positive effects seen with the vertebral column, which is mostly cancellous bone, are not seen in the appendicular skeleton, which is mostly cortical bone. Indeed, fracture rates in the appendicular skeleton have actually been shown to increase with intensive F treatment.[144] Although an international conference in 1988 recommended F treatment for vertebral crush syndrome,[75] high-dose F treatment (up to 80 mg F/day) for bone fragility conditions is no longer recommended in the United States,[70, 77, 84] nor is F therapy seen as a measure that can prevent fractures resulting from osteoporosis.[126]

A more immediate issue in dentistry is the effect of fluoridated water on bone fracture experience. Day-to-day use of fluoridated water obviously results in much lower daily intakes (1 to 3 mg F/day for adults, see previously) than those seen in the therapeutic doses just described.

As mentioned earlier, McClure studied self-reported bone fracture experience relative to fluoridated waters among young men during World War II and reported no association. Like other early studies,[11, 66] McClure's study did not consider confounders such as body mass, medications, and dietary factors; and the radiographic techniques of the time were less sensitive than today's. In more recent times, a series of ecologic studies (Chapter 12) to assess the risk of bone fracture relative to fluoridated water have produced mixed results: decreased risk,[85, 156] no association,[5, 90, 109, 170] and increased risk.[26, 29, 86, 87] The extent of increased risk in the latter group of studies was generally low, with relative risks in the range of 1.08 to 1.41. Given the lack of precision that is inherent in ecologic studies, it is not surprising that this body of research does not yield clear conclusions for either increased risk or a protective F effect. Extensive reviews of literature have also reached the conclusion that no relationship can be discerned between bone fracture experience and water with 1.0 ppm F.[77, 94]

Research based on data from individual study participants is more likely to be internally valid than that from ecological studies. Results from several rural Iowa communities found reduced radial bone mass and slightly higher fracture experience in a town where the drinking water contained 4.0 ppm F.[164, 165]

At lower F levels, however, a study of 2000 women in western Pennsylvania found no association between long-term exposure to fluoridated water (1.0 ppm F) and bone mineral density and fracture experience.[21]

This issue has been the subject of extensive reviews,[130, 177] all of which have found no clear relationship between bone fracture experience and fluoridated water. In summary, although there does not appear to be any protective effect from fluoridated water, neither is there evidence that bone fracture experience is associated with drinking water containing 1.0 ppm F.

Child Development

An important study of F's effect on children came with the Newburgh-Kingston fluoridation project, one of the original fluoridation field trials that began in 1945. Participating children received a complete physical examination, selected physical measurements, and laboratory and radiographic studies. No significant differences in general health or body processes between children in the two cities were seen, and no radiographic differences in bone density could be demonstrated. There was essential similarity in vision and hearing tests and in findings for skeletal maturation, hemoglobin level, erythrocyte and leukocyte counts, and quantity of sugar, albumin, red blood cells, and casts in urine. At the final examination, 19 of 476 children in Newburgh (4.0%) and 20 of 405 children in Kingston (4.9%) were referred to the family physician for conditions including such minor ailments as a plantar wart or ringworm. Long-term downward trends in stillbirth and maternal and infant mortality rates continued in each of the cities. The overall conclusion was that no differences of medical significance could be found between the two groups of children.[153]

As part of the main health study in the Newburgh-Kingston fluoridation project, 100 boys, aged 12 at final examinations, were selected from the 881 participants in both cities for a substudy of specific urinary components.[152] Children who had recently been ill were excluded because results could otherwise have been confounded by a variety of unrelated conditions. No difference between the two populations could be found.

FLUORIDE TOXICITY

There is a world of difference between a single intake of 5.0 g F and constant intake of

1 to 3 mg F daily. F is thus like many other nutrients: beneficial in small amounts, toxic in high amounts. This gradation in response with variations in dose is a common pharmaceutical phenomenon and is known as a *dose-response* relationship.

Information on F toxicity levels cannot be gathered from controlled studies with humans. Available data are from a mix of case studies of various kinds and research on workers in certain industrial processes. The classic work in occupational F toxicity is that of the Danish scientist Kaj Roholm, who studied cryolite workers in aluminum plants during the 1930s. Their daily absorption was estimated at 0.2 to 1.0 mg F/kg body weight (about 14 to 68 mg F per day for a 150-lb person). Some workers had been employed as long as 31 years. Under these conditions, a number of toxic effects were observed, principally gastric complaints and osteosclerosis.

Ingestion of a single dose of 5 to 10 g of sodium fluoride by an adult male (32 to 64 mg F/kg body weight) results in a rather unpleasant death in 2 to 4 hours if first aid is not applied immediately. From that lower limit of 32 mg F/kg body weight, the estimated equivalent dose for a 10-kg child (12 to 18 months old) is 320 mg F.[76] Crippling skeletal fluorosis can eventually occur in an adult if 10 to 20 mg F is ingested or inhaled daily for 10 to 20 years.[130] The evidence on known toxic effects of F ingestion are summarized in Table 23-2.

If an individual is known or suspected to have taken a potentially toxic amount of F, first aid is to induce vomiting as quickly as possible, or to ingest a material to bind F. Milk is usually the most readily available.[76] The American Dental Association recommends, as a safety precaution, that F materials for home use contain no more than 264 mg F if packaged in a bulk container (tablets, mouthwash) or up to 300 mg F if the F material is individually packaged.

At the other end of the toxicity spectrum, there are many instances of remarkable toleration of high quantities of F without ill effects,

Table 23-2. DEGREES OF POTENTIALLY TOXIC INGESTION OF FLUORIDE

EFFECT	FLUORIDE INTAKE, TIME*
Acute fatal poisoning, adults[a]	2.5–5.0 g, 2–4 hr
Acute fatal poisoning, 10 kg child[b]	320 mg, 2–4 hr
Acute fatal poisoning, 3-year-old child[c]	Approx. 435 mg, approx. 3 hr
Acute fatal poisoning, adult renal dialysis patient[d]	Dialysate fluid 35–50 ppm F, for 3 hr
Acute fatal poisoning, adult male[e]	17.9 mg F/kg body weight for 24 hr
Short-term nonserious nausea in elementary schoolchildren[f]	93–375 ppm F in drinking water, small amounts; symptoms within 30 minutes
Nausea and vomiting in adults[g]	Nausea with ingestion of an estimated 80 mg F over a few hours, vomiting from ingestion of an estimated 143 mg F over a few hours
Severe skeletal fluorosis[h]	10–20 mg F daily, 10–20 yr
Osteosclerosis, radiographic changes in human bone[i]	8–14 ppm F in drinking water, lifetime exposure
Dental fluorosis[j]	0.1 mg F/kg body weight/day during tooth development (i.e., the first 8 years)
Acute fatal poisoning in animals[a]	Approx. 50 mg F/kg body weight
Interference with reproduction, thyroid disturbance, loss of body weight, and lameness in cattle[a]	40–60 ppm F in feed daily for several years

*With drinking water fluoridated at 1.0 ppm, an adult would have to drink 660 gallons in 2–4 hours to reach the lower limit of a fatal dose. A 10 kg child (12–18 months old) would have to drink 85 gallons in 2–4 hours. Severe skeletal fluorosis could only result from drinking 2.6–6.6 gallons of water daily for 10–20 years if none of the fluoride was excreted.

Data from:
a) Hodge[78]
b) Heifetz and Horowitz[76]
c) Horowitz[82]
d) Fluoride intoxication[61]
e) Gessner et al.[65]
f) Hoffman et al.[80]
g) Vogt et al.[180]
h) National Research Council[130]
i) Hodge and Smith[79]
j) Fejerskov et al.[59]

such as the osteoporosis patients mentioned earlier. Adverse effects in these patients are reported to be usually no worse than nausea, stomach pains, and occasional diarrhea. The greatly elevated levels of plasma F may also be associated with some arthritic-type joint pain, but it is not certain whether these pains come from the treatment or the disease itself.[89]

Dental Fluorosis

Dental fluorosis is a permanent hypomineralization of enamel, characterized by greater surface and subsurface porosity than in normal enamel. It results from excess F reaching the developing tooth during developmental stages.[58] Its distribution and risk factors are described in Chapter 21.

FLUORIDE AND CARIES CONTROL: MECHANISMS OF ACTION

F works best to prevent caries when a constant, low ambient level of F is maintained in the oral cavity.[24] Its most important caries-inhibitory action is posteruptive, though a pre-eruptive role continues to be suggested.[69, 129] F's action in preventing caries is multifactorial; its effect comes from a combination of several mechanisms. Three major mechanisms of action have been identified (Table 23–3), although some possible additional mechanisms have been hypothesized.

It has long been held that pre-eruptive F exerts some degree of caries inhibition. In this model, F is thought to act by being incorporated into the developing enamel hydroxyapatite crystal and thus reducing enamel solubility. It has been argued that pre-eruptive benefits are especially important for reducing pit-and-fissure lesions.[69] This is the "pre-eruptive" model of F's caries-preventive action assumed to be the primary effect for many years, but for which the actual supportive evidence is thin. If there is a pre-eruptive effect on caries inhibition, it is likely to be minor; the evidence for posteruptive F action is much stronger.

Fluoride and Plaque

The topical effect of a constant infusion of low-concentration F into the oral cavity, such as occurs with drinking fluoridated water or regular brushing with an F toothpaste, is to enhance remineralization during the repeated cycles of demineralization and remineralization (often shortened to *demin-remin*) in the early stages of the carious process.[98] F introduced into the mouth is partly taken up by dental plaque,[157] where 95% of it is held in bound form rather than as ionic F. Plaque contains 5 to 10 mg F/kg wet weight in low F areas and 10 to 20 mg F/kg wet weight in fluoridated areas. The bound F can be released in response to lowered pH,[171] and F is taken up more readily by demineralized enamel than by sound enamel.[184] The availability of plaque F to respond to the acid challenge leads to the gradual establishment of a well-crystallized and more acid-resistant apatite in the enamel surface during demin-remin.[22, 54, 93, 174, 175]

F in plaque also inhibits glycolysis, the process by which fermentable carbohydrate is metabolized by cariogenic bacteria to produce acid. F from drinking water and toothpaste concentrates in plaque, which contains higher levels of F than does saliva.[74, 159] There is also some evidence that plaque F can inhibit the production of extracellular polysaccharide by cariogenic bacteria, a necessary process for plaque adherence to smooth enamel surfaces.[74]

In addition to these mechanisms, high-concentration F gels may have a specific bactericidal action on cariogenic bacteria in plaque.[15] These gels also leave a temporary layer of CaF_2 on the enamel surface, which is available for release when the pH drops at the enamel surface.[100] At lower concentrations, *Streptococcus mutans* has been shown, in laboratory conditions, to become less acidogenic through adaptation to an environment where F is constantly present.[15, 16, 112, 147] It is

Table 23–3. THREE PRINCIPAL MECHANISMS BY WHICH FLUORIDE IS CONSIDERED TO INHIBIT DENTAL CARIES

POSTERUPTIVE

1. Promoting remineralization and inhibiting demineralization of early carious lesions.
2. Inhibition of glycolysis, the process by which cariogenic bacteria metabolize fermentable carbohydrates.

PRE-ERUPTIVE

3. Some reduction in enamel solubility in acid by pre-eruptive incorporation of fluoride into the hydroxyapatite crystal.

not yet known whether this ecologic adaptation reduces the cariogenicity of acidogenic bacteria in humans.[178]

Fluoride and Enamel

Practically from the beginning of F research, it was assumed that F's inhibition of caries depended on its pre-eruptive incorporation into developing dental enamel, thus reducing enamel solubility in demineralizing acids.[36, 120] In most of the early fluoridation studies, greater caries reductions were found in children who were born as fluoridation began when compared with those for whom fluoridation began after birth.[20, 62, 67, 83, 91] It was also clear from these early days, however, that there was caries inhibition in teeth already erupted when fluoridation began,[6, 7, 96, 97, 148] or in first molars that were erupting when fluoridation began.[8, 10, 150]

It became evident to researchers as early as the mid-1970s that a higher concentration of enamel F could not by itself explain the extensive reductions in caries that F produced.[104] The concentration of F in enamel is actually rather low. From a depth of 2.0 microns, enamel F concentrations averaged 1700 ppm in nonfluoridated areas and 2200–3200 in areas fluoridated at 1.0 ppm. Even in 5 to 7 ppm F areas, enamel F concentrations were only as high as 4800 ppm,[1] showing that enamel F is poorly correlated with water F levels. If the pre-eruptive hypothesis was true (i.e., that pre-eruptive F uptake by developing enamel was the major factor in F's cariostatic effects), one would expect caries experience in a population to be inversely related to enamel F concentrations, but such is not the case.[24] The converse also holds (i.e. it has been observed that higher concentrations of enamel F do not necessarily mean that caries will not occur).[3] The theoretical concentration of F in pure fluorapatite that would reduce its acid solubility is 38,000 ppm,[181] a concentration not even approached in human dental enamel. Thus, although some pre-eruptive effect of F can be inferred from field studies,[19, 45] any such action is likely to be a minor part of the overall impact of F.

Perhaps the most revealing study on the action of F in inhibiting dental caries came from the Tiel-Culemborg fluoridation study in the Netherlands.[68] Although there were considerably fewer dentinal lesions in fluoridated Tiel than in nonfluoridated Culemborg after 15 years of fluoridation, as would be expected, there was no difference between the two communities in initial enamel lesions. This finding means that fewer enamel lesions progress to dentinal caries in a fluoridated area than in a nonfluoridated area. F, therefore, does not prevent the initial carious attack, which would be expected if its presence in the enamel crystal increased enamel resistance to acid dissolution. The Tiel-Culemborg findings mean than F in the oral cavity inhibits further demineralization of the lesion and promotes its remineralization.

We can speculate on why the pre-eruptive view of F's action became dominant[151] in the United States, despite the evidence for both pre-eruptive and posteruptive effects even in the 1950s and 1960s. One likely explanation is that because the adverse effect of F ingestion, fluorosis, was investigated first and shown to be a systemic condition, it was understandable that the beneficial effects came to be seen the same way.[103] The early days of F research were also the time in history when the role of vitamins were being discovered, so there could have been some linkage of mechanisms in the minds of researchers.

Fluoride and Saliva

Salivary F concentrations are low, although they are 3 times higher in fluoridated than in nonfluoridated areas. In a fluoridated area, salivary F levels have averaged 0.016 ppm; in a nonfluoridated area, they were 0.006 ppm.[135] These levels are considered to be too low to have any impact on caries. Fluctuation of salivary F levels is normal, and after toothbrushing with an F toothpaste or mouthrinsing with an F solution, salivary F levels can rise 100- to 1000-fold. This level rapidly returns to normal, and the saliva is likely to be an important source of plaque F during this time.[146]

Effects on Different Tooth Surfaces

One of the observations from early fluoridation studies in the Netherlands and New Zealand was that of greater proportional caries reductions on the free smooth and proximal surfaces than on pit-and-fissure surfaces.[10, 108] Murray's study of 15-year-olds in naturally fluoridated Hartlepool and nonfluoridated York, England, found that those in Hartlepool averaged 4.96 decayed, missing, or filled (DMF) teeth, whereas those in York had a mean DMFT of 8.95. However, the number of carious approximal surfaces of molars was 11 times greater in York.[128] This pattern of more pronounced effect on smooth surfaces compared to pit-and-fissure surfaces has become a standard finding in studies where caries was recorded by tooth surface.[9] Although F reduces caries on both types of surface, the greatest relative effect is on smooth and proximal surfaces. Therefore, it follows that when DMFS scores are declining in a population, the *proportion* of all decayed surfaces that are pit-and-fissure surfaces will increase, even as their absolute number diminishes.

EFFECTIVE USE OF FLUORIDE

Categorizing F compounds into systemic fluorides and topical fluorides is not easy because the line between these categories gets blurred: systemic vehicles such as water fluoridation and F supplements have been shown to have topical cariostatic action, and some topical vehicles such as F toothpaste can be swallowed inadvertently and have systemic effects (fluorosis). As stated earlier, the evidence shows that the most effective community-wide use of F is in frequent, low-concentration intraoral exposures such as in drinking water or toothpaste.[3, 57, 111, 182] Less frequent application of high-concentration gels has its place in the care of caries-susceptible patients.

The most cost-effective way of reaching an entire community with regular, low-concentration F is through water fluoridation. This is true public health action, and it is also one that has stirred public controversy. The unique position of water fluoridation as a public health action is the subject of the next chapter.

REFERENCES

1. Aasenden R. Fluoride concentrations in the surface tooth enamel of young men and women. Arch Oral Biol 1974;19:697-701.
2. Ainsworth, NJ. Mottled teeth. Br Dent J 1933; 55:233-50.
3. Arends J, Christoffersen J. Nature and role of loosely bound fluoride in dental caries. J Dent Res 1990;69(Special Issue):601-5.
4. Armstrong WD. Mechanisms of fluoride homeostasis. Arch Oral Biol 1961;4:156-9.
5. Arnala I, Alhava EM, Kivivuori R, Kauranen P. Hip fracture incidence not affected by fluoridation. Osteofluorosis studies in Finland. Acta Orthop Scand 1986;57:344-8.
6. Arnold FA Jr, Dean HT, Knutson JW. Effect of fluoridated public water supplies on dental caries incidence. Results of the seventh year of study at Grand Rapids and Muskegon, Mich. Public Health Rep 1953;68:141-8.
7. Ast DB, Chase HC. The Newburgh-Kingston caries fluorine study. IV. Dental findings after six years of fluoridation. Oral Surg 1953;6:114-23.
8. Backer Dirks O. The relation between the fluoridation of water and dental caries experience. Int Dent J 1967;17:582-605.
9. Backer Dirks O. The benefits of water fluoridation. Caries Res 1974;8 (Suppl 1):2-15.
10. Backer Dirks O, Houwink B, Kwant GW. The result of 6½ years of artificial drinking water in the Netherlands: The Tiel-Culemborg experiment. Arch Oral Biol 1961;5:284-300.
11. Bernstein DS, Sadowsky N, Hegsted DM, et al. Prevalence of osteoporosis in high-and low-fluoride areas in North Dakota. JAMA 1966;198:499-504.
12. Berry WTC. A study of the incidence of mongolism in relation to the fluoride content of water. Am J Ment Deficiency 1958;62:634-6.
13. Black GV, McKay FS. Mottled teeth—an endemic developmental imperfection of the teeth heretofore unknown in the literature of dentistry. Dent Cosmos 1916;58:129-56.
14. Boring CC, Squires TS, Tong T, Montgomery S. Cancer statistics, 1994. CA 1994;44:7-26.
15. Bowden GHW. Effects of fluoride on the microbial ecology of dental plaque. J Dent Res 1990;69(Special Issue):653-9.
16. Bowden GHW, Odlum O, Nolette N, Hamilton IR. Microbial populations growing in the presence of fluoride at low pH isolated from dental plaque of children living in an area with fluoridated water. Infect Immun 1982;36:247-54.
17. Burk D, Yiamouyiannis J. Fluoridation and cancer. 94th Congress, first session. Congress Record 1975 July 21;121:7172-6.
18. Burt BA. The changing patterns of systemic fluoride intake. J Dent Res 1992;71:1228-37.
19. Burt BA, Eklund SA, Loesche WJ. Dental benefits of limited exposure to fluoridated water in childhood. J Dent Res 1986;61:1322-5.
20. Carlos JP, Gittelsohn AM, Waddon W Jr. Caries in deciduous teeth in relation to maternal ingestion of fluoride. Public Health Rep 1962;77:658-60.
21. Cauley JA, Murphy PA, Riley TJ, Buhari AM. Effects of fluoridated drinking water on bone mass and fractures: the study of osteoporotic fractures. J Bone Miner Res 1995;10:1076-86.
22. Chow LC. Tooth-bound fluoride and dental caries. J Dent Res 1990;69(Special Issue):595-600.
23. Churchill HV. Occurrence of fluorides in some waters of the United States. J Ind Eng Chem 1931;23:996-98.
24. Clarkson BH, Fejerskov O, Ekstrand J, Burt BA. Rational use of fluorides in caries control. In: Fejerskov O, Ekstrand J, Burt BA, eds: Fluorides in dentistry. 2nd ed. Copenhagen: Munksgaard, 1996:347-57.
25. Clovis J, Hargreaves JA. Fluoride intake from beverage consumption. Community Dent Oral Epidemiol 1988;16:11-5.
26. Cooper C, Wickham CA, Barker DJ, Jacobsen SJ. Water fluoridation and hip fracture [letter]. JAMA 1991;266:513-4.

27. Cremer H-D, Buttner W. Absorption of fluorides. In: World Health Organization. Fluorides and human health. Geneva: WHO, 1970:75-91.

28. Dabeka RW, McKenzie AD, Lacroix GM. Dietary intakes of lead, cadmium, arsenic and fluoride by Canadian adults: A 24-hour duplicate diet study. Food Addit Contam 1987;4:89-101.

29. Danielson C, Lyon JL, Egger M, Goodenough GK. Hip fractures and fluoridation in Utah's elderly population. JAMA 1992;268:746-8.

30. Dean HT. Distribution of mottled enamel in the United States. Public Health Rep 1933;48:703-34.

31. Dean HT. Classification of mottled enamel diagnosis. J Am Dent Assoc 1934;21:1421-6.

32. Dean HT. Chronic endemic dental fluorosis (mottled enamel). JAMA 1936;107:1269-72.

33. Dean HT. Endemic fluorosis and its relation to dental caries. Public Health Rep 1938;53:1443-52.

34. Dean HT. The investigation of physiological effects by the epidemiological method. In: Moulton FR, ed: Fluorine and dental health. Washington DC: American Association for the Advancement of Science, 1942:23-31.

35. Dean HT, Arnold FA Jr, Elvove E. Domestic water and dental caries. V. Additional studies of the relation of fluoride domestic waters to dental caries experience in 4,425 white children aged 12–14 years of 13 cities in 4 states. Public Health Rep 1942; 57:1155-79.

36. Dean HT, Dixon RM, Cohen C. Mottled enamel in Texas. Public Health Rep 1935;50:424-42.

37. Dean HT, Elvove E. Studies on the minimal threshold of the dental sign of chronic endemic fluorosis (mottled enamel). Public Health Rep 1935;50:1719-29.

38. Dean HT, Elvove E. Some epidemiological aspects of chronic endemic dental fluorosis. Am J Public Health 1936;26:567-75.

39. Dean HT, Elvove E. Further studies on the minimal threshold of chronic endemic dental fluorosis. Public Health Rep 1937;52:1249-64.

40. Dean HT, Elvove E, Poston RF. Mottled enamel in South Dakota. Public Health Rep 1939;54:212-28.

41. Dean HT, Jay P, Arnold FA Jr, Elvove E. Domestic water and dental caries. II. A study of 2,832 white children aged 12-14 years, of eight suburban Chicago communities, including L. acidophilus studies of 1,761 children. Public Health Rep 1941;56:761-92.

42. Dean HT, Jay P, Arnold FA Jr, McClure FJ, Elvove E. Domestic water and dental caries, including certain epidemiological aspects of oral L. acidophilus. Public Health Rep 1939;54:862-88.

43. Dean HT, McKay FS. Production of mottled enamel halted by a change in common water supply. Am J Public Health 1939;29:590-6.

44. Doll R, Kinlen L. Fluoridation of water and cancer mortality in the U.S.A. Lancet 1977;1:1300-2.

45. Driscoll WS, Heifetz SB, Brunelle JA. Caries preventive effects of fluoride tablets in school children four years after discontinuation of treatments. J Am Dent Assoc 1981; 103:878-81.

46. Ehrnebo M, Ekstrand J. Occupational fluoride exposure and plasma fluoride levels in man. Int Arch Occupational Environ Health 1986;58:179-90.

47. Ekstrand J. Relationship between fluoride in the drinking water and the plasma fluoride concentration in man. Caries Res 1978;12:123-7.

48. Ekstrand J. Fluoride metabolism. In: Fejerskov O, Ekstrand J, Burt BA, eds: Fluoride in dentistry. Copenhagen: Munksgaard, 1996:55-68.

49. Ekstrand J, Ehrnebo M. The relationship between plasma fluoride, urinary excretion rate and urine fluoride concentration in man. J Occup Med 1983;25:745-8.

50. Ekstrand J, Koch G, Lindgren LE, Petersson LG. Pharmacokinetics of fluoride gels in children and adults. Caries Res 1981;15:213-20.

51. Erickson JD. Mortality in selected cities with fluoridated and nonfluoridated water supplies. N Engl J Med 1978;298:112-6.

52. Erickson JD. Down syndrome, water fluoridation, and maternal age. Teratology 1980;21:177-80.

53. Erickson JD, Oakley GP Jr, Flynt JW Jr, Hay S. Water fluoridation and congenital malformations: No association. J Am Dent Assoc 1976;93:981-4.

54. Ericsson Y. Cariostasis mechanisms of action of fluorides; clinical observations. Caries Res 1977; 11(Suppl 1):2-23.

55. Ericsson Y, Malmnas C. Placental transfer of fluorine investigated with F^{18} in man and rabbit. Acta Obstet Gynecol Scand 1962;41:144-58.

56. Farkas CS, Farkas EJ. Potential effect of food processing on the fluoride content of infant foods. Science Total Environ 1974;2:399-405.

57. Featherstone JDB, Glena R, Shariati M, Shields PC. Dependence of in vitro demineralization of apatite and remineralization of dental enamel on fluoride concentration. J Dent Res 1990;69(Special Issue): 620-5.

58. Fejerskov O, Manji F, Baelum V. The nature and mechanisms of dental fluorosis in man. J Dent Res 1990;69(Special Issue):692-700.

59. Fejerskov O, Stephen KW, Richards A, Speirs R. Combined effect of systemic and topical fluoride treatments on human deciduous teeth—case studies. Caries Res 1987;21:452-9.

60. Filippo FA, Battistone GC. The fluoride content of a representative diet of the young adult male. Clin Chim Acta 1971;31:453-7.

61. Fluoride intoxication in a dialysis unit—Maryland. MMWR 1980;29:134-6.

62. Forrest JR, James PMC. A blind study of enamel opacities and dental caries prevalence after eight years of fluoridation of water. Br Dent J 1965; 119:319-22.

63. Freni SC, Gaylor DW. International trends in the incidence of bone cancer are not related to drinking water fluoridation. Cancer 1992;70:611-8.

64. Gelberg KH, Fitzgerald EF, Hwang S, Dubrow R. Fluoride exposure and childhood osteosarcoma: A case-control study. Am J Public Health 1995; 85:1678-83.

65. Gessner BD, Beller M, Middaugh JP, Whitford GM. Acute fluoride poisoning from a public water system. N Engl J Med 1994;330:95-9.

66. Goggin JE, Haddon W Jr, Hambly GS, Hoveland JR. Incidence of femoral fractures in postmenopausal women. Public Health Rep 1965;80:1005-11.

67. Grainger RM, Coburn CI. Dental caries of the first molars and the age of children when first consuming naturally fluoridated water. Can J Public Health 1955;46:347-54.

68. Groeneveld A. Longitudinal study of the prevalence of enamel lesions in a fluoridated and a non-fluoridated area. Community Dent Oral Epidemiol 1985;13:159-63.

69. Groeneveld A, Van Eck AAMJ, Backer Dirks O. Fluoride in caries prevention: Is the effect pre- or post-eruptive? J Dent Res 1990;69(Special Issue): 751-5.

70. Gruber HE, Baylink DJ. The effects of fluoride on bone. Clin Orthop 1991;(267):264-77.

71. Guy WS. Inorganic and organic fluoride in human blood. In: Johansen E, Taves DR, Olsen TO, eds.: Continuing evaluation of the use of fluorides. AAAS Selected Symposium No 11. Boulder CO: Westview, 1979:125-47.

72. Hagan TL, Pasternack M, Scholz G. Waterborne fluorides and mortality. Public Health Rep 1954; 69:450-4.

73. Haikel Y, Voegel JC, Frank RM. Fluoride content of water, dust, soils and cereals in the endemic dental fluorosis area of Khouribga (Morocco). Arch Oral Biol 1986;31:279-86.

74. Hamilton IR. Biochemical effects of fluoride on oral bacteria. J Dent Res 1990;69(Special Issue):660-67.

75. Heaney RP, Baylink DJ, Johnston CC Jr, et al. Fluoride therapy for the vertebral crush fracture syndrome. A status report. Ann Intern Med 1989;111:678-80.

76. Heifetz SB, Horowitz HS. Amounts of fluoride in self-administered dental products: Safety considerations for children. Pediatrics 1986;77:876-82.

77. Hillier S, Inskip H, Coggon D, Cooper C. Water fluoridation and osteoporotic fracture. Community Dent Health 1996;13(Suppl 2):63-8.

78. Hodge HC. The safety of fluoride tablets or drops. In: Johansen E, Taves DR, Olsen TO, eds.: Continuing evaluation of the use of fluorides. AAAS Selected Symposium No. 11. Boulder: Westview, 1979:253-74.

79. Hodge HC, Smith FA. Fluorine chemistry. Vol 4 of a series, Simons JH, ed. New York: Academic Press, 1965.

80. Hoffman R, Mann J, Calderone J, et al. Acute poisoning in a New Mexico elementary school. Pediatrics 1980;65:89-900.

81. Hoover RN, McKay FW, Fraumeni JF. Fluoridated drinking water and the occurrence of cancer. J Natl Cancer Inst 1976;57:757-68.

82. Horowitz HS. Abusive use of fluoride [editorial]. J Public Health Dent 1977;37:106-7.

83. Horowitz HS, Heifetz SB. Effects of prenatal exposure to fluoridation on dental caries. Public Health Rep 1967; 82:297-304.

84. Inkovaara JA. Is fluoride treatment justified today? Calcif Tissue Int 1991;49 (Suppl):S68-9.

85. Jacobsen SJ, O'Fallon WM, Melton LJ 3rd. Hip fracture incidence before and after the fluoridation of the public water supply, Rochester, Minnesota. Am J Public Health 1993;83:743-5.

86. Jacobsen SJ, Goldberg J, Cooper C, Lockwood SA. The association between water fluoridation and hip fracture among white women and men aged 65 years and older. A national ecologic study. Ann Epidemiol 1992;2:617-26.

87. Jacobsen SJ, Goldberg J, Miles TP, et al. Regional variation in the incidence of hip fracture: US white women aged 65 years and older. JAMA 1990; 264:500-2.

88. Johnson WJ, Taves DR, Jowsey J. Fluoridation and bone disease in renal patients. In: Johansen E, Taves DR, Olsen TO, eds.: Continuing evaluation of the use of fluorides. AAAS Selected Symposium No 11. Boulder CO: Westview, 1979:275-93.

89. Jowsey J, Riggs BL, Kelly PJ. Fluoride in the treatment of osteoporosis. In: Johansen E, Taves DR, Olsen TO, eds.: Continuing evaluation of the use of fluorides. AAAS Symposium No 11. Boulder CO: Westview, 1979:111-23.

90. Karagas MR, Baron JA, Barrett JA, Jacobsen SJ. Patterns of fracture among the United States elderly: Geographic and fluoride effects. Ann Epidemiol 1996;6:209-16.

91. Katz S, Muhler JC. Prenatal and postnatal fluoride and dental caries experience in deciduous teeth. J Am Dent Assoc 1968;76:305-11.

92. Keshiviah P. Water treatment for hemodialysis. In: Henderson LW, Thuma RS, eds: Quality assurance in dialysis. Dordrecht: Kluwer, 1994:85-107.

93. Kidd EA, Thylstrup A, Fejerskov O, Bruun C. Influence of fluoride in surface enamel and degree of dental fluorosis on caries development in vitro. Caries Res 1980;14:196-202.

94. Kleerekoper M. Fluoride and the skeleton. Crit Rev Clin Lab Sci 1996;33:139-61.

95. Kleerekoper M, Mendlovic DB. Sodium fluoride therapy of postmenopausal osteoporosis. Endocr Rev 1993;14:312-23.

96. Klein H. Dental caries in relocated children exposed to water containing fluorine. I. Incidence of new caries after 2 years of exposure among previously caries-free permanent teeth. Public Health Rep 1945;60:1462-7.

97. Klein H. Dental caries (DMF) experience in relocated children exposed to water containing fluorine. II. J Am Dent Assoc 1946;33:1136-41.

98. Koulourides T. Summary of session II: Fluoride and the caries process. J Dent Res 1990;69(Special Issue):558.

99. Kramer L, Osis D, Wiatrowski E, Spencer H. Dietary fluoride in different areas of the United States. Am J Clin Nutr 1974;27:590-4.

100. LeGeros RZ. Crystal and crystallographic events in the caries process. J Dent Res 1990;69(Special Issue):567-74.

101. Leone NC, Geever IF, Moran NC. Acute and subacute toxicity studies of sodium fluoride in animals. Public Health Rep 1956;71:459-67.

102. Leone NC, Shimkin MB, Arnold FA, et al. Medical aspects of excessive fluoride in the water supply. Public Health Rep 1954;69:925-36.

103. Leverett D. Appropriate use of systemic fluoride: considerations for the '90s. J Public Health Dent 1991;51:42-7.

104. Levine RS. The action of fluoride in caries prevention; a review of current concepts. Br Dent J 1976;140:9-14.

105. Levy SM, Kiritsy MC, Warren JJ. Sources of fluoride intake in children. J Public Health Dent 1995;55:39-52.

106. Levy SM, Kohout FJ, Guha-Chowdbury N, et al. Infants' fluoride intake from drinking water alone, and from water added to formula, beverages, and food. J Dent Res 1995;74:1399-407.

107. Likins RC, Scow R, Zipkin I, Steere AC. Deposition and retention of fluoride and radiocalcium in the growing rat. Am J Physiol 1959;197:75-80.

108. Ludwig TG. The Hastings Fluoridation Project. V. Dental effects between 1954 and 1964. N Z Dent J 1965;61:175-9.

109. Madans J, Kleinman JC, Cornoni-Huntley J. The relationship between hip fracture and water fluoridation: An analysis of national data. Am J Public Health 1983;73:296-8.

110. Manji F, Kapila S. Fluorides and fluorosis in Kenya. Part I. The occurrence of fluorides. Odont-Stomatol Trop 1986;9:15-20.

111. Margolis HC, Moreno EC. Physicochemical perspec-

tives on the cariostatic mechanisms of systemic and topical fluorides. J Dent Res 1990;69(Special Issue):606-13.

112. Marquis RE. Diminished acid tolerance of plaque bacteria caused by fluoride. J Dent Res 1990;69(Special Issue):672-75.

113. McCann HG, Bullock FA. The effect of fluoride ingestion on the composition and solubility of mineralized tissues of the rat. J Dent Res 1957;36:391-8.

114. McClure FJ. A review of fluorine and its physiological effects. Physiol Rev 1933;13:277-300.

115. McClure FJ. Ingestion of fluoride and dental caries. Quantitative relations based on food and water requirements of children 1 to 12 years old. Am J Dis Child 1943;66:362-9.

116. McClure FJ. Fluoride domestic waters and systemic effects. I. Relation to bone-fracture experience, height and weight of high school boys and young selectees of the armed forces of the United States. Public Health Rep 1944;59:1543-58.

117. McClure FJ. Water fluoridation: The search and the victory. Bethesda, MD: National Institutes of Health, 1970:12-29.

118. McClure FJ, Kinser CA. Fluoride domestic waters and systemic effects. II. Fluorine content of urine in relation to fluorine in drinking water. Public Health Rep 1944;59:1575-91.

119. McClure FJ, Kornberg A. Blood hemoglobin and hematocrit results on rats ingesting sodium fluoride. J Pharmacol Exp Ther 1947;89:77-80.

120. McClure FJ, Likins RC. Fluorine in human teeth studied in relation to fluorine in the drinking water. J Dent Res 1951;30:172-6.

121. McClure FJ, Mitchell HH. The effect of fluorine on the calcium metabolism of albino rats and the composition of the bones. J Biol Chem 1931;60:297-320.

122. McClure FJ, Mitchell HH, Hamilton TS, Kinser CA. Balances of fluorine ingested from various sources in food and water by five young men. Excretion of fluorine through the skin. J Indust Hygiene Toxicol 1945;27:159-70.

123. McGuire SM, Vanable ED, McGuire MH, et al. Is there a link between fluoridated water and osteosarcoma? J Am Dent Assoc 1991;122:38-45.

124. McKay FS. The relation of mottled enamel to caries. J Am Dent Assoc 1928;15:1429-37.

125. McKay FS. Mottled enamel: The prevention of its further production through a change of water supply at Oakley, Idaho. J Am Dent Assoc 1933;20:1137-49.

126. Melton LJ 3rd. Fluoride in the prevention of osteoporosis and fractures. J Bone Miner Res 1990;5 (Suppl 1):S163-7.

127. Moss ME, Kanarek MS, Anderson HA, et al. Osteosarcoma, seasonality, and environmental factors in Wisconsin, 1979-1989. Arch Environ Health 1995;50:235-41.

128. Murray JJ. Caries experience of 15-year-old children from fluoride and non-fluoride communities. Br Dent J 1969; 127:128-31.

129. Murray JJ. Systemic fluorides: water fluoridation. Caries Res 1993;27(Suppl 1):2-8.

130. National Research Council. Health effects of ingested fluoride. Washington DC: National Academy Press, 1993.

131. National Research Council, Food and Nutrition Board. Recommended dietary allowances. 8th ed. Washington DC: National Academy of Sciences, 1974:98-9.

132. National Research Council, Food and Nutrition Board. Recommended dietary allowances. 10th ed. Washington DC: National Academy of Sciences, 1989:235-40.

133. Needleman HL, Pueschel SM, Rothman KJ. Fluoridation and the occurrence of Down's syndrome. N Engl J Med 1974;291:821-3.

134. Oldham PD, Newell DJ. Fluoridation of water supplies and cancer: A possible association? Appl Statistics 1977;26:125-35.

135. Oliveby A, Twetman S, Ekstrand J. Diurnal fluoride concentration in whole saliva in children living in a high- and a low-fluoride area. Caries Res 1990;24:44-7.

136. Ophaug RH, Singer L, Harland BF. Estimated fluoride intake of average two-year-old children in four dietary regions of the United States. J Dent Res 1980;59:777-81.

137. Ophaug RH, Singer L, Harland BF. Estimated fluoride intake of 6-month-old infants in four dietary regions of the United States. Am J Clin Nutr 1980;33:324-7.

138. Osis D, Kramer L, Wiatrowski E, Spencer H. Dietary fluoride intake in man. J Nutr 1974;104:1313-8.

139. Pak CY, Sakhaee K, Piziak V, et al. Slow-release NaF in the management of postmenopausal osteoporosis. A randomized controlled trial. Ann Intern Med 1994;120:625-32.

140. Pang DTY, Phillips CL, Bawden JW. Fluoride intake from beverage consumption in a sample of North Carolina children. J Dent Res 1992;71:1382-8.

141. Rapaport I. Contribution a l'étude du mongolisme. Role pathogenique du fluor. Bull Acad Natl Med 1956;140:529-31.

142. Rapaport I. Nouvelles récherches sur le mongolisme. A propos du role pathogenique du fluor. Bull Acad Natl Med 1959;143:367-70.

143. Rapaport I. Oligophrénie mongolienne et caries dentaires. Rev Stomatol 1963;46:207-18.

144. Riggs BL, O'Fallon WM, Lane A, et al. Clinical trial of fluoride therapy in postmenopausal osteoporotic women: extended observations and additional analysis. J Bone Miner Res 1994;9:265-75.

145. Rogot E, Sharrett AR, Feinleib M, Fabsitz RR. Trends in urban mortality in relation to fluoridation status. Am J Epidemiol 1978;107:104-12.

146. Rölla G, Ekstrand J. Fluoride in oral fluids and dental plaque. In: Fejerskov O, Ekstrand J, Burt BA, eds: Fluoride in dentistry. Copenhagen: Munksgaard, 1996:215-29.

147. Rosen S, Frea JI, Hsu SM. Effect of fluoride-resistant microorganisms on dental caries. J Dent Res 1978;57:180.

148. Russell AL. Dental effects of exposure to fluoride-bearing Dakota sandstone waters at various ages and for various lengths of time. II. Patterns of dental caries inhibition as related to exposure span, to elapsed time since exposure, and to periods of calcification and eruption. J Dent Res 1949;28:600-12.

149. Russell AL. Letters to Dr. Rapaport and Dr. Forrest. In: Crisp P. Report of the Royal Commission on the fluoridation of public water supplies. Hobart, Australia: Tasmanian Government Printing Office, 1968:262-5.

150. Russell AL, Hamilton PM. Dental caries in permanent first molars after eight years of fluoridation. Arch Oral Biol 1961;6:50-7.

151. Russell AL, White CL. Dental caries in Maryland children after seven years of fluoridation. Public Health Rep 1961;76:1087-93.

152. Schlesinger ER, Overton DE. Study of children drinking fluoridated and nonfluoridated water. JAMA 1956;160:21-4.

153. Schlesinger ER, Overton DE, Chase HE, Cantwell KT. Newburgh-Kingston caries-fluorine study. XIII. Pediatric findings after ten years. J Am Dent Assoc 1956;52:296-306.

154. Schneiderman MA. Fluoridation and health: A short review of some evidence from the United States. Bethesda MD: National Cancer Institute, 1979.

155. Sheridan P. National Institute of Dental Research: 40 years of progress. J Am Dent Assoc 1988;116:837-44.

156. Simonen O, Laitenen O. Does fluoridation of drinking water prevent bone fragility and osteoporosis? Lancet 1985;2(8452):432-4.

157. Singer L, Jarvey BA, Venkateswarlu P, Armstrong WD. Fluoride in plaque. J Dent Res 1970;49:455.

158. Singer L, Ophaug RH, Harland BF. Fluoride intake of young adult males in the United States. Am J Clin Nutr 1980;33:328-32.

159. Singer L, Ophaug RH, Harland BF. Dietary fluoride intake of 15-19-year-old male adults residing in the United States. J Dent Res 1985;64:1302-5.

160. Smith FA, Gardner DE. Determination of fluoride in soft tissues following prolonged ingestion of fluoride at various levels. Arch Industr Health 1960; 21:330-2.

161. Smith GE. Toxicity of fluoride-containing dental preparations: A review. Sci Total Environ 1985; 43:41-61.

162. Smith MC, Lantz EM, Smith HV. The cause of mottled enamel, a defect of human teeth. J Dent Res 1932, 12:149-59. [Reprinted from: Tech Bull No 32. Tucson: University of Arizona College of Agriculture, 1931].

163. Sognnaes RF. Historical perspectives. In: Johansen E, Taves DR, Olsen TO, eds: Continuing evaluation of the use of fluorides. AAAS Selected Symposium No 11. Boulder, CO: Westview, 1979:5-31.

164. Sowers MF, Clark MK, Jannausch ML, Wallace RB. A prospective study of bone mineral content and fracture in communities with differential fluoride exposure. Am J Epidemiol 1991;133:649-60.

165. Sowers MF, Wallace RB, Lemke JH. The relationship of bone mass and fracture history to fluoride and calcium intake: A study of three communities. Am J Clin Nutr 1986;44:889-98.

166. Spak CJ, Berg U, Ekstrand J. Renal clearance of fluoride in children and adolescents. Pediatrics 1985;75:575-9.

167. Spencer H, Osis D, Lender M. Studies of fluoride metabolism in man. A review and report of original data. Sci Total Environ 1981;17:1-12.

168. Stewart WK. The composition of dialysis fluid. In: Maher JF, ed: Replacement of renal function by dialysis. 3rd ed. Dordrecht: Kluwer, 1989:199-217.

169. Strassburg MA, Greenland S. Methodologic problems in evaluating the carcinogenic risk of environmental agents. J Environ Health 1979;41:214-7.

170. Suarez-Almazor ME, Flowerdew G, Saunders LD, et al. The fluoridation of drinking water and hip fracture hospitalization rates in two Canadian communities. Am J Public Health 1993;83:689-93.

171. Tatevossian A. Fluoride in dental plaque and its effects. J Dent Res 1990;69(Special Issue):645-52.

172. Taves DR. Is fluoride intake in the United States changing? In: Johansen E, Taves DR, Olsen TO, eds: Continuing evaluation of the use of fluorides. AAAS Selected Symposium No 11. Boulder, CO: Westview, 1979:149-57.

173. Taves DR. Dietary intake of fluoride ashed (total fluoride) v. unashed (inorganic fluoride) analysis of individual foods. Br J Nutr 1983;49:295-301.

174. Thylstrup A. Clinical evidence of the role of pre-eruptive fluoride in caries prevention. J Dent Res 1990;69(Special Issue):742-50.

175. Thylstrup A, Fejerskov O, Bruun C, Kann J. Enamel changes and dental caries in 7-year-old children given fluoride tablets from shortly after birth. Caries Res 1979;13:265-76.

176. US Public Health Service. NTP technical report on on the toxicity and cariogenesis studies of sodium fluoride in 344/N rats and B6C3F1 mice (drinking water studies). NIH Rep No 90-2848. Washington DC: Government Printing Office, 1990.

177. US Public Health Service, Ad Hoc Subcommittee on Fluoride. Review of fluoride benefits and risks. Washington DC: Government Printing Office, 1991.

178. Van Loveren C. The antimicrobial action of fluoride and its role in caries inhibition. J Dent Res 1990;69 (Special Issue):676-81.

179. Velu H, Balozet L. Darmous (dystrophic dentaire) du mouton et solubilité du principé actif des phosphates naturels qui le provique. Bull Soc Pathol Exot 1931;24:848-51.

180. Vogt RL, Witherell L, LaRue D, Klaucke DN. Acute fluoride poisoning associated with an on-site fluoridator in a Vermont elementary school. Am J Public Health 1982;72:1168-9.

181. Wefel JS, Maharry G, Jensen ME, et al. In vivo demineralisation and remineralisation of enamel and root surfaces. In: Leach SA, ed.: Factors relating to demineralisation and remineralisation of the teeth. Oxford, England: IRL Press, 1986:181-90.

182. Wefel JS. Effects of fluoride on caries development and progression using intra-oral models. J Dent Res 1990;69 (Special Issue):626-33.

183. Weidmann SM, Weatherell JA. Distribution in hard tissues. In World Health Organization. Fluorides and human health. Geneva: WHO, 1970:104-28.

184. White DJ, Nancollas GH. Physical and chemical considerations of the role of firmly and loosely bound fluoride in caries prevention. J Dent Res 1990;69 (Special Issue):587-94.

185. Whitford G. Fluoride metabolism. In: Newbrun E, ed: Fluorides and dental caries. 3rd ed. Springfield IL: Thomas, 1986:174-98.

186. Whitford GM. The metabolism and toxicology of fluoride. 2nd ed. Monogr Oral Sci vol. 16. Basel: Karger, 1996.

187. World Health Organization. Fluorides and oral health. Tech Rep Series No 846. Geneva: WHO, 1994.

188. Yiamouyiannis J, Burk D. Fluoridation and cancer: Age-dependence of cancer mortality related to artificial fluoridation. Fluoride 1977; 10:102-23.

189. Zipkin I, Likins RC. The absorption of various fluorine compounds from the gastrointestinal tract of the rat. Am J Physiol 1957;191:549-50.

190. Zipkin I, McClure FJ. Cariostatic effect and metabolism of ammonium fluosilicate. Public Health Rep 1954;69:730-3.

191. Zipkin I, Scow RO. Fluoride deposition in different segments of the tibia of the young growing rat. Am J Physiol 1956;185:81-4.

24

Fluoridation
of Drinking Water

Optimal Fluoride Concentrations in Drinking Water ◆
Early Studies ◆ World Status of Fluoridation ◆
Fluoridation in the United States ◆ Federal, State, and
Local Government Roles ◆ Drinking Water
Standards ◆ Caries Reductions from Fluoridation in
Children and Adults ◆ Prenatal Benefits ◆ Effects
on the Primary Dentition ◆ Partial Exposure to
Fluoridated Water ◆ Fluoridation in the Age of
Multiple Fluoride Exposure ◆ Economics of
Fluoridation ◆ Savings in Treatment Costs ◆ Effects
on Dental Practice ◆ The Politics of Fluoridation ◆
Public Attitudes and Knowledge ◆ Opposition to
Fluoridation ◆ Court Decisions ◆ Fluoridation
Decisions at Community Level ◆ The Future of
Fluoridation

Fluoridation is defined as the controlled addition of a fluoride (F) compound to a public water supply to bring its F concentration up to an optimal level to prevent dental caries. A related public health measure is defluoridation, the process of removing excess F naturally present in a water supply to prevent dental fluorosis (or even skeletal fluorosis, in some parts of the world, if the naturally occurring F concentration is high enough).

In our studies of F and its influence on dental caries, water fluoridation deserves special attention because the F-caries relationship was first discovered from studies in communities with naturally fluoridated water, and because water fluoridation is the purest public health use of F. Fluoridation is not a "targeted" approach to caries prevention; its use means that F reaches everyone in a community. This feature is probably the measure's greatest strength, although at the same time it is the source of its greatest problems in terms of social policy. This chapter describes the various issues specific to water fluoridation as a means of controlling caries at a community level.

The unit usually used in the United States for expressing the F concentration in drinking water is parts per million (ppm), although countries using metric measurements usually express this concentration in milligrams per liter (mg/L). It is convenient that the numerical values are the same in both measuring units, that is, 1.2 ppm is the same as 1.2 mg/L.

OPTIMAL F CONCENTRATIONS IN DRINKING WATER

Public policy for controlled water F levels in the United States comes mostly in the form of nonenforceable guidelines set by the US Public Health Service. Current policy is that these levels, for the United States, should be between 0.7 ppm F and 1.2 ppm F, depending on mean annual temperature of the locality.[119] These guidelines, based on the assumption that people will drink more water in a hotter climate than they will in a cooler one, are shown in Table 24–1.

These temperature-related guidelines

Table 24–1. FLUORIDE LEVELS RECOMMENDED BY US PUBLIC HEALTH SERVICE FOR COOL AND WARM CLIMATES

ANNUAL AVERAGE OF MAXIMUM DAILY AIR TEMPERATURES (Degrees F)*	RECOMMENDED CONTROL LIMITS OF F CONCENTRATIONS (ppm)		
	LOWER	*OPTIMUM*	*UPPER*
50.0–53.7	0.9	1.2	1.7
53.8–58.3	0.8	1.1	1.5
58.4–63.8	0.8	1.0	1.3
63.9–70.6	0.7	0.9	1.2
70.7–79.2	0.7	0.8	1.0
79.3–90.5	0.6	0.7	0.8

*Based on temperature data obtained for a minimum of 5 years.

From US Public Health Service, Public Health Service drinking water standards 1962. PHS Publ No 956. Washington DC: Government Printing Office, 1962.

were developed from a series of epidemiologic studies conducted in the American west during the 1950s.[56-59] They were well-conducted studies, and they produced an algebraic formula for determining the temperature-related optimum water F level for a community. This formula is based on Dean's conclusion (Chapter 23) that 1.0 ppm F was the optimum concentration for the Chicago area. Regardless of how appropriate Dean's conclusion was in his time, its appropriateness for the 21st century is less clear in view of today's greater exposure to F from multiple sources than was the case in the 1930–1950 period.

The temperature-related guidelines in Table 24–1, developed under American dietary and cultural conditions, have been found questionable for Asian and African conditions. Hong Kong, for example, reduced its water F levels to 0.5 ppm F by the mid-1990s, and an expert committee of the World Health Organization (WHO) has recommended a range of 0.5 to 1.0 ppm F for all parts of the world.[122] The recommended levels for the United States have stood since 1962, and much in our lifestyles and exposure to F has changed since then. As examples, air-conditioning is widespread and has made life in hotter parts of the country more appealing. There has been a huge increase in consumption of soft drinks and bottled waters, and in F exposure from toothpastes, other dental products, and processed foods and beverages. There has also been an increase in the prevalence of fluorosis since the time the guidelines were developed (Chapter 23). Like all guidelines for F use, the temperature-related recommended F levels in drinking water need

periodic monitoring in a world which has changed from the time when they were developed.

EARLY STUDIES WITH FLUORIDATED WATER

The most important early studies have been described in Chapter 23. All the early research on the safety of F use, and its impact on human health and function, was carried out with fluoridated water. By the time that the first controlled fluoridation trials were begun in 1945, research had established these facts:

- The healthy human body possessed a prompt and efficient excretory mechanism for F, at least at the low levels usually found naturally in the United States, that minimized the danger of long-term accumulation.
- Although ingested F was partly deposited in bone, and although skeletal F concentrations increased with age, skeletal damage could not be demonstrated in users of F-bearing domestic waters in the United States.
- No impairment to general health could be found among people who had drunk waters up to 8.0 ppm F for long periods.

Four independent studies in controlled fluoridation, in which the F concentration in the water supplies of the communities was brought up from negligible to 1.0 to 1.2 ppm, were begun in 1945 and 1946. They followed a long series of epidemiologic studies of caries experience related to F concentration in drinking waters, which were summarized in Chapter 23. These original 4 studies were:

- Grand Rapids, Michigan, with nearby Muskegon as the control city. This study was directed by Dean and his colleagues.[29]
- Newburgh, New York, with Kingston as the control city.[5]
- Evanston, Illinois, with Oak Park as control.[13]
- Brantford, Ontario, with Sarnia as control. Naturally fluoridated Stratford, Ontario, was also included in this study.[69]

At the end of terms ranging up to 15 years, caries experience was shown to be sharply reduced in each of the study populations, despite some differences in study design and examination criteria.[3, 6, 12, 70] These pioneer studies also found that dental fluorosis occurred at about the same extent[7, 104] as Dean had described earlier,[27] namely that some 7% to 16% of the population, at that time, were found to have mild to very mild fluorosis when their F exposure came from drinking waters containing 1.0 ppm F.

The 4 original studies in which F was added to drinking water are sometimes called *classic* studies, but *pioneering* might be a better term. By present-day standards of field trials they were rather crude. Although they are often referred to as *longitudinal* studies, none of them were; all were of sequential cross-sectional design. Sampling methods and dental examiners tended to vary from one year to another,[2] thereby risking bias and unnecessary random error. Methods of statistical analysis, by today's standards, were primitive; data from the control communities were largely neglected after the initial reports, with conclusions based on the much weaker before-after analysis. (Among the early studies, the only true longitudinal study of fluoridation's effects was the Tiel-Culemborg study in the Netherlands.[9, 10])

Perhaps too much emphasis has been ascribed to these 4 pioneering studies, for they really only confirmed prospectively what had already been demonstrated through Dean's research, which still stands as a model of how to apply the epidemiologic method. Despite the design flaws in the "original 4," however, it is difficult for an open-minded observer to reject their conclusions that fluoridation was effective in reducing the prevalence and severity of caries.

WORLD STATUS OF FLUORIDATION

Because there is no central compendium for international data on populations receiving fluoridated water, information on the current global status of fluoridation is not reliable. The World Dental Federation, formerly known as the Fédération Dentaire Internationale and hence still known as the FDI, compiles information supplied by the dental associations of member countries, but there is only moderate response to the FDI surveys. According to the FDI, in 1990 there were 24 countries reporting fluoridation projects reaching some 275 million people, not including naturally occurring F in drinking waters.[52] Some summary statements about the global distribution of fluoridation are shown in Table 24–2.

Ireland is the only nation to have a mandatory fluoridation law. Enacted in 1960, it subsequently withstood a legal challenge that went to the Irish High Court. Most large urban communities fluoridated in the period 1964–1972; 67% of Ireland's population resided in fluoridated areas by 1996.[92]

At the other end of the spectrum, fluoridation has made little headway in Europe, and it is not technically feasible for much of Asia and Africa because of the relative absence of municipal water systems there. The status of reported fluoridation projects in

Table 24–2. SUMMARY OF GLOBAL DISTRIBUTION OF WATER FLUORIDATION IN 1997

- In 1984, the FDI reported 34 countries had some fluoridation projects that reached a total of 246 million people.
- In the city-states of Hong Kong and Singapore, fluoridation in the mid-1990s reached virtually 100% of the population.
- Fluoridation reaches more than 50% of the population in Australia, Ireland, Malaysia, New Zealand, and the United States.
- There is little water fluoridation in Europe outside Basel, Switzerland, and Seville, Spain.
- Previously-reported fluoridation projects in eastern European countries are of uncertain status since the breakup of the Soviet Union in the period 1989–1991. Those in the former East Germany are known to have ceased since German reunification in 1989.
- Extensive water fluoridation projects previously reported from South and Central America are of uncertain status.

Data from Fédération Dentaire Internationale. Basic facts 1990; Dentistry around the world. London: FDI, 1990.

Latin America is uncertain. In Europe, fluoridation in the socialist countries of Eastern Europe is thought to have ended with the demise of the former Soviet Union in the early 1990s. Birmingham, the second largest city in Britain, has been fluoridated since 1964, and there is a belt of fluoridated communities near Birmingham in the West Midlands. On the other hand, there is no water fluoridation at all in Austria, Belgium, Denmark, France, Germany, Italy, Norway, and Sweden. Specific bans are in place in Sweden and Denmark (where a law on additives is interpreted to exclude fluoridation), and for various reasons fluoridation is a dead political issue in the others.

A notable setback in Europe, as opposed to lack of progress, came in the Netherlands, where fluoridated water at one point reached 3 million people. The Netherlands' government ended all fluoridation in 1976. The background to this action has been described in *Consumer Reports*.[1] The long-fluoridated Finnish city of Kuopio also ceased fluoridating in 1992.

FLUORIDATION IN THE UNITED STATES

The Division of Oral Health of the Centers for Disease Control and Prevention in Atlanta (CDC) maintains fluoridation information for the United States. A voluntary reporting system forwards data from the states to CDC, which then publishes it periodically on its website.

At the end of 1992, CDC estimated that fluoridated water was reaching 145 million people in the United States, 56% of the total population and 62% of those receiving municipal water. About 10 million of these people were receiving water naturally fluoridated at 0.7 ppm F or more; the greatest concentration of naturally fluoridated communities is found in Texas, Illinois, and New Mexico.[120] There were more than 14,000 water systems with controlled or natural fluoride levels of 0.7 ppm F or more, representing 24% of all public water systems in the country. This may not sound like much, but a large majority of public water systems serve communities with fewer than 1000 people, where fluoridation is not cost-effective. Drinking water is fluoridated in 42 of the 50 largest American cities. There are over 700 communities in the United States that have been fluoridating for 25 years or more, and many of the naturally fluori-

dated communities have been using the same water source for more than 3 generations. The proportion of state populations reached by fluoridation ranges from close to 100% in Georgia, Maryland, Wisconsin, and Tennessee (plus the District of Columbia) to 2% to 4% in Utah and Nevada.

Federal, State, and Local Government Roles in Fluoridation

The decision to fluoridate is usually made by the local community, although a number of jurisdictions can be involved when water service district boundaries do not coincide with city and county boundaries. State laws requiring fluoridation now stand in 9 states; at the other end of the spectrum, 5 states have laws requiring referenda. These states are shown in Table 24-3. The fluoridation laws have been generally successful, because in states that have them, a high proportion of their population receive fluoridated water. Some of these states, however, have provisions in their laws that can frustrate progress. These provisions are the result of the political compromises necessary to get the law passed. For example, the California law, passed after a vigorous political battle in 1996, cannot be enforced unless outside funds (i.e., state or federal funds) are made available to the local community for the purchase, installation, and operation of the fluoridation system.

The US Public Health Service, initially through its Division of Dental Health (now defunct) and later through CDC, has provided funds and consultative expertise to promote fluoridation through several mechanisms. Federal funds were available through the Division of Dental Health in 1965–1967, and 13 states used them to begin fluoridation projects. These funds were specifically earmarked for fluoridation, whereas some federal contract funds had previously been used for demonstration projects.[114] These earmarked grants in the mid-1960s were cut as the cost of the Vietnam War increased. They were revived from 1978–1981, when CDC had a budget of up to $9 million per year for distribution to states and communities for fluoridation. A total of 765 communities, with a population of nearly 11 million, benefited directly[50] during this period.

In 1981, 7 block grants were initiated as a method of distributing federal health funds to the states.[17] The philosophy of block grants

Table 24-3. STATES WITH FLUORIDATION LAWS IN 1997*

STATE	YEAR STARTED	SIZE OF COMMUNITY AFFECTED	EXEMPTION PROVISION?	MAXIMUM NATURAL F LEVEL (ppm)	F LEVEL TO BE MAINTAINED
CT	1965	20,000+	No	0.8	0.8–1.2
MN	1967	All	No	—	0.9–1.5
IL	1967	All	No	0.8	0.9–1.2
MI	1968	1000+	By local governing body within 5 years	0.9	0.9–1.2
SD	1969	500+	No	0.9	0.9–1.7
OH	1969	5000+	No	—	0.8–1.3
GA	1973	All incorporated	Public vote	—	No greater than 1.0 ppm
NE	1973	All political subdivisions	Public vote	0.7	0.8–1.5
CA	1996	10,000+	No	0.7	0.7–1.2

*Five states have laws that require a favorable vote of the local community before fluoridation can be implemented: DE (1974), ME (1957), NH (1959), NE (1967), UT (1976).
From Centers for Disease Control and Prevention, Division of Oral Health, personal communication 1997.

is that a host of federal categorical programs, which had grown up over the years, were lumped together in specific "blocks," and recipient states could determine for themselves to which programs they would allocate the funds. The prevention block grant includes fluoridation, but it then has to compete at the intrastate level against other worthy prevention causes such as hypertension control and emergency medical services. Although the concept of letting states make their own decisions on funding prevention programs has appeal, it requires a strong state dental director to secure fluoridation funds against the competition of other popular programs. Unfortunately the block grant concept has come with deep cuts in the funds themselves, so fluoridation has not done well under block grants in many states. The preoccupation with reducing the federal deficit that dominated politics in the late 1990s makes the provision of more federal funds for fluoridation uncertain.

Drinking Water Standards

The US Environmental Protection Agency (EPA) has the responsibility for setting national standards for acceptable drinking water under the Safe Drinking Water Act (PL 93-523), first passed in 1974 and renewed several times since. Most of these standards deal with defining acceptable levels of bacterial and chemical contaminants. In the 1975–1976 National Interim Primary Drinking Water Regulations, the standards promulgated soon after passage of the legislation, the EPA referred to naturally-occurring F above 2.0 ppm as a "contaminant" requiring removal from drinking waters. This latter requirement was intended to reduce dental fluorosis in affected areas, but it was heavily criticized by many public authorities on cost grounds (defluoridation is a more expensive process than fluoridation). Many communities that use drinking water naturally fluoridated at more than 2.0 ppm are small and could not afford the cost of meeting the standard. In addition, few of them seemed interested in defluoridating: Their fluorosis did not concern them and they were not aware of any other ill effects, so why bother?

The Interim Primary Drinking Water Regulations of 1980[43] left the recommended maximum contaminant level (RMCL) at 2.0 ppm F, but included an explanatory statement that this standard did not contradict the beneficial effects of F in reducing dental decay. Whether this statement really helped clarify things, especially as the unfortunate word "contaminant" was retained, is doubtful. Public discussion on establishing the final standards became intense during the mid-1980s; the EPA was deluged with demands from both proponents and opponents of fluoridation. The state of South Carolina, for which compliance with the 2.0 ppm F RMCL would have been highly expensive, brought suit against the EPA to revoke the interim RCML in 1981. The EPA, in response, promised to rule on the issue when its studies were complete. These took some time, which was not all the fault of the EPA, because this whole debate illustrated the difficulty of establishing public policy in areas in which effects are not clear-cut. South Carolina sued again in 1984, seeking faster action from the EPA, and this led to a consent decree in January 1985.[44]

Eventually the EPA settled this seemingly irresolvable issue by ducking underneath it. Concluding after its studies that dental fluorosis in the United States was a cosmetic rather than a health defect, the EPA proposed the RMCL for F at 4.0 ppm F, on the grounds that this level was sufficiently low to protect against crippling skeletal fluorosis.[45] By late 1986, this RMCL became an MCL (maximum contaminant level) of 4.0 ppm F, meaning that after all the debate the EPA now had a standard to enforce. The original 2.0 ppm F became a secondary standard, meaning that it was a nonenforceable recommended maximum, in effect a guideline.[46] This secondary standard was justified on the grounds that: "2 mg/L would prevent the majority of cases of water-related cosmetically objectionable dental fluorosis while still allowing for the beneficial effects of F (prevention of dental caries)."[46]

Although some aspects of this debate resembled a Gilbert and Sullivan operetta, it illustrated some serious issues:

- Should the control of dental fluorosis be a subject for national standards, or should it be left to states or localities?
- Is there any rationale for saying a community with 4.1 ppm F in its drinking water must defluoridate, while a community with 3.9 ppm F does not have to? Especially when temperature considerations are not included in the National Primary Drinking Water Regulations?

Not all state dental directors were happy with the requirement that local communities had to be notified when their F levels were between 2 and 4 ppm, especially because the EPA mandate is for that persistent word *contaminant* to appear in the letters of notification.[47]

Standards of this sort quite properly need reexamination from time to time. In 1992, the EPA requested the National Research Council to review the issue of primary and secondary standards for F in drinking waters. An expert committee from a variety of backgrounds (most were from outside dentistry) worked for more than a year, and concluded that there was no current evidence to justify change in the standards.[88] The one area noted by the committee where more evidence was particularly needed was in the relationship between fluoridated water and osteoporosis (Chapter 23). The committee recommended that the issue of F's relationship to health needed to be revisited at regular intervals because new evidence was coming out all the time. Following this report, the EPA decided in late 1993 not to change what was now called the maximum contaminant level goal (MCLG) of 4.0 ppm F.[48]

CARIES REDUCTIONS FROM FLUORIDATION

Caries Reductions in Children

The many fluoridation studies conducted in different parts of the world have varied in the quality of their design and operation, but their results have still been remarkably uniform. In Britain, where water fluoridation is not widespread, reductions of 50% are still found in primary and mixed dentitions. Where fluoridation is more widespread, such as in Australia, New Zealand, Canada, Ireland, and the United States, differences in caries experience between children in fluoridated and nonfluoridated communities is now more in the order of 18% to 35%.[18, 26, 90] This apparent anomaly is explained by the so-called "halo effect" of processed food and beverages, which indirectly spreads some effect of fluoridated water to nonfluoridated communities.

For many years, the statement that "fluoridation reduces dental caries experience by half" was hardly questioned within dentistry. At a time when drinking water was the only significant source of F, that statement was probably true. Its basis was Dean's 21 Cities epidemiologic study of naturally fluoridated areas,[28, 30] supplemented by the results of the initial 4 controlled fluoridation projects begun in 1945–1946. (A summary of the results of these 4 pioneering studies is shown in Table 24–4.) The table shows that after 13 to 15 years of fluoridation, DMF scores in 12 to 14 year-old permanent-resident children favored fluoridation by 48% to 70%. In absolute terms, DMF levels in the fluoridated communities dropped from more than 7 teeth at the start

Table 24–4. DMF TEETH PER CHILD AGED 12 TO 14 YEARS, AND MISSING TEETH PER CHILD, AT THE END OF THE STUDY TERM IN 4 PIONEER FLUORIDATION COMMUNITIES. FLUORIDATED COMMUNITIES ARE DESIGNATED BY (F), NONFLUORIDATED BY (NON-F), AFTER CITY NAME

COMMUNITY	YEAR	MEAN DMF TEETH PER CHILD	PERCENT DIFFERENCE	MISSING TEETH PER CHILD	PERCENT DIFFERENCE
Grand Rapid (F)	1944–1945	9.58	55.5	0.84	65.6
	1959	4.26		0.29	
Evanston (F)	1946	9.03	48.4	0.19	68.4
	1959	4.66		0.06	
Sarnia (Non-F)	1959	7.46		0.75	
Brantford (F)	1959	3.23	56.7	0.22	70.7
Kingston* (Non-F)	1960	12.46		0.92	
Newburgh* (F)	1960	3.73	70.1	0.10	89.1

*Children in Kingston and Newburgh were aged 13–14 years.
From Ast DB, Fitzgerald B. Effectiveness of water fluoridation. J Am Dent Assoc 1962;65:581–5.

of the studies to 3 to 4 teeth per child after 13 to 15 years.

Results of studies with controlled fluoridation, which began around the 1950s to the early 1960s in other countries, were similar to those from the United States. Caries reductions of 44% to 60% were reported from Canada, Australia, Britain, New Zealand, the Netherlands, and from what was then the German Democratic Republic (East Germany) before German reunification.[89]

Caries Reductions in Adults

The caries-inhibitory effects of F are not confined to childhood. Contrary assumptions were surprisingly common (in view of the evidence in Chapter 23), and stemmed from beliefs that (a) F's primary cariostatic action was pre-eruptive, and (b) caries was primarily a disease of childhood. Over a lifetime, fluoridation has been estimated to reduce coronal and root caries by about 20% to 40%.[90] In an age of multiple F exposure, however, it is questionable whether that statement has much meaning, because separating out the caries reductions attributable to various different forms of F is extremely difficult.

Studies on fluoridation's effects in adulthood began early. McKay,[83] for example, observed that 45-year-old adults benefitted from consuming fluoridated water. Adults born and raised in Colorado Springs had 60% lower mean DMF scores than their counterparts in nonfluoridated Boulder.[105] Residents of Colorado Springs also had far fewer teeth missing, and lower caries experience in all

tooth-types was evident.[103, 105] Similar findings among adults came from Aurora, Illinois, a city with naturally occurring 1.2 ppm F in its drinking water.[42] Both the Colorado Springs and the Aurora studies went to considerable lengths to confine the analysis to permanent residents to assess lifetime effects of fluoridated water. In light of today's questions about pre-eruptive and posteruptive cariostatic effects of F, it is a pity that the deliberate exclusion of persons who moved into the fluoridated areas after childhood precluded any consideration of F's solely posteruptive effects. It is also unfortunate that neither study assessed socioeconomic status (SES) of the people concerned. In fairness, today's sensitivity to the impact of SES on health status (Chapters 19 and 20) was not as sharp at the time of these studies, but the net effect is to diminish their value in the perspective of history.

A later study did involve more detailed statistical analysis with data from Lordsburg (3.5 ppm F) and Deming (0.7 ppm F), New Mexico, where SES status was higher in Deming. Results still favored the higher-F community. After controlling for other important variables, Deming adults had 2 more restored teeth per person than did those in Lordsburg, although fluorosis was naturally more severe in Lordsburg.[39] The DMFT data for these two communities is shown in Figure 24–1.

Root caries is also less prevalent in fluoridated areas compared with nonfluoridated.[21, 112] This finding is important, because with increasing tooth retention in an aging population, the amount of root caries would

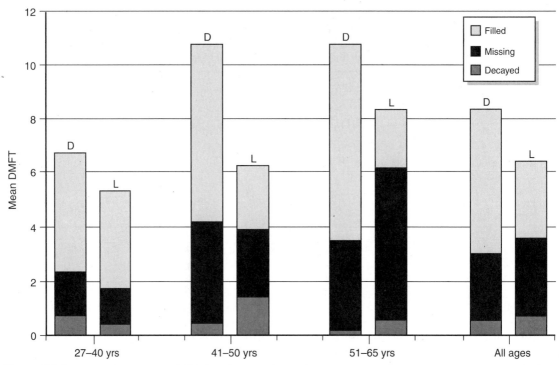

Figure 24–1. Decayed, missing, and filled teeth in adults aged 27-65 in Deming (column D; 0.7 ppm F in drinking water) and Lordsburg (column L; 3.5 ppm F in drinking water), NM. (From Eklund SA, Burt BA, Ismail AI, Calderone JJ. High-fluoride drinking water, fluorosis and dental caries in adults. JA Dent Assoc 1987;114:324-28.)

otherwise be expected to increase and become a greater treatment problem in the future. It is not yet clear whether F's protective effect against root caries is due to topical action on exposed root surfaces, to incorporation of F into cementum before root exposure in the oral cavity, or to a combination of both.

Prenatal Benefits

The policy issue on whether prenatal F actively promotes caries resistance in the offspring is related to the use of supplements (Chapter 25). F ingested by the mother crosses the placenta and enters the fetal circulation.[93, 110, 111] The fetal plasma F level is correlated with the maternal level, although it is somewhat lower, probably because much of the F is taken up by the rapidly mineralizing skeleton and teeth of the fetus.[93] The pertinent question is whether the developing primary dentition has enhanced resistance to caries because of this additional F.

Support for a prenatal benefit came from the Evanston fluoridation study, where children who received fluoridated water in utero, as well as postnatally, were reported to have fewer carious lesions than those who received

it only postnatally.[11] Other authorities, however, did not find this effect.[9, 68] A comprehensive 1981 review concluded that there was probably no benefit in prenatal F, although it was not ruled out completely.[35] If the offspring derives any benefit at all from prenatal F, however, such benefit would be marginal.[35, 110, 111]

The absence of prenatal benefits is a part of the pre-eruptive versus posteruptive discussion on how F works. Benefits or lack of them aside, it is clear that fluoridation is quite safe for the developing fetus.[110] No special precautions are therefore necessary for expectant mothers in a fluoridated area.

Effects on the Primary Dentition

Early fluoridation studies reported caries reductions in the primary dentition of about the same range as was found in the permanent dentition.[6, 67, 116] More recent British data show that this range of caries reduction attributable to fluoridation is being maintained.[15, 16, 24, 25, 36, 55, 74, 86, 102] The data are clear that the primary dentition benefits from fluoridated drinking water.

Partial Exposure to Fluoridation

Because a concentration of about 1.0 ppm F, depending on climate, is regarded as optimal for maximum caries reduction with minimum fluorosis, what happens in communities with water naturally fluoridated at suboptimal levels, such as 0.4 to 0.7 ppm F? Some benefits still accrue in such instances, and dental benefits are generally proportional to the F concentration.[40] A decision on whether it is worth fluoridating a community whose water contains, for example, 0.6 ppm F, is not easily made, for it is not certain whether the cost of fluoridating is worth the additional dental benefits expected.

Evidence that cariostatic efficacy of fluoridated water depends on constant exposure, rather than permanent benefits accruing from partial exposure in childhood, comes from 4 communities where fluoridation started and stopped some years later. Two of the four communities are in Scotland, one is in Germany, and one is in Wisconsin.[31, 78, 80, 113] In each instance, a decline in caries prevalence was seen in young children after fluoridation began, but this decline did not continue after fluoridation stopped. In Wick, Scotland, there was a noticable increase in caries prevalence after fluoridation ceased in 1979.[113] It should be noted that in each community, the drinking water was the only substantial exposure to F at the time of the studies. Trends in the German cities in which caries rose after cessation of fluoridation have been followed for more than 30 years. Caries levels did indeed rise after fluoridation ended, but since 1987 have declined again with greater use of F toothpastes.[79]

Fluoridation ended in 1973 in Tiel, the test city in the landmark Tiel-Culemborg study in the Netherlands. At the time, caries experience was far more favorable in fluoridated Tiel. However, 15 years after fluoridation ended in Tiel, the caries experience of Culemborg children was more favorable.[76] This finding illustrates the importance of constant exposure to F (in this case through fluoridated water) for full dental benefits, as well as the effectiveness of other F exposures, most notably the widespread use of fluoridated toothpaste that has developed since the mid-1970s. (Because Culemborg was of higher SES than Tiel, it would be expected that its use of fluoridated toothpaste was better.) These changes in caries among children in Tiel and Culemborg, relative to fluoridation and subsequent exposure to F toothpaste, are shown in Figure 24–2. Had water fluoridation continued in Tiel, we would expect caries experience in that city to look better than in Culemborg.

The United States and Canada are highly mobile societies. Many people, therefore, have spent part of their lives in a fluoridated area and part in a nonfluoridated area. The benefit of partial exposure to fluoridated water in adulthood has not been documented, but there is evidence that partial exposure in childhood reduces caries experience proportional to the length of exposure. This effect was found in the interim and final reports of the Newburgh-Kingston study.[6, 7] In nonfluoridated Coldwater, Michigan, children who had moved to Coldwater after some residence in a fluoridated area had less caries experience than did those who had lived in Coldwater all their lives.[20] In addition to these North American reports, a well-conducted British study demonstrated a 27% reduction in caries incidence among children who were 12 years old when fluoridation began in their community, relative to the incidence in controls of the same age in nonfluoridated areas.[65] This study also clearly demonstrated that fluoridated water has posteruptive effects.

The evidence on partial exposure to fluoridated water is that cariostatic benefit will be received in proportion to the extent of the exposure. Maximum benefit comes with lifetime exposure.

FLUORIDATION IN THE AGE OF MULTIPLE FLUORIDE EXPOSURE

Caries experience in the populations of the United States, Canada, western European nations, Australia, and New Zealand continue to diminish, although caries-preventive effects directly attributable to water fluoridation are not as high as they once were. The pioneering 4 studies reported caries reductions of 50% to 70% (Table 24–4), whereas more recent studies of fluoridation's effects often produce smaller differences.[34, 71, 81, 98] The reason for reduced effects attributable to water fluoridation is the increase in exposure to F from other sources. The main such exposure is F toothpaste, but there are also other dental products and a variable but possibly significant amount of F in processed foods and beverages. The rise in the prevalence of fluorosis

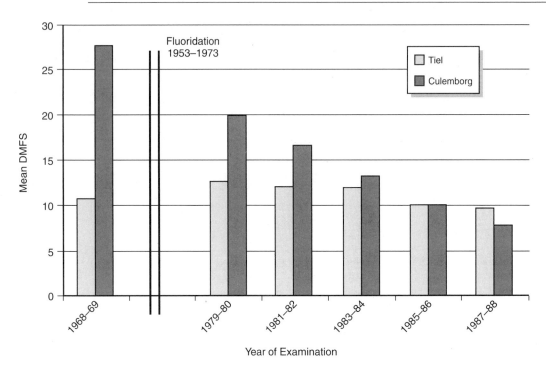

Figure 24–2. Caries experience among 15-year-old children in Tiel and Culemborg, the Netherlands, when fluoridation ended in Tiel and for 15 years subsequently. The drinking water of Tiel was fluoridated between 1953 and 1973. (From Kalsbeek H, Kwant Gw, Groeneveld A, et al. Caries experience of 15-year-old children in the Netherlands after discontinuation of water fluoridation. Caries Res 1993;27:201-5.)

(Chapter 21) also attests to a broad increase in F exposure.

On the other hand, some recent studies of fluoridation's effects in Britain and Australia have yielded results that still show caries experience to be significantly lower in fluoridated communities.[41, 49, 97, 108] One theory put forward to explain these mixed results is that the clear benefits of water fluoridation tend to be seen more in places where fluoridation is less common, thus reducing the "halo effect" and emphasizing the impact from water fluoridation. (The "halo effect" is the name given to the impact of F coming indirectly from water fluoridation, as in processed foods and drinks. The impact of these sources cannot be documented precisely, but is thought to be greater in the United States than in other countries because of the wider extent and complexity of food processing and distribution in the United States. A strong "halo effect" reduces the caries-preventive effect attributable to water fluoridation.) However, the data are not sufficiently distinct between highly-fluoridated and less-fluoridated countries to support this theory, and it is just as likely that the differences seen are due to methodologic differences in the studies.

The standard method of measuring exposure to fluoridated water has traditionally been ecologic (i.e., if you live in a fluoridated community you drink fluoridated water, if you live in a nonfluoridated community you don't). That may have been adequate in other days, but in today's world of high mobility, heavy consumption of soft drinks and bottled water, extensive use of water softeners (which can take F from water), and high consumption of processed foods, it becomes increasingly questionable as a research design. Studies of the effects of fluoridated water in the modern world require increasingly sophisticated methods for measuring F exposure,[101] and hence are not likely to be done all that often.

With the caries experience between fluoridated and nonfluoridated communities increasingly blurred, the decision to fluoridate a water supply is not always as automatic as it once was.[72] It can be argued that if caries experience is already low, good F exposure comes from other sources, and the economic cost of installing fluoridation is high, then fluoridation is unnecessary. However, there are two good reasons to argue for fluoridation except in the most exceptional circumstances.

One is the cost-effectiveness of the measure compared with other methods of caries control (next section), and the second is the social equity benefits of fluoridation. People who live in lower-SES areas are the hardest ones to reach with traditional public health programs, but fluoridation reaches everybody in the community. A major social advantage of water fluoridation is that it benefits lower socioeconomic areas relatively more than higher socioeconomic areas; it has been clearly demonstrated to reduce the strong SES gradient (Chapter 19) usually seen with caries distribution.[25, 75, 87, 95, 109, 117, 118] Caries is still more prevalent and severe in lower-SES groups than in the higher-SES groups in fluoridated areas, but the differences are much less marked than they are in nonfluoridated communities. This factor alone is a strong argument for fluoridating a community's drinking water.

ECONOMICS OF FLUORIDATION

People look at the costs of fluoridation in different ways. A city manager will be concerned about the impact of equipment and operating costs on the city's budget—a subject that can make any city council nervous. Proponents of fluoridation want to stress the impressive cost-effectiveness of the measure over the long term. Dental practitioners usually support fluoridation because it is the right thing to do, even though some have had reservations about diminished practice income as a result. Those opposed to fluoridation may claim that "costs" include social costs such as ill health and environmental damage.

A 1989 workshop at the University of Michigan examined the economics of water fluoridation and other prevention programs. Water fluoridation in the United States in 1989 was estimated to cost 51 cents per person per year on average, although in any one community the annual cost ranged from 12 cents to $5.41 per person per year.[96] These factors were found to influence the per capita cost:

- The size of the community: the bigger the population to be reached, the lower the per capita cost
- The number of F injection points required
- The amount and type of equipment to be used
- The amount and type of F chemical used,

its price, plus the cost of transportation and storage
- Probably the expertise of water plant personnel

Although city managers may well be impressed by the low per capita cost, they will be more immediately interested in the front-end total expenditure. This information would best come from the state health department's water supply division, because each community has its own characteristics. CDC has an expert water engineering staff who can also give estimates of likely cost for a community. Per capita cost is generally inversely proportional to the population to be served, although total expenditures on equipment and material are naturally greater in larger communities.[33, 61]

F compounds used in fluoridation are sodium fluoride and sodium silicofluoride, both solids, and hydrofluosilicic acid, a liquid. The availability, and hence price, of all 3 is highly variable, and prices can also be greatly affected by fluctuations in transportation costs. If a water system has several sources, such as a river plus a number of wells, separate sets of fluoridation equipment may be required for each. Where natural F content is relatively high, less F needs to be added, thus reducing cost of supplies. The US Public Health Service recommendations on F concentrations in various temperature ranges (Table 24–1) mean that less F will be used in a warmer climate, other things being equal.

Although additional personnel costs for fluoridation are virtually negligible in a large city's water treatment plant, they can be a significant factor in the running costs of fluoridating a small community.[96] The water engineers at CDC recommend that water plant operators receive at least 1 day per year of training to allow them to remain efficient and up-to-date. This training may be given by health department water supply personnel or university faculty.

Savings in Treatment Costs

Health economists at the 1989 Michigan workshop[96] concluded that water fluoridation was one of the very few public health measures to demonstrate true cost savings, meaning that it actually saved more money than it cost to operate. Estimates from the workshop were that fluoridation cost $3.35 per carious surface saved, an estimate far less than the fee for any restoration.

Data have been available for years to show that costs of restorative care for children are sharply reduced by fluoridation. In the Newburgh-Kingston study, initial dental care for 6-year-old children cost 58% less in fluoridated Newburgh than in nonfluoridated Kingston.[4] These savings came from fewer extractions needed, fewer restorations, and a smaller proportion of complex restorations. Comparable findings from British studies, which reported a 49% saving for children aged 4 to 5 years and 54% for children aged 11 to 12 years, have been maintained even after the caries decline was recognized.[8]

Some caveats are required, however, in interpreting these findings on cost savings. First, whereas children's restorative costs are certainly cut, fluoridation's effect on costs of adult dental care is less clear. It could be hypothesized, for example, that dollar savings achieved early in life are lost in later life, because greater tooth retention will increase the requirement for periodontal treatment and crowns and bridges in later years. In terms of direct expenditures only, total neglect and complete removal of remaining teeth at an early age are the cheapest forms of dental care.[22] (This profound statement is equivalent to saying the cheapest form of medical care is to let sick people die, and thereby avoid the cost of emergency services, intensive care units, and chronic care facilities. We are not advancing the argument that dentistry should go in for early extractions, but the cold economic fact is that it is the cheapest form of care.) The greater the degree of tooth retention, the more that dental services are likely to be needed in the later years of life. Of course, this argument applies to monetary expenditures only. The worth of a healthy dentition throughout life will vary from one individual to another; virtually beyond price for some, of little consequence to others.

A second caveat concerns the provision of diagnostic and preventive services to children in a fluoridated area. If many of these services are only marginally necessary, their provision will add to the cost of services without providing much in the way of benefits. With declining caries and the associated diminished need for restorations, diagnosis and prevention assume a greater proportion of total cost of dental care. Children with an obviously low caries attack rate in a fluoridated area do not need to visit the dentist as often as they used to, and they require bitewing radiographs less frequently. Whether they need professional F gel applications at all is debatable, especially if they are using F toothpaste and perhaps mouthrinsing with F solutions. If dentists continue to see such children twice a year and apply the full battery of diagnostic and preventive services each time (all in the name of "good preventive dentistry"), however, the substantial savings that can be realized in the cost of restorative treatment will be drastically reduced.[19, 123]

Effects on Dental Practice

A study in the mid-1960s, comparing dental practices in naturally fluoridated and nonfluoridated communities in the Midwest, found little difference in dentist/population ratios between them and also little difference in dentists' incomes.[32] There were differences in the types of treatment provided, and the dentists in the fluoridated areas reported getting more satisfaction out of their practices. The application of these findings to dental practice in the 1990s is uncertain, but the similarities between fluoridated and nonfluoridated areas in dentist/population ratios and dentists' incomes, even in the high-caries days of the 1960s, suggested that fluoridation had little impact on the overall cost of dental care. The shrinking gap in total caries experience between fluoridated and nonfluoridated areas in the 1990s, plus the growth in dental services unrelated to caries, such as cosmetic dentistry, reduces even further the likelihood of a cost differential.

Fluoridation's impact on dental practice, however, is more subtle than mere direct monetary cost. It changes the nature of the services provided away from "drill-and-fill" toward better maintenance, and of course the quality of community oral health is greatly improved. The overall impact of fluoridation on society is perhaps best thought of as raising the quality of life.

Certainly the practice of dentistry for children has changed in the era of the caries decline. The dentists in one pediatric dental practice analyzed their patient records and found, over a 2-year period, that 86% of patients entering before the community's fluoridating needed restorative care, and 41% required treatment of the pulp. By contrast, after the community fluoridated, less than 40% needed restorative care, and less than 10% required treatment of the pulp.[38]

A relatively low demand for restorative care among children who are regular dental attenders became a norm during the 1990s. Need for restorative care has also become concentrated in pit-and-fissure lesions. In the 1986–1987 National Survey of US School Children aged 5 to 17 years, only 9% of children with lifelong fluoridation exposure had mesial or distal surfaces affected by caries. Among those with no fluoridation exposure, the rate was 14%.[18]

THE POLITICS OF FLUORIDATION

Despite the powerful evidence to favor fluoridation as public policy, its implementation has been sporadic in the United States and even slower in most other countries. Frequently it has been the subject of vigorous opposition. Although the major arguments of opponents have varied, opposition remains a persistent fact of life.

Whose job is it to see that fluoridation is implemented in a community where the conditions are right for it? Because that is a political question, the ultimate decision is made by mayors, town councils, state legislatures, or the electorate. Those decisions don't just happen by themselves. Dental professionals carry the main commitment for promoting fluoridation, for without their support, the issue will almost certainly fail.[51, 54] The inherent problem, however, is that this commitment can demand a kind of leadership with which dental professionals are often not comfortable: political action, public speaking, and a level of visibility that can have troubling ethical undertones. Dental and dental hygiene schools do not train their graduates for political action. The detailed role of dental professionals in promoting fluoridation is discussed in Chapter 5.

Public Attitudes and Knowledge

Polls of public opinion have shown that opposition to fluoridation is reported by 10% to 20% of the US population. The most recent national Gallup Poll in 1991 found that 78% approved of fluoridation, although the sample was confined to parents.[91] The 1990 National Health Interview Survey found that 76% of those with more than 12 years of education knew what water fluoridation was for, compared with 36% of those with less than 12 years.[62] Approval ratings vary considerably in different regions and communities, often according to whether or not fluoridation has been a recent local issue. Although all national and local studies find that opponents of fluoridation constitute a minority,[53] history has shown repeatedly that even a small single-issue group, when dedicated and well-organized, can sway political decisions. Many of those who say they are in favor are really passively so, and a sizable proportion of people in public opinion surveys are just not particularly interested in fluoridation one way or the other.[53] This factor immediately evens out the numbers in most political campaigns.

Social scientists were first attracted to the fluoridation issue by the community conflict it generated, and much of their research dates from the 1960s. Since then the volume of social science research has diminished sharply. That is to be regretted, for common sense tells us that some issues that dictate today's attitudes to fluoridation, such as environmental concerns, must have changed since the 1960s.

Some of this social science research attempted to "profile" the various antifluoridationists, the rationale being that opposition could then be predicted and countered during promotional efforts. Unfortunately, the infinite complexities of human beliefs and behavior resulted in a picture that is anything but clear. Some of the studies on the attitudes of persons who voted against fluoridation in referenda, for example, concluded that opponents felt a sense of deprivation or powerlessness, and that they held a grudge against "them," the people whom they saw to be directing society. In this view, a general discontent with society at large can be conveniently expressed by opposing fluoridation.[63, 64, 94, 107] Alienation may still be driving some present-day antifluoridation leaders,[66] a view that perceives these individuals as "true believers" who are not influenced by scientific arguments.

Although opponents of fluoridation have been characterized as more likely to be older, childless people of lower than median income and education, a referendum can also fail in a young, high-income, and highly educated community.[106] The prevailing image of the profluoridationist, from the 1960s research, is one of a younger married person with small children and with above-median income and education.[82] Even at that time, however, this image was confused by a finding of support in all SES groups,[60] and by a Californian study that found greater opposition to fluoridation among nonmanual than among manual workers.[64]

This confused picture of attitudes to fluoridation still pertained in more recent times. A study in Norway, where there is no water fluoridation, found a 20% rise in public opposition to fluoridated water between 1973 and 1983. Pinpointing the cause was difficult, but it was thought to stem from a perception that dental health was improving anyway so that fluoridation was an unnecessary risk.[99] A Massachusetts study found that 60% of the state's voters said they favored fluoridation in a telephone survey, but this percentage was at odds with the 61% who voted against it in referenda.[121]

Some have always opposed fluoridation on the freedom-of-choice issue, meaning that they believe that the dichotomous nature of fluoridation (the community either fluoridates or it doesn't) removes individual choice. This issue remains alive and well,[51, 73] as some would argue it should in a healthy society. However one looks at it, the evidence is that public attitudes toward fluoridating water have become a little more accepting since opinions were first measured in the 1950s.

Opposition to Fluoridation

The dichotomous nature of fluoridation ensures that there will be organized political opposition to its adoption. Even apart from specific arguments on effectiveness and health effects, skilled opponents can easily exploit the issues of overregulation, increasing environmental sensitivity, and cynicism about governmental policies and officials.

Tactics of those opposed to fluoridation have become more sophisticated in recent years. Opponents, although small in number, have learned to exploit society's concerns about health, whether real or imagined, and how to work effectively with legislatures and city councils.[37] Most states have small "Pure Water Councils," loosely affiliated with each other, which spring to life to oppose fluoridation when the question arises in a community. There is also a handful of PhDs, physicians, and dentists, who tend to appear anywhere in the country (or in the world for that matter) to support a local antifluoridation group.

Court Decisions on Fluoridation

Many communities that have begun fluoridation have had legal suits brought against them in an effort to stop it. Although lower courts have ruled against fluoridation in a few of these suits, fluoridation has never been ruled against in appellate court.[14] Lower courts that have ruled against fluoridation have usually done do on the issues of personal liberty and religious beliefs.[14, 23, 115]

As early as 1965, state Supreme Courts had upheld the legality and constitutionality of fluoridation 13 times.[100] By 1984, 13 appeals had reached the US Supreme Court, which on every occasion either dismissed appeals or refused review.[14] No American court of last resort has ever ruled against fluoridation for any reason.

The most searching courtroom scrutiny of water fluoridation, especially in respect to its impact on human health, came from Glasgow, Scotland, in 1983.[84] Known as the Strathclyde case, this was the longest court case in British legal history. The presiding judge, Lord Jauncey, ruled that the evidence for fluoridation's safety was convincing.

Fluoridation Decisions at Community Level

Unless state law dictates otherwise, fluoridation is adopted by the local community under whose jurisdiction the water supply falls. This is usually a city council. Even when a city provides water to suburban areas and surrounding townships, the decision remains that of the city council, although the issue becomes more complicated. Where the issue is volatile, however, many councils do not want to make the decision without a clear indication of public feeling, and that often means a referendum.

The first referendum on fluoridation was in 1950, in Stevens Point, Wisconsin.[85] It lost. McNeil's entertaining description of that campaign shows how quickly fluoridation can flare up into a major issue in a community, and how an unprepared dental community, no matter how well-intentioned, can make some serious political errors. It was estimated in 1970 that two-thirds of the first 900 referenda were lost,[77] and 33 of the 41 held in 1980 were also lost.[51]

THE FUTURE

Chapters 23 and 24 have examined the F issue from many perspectives. It all began with Colorado brown stain and it led to water fluoridation, dentistry's greatest contribution to the public's health. F has changed the face of America (literally!), banished childhood toothache agonies for millions, and presented the prospects of an uneventful lifetime dental history for millions more. Its controlled use has improved the quality of life for all it reaches, and good oral health is primarily a quality-of-life issue. It is the most cost-effective method of bringing F to a community, and it benefits the socially-deprived relatively more than the socially-advantaged. F has also probably done more to change the nature of dental practice over the last generation than any other single factor.

Despite all those benefits, and despite reaching more than 55% of the American population, recent progress has been slow, and water fluoridation continues to struggle for public acceptance. Society changes, and issues that were not thought of during the time of Dean and McClure, nor during the steady progress made in implementing fluoridation during the 1950s and 1960s, have to be dealt with if progress is to continue. Social science research on public acceptance of fluoridation has not continued much from the 1960s, and some believe that dental, medical, and social researchers have at least partly failed to carry on that superb start that the Dean-McClure generation gave us. Fluoridation proponents have also made honest mistakes in promoting it. What can appear to some, in retrospect, as arrogance and complacency in past years can still present problems in promoting fluoridation today. In a free society, water fluoridation can continue as public policy only if the public accepts it.

REFERENCES

1. A two-part report on fluoridation. Part 1: The cancer scare. Consumer Rep 1978;43:392-6.
2. Arnold FA Jr, Dean HT, Knutson JW. Effect of fluoridated public water supplies on dental caries incidence. Results of the seventh year of study at Grand Rapids and Muskegon, Mich. Public Health Rep 1953;68:141-8.
3. Arnold FA Jr, Likins RC, Russell AL, Scott DB. Fifteenth year of the Grand Rapids fluoridation study. J Am Dent Assoc 1962;65:780-5.
4. Ast DB, Cons NC, Pollard ST, Garfinkel J. Time and cost factors to provide regular periodic dental care for children in a fluoridated and nonfluoridated area: Final report. J Am Dent Assoc 1970;80:770-6.
5. Ast DB, Finn SB, McCaffrey I. The Newburgh-Kingston caries-fluorine study. I. Dental findings after three years of water fluoridation. Am J Public Health 1950;40:716-24.
6. Ast DB, Fitzgerald B. Effectiveness of water fluoridation. J Am Dent Assoc 1962;65:581-5.
7. Ast DB, Smith DJ, Wachs B, Cantwell KT. The Newburgh-Kingston caries-fluorine study. XIV. Combined clinical and roentgenographic dental findings after ten years of fluoride experience. J Am Dent Assoc 1956;52:314-25.
8. Attwood D, Blinkhorn AS. Reassessment of the effect of fluoridation on cost of dental treatment among Scottish schoolchildren. Community Dent Oral Epidemiol 1989;17:79-82.
9. Backer Dirks O. The relation between the fluoridation of water and dental caries experience. Int Dent J 1967;17:582-605.
10. Backer-Dirks O, Houwink B, Kwant GW. The results of 6½ years of artificial drinking water in the Netherlands: The Tiel-Culemborg experiment. Arch Oral Biol 1961;5:284-300.
11. Blayney JR, Hill IN. Evanston dental caries study. XXIV. Prenatal fluorides: Value of waterborne fluorides during pregnancy. J Am Dent Assoc 1964;69:291-4.
12. Blayney JR, Hill IN. Fluorine and dental caries. J Am Dent Assoc 1967;74(Special Issue):233-302.
13. Blayney JR, Tucker WH. The Evanston dental caries study. J Dent Res 1948;27:279-86.
14. Block LE. Antifluoridationists persist: The constitutional basis for fluoridation. J Public Health Dent 1986;46:188-98.
15. Booth IM, Mitropoulos CM, Worthington HV. A comparison between the dental health of 3-year-old children living in fluoridated Huddersfield and non-fluoridated Dewsbury in 1989. Community Dent Health 1992;9:151-7.
16. Bradnock G, Marchment MD, Anderson RJ. Social background, fluoridation and caries experience in a 5-year-old population in the West Midlands. Br Dent J 1984;156:127-31.
17. Brandt EN Jr. Block grants and the resurgence of federalism. Public Health Rep 1981;96:495-97.
18. Brunelle JA, Carlos JP. Recent trends in dental caries in U.S. children and the effect of water fluoridation. J Dent Res 1990;69(Special Issue):723-7.
19. Burt BA. Diagnostic and preventive services in a national incremental dental plan for children. J Public Health Dent 1977;37:31-46.
20. Burt BA, Eklund SA, Loesche WJ. Dental benefits of limited exposure to fluoridated water in childhood. J Dent Res 1986;61:1322-5.
21. Burt BA, Ismail AI, Eklund SA. Root caries in an optimally fluoridated and a high fluoride community. J Dent Res 1986;65:1154-8.
22. Burt BA, Warner KE. Prevention of oral disease: Its potential for containing the cost of dental care. In: Kudrle RT, Meskin LH, eds. Opportunities for cost-containment in dentistry. Minneapolis: University of Minnesota Press, 1980:132-61.
23. Butler HW. Legal aspects of fluoridating community water supplies. J Am Dent Assoc 1962;65:653-8.
24. Carmichael CL, French AD, Rugg-Gunn AJ, Furness JA. The relationship between social class and caries experience in five-year-old children in Newcastle and Northumberland after twelve years' fluoridation. Community Dent Health 1984;1:47-54.
25. Carmichael CL, Rugg-Gunn AJ, Ferrell RS. The relationship between fluoridation, social class and caries experience in 5-year-old children in Newcastle and Northumberland in 1987. Br Dent J 1989;167:57-61.
26. Clark DC, Hann HJ, Williamson MF, Berkowitz J. Effects of lifelong consumption of fluoridated water or use of fluoride supplements on dental caries

prevalence. Community Dent Oral Epidemiol 1995;23:20-4.

27. Dean HT. The investigation of physiological effects by the epidemiological method. In: Moulton FR, ed. Fluorine and dental health. Washington DC: American Association for the Advancement of Science, 1942:23-31.

28. Dean HT, Arnold FA Jr, Elvove E. Domestic water and dental caries. V. Additional studies of the relation of fluoride domestic waters to dental caries experience in 4,425 white children aged 12–14 years of 13 cities in 4 states. Public Health Rep 1942;57:1155-79.

29. Dean HT, Arnold FA Jr, Jay P, Knutson JW. Studies on mass control of dental caries through fluoridation of the public water supply. Public Health Rep 1950;65:1403-8.

30. Dean HT, Jay P, Arnold FA Jr, Elvove E. Domestic water and dental caries. II. A study of 2,832 white children aged 12-14 years, of eight suburban Chicago communities, including L. acidophilus studies of 1,761 children. Public Health Rep 1941;56:761-92.

31. Department of Health and Social Security (Great Britain). The fluoridation studies in the United Kingdom and the results achieved after eleven years. London: Her Majesty's Stationery Office, 1969:33-44.

32. Douglas BL, Wallace DA, Lerner M, Coppersmith SB. Impact of water fluoridation on dental practice and dental manpower. J Am Dent Assoc 1972;84:355-67.

33. Dowell TB. The economics of fluoridation. Br Dent J 1976; 140:103-6.

34. Downer MC, Blinkhorn AS, Holt RD, et al. Dental caries experience and defects of dental enamel among 12-year-old children in north London, Edinburgh, Glasgow, and Dublin. Community Dent Oral Epidemiol 1994;22:283-5.

35. Driscoll WS. Review of clinical research on prenatal fluorides. J Dent Child 1981;48:109-17.

36. Duxbury JT, Lennon MA, Mitropoulos CM, Worthington HV. Differences in caries levels in 5-year-old children in Newcastle and North Manchester in 1985. Br Dent J 1987;162:457-8.

37. Easley MW. The new antifluoridationists: who are they and how do they operate? J Public Health Dent 1985;45:133-41.

38. Eichenbaum IW, Dunn NA, Tinanoff N. Impact of fluoridation in a private pedodontic practice: Thirty years later. J Dent Child 1981;48:211-4.

39. Eklund SA, Burt BA, Ismail AI, Calderone JJ. High-fluoride drinking water, fluorosis and dental caries in adults. J Am Dent Assoc 1987;114:324-8.

40. Eklund SA, Striffler DF. Anticaries effect of various concentrations of fluoride in drinking water: Evaluation of empirical evidence. Public Health Rep 1980;95:486-90.

41. Ellwood RP, O'Mullane DM. The association between area deprivation and dental caries in groups with and without fluoride in their drinking water. Community Dent Health 1995;12:18-22.

42. Englander HR, Wallace DA. Effects of naturally fluoridated water on dental caries in adults. Public Health Rep 1962;77:887-93.

43. Environmental Protection Agency. Interim primary drinking water regulations. Fed Register 1980 Feb 17;45:57332-57.

44. Environmental Protection Agency. National primary drinking water regulations; fluoride. Fed Register 1985 May 14;50:20164-75.

45. Environmental Protection Agency. National primary drinking water regulations; fluoride. Fed Register 1985 Nov 14;50:47142-71.

46. Environmental Protection Agency. National primary and secondary drinking water regulations: fluoride; final rule. Fed Register 1986 Apr 18;51:11396-412.

47. Environmental Protection Agency. Drinking water regulations; public notification. Fed Register 1987 Oct 28;52:41534-50.

48. Environmental Protection Agency. Drinking water maximum contaminant level goal; fluoride. Fed Register 1993 Dec 29;58:68826-7.

49. Evans DJ, Rugg-Gunn AJ, Tabari ED. The effect of 25 years of water fluoridation in Newcastle assessed in four surveys of 5-year-old children over an 18-year period. Br Dent J 1995;178:60-4.

50. Expiring fluoridation program success despite short lifespan. ADA News 1981; Nov 23:1, 13.

51. Faine RC, Collins JJ, Daniel J, et al. The 1980 fluoridation campaigns: A discussion of results. J Public Health Dent 1981;41:138-42.

52. Fédération Dentaire Internationale. Basic facts 1990: Dentistry around the world. London: FDI, 1990.

53. Frazier PJ. Public and professional adoption of certain measures to prevent dental decay. In: Cohen LK, Bryant PS, eds: Social sciences and dentistry: A critical bibliography vol II. London: Quintessence and Federation Dentaire Internationale, 1984:84-144.

54. Frazier PJ. Priorities to preserve fluoride uses: rationales and strategies. J Public Health Dent 1985; 45:149-76.

55. French AD, Carmichael CL, Rugg-Gunn AJ, Furness JA. Fluoridation and dental caries experience in 5-year-old children in Newcastle and Northumberland in 1981. Br Dent J 1984;156:54-7.

56. Galagan DJ. Climate and controlled fluoridation. J Am Dent Assoc 1953;47:159-70.

57. Galagan DJ, Lamson GG Jr. Climate and endemic dental fluorosis. Public Health Rep 1953;68:497-508.

58. Galagan DJ, Vermillion JR. Determining optimum fluoride concentrations. Public Health Rep 1957;72:491-93.

59. Galagan DJ, Vermillion JR, Nevitt GA, et al. Climate and fluid intake. Public Health Rep 1957;72:484-90.

60. Gamson WA, Irons PH. Community characteristics and fluoridation outcome. J Soc Issues 1961;17:66-74.

61. Garcia AI. Caries incidence and cost of prevention programs. J Public Health Dent 1989;49(Special Issue):259-71.

62. Gift HC, Corbin SB, Nowjack-Raymer RE. Public knowledge of prevention of dental disease. Public Health Rep 1994;109:397-404.

63. Green AL. The ideology of anti-fluoridation leaders. J Social Issues 1961;17:13-25.

64. Hahn HD. Fluoridation and patterns in community politics. J Public Health Dent 1965;25:152-7.

65. Hardwick JL, Teasdale J, Bloodworth G. Caries increments over 4 years in children aged 12 at the start of water fluoridation. Br Dent J 1982;153:217-22.

66. Hastreiter RJ. Fluoridation conflict: A historical and conceptual synthesis. J Am Dent Assoc 1983;106:486-90.

67. Hill IN, Blayney JR, Wolf W. The Evanston dental caries study. XVI. Reduction in dental caries attack rates in children six to eight years old. J Am Dent Assoc 1956;53:327-33.

68. Horowitz HS, Heifetz SB. Effects of prenatal exposure to fluoridation on dental caries. Public Health Rep 1967;82:297-304.

69. Hutton WL, Linscott BW, Williams DB. The Brantford fluorine experiment. Interim report after five years of water fluoridation. Can J Public Health 1951;42:81-7.

70. Hutton WL, Linscott BW, Williams DB. Final report of local studies on water fluoridation in Brantford. Can J Public Health 1956;47:89-92.

71. Ismail AI. What is the effective concentration of fluoride? Community Dent Oral Epidemiol 1995; 23:246-51.

72. Ismail AI, Shoveller J, Langille D, et al. Should the drinking water of Truro, Nova Scotia, be fluoridated? Water fluoridation in the 1990s. Community Dent Oral Epidemiol 1993;21:118-25.

73. Isman R. Public views on fluoridation and other preventive dental practices. Community Dent Oral Epidemiol 1983;11:217-23.

74. Jackson D, James PM, Thomas FD. Fluoridation in Anglesey 1983: A clinical study of dental caries. Br Dent J 1985;158:45-9.

75. Jones CM, Taylor GO, Whittle JG, et al. Water fluoridation, tooth decay in 5 year olds, and social deprivation measured by the Jarman score: Analysis of data from British dental surveys. Br Med J 1997;315:514-7.

76. Kalsbeek H, Kwant GW, Groeneveld A, et al. Caries experience of 15-year-old children in the Netherlands after discontinuation of water fluoridation. Caries Res 1993;27:201-5.

77. Knutson JW. Water fluoridation after 25 years. J Am Dent Assoc 1970;80:765-9.

78. Künzel W. Effect of an interruption in water fluoridation on the caries prevalence of the primary and secondary dentition. Caries Res 1980;14:304-10.

79. Künzel W, Fischer T. Rise and fall of caries prevalence in German towns with different F concentrations in drinking water. Caries Res 1997;31:166-73.

80. Lemke CW, Doherty JM, Arra MC. Controlled fluoridation: The dental effects of discontinuation in Antigo, Wisconsin. J Am Dent Assoc 1970;80:782-6.

81. Lewis DW, Banting DW. Water fluoridation: Current effectiveness and dental fluorosis. Community Dent Oral Epidemiol 1994;22:153-8.

82. Mausner B, Mausner, J. The anti-scientific attitude. Sci Am 1955;192:35-9.

83. McKay FS. Mass control of dental caries through the use of domestic water supplies containing fluorine. Am J Public Health 1948;38:828-32.

84. McKechnie R. The Strathclyde fluoridation case. Community Dent Health 1985;2:63-8.

85. McNeil DR. The fight for fluoridation. New York: Oxford University Press, 1957.

86. Mitropoulos CM, Lennon MA, Langford JW, Robinson DJ. Differences in dental caries experience in 14-year-old children in fluoridated South Birmingham and in Bolton in 1987. Br Dent J 1988;164:349-50.

87. Murray JJ, Breckon JA, Reynolds PJ, et al. The effect of residence and social class on dental caries experience in 15–16-year-old children living in three towns (natural fluoride, adjusted fluoride, and low fluoride) in the north east of England. Br Dent J 1991;171:319-22.

88. National Research Council. Health effects of ingested fluoride. Washington DC: National Academy Press, 1993.

89. Newbrun E. Cost-effectiveness and practicality issues in the systemic use of fluorides. In: Burt BA, ed: The relative efficiency of methods of caries prevention in dental public health. Ann Arbor, MI: University of Michigan, 1979.

90. Newbrun E. Effectiveness of water fluoridation. J Public Health Dent 1989;49(Special Issue):279-89.

91. Newbrun E. The fluoridation war: A scientific dispute or a religious argument? J Public Health Dent 1996;56(Special Issue):246-52.

92. O'Mullane DM, Whelton H, Costelloe P, et al. The results of water fluoridation in Ireland. J Public Health Dent 1996;56(Special Issue):259-64.

93. Parker PR, Bawden JW. Prenatal fluoride exposure: Measurement of plasma levels and enamel uptake in the guinea pig. J Dent Res 1986;65:1341-5.

94. Pinard M. Structural attachments and political support in urban politics: The case of fluoridation referendums. Am J Sociol 1963;68:513-26.

95. Provart SJ, Carmichael CL. The relationship between caries, fluoridation and material deprivation in five-year-old children in County Durham. Community Dent Health 1995;12:200-3.

96. Results of the workshop. J Public Health Dent 1989;49(Special Issue):331-7.

97. Riordan PJ. Dental caries and fluoride exposure in Western Australia. J Dent Res 1991;70:1029-34.

98. Ripa LW. A half-century of community water fluoridation in the United States: Review and commentary. J Public Health Dent 1993;53:17-44.

99. Rise J, Kraft P. Opinions about water fluoridation in Norwegian adults. Community Dent Health 1986;3:313-20.

100. Roemer R. Water fluoridation: Public health responsibility and the democratic process. Am J Public Health 1965;55:1337-48.

101. Rozier RG. The effectiveness of community water fluoridation: beyond dummy variables for fluoride exposure [editorial]. J Public Health Dent 1995; 55:195.

102. Rugg-Gunn AJ, Carmichael CL, Ferrell RS. Effect of fluoridation and secular trend in caries in 5-year-old children living in Newcastle and Northumberland. Br Dent J 1988;165:359-64.

103. Russell AL. The inhibition of approximal caries in adults with lifelong fluoride exposure. J Dent Res 1953;32:138-43.

104. Russell AL. Dental fluorosis in Grand Rapids during the seventeenth year of fluoridation. J Am Dent Assoc 1962;65:608-12.

105. Russell AL, Elvove E. Domestic water and dental caries. VII. A study of the fluoride-dental caries relationship in an adult population. Public Health Rep 1951;66:1389-401.

106. Shaw CT. Characteristics of supporters and rejectors of a fluoridation referendum and a guide for other community programs. J Am Dent Assoc 1969;78:339-41.

107. Simmel A. A signpost for research on fluoridation conflicts: The concept of relative deprivation. J Social Issues 1961;17:26-36.

108. Slade GD, Davies MJ, Spencer AJ, Stewart JF. Associations between exposure to fluoridated drinking water and dental caries experience among children in two Australian states. J Public Health Dent 1995;55:218-28.

109. Slade GD, Spencer AJ, Davies MJ, Stewart JF. Influence of exposure to fluoridated water on socioeconomic inequalities in children's caries experience. Community Dent Oral Epidemiol 1996;24:89-100.

110. Speirs RL. The value of prenatally administered fluoride. Dent Update 1983;10:43-6, 49-51.

111. Stamm JW. Perspectives on the use of prenatal fluorides: a reactor's comments. J Dent Child 1981;48:128-33.

112. Stamm JS, Banting DW, Imrey PB. Adult root caries survey of two similar communities with contrasting natural fluoride levels. J Am Dent Assoc 1990; 120:143-9.

113. Stephen KW, McCall DR, Tullis, JI. Caries prevalence in northern Scotland before, and 5 years after, water fluoridation. Br Dent J 1987;163:324-6.

114. Striffler DF, Atkins WD, Caldwell CG, et al. Fluoridation of water supplies in small rural communities. Public Health Rep 1965;80:25-32.

115. Strong GA. Liberty, religion, and fluoridation. J Am Dent Assoc 1968;76:1398-409.

116. Tank G, Storvick CA. Caries experience of children one to six years old in two Oregon communities (Corvallis and Albany). I. Effect of fluoride on caries experience and eruption of teeth. J Am Dent Assoc 1964;69:749-57.

117. Treasure ET, Dever JG. The prevalence of caries in 5-year-old children living in fluoridated and nonfluoridated communities in New Zealand. N Z Dent J 1992;88:9-13.

118. Treasure ET, Dever JG. Relationship of caries with socioeconomic status in 14-year-old children from communities with different fluoride histories. Community Dent Oral Epidemiol 1994;22:226-30.

119. US Public Health Service. Public Health Service drinking water standards 1962. PHS Publ No 956. Washington DC: Government Printing Office, 1962.

120. US Public Health Service, Division of Dental Health. Natural fluoride content of community water supplies 1969. Washington DC: Government Printing Office, undated.

121. Weintraub JA, Connolly GN, Lambert CA, Douglass CW. What Massachusetts residents know about fluoridation. J Public Health Dent 1985;45:240-46.

122. World Health Organization. Fluorides and oral health. WHO Tech Rep 846. Geneva: WHO, 1994.

123. Young WO, Pelton WJ. Planning a dental prepayment program for children in an area of low caries prevalence. J Am Dent Assoc 1956;53:38-46.

25

Other Uses of Fluoride in Caries Prevention

Fluoridated Salt ◆ Fluoridated School Drinking
Water ◆ Milk Fluoridation ◆ Dietary Fluoride
Supplements ◆ Professionally Applied Fluoride Gels ◆
Fluoride Varnishes ◆ Self-Applied Fluorides ◆
Fluoride Mouthrinses ◆ Fluoride Toothpastes ◆
Multiple Fluoride Exposure

Fluoride (F) was first used to prevent dental caries by adding it to drinking water, but it was not long before alternative uses were put into practice. The result today is that F is used in a variety of ways to control caries in public health, individual patient care, and in self-care. Any deliberate use of F by dental professionals today must be made in the knowledge that there is extensive "background" exposure to F through drinking water, toothpaste, mouthrinses, and in processed food and drink. We stated in Chapter 23 that F works best to control caries when low ambient levels are constantly present in the oral cavity (plaque, saliva, enamel surface, soft tissues). Any use of F rinses, professionally applied gels, or F dietary supplements should be aimed toward achieving that condition, either for the individual patient or for the public.

We also discussed the pre-eruptive and posteruptive action of F in Chapter 23. In the light of F's predominantly posteruptive action in caries prevention, the traditional categorization of F measures into systemic and topical fluorides is no longer appropriate because systemic vehicles have topical effects, and if young children inadvertently swallow enough of a topical vehicle, the systemic outcome can be fluorosis.

This chapter examines the evidence for F use in salt, school drinking water, milk, dietary supplements, professionally applied gels and varnishes, self-applied gels, and F mouthrinses; recommendations are made for

their use. The chapter closes with an assessment of multiple F use.

FLUORIDATED SALT

Salt fluoridation is the controlled addition of F to domestic salt for the purpose of preventing dental caries. Fluoridated salt uses the same public health principle as water fluoridation, namely that a small amount of fluoride in a dietary staple serves to inhibit dental caries with little conscious action by the individual. The concept of adding F to salt followed the success of iodized salt, which had been initiated in Switzerland in 1922 to prevent goiter, the thyroid condition that was endemic in the Swiss Alpine region through the early years of the 20th century.

Fluoridated salt was first used in Switzerland in 1955. Water fluoridation in Switzerland is confined to the city of Basel, and the nation has only one salt processing and distribution company. Switzerland is a prosperous, highly-developed country, and there have been few problems with safety and control of the procedure. The reduction in caries incidence in Swiss communities using fluoridated salt, measured only in before-after designs, appears similar to that found with water fluoridation.[42, 127, 173] Fluoridated salt has been well accepted by the Swiss public, now holding 75% of the table salt market. The effects of fluoridated salt have also been studied in Colombia[73] and Hungary,[188, 189] with generally favorable results, although neither country now markets fluoridated salt. Although the evidence for salt fluoridation is consistent, it is based only on a limited number of observational studies rather than clinical trials, and a clear mechanism for the beneficial action of fluoridated salt has not been established.

The concentration of F in salt is based on estimates of salt consumption and evaluated by studies of urinary F concentration. The material most commonly used to fluoridate salt is potassium fluoride (KF), although sodium fluoride (NaF) is also used. The early Swiss studies began with salt fluoridated to 90 parts per million (ppm), but it became clear that this level was too low. In the early 1970s, the concentration was increased to 250 mg KF/kg salt (or 225 mg NaF/kg salt), which was based on adult salt consumption estimates of some 8 to 10 g/day. Even though patterns of salt consumption vary from one country to another,[95] 250 mg KF/kg salt now appears to be the standard in countries other than Switzerland as well.

Salt fluoridation has political appeal because it gives consumers a choice in a way that fluoridation of water does not. In most places in which fluoridated salt is available, it appears alongside nonfluoridated salt on supermarket shelves, and purchasers can make their choice. The Swiss Canton of Vaud, interestingly enough, removes that choice by fluoridating all salt on the supermarket shelves as well as the salt delivered in bulk to restaurants, bakeries, food processors, hospitals, and other institutions. Oral health should benefit as a result, although consumer choice is curtailed.

Some concerns have been expressed that use of fluoridated salt may promote increased salt consumption with possibly detrimental effects on hypertension, although there is no evidence that this has happened. Nothing in salt fluoridation encourages people to consume more salt than usual.

By the mid-1990s salt fluoridation had become established in France and Germany as well as Switzerland. In the western hemisphere, it was established in Costa Rica, Mexico, and Jamaica. Further growth in Latin America is likely. It has never been used in the United States or Canada, and given the mass distribution of food, multiple salt production companies, and the extent of water fluoridation, salt fluoridation would not be appropriate in either country.

FLUORIDATION OF SCHOOL DRINKING WATER

In rural areas where community water fluoridation is not possible, the approach of fluoridating a school's drinking water was promoted for years. The procedure was reported to reduce dental caries among schoolchildren by about 40%,[89] although none of these studies was conducted in a blind fashion, and there were no concurrent controls.

Relative to community water fluoridation, the disadvantages of school fluoridation were that children did not receive the benefits until they were old enough to begin school, and they drank the water only when school was in session. To compensate for this reduced exposure, the recommended concentration was 4.5 times the optimum for water fluoridation for the locality. At its peak, school water fluoridation was introduced in 13 states in the United States; data reported by states to the Division of Oral Health of the Centers for Disease Control (CDC) showed that in 1981, it was established in 470 schools, serving 170,000 children. Its current extent is not known. There is no record of the procedure being used in countries outside the United States.

Despite CDC safety guidelines, a number of overspill mishaps have occurred, fortunately without lasting ill effects.[3, 84, 193] CDC no longer promotes school water fluoridation.

MILK FLUORIDATION

Milk fluoridation is the addition of a measured quantity of F to bottled or packaged milk to be drunk by children. The rationale is that this procedure "targets" F directly to children, and thus should theoretically be more efficient than fluoridating the drinking water. Having both fluoridated and nonfluoridated milk available also maintains consumer choice.

Only one randomized double-blind trial has been conducted to test the efficacy of fluoridated milk,[174] although a test of fluoridated milk readily fits the randomized design. Other studies testing the efficacy of fluoridated milk have been seriously flawed. There are questions about the mechanism for efficacy, because F is incompletely ionized in milk,[64] which means that limited posteruptive effect can take place. There are also practical concerns, such as the considerable number of children who do not drink milk for one reason or another. Few public health programs using fluoridated milk have become established, although there are reports of such programs in Bulgaria[136] and another in St. Helens, near Liverpool.[114] However, it is hard to recommend further research into milk fluoridation in view of the large number of F vehicles available today and the restricted posteruptive effects from F in milk.

DIETARY FLUORIDE SUPPLEMENTS

Because it was assumed in the 1940s that the effect of fluoridated water was mainly pre-eruptive, dietary supplements were intended to mimic the observed action of fluoridated water. F supplements in the form of tablets, lozenges, drops, liquids, and F-vitamin preparations have been used around the world since the 1940s, and still are extensively used.

F supplements have F quantities of 1.0, 0.5, or 0.25 mg. They were originally made as a 1.0 mg F pill to be dissolved in a liter of the infant's drinking water,[11] an approach that in time gave way to the simpler once-a-day ingestion of the tablet. Later, chewable tablets and lozenges were manufactured for older children to be chewed or sucked a minute or two before swallowing, the intent here being to get both topical and systemic effects. Most tablets contain neutral sodium fluoride (NaF), although acidulated phosphate F tablets have been tested. There are also F-vitamin drops for infants, often prescribed by pediatricians.

Caries Prevention by Fluoride Supplements

Early studies of the pre-eruptive caries-preventive effects of F supplements in children often were seriously deficient, thus yielding questionable results. Reports of 50% to 80% caries reductions in the primary and the permanent dentitions,[22] for example, included some flawed studies from the United States, Europe, and Australia from the 1960s and early 1970s. Some of the highest caries reduction rates, 80% over several years, were reported from American studies in the mid-1970s,[2, 123] but there were design flaws in many of these studies. These included self-selection into test and control groups or the absence of concurrent controls, high attrition rates, and nonblinded examiners. The association that practitioners have observed between

conscientious use of F supplements and freedom from caries also cannot be taken as evidence of efficacy, because compliance with the F supplement regimen is naturally higher among dentally aware people who also have other good oral health habits.

Subsequent evidence to favor a pre-eruptive benefit from F supplements remains limited to retrospective analyses, which are inherently biased by self-selection. Positive retrospective results have been reported,[5, 35, 44, 45, 66, 125, 198, 199] but self-selection bias was evident in all of these studies. In addition, these reports are counterbalanced by other retrospective studies which found no difference in caries experience between those children who reported using fluoride supplements and those who did not.[15, 17, 71, 88, 101, 185]

Although the evidence for pre-eruptive benefits from F supplements is weak, well-conducted randomized clinical trials with placebos and blind examiners have shown that they can have posteruptive benefits in school-aged children. Studies in which the supplements were chewed, swished and swallowed under supervision have reported caries reductions of 20% to 28% over 3 to 6 years.[47, 55] Caries reductions of 81% were reported from a Glasgow study in which children initially aged 5.5 years, from lower socioeconomic groups, sucked a 1.0 mg fluoride tablet, or a placebo, under supervision in schools every school day for 3 years.[175]

In summary, F supplements have a demonstrated posteruptive effect because they meet the goal of maintaining ambient F in the oral cavity. However, there is no good evidence to demonstrate a pre-eruptive benefit.

Dosage Schedules

F supplements in the United States and Canada require prescription by a dentist or physician; both the American Dental Association (ADA) and the American Academy of Pediatrics (AAP) maintain schedules of recommended dosage for F supplements. Before 1979 the two schedules did not coincide: AAP had first recommended 0.5 mg/day[6] for children under 2 years of age, whereas the ADA recommended 0.25 mg/day. The AAP, however, altered its earlier recommendations in 1979[7] to bring them into line with those of the ADA and reaffirmed them in 1986.[8] In response to the growing evidence that F supplements were a risk factor for fluorosis, the ADA revised its schedule in 1994 to reduce the amount of F ingested by young children, and the AAP accepted this schedule a year later.[9] The current ADA-recommended schedule, based on the age of the child and the concentration of F in the water supply, is shown in Table 25–1. Note that supplements are not recommended for infants under 6 months old. A Canadian workshop in 1992 recommended a more conservative schedule,[147] as did a European Community group in 1991 which advocated that a supplement of 0.5 mg F should be used only for "at-risk" individuals from the age of 3 years on, and that supplements had no place as a public health measure.[37] After another conference on F supplements in 1997, the 1992 Canadian schedule was replaced by one that was virtually the same as the ADA schedule shown in Table 25–1. The Canadian schedule, however, was intended to apply only to high-risk children who did not use F toothpaste and received drinking water with less than 0.3 ppm F.

Fluorosis Risk from Fluoride Supplements

The major concern now associated with supplements is that of dental fluorosis. Although fluorosis can develop at any pre-eruptive stage under certain conditions, late secretion and early maturation have been identified as the developmental times when dental enamel is especially sensitive to ingested fluoride.[46, 65, 110] Some studies found no association between supplement use and the development of fluorosis,[17, 178] but consider-

Table 25–1. RECOMMENDED DOSAGE LEVELS OF SUPPLEMENTAL FLUORIDE, AS ESTABLISHED BY THE AMERICAN DENTAL ASSOCIATION IN 1994 (in mg F/day)

AGE	CONCENTRATION OF FLUORIDE IN WATER (ppm)		
	<0.3	0.3–0.6	>0.6
Birth–6 months	—	—	—
6 months–3 years	0.25	—	—
3–6 years	0.50	0.25	—
6 + years	1.00	0.5	—

From American Dental Association, Council on Dental Therapeutics. New fluoride schedule adopted: Therapeutics council affirms workshop outcome. ADA News 1994 May 16;25:12, 14.

ably more have reported a clear association.[2, 43-45, 88, 101, 109–111, 152, 181, 185, 201, 202] A series of excellent case-control studies has provided strong evidence for a cause-and-effect relation between F supplements and dental fluorosis.[138–140] The weight of evidence is that fluoride supplements, when ingested before tooth eruption, are a risk factor for dental fluorosis in both fluoridated and nonfluoridated areas.

Medical practitioner adherence to the early AAP recommendation of 0.5 mg/day for children under 2 years old probably led to a lot of fluorosis, and the problem is exacerbated when F supplements are inappropriately prescribed for children in fluoridated areas. A 1980 national survey of pediatricians found that 20% of them who practiced in fluoridated areas were prescribing F supplements for child patients who lived in the same communities,[122] a clearly inappropriate action that inadvertently increases the risk of dental fluorosis. Things were no better 15 years later.[141] These studies have emphasized the need for continuing education of both physicians and dentists. If supplements are prescribed at all, they should not be prescribed for patients who consume fluoridated water.

How Should Fluoride Supplements be Used?

Although F supplements are still being used by 16% of American children under 2 years of age,[134] their continued prescription in the United States and Canada needs to be thoughtfully reviewed. As often is the case in public health, their use requires trade-off decisions: F supplements have some beneficial impact on oral health, but there is also the hazard of fluorosis when they are used in an age of wide exposure to fluoride.[183] The reasons why prescription of F supplements for infants and young children needs to be considered carefully are as follows:

- Any pre-eruptive action of F is relatively minor.
- Evidence to support a pre-eruptive effect specifically for F supplements is weak.
- F supplements have been identified as a risk factor for dental fluorosis, and the prevalence of fluorosis is increasing.
- The prevalence of caries continues to decline, which reduces the need to pursue a strategy that carries documented risks with little counterbalancing benefit.

In light of the advantages and disadvantages of F supplements in a time of widespread F exposure, calls have been made for a re-evaluation of their use among young children.[15, 96, 151] They have a place when used for a posteruptive effect in children older than 7 years, and it is likely that they would be useful in the growing population of older dentate people who are at risk of both coronal and root caries, although no trials have yet been conducted for this purpose. However, the use of F supplements in infants and young children should be reconsidered because the risks of fluorosis outweigh the likely preventive benefits. At the very least, parents being given a prescription for F supplements for an infant should be fully informed of the fluorosis risk as well as the presumed benefit.

Prenatal Fluoride Supplementation

The question of whether to prescribe F supplements for an expectant woman to increase caries resistance in the offspring has been around for years. As a corollary to the discussion on dietary F supplements in general, it is not surprising that current views are that any enhanced resistance to caries will be, at best, only minor. Prenatal supplements, therefore, are not recommended. There are dissenting views, however, and contrary arguments at times have been spirited.[75] The only prospective randomized trial for prenatal supplements found no significant difference in the caries experience of the offspring.[117]

F can cross the placental barrier and enter the fetal circulation.[33, 137, 171] Fetal plasma F levels are correlated with maternal levels, although generally they are lower.[137] F is taken up in the mineralizing tissues of the fetus; fetal enamel levels increase with an increase in maternal plasma F levels.[137] Research on fluorosis supports the view that the most critical time for F uptake in enamel is the postsecretory maturation phase, meaning the immediate pre-eruptive and early posteruptive period.[46, 149] As a result, prenatal F will have little effect, especially as mineralization, even of primary teeth, is not far advanced at birth.[184] Some reports claim that primary teeth have better crystal formation and generally better morphology when supplementation is begun early in pregnancy,[74, 113] although aspects of these reports can be questioned.

Collectively, research evidence suggests that prenatal F administration cannot be supported. As long ago as 1966, the US Food and Drug Administration banned advertisements claiming that prenatal F administration would increase the caries resistance of offspring.[192] No convincing research has emerged since then to change that picture, and hence that ban still applies. Although there is nothing to suggest that prenatal F supplementation will harm either fetus or mother, the evidence is just not strong enough to support claims of prenatal benefit.

PROFESSIONALLY-APPLIED FLUORIDE GELS

The F compounds that dental professionals routinely use in tray applications are highly concentrated and require careful attention to technique and the amounts used. Table 25–2 shows the quantities and concentrations of the most frequently used F compounds in dental practice, as well as those employed in public health programs and self-applied by individuals. Tables 25–3 and 25–4 are included as guides to estimating if inadvertently ingested fluoride presents a health hazard to the individual.

Early work with professionally-applied NaF solutions began even before the first water fluoridation projects.[21, 106] This led to the Knutson technique, in which an NaF solution was applied 4 times over a week after an initial prophylaxis.[105] In the 1950s, the annual application of 8% stannous fluoride (SnF_2) was reported to give beneficial results similar to those achieved with NaF, but staining problems were reported, and the material had an unpleasant taste.[29] Since the early 1960s, acidulated phosphate fluoride (APF) has become the most widely used F compound for professional application.[155] This material has a pH of about 3.0. It was developed following experimental work in the early 1960s that showed that enamel's uptake of F was greater in an acid environment.[30] It has been tested in several concentrations, the most common being 1.23% F, usually as NaF, in orthophosphoric acid. APF has been successfully tested in both solution and gel form, but the gel is by far the most widely used today. The material is nonirritating and nonstaining, will tolerate the addition of flavorings, and is acceptable to patients.

Professionally-applied F procedures were

Table 25–2. CONCENTRATION AND QUANTITY OF FLUORIDE IN COMMONLY USED TOPICAL FLUORIDE COMPOUNDS

COMPOUND	CONCENTRATION (ppm)	QUANTITY
TOPICALLY APPLIED		
2.00% NaF	9050	45.0 mg in 5 ml*
1.23 APF solution, gel, or prophylaxis paste	12,300	62.0 mg in 5 g
8.00% SnF$_2$ solution	19,363	97.0 mg in 5 ml
0.4% SnF$_2$ gel	968	4.9 mg in 5 g
5.0% NaF varnish (2.26% F)	22,600	51.0 mg in 5 ml
MOUTHRINSES		
0.2% NaF weekly	905	9.0 mg in 10 ml†
0.05% NaF daily	226	2.0 mg in 10 ml
0.1% SnF$_2$ daily	242	2.0 mg in 10 ml
APF rinse (0.1% fluoride) weekly	1000	10.0 mg in 10 ml
APF rinse (0.022% fluoride) daily	200	2.0 mg in 10 ml
		1.0 mg in 5 ml of oral rinse supplement ("rinse and swallow")
TOOTHPASTES		
0.76% Sodium monofluorophosphate	1000	1.0 mg per g‡
0.243% Sodium fluoride	1105	1.1 mg per g
1.14% Sodium monofluorophosphate	1500	1.5 mg per g
0.332% Sodium fluoride	1500	1.5 mg per g
0.4% Stannous fluoride	966	1.0 mg per g
0.4% Sodium monofluorophosphate§	526	0.5 mg per g
0.304% Sodium monofluorophosphate§	401	0.4 mg per g

Note: Some figures are rounded.
*A topical application or prophylaxis uses about 5 ml or 5 g of material.
†Amounts of 5 and 10 ml are used in supervised mouthrinsing.
‡An average load of toothpaste on the brush is about 1 g.
§Not marketed in the United States.

developed on the basis that the F would form a fluorapatite in the crystalline structure of the enamel; a prophylaxis was thus considered mandatory before the application of the F to maximize this reaction. Subsequent research, however, showed that high-concentration F such as that in APF gels tends to form a CaF$_2$-like material on the enamel surface,[50] thus forming a "reservoir" of F that becomes available for remineralization when pH drops.[112] As a result, the prophylaxis before a professional F application is unnecessary; it

Table 25–3. HOW TO ESTIMATE THE AMOUNT OF FLUORIDE IN A DENTAL PRODUCT

Basic Information:
1 ounce = 28.4 g
"Percent" means g or ml per 100 g or ml, e.g., 2% NaF solution means 2 g NaF per 100 ml
Atomic weights: Na = 23; F = 19; Sn = 119; P = 31; O = 16
Fluoride compounds most often used are NaF, SnF$_2$, Na$_2$FPO$_3$

Example 1: How much F is in 10 ml of 0.05% NaF mouthrinse?
The mouthrinse has 0.05 g of NaF per 100 ml of rinse
= 50 mg of NaF, or 5 mg of NaF per 10 ml
Amount of F = 5 mg × 19/42 = 2.26 mg

Example 2: How much F is in a 6.4 oz tube of Colgate MFP toothpaste? (6.4 oz = 181.8 g)
Colgate with MFP is 0.76% Na$_2$FPO$_3$, so it has 0.76 g of MFP per 100 ml toothpaste
Grams of Na$_2$FPO$_3$ in a 6.4 oz tube = 0.76 × 181.8/100 = 1.38 g, which is 1380 mg Na$_2$FPO$_3$
So mg F in the tube = 1380 mg × 19/144 = 182.1 mg

Example 3: How much F is in an 8.2 oz tube of Crest toothpaste? (8.2 oz = 232.9 g)
Crest contains 0.243% NaF, so it has 0.243 g of NaF per 100 ml toothpaste
Grams of NaF in an 8.2 oz tube = 0.243 × 232.9/100 = 0.566 g, which is 566 mg NaF
So mg F in the tube = 566 mg × 19/42 = 256.0 mg

Table 25–4. DATA ON TOXIC INTAKE LEVELS IN HUMANS

- Certainly Lethal Dose (CLD) = 32–64 mg F/kg body weight.
- Death is likely in a child who ingests more than 15 mg F/kg body weight.
- Probably toxic dose (PTD), defined as the minimum dose that could cause toxic signs and symptoms, including death, and the ingestion of which should trigger immediate intervention and hospitalization = 5 mg F/kg body weight.

The 10th and 90th percentiles of weight for children at various ages are:

Age	Weight
1 year	8–12 kg
2 years	10–15 kg
3 years	12–17 kg
4 years	14–20 kg
6 years	17–27 kg
8 years	22–34 kg

For a child about 7 years, who would weigh approx. 20 kg, the PTD would be approximately 100 mg F.

Data from Burt BA. The changing patterns of systemic fluoride intake. J Dent Res 1992;71:1228–37; Heifetz SB, Horowitz HS. Amounts of fluoride in self-administered dental products: Safety considerations for children. Pediatrics 1986;77:876–82.

has been shown to be no more beneficial than self-toothbrushing and flossing.[94, 159] This finding results in considerable time-saving in office F applications. Professional gel-tray applications have long been considered not cost-effective for public health programs, although they might be a reasonable approach for highly susceptible special groups in targeted programs.

F-containing prophylaxis pastes are widely used in dentistry; the reasoning behind their development was that the prophylaxis and the professional F application could be carried out at one time. Results from clinical trials that tested this procedure, however, were disappointing. When a prophylaxis paste is to be used, it should routinely be an F-containing paste, but such use is not by itself a substitute for an F gel professional application.

FLUORIDE VARNISHES

F varnish is not intended to be as permanent as a fissure sealant (Chapter 26); rather it is a vehicle for holding F in close contact with the tooth for a period of time. A theoretical advantage for varnishes over other methods of professional F application is that varnishes are adhesive, and hence should maximize F contact with the tooth surface. Varnishes are a way of using high F concentrations in small amounts of material. F varnishes are widely used in Europe and Canada and were accepted for use in the United States in 1994.[121] Despite their recent introduction to the United States, a use for F varnishes in treating early childhood caries has been reported.[196]

Early European clinical trials on the efficacy of F varnishes produced mixed results.[34, 87, 108, 133] A large clinical trial in Quebec, which ran for nearly 5 years in communities chosen for their high caries experience, reported moderate efficacy.[36] As with most modern clinical trials in North America, the study was conducted in an environment of extensive F exposure from toothpaste and supplements, which always makes the impact of any one F vehicle difficult to discern. More recent studies in Europe have demonstrated the efficacy of F varnishes.[40, 83] They have been shown to slow the progression of existing enamel lesions,[144] and to be at least as effective as APF gel when applied semiannually.[164] There is evidence that lower fluoride levels in the varnish may not reduce their cariostatic effects.[41, 78, 165]

Varnishes need to be reapplied at regular intervals to maintain their cariostatic effect,[40, 163] although application 4 times per year seems no more effective than twice per year.[166] Investigations continue into the optimum application frequency. Intensive use, meaning applications 3 times in a week each year, may be more effective than the conventional twice-per-year regimen.[142, 169] Varnishes are clearly effective, although as a professionally-applied procedure, they are inherently more expensive than self-applied methods. Cost-effectiveness has been claimed in a Swedish study.[143] They may well be cost-effective in Scandinavian countries with their highly developed school dental services, where dental professionals see individual patients regularly. It is not yet clear whether varnishes would be most efficiently used in clinical programs with high-caries populations, or whether their use is best reserved for individual patients on an ad hoc basis. In any event, they are a useful addition to the dental practitioner's F armamentarium for use in caries-susceptible patients. For example, they have been found effective in preventing decalcification beneath orthodontic bands.[4]

Research into F varnishes (F concentrations, most effective application protocols, efficacy relative to other uses of F) is likely to continue both in Europe and North America, and we can expect that the use of F varnishes will increase.

SELF-APPLIED FLUORIDES

The methods for using F described so far are all for application by public health personnel or dental practitioners. Numerous methods have also been devised for F self-application, methods that can be used by an individual at home or by supervised groups in school-based programs. Some self-applied methods have come and gone, usually because they were logistically cumbersome, and more efficient methods have replaced them. Examples include individualized gel-tray applications,[62] an effective but highly expensive procedure, and supervised toothbrushing programs. The latter were popular in the Scandinavian countries for many years, but gave way to logistically simpler procedures that are probably more cost-effective as well.[160] F toothpaste and F mouthrinsing, however, are two self-applied procedures still very much in use. Indeed, most authorities consider F toothpaste the principal factor in the global decline in caries.

FLUORIDE MOUTHRINSES

The idea of preventing caries by mouthrinsing with dilute F solutions has been around for decades,[21, 197] but it was some years before it became a standard procedure in preventive dentistry. A Swedish report in 1965 that found nearly 50% reduction in caries increment over 2 years[187] naturally sparked interest in the procedure. Since then, NaF rinses have been extensively tested; others tested to a lesser extent include APF, SnF$_2$, ammonium fluoride, and amine fluoride. Its low cost, convenience in handling, and pleasant taste have led to NaF becoming the most widely used of these products.

NaF has been tested as a weekly rinse at 0.2% F and for daily rinsing at 0.05%. School-based public programs have found the weekly regimen to be the most convenient; daily rinsing is most appropriate for individual use. The caries reductions from daily rinsing are only slightly greater than those from weekly rinsing[57, 82]; the slight differences do not compensate for the greater practicality and lower cost of weekly rinsing in a school-based program. For home use, dentists can advise patients to buy an F mouthrinse from the drugstore or supermarket. The number of home-use nonprescription rinses on the market grew considerably through the 1990s; a list of available products that have received ADA approval is available on the ADA's website.

Because mouthrinsing with F solutions is a convenient way of maintaining a constant level of ambient F in the mouth, it is not surprising that clinical trials have mostly given positive results. Most studies are with NaF rinses and date from the 1970s. Collectively, they show that regular use of NaF mouthrinses reduces caries increments in children by 20% to 35% over 2 to 3 years.[24, 48, 70, 91, 158, 162] Positive benefits were also reported in the primary dentition.[156] Several studies using APF rinse, 1.23% F at pH 4.0, have reported reductions on the order of 20% to 30%.[24] APF "rinse-and-swallow" rinse has also been shown to be beneficial,[1] although with the potential for fluorosis from systemic absorption this product should be prescribed with caution in younger children. A limited number of tests with 0.1% SnF$_2$ rinse have given positive caries reductions,[128, 145] and SnF$_2$ has also demonstrated antibacterial properties not possessed by NaF.[182, 186] Other rinse compounds tested, with results generally similar to those for NaF and SnF$_2$, are ammonium fluoride[48] and amine fluoride.[150] Literature reviews from around the late 1970s on the efficacy of F mouthrinsing were favorable.[24, 153] Continuing caries reductions over long-term use of 10 years were reported,[23] and retained benefits have also been demonstrated in children some years after they completed a school rinsing program.[77, 115] A more recent study, however, found that the benefits from 6 years of mouthrinsing in a school-based program were lost 4 years after the program ended.[85]

F mouthrinsing soon became established as a major caries-preventive public health program in the United States, Canada, and other countries. A 1984 survey found that 3.2 million American children were participating in F mouthrinsing programs in 48 states.[18] According to the CDC, there were 3.25 million American schoolchildren in F mouthrinsing programs in 1988 in more than 11,683 sites.

A major attraction of F mouthrinsing in

public health programming has been its presumed cost-effectiveness. In many school districts, weekly rinsing is held in the classroom with supervision provided by the teacher at no additional cost to the public health program. In others, supervision is provided by volunteer mothers or inexpensive hourly workers. Costs of around $1 per child per year have been given by program administrators,[72] but these almost certainly are underestimates.[53, 104] When the true costs of volunteer labor and promotion are included, the annual costs come closer to $8 per child in 1978 dollars,[53] which would probably be at least doubled by the 1990s. Even so, these costs would probably still be acceptable if the procedure is as effective as the early studies suggested.

During the 1970s, the National Institute of Dental Research* (NIDR) conducted a demonstration program, intended to show the effectiveness of F mouthrinsing as a routine procedure, in 17 different public health jurisdictions. Unfortunately the outcome of this program was reported only in generalized, summary terms,[129] and given the nonexperimental nature of the demonstration projects (e.g., no concurrent controls, no placebos, variable blindness of examiners, uncertain procedural control), some of the conclusions reached from the demonstration were unjustified. Even active researchers who carried out mouthrinsing studies without concurrent controls around this time were questioning the validity of their own results.[118] However, it was the results of the National Preventive Dentistry Demonstration Program (NPDDP), a large program conducted in 10 US cities during the 1976–1981 period to compare the costs and effectiveness of a series of preventive mechanisms, that really brought F mouthrinsing under strong scrutiny in the late 1980s.

The NPDDP found that the effectiveness of F mouthrinsing was poor, both in overall results[104] and when assessed separately in first-grade children with high and low caries increments.[52] Earlier reviews by the NPDDP researchers had reported serious flaws with the conduct of many earlier studies which did not use concurrent control groups,[26] and with some of the economic analyses which led to the assumption of cost-effectiveness,[172] especially in fluoridated communities.[27] Strong criticism was also leveled at the way in which NIDR had used its data to promote

the use of F mouthrinses in public health.[51] At the same time, the NPDDP itself was criticized for faulty design and analysis.[68] The atmosphere of uncertainty was settled to some extent at a workshop on cost-effectiveness of preventive procedures in 1989, where Leverett's comprehensive review concluded that F mouthrinsing was a reasonable procedure to use for high-risk individuals or groups, although of questionable cost-effectiveness as a population-based strategy.[116]

This debate emphasizes the need for clinical trials with due regard to the principles of experimental studies (Chapter 12), and the dangers in extrapolating data from demonstrations and other noncontrolled projects into public policy. F mouthrinsing continues to be used in public health, although program directors are taking more care with selection of communities in which to conduct them. For example, they are no longer promoted in fluoridated communities. F mouthrinsing is seen now as appropriate for high-risk groups as a "targeted" procedure rather than a population strategy.

FLUORIDE TOOTHPASTES

Toothpastes without active ingredients, meaning those that contain abrasive and flavoring agents only and are thus intended for oral hygiene and cosmetic benefits, have no anticaries action by themselves. Because toothbrushing is an established practice in the developed world, however, a variety of preventive and therapeutic agents (both known and hypothetical) have been added to toothpastes over the years. Early efforts to produce therapeutic toothpastes included the addition of ammonia,[79, 103] antibiotics,[67] chlorophyll, and various other additives. None were effective. To date, F is the only nonprescription toothpaste additive that has been shown to prevent caries.

The earliest attempts to add F to toothpaste were unsuccessful because of the incompatible abrasives used in the products that bound the F and thus made it biologically unavailable. The first successful clinical trials of an F additive used SnF_2 with a calcium pyrophosphate abrasive.[132] These positive results were replicated during the 1960s in other American and British studies with the same formulation, which reported a 15% to 30% rate of caries reductions in children over 2 to 3 years.[92, 97, 100, 131, 170] Clinical trials of F toothpastes in fluoridated areas have demonstrated an additive effect,[119, 126, 195] and there

---

*Now the National Institute of Dental and Craniofacial Research (NIDCR).

is some evidence that F toothpaste prevents root caries in older adults.[98]

In all, more than 90 clinical trials have been conducted with various F compounds as the active ingredient: SnF_2, NaF, sodium monofluorophosphate (MFP), and amine fluoride have all been successfully tested.[38] Even more abrasives have been developed and tried; insoluble metaphosphate, sodium trimetaphosphate, hydrated silica gel, calcium carbonate, dicalcium dihydrate, and calcium pyrophosphate are the main ones. New formulations are constantly under investigation and are soon marketed when found effective.

There is some laboratory evidence that toothpastes with NaF may be more efficacious than those with MFP,[31, 58] although clinical data on this subject are hard to interpret. Analyses of data available in the early 1990s were split on the issue, and discussions were often pedantic.[86, 99, 179, 194] Subsequent clinical trials that gave a slight edge to NaF required large groups to show statistical significance,[124, 176] and another trial found no difference between the products.[49] Given the size of the market, this form of dueling is likely to continue. Whether there is very much difference between the products in effectiveness at the population level is difficult to gauge.

Serious marketing of F toothpastes was underway by the early 1970s, and public acceptance was immediate in virtually all of the economically developed nations. By the 1990s, F toothpastes accounted for well over 90% of the toothpaste market in the United States, Canada, and other developed countries. Their use in the developing world, where F toothpastes could potentially fill an important preventive role, is inhibited by their relatively high cost, poor distribution, and often by the relative absence of the oral hygiene culture taken for granted in the developed world. The development of the F toothpaste market in developing countries is a challenge to the manufacturers and to dental public health in general.

Quality of the Fluoride Toothpaste Trials

Many of the clinical trials for F toothpaste are among the most elegant trials in dentistry, or in biomedicine in general, to demonstrate the efficacy of a product. All of the essential features of the best clinical trials (Chapter 12) can be found in many of these studies: randomized groups, double-blind designs, placebo controls, meticulous procedural protocols. Because the water fluoridation field trials have inherent design limitations (Chapter 24), opponents of fluoride can attack their validity. If the issue is the efficacy of fluoride, however, the fluoride toothpaste trials collectively include many studies that meet the "gold standard" for such trials. Taken together, the toothpaste trials are the strongest evidence we have that F is efficacious in controlling caries.

Fluoride Concentrations in Toothpastes

As seen in Table 25–2, the F toothpastes that first became widely tested and marketed contained about 1000 to 1100 ppm F. When introduced into the oral cavity, F in toothpaste is taken up directly by demineralized enamel,[146, 180] although its retention on sound enamel is thought to be of relatively minor importance.[31] It also increases the F concentration in dental plaque,[60, 61, 167] thus leaving a store of F available for remineralization when pH drops. Salivary F levels, normally low in resting saliva, rise 100- or even 1000-fold after toothbrushing with an F toothpaste.[161] This level drops over the next 1 to 2 hours, with some of the salivary F being taken up by plaque. Postbrushing levels of intraoral F are affected by the amount and vigor of rinsing after brushing,[59, 168] with the best advice for adults being to rinse gently after brushing.

Because laboratory studies showed that the uptake of F into demineralized enamel and into plaque was proportional to the concentration of F in the toothpaste, a natural consequence was the testing of toothpastes with concentrations higher than the original 1000 to 1100 ppm F. Toothpastes with 1500 ppm F have been found slightly more efficacious in studies in Europe and the United States.[39, 69, 76, 135] The review by Ripa[154] of the action of these higher-concentration toothpastes concluded that an MFP toothpaste at 1500 ppm F reduced the caries increment by another 12% over that achieved by the standard F toothpastes of 1000 to 1100 ppm F, although the results of studies with toothpastes containing mixed fluorides were more equivocal. Clinical trials have also been conducted with toothpastes of 2500 ppm F or more with rather mixed results. Studies in Scotland, testing several products, found that caries reductions were proportional to the F concentration in the toothpaste,[177] but two North American studies found no difference between the high-F (2500 ppm F) MFP products and standard-strength F toothpastes.[120, 157]

At the other end of the spectrum, concerns about the fluorosis risk from children swallowing toothpaste have led to lower-than-standard F toothpastes being tested. The first clinical trials compared products with 250 ppm F against 1000 ppm F toothpastes and yielded conflicting results.[107, 130] Findings from later studies of 500 to 550 ppm F products, however, suggested that they may be no less efficacious than 1000 ppm F toothpastes.[191, 200] Because children have been reported to swallow between 0.12 and 0.38 mg of toothpaste per brushing,[20] the marketing of lower-F toothpastes is likely to reduce the risk of fluorosis while substantially retaining caries-preventive benefits. Toothpastes containing 400 ppm F have been available in Europe, Australia, and New Zealand for years, although these products have not yet been tested in clinical trials. They are not available in the United States and Canada, despite strong calls to market these child-strength toothpastes in North America.[90]

F toothpastes have practically been institutionalized in the United States and in many other countries. It is hard to find a toothpaste that does not contain F, and manufacturers no longer bother to use F content as part of their advertising. Further research can be expected to focus on the most favorable F/abrasive formulations and the most appropriate F concentrations. A welcome development, alluded to already, would be the marketing of "children's toothpastes" of 500 to 550 ppm F separately from "adult strength" products, which might be 1500 to 2500 ppm F. Because the swallowing of F toothpaste by children is a risk factor for fluorosis (Chapter 21), if those children swallow higher-F toothpaste, the prevalence and severity of fluorosis could get worse (none of the high-F toothpaste trials have been designed to examine the development of fluorosis). On the other hand, higher-F toothpastes are likely to be more beneficial for preventing coronal and root caries in adults than the first-generation products. Perhaps the market could manage both forms of toothpaste with appropriate color-coding and warning labels on the high-F products.

Standards for Toothpaste Efficacy

The toothpaste market is a multibillion dollar industry in the United States, so competition between major manufacturers is keen. Companies spend much time and money on research to secure the ADA's Seal of Approval for their products; the logo on the package improves marketing and is a guide for consumers as well. With the multitude of F/abrasive formulations that are available, the ADA developed guidelines for use in judging applications for its Seal of Approval for F toothpastes.[10] With newer formulations replacing earlier products, and advertising claims of superiority over rival products, the ADA went further in 1988 with a workshop to determine what evidence would be adequate to substantiate claims of equivalency or superiority of a particular formulation (i.e., fluoride ingredient with compatible abrasives) relative to other formulations.[12] The workshop determined that such claims always required rigorous clinical trials in human populations, and trials would require a positive control of the rival product. The trials would have to be designed to show a 10% difference in caries increment with a power of 80% (Chapter 12). The ADA's Seal of Approval goes to particular formulations rather than to products. The list of toothpastes that carry the seal, to be found on the ADA website, is now quite long and continues to grow.

Global Impact of Fluoride Toothpastes

The impact of F toothpastes on global caries experience has been profound. F exposure is accepted as the main reason for the decline of dental caries over recent years, and most authorities believe that F toothpaste has been the most important F vehicle on a global scale.[28] The caries reductions of 15% to 30% achieved in most clinical trials may appear modest when compared with water fluoridation, but it must be remembered that these were trials of 2 to 3 years' duration, whereas water fluoridation studies usually measured lifetime exposure. Knowing that F works most effectively to prevent caries when small amounts are in the oral cavity at all times, there is no reason why regular lifetime use of F toothpaste should not give results that are similar to those of lifetime use of fluoridated water. The catch, in terms of community-wide impact, is that not everyone brushes their teeth, whereas the whole community is exposed to fluoridated water.

MULTIPLE FLUORIDE EXPOSURE

The majority of clinical trials with F products test only a single agent. In the modern world, however, exposure to multiple sources of F is the rule rather than the exception. People who live in fluoridated areas brush their teeth with F toothpastes and are periodically given professional applications by their dentists. F mouthrinsing is a common procedure in public health programs, and some cosmetic mouthwashes contain F. There are also dietary supplements, whether used appropriately or not, as well as the poorly-defined F exposures from food and drink. When added together, it becomes readily apparent that people in most developed countries are being exposed to much more F today than previously. This is likely to be especially true in highly-fluoridated countries such as the United States, as many processed foods and drinks are made with fluoridated water.

This phenomenon of multiple F exposure can be looked at from several viewpoints. In one way it is beneficial, because with the several different anticaries actions of F (Chapter 23) fuller advantage is being taken of F's potential. On the other hand, the increasing prevalence of fluorosis (Chapter 21) is almost certain to be a product of this multiple and poorly-controlled F exposure. Dentistry's goal, although not easy for either an individual patient or the community, is to maximize the benefits from F exposure while avoiding an unacceptable level of the undesirable side effects.

Multiple F therapy, whether in fluoridated or nonfluoridated areas, is clearly beneficial for patients who are especially suscepti-ble to caries. For example, Dreizen and colleagues[54] reported excellent results in preventing caries among patients who had received radiation treatment for oral cancer, a treatment that produces dysfunction of the salivary glands and hence loss of salivary buffering capacity. The therapy included F gel-tray applications, daily F mouthrinsing, and routine use of an F toothpaste.

Caries reductions above those expected from fluoridated water alone have been found among children in fluoridated areas who received: (a) annual topical applications of SnF_2,[91] (b) F mouthrinses and gel-tray applications in combination,[80] and (c) intensive self-application of F in custom-made trays.[63] An 11-year demonstration, begun by NIDR in 1972, provided F supplements, F mouthrinses, and F toothpaste to children in a poor rural area. The intention was to show that school-based combined F programs could reduce caries experience in rural areas.[93] Cohorts of 1983 participants had DMF scores that were 65% lower than those in baseline cohorts in 1972. (The demonstration was not designed to permit identification of the individual effects of the different F regimens, and the absence of concurrent controls made interpretation of the caries reductions difficult.)

In the context of cost-effectiveness, the data on the use of F mouthrinses in fluoridated areas is worth examining in detail. Table 25–5 presents these data for five North American studies. There is a beneficial effect in each case, although even in the earlier studies, the effects were limited in terms of absolute caries reductions. A later study of multiple F use compared the impact of F tablets and F rinses.[56] After 8 years, children who

Table 25–5. SUMMARIZED RESULTS OF STUDIES OF FLUORIDE MOUTHRINSES IN FLUORIDATED AREAS

MATERIAL	AGE GROUP STUDIED	DURATION	PERCENT REDUCTION	DMFS REDUCTION	REFERENCE
0.1% SnF_2 daily	8–13 years	20 months	33.1* 43.3†	1.00 1.22	Radike et al.[145]
0.05% NaF daily	12 years	30 months	27.9* 49.7†	0.72 0.94	Driscoll et al.[57]
0.25% NaF weekly	12 years	30 months	22.1* 55.0†	0.57 1.04	Driscoll et al.[57]
0.2% NaF weekly	9 years	24 months	33.8	0.52	Kawall et al.[102]
0.2% NaF weekly	Grades 1–2 Grade 5	48 months 24 months	not given‡ not given‡	0.29 0.03	Bell et al.[19]

*First of two examiners.
†Second of two examiners.
‡Could not be determined from data given.

Table 25–6. SUMMARIZED RESULTS OF STUDIES OF ADDITIVE EFFECTS OF FLUORIDE MOUTHRINSING AND SUPERVISED BRUSHING WITH FLUORIDE TOOTHPASTES

AGE GROUPS	DURATION	DMFS INCREMENTS			PLACEBO	REFERENCE
		F RINSE*	F TOOTHPASTE†	RINSE + TOOTHPASTE‡		
Approx 13 years	24 months	4.81	4.44	4.12	5.61	Ashley et al.[14]
		(13.1%)§	(17.9%)§	(22.7%)§		
11 years	30 months	4.79	5.14	5.30	6.51	Ringelberg et al.[150]
		(23.4%)§	(17.8%)§	(15.2%)§		
10–13 years	30 months	none	6.30	5.60	none	Triol et al.[190]
				(11.1%)‖		
11–12 years	36 months	4.72	4.60	4.76	6.25	Blinkhorn et al.[25]
		(24.5%)§	(26.3%)§	(26.8%)§		

*0.05% NaF daily at school.
†0.76% sodium monofluorophosphate except for Ringelberg et al[150] (0.4% stannous fluoride, unsupervised).
‡All conducted supervised rinse immediately after brushing.
§Percentage reduction compared with placebo control.
‖Percentage reduction compared to monofluorophosphate toothpaste alone.

both ingested the F tablet (after chewing) and rinsed weekly with neutral 0.2% NaF solution had a caries increment that was 33% lower than that for children who rinsed only, and 15% lower than for those who took the supplements only. In the age of low caries experience, however, the largest absolute difference between groups was only 1.17 DMFS over the 8 years. Cost-effectiveness issues arise from these results. When a new F program is instituted among children who already have some F exposure and low caries experience, is the additional benefit worth the cost?

The NPDDP data[19] in Table 25–5 provoked the subsequent criticisms of F mouthrinsing mentioned earlier in this chapter. Table 25–6 gives results of studies in which supervised brushing with an F toothpaste was combined with supervised daily F mouthrinsing at school, and the results compared against each procedure alone. The results of the combined procedures are only slightly superior to the use of either procedure alone. Scandinavian studies, not included in Table 25–6 because they tested weekly or 2-weekly rinsing and unsupervised home use of an F toothpaste, also reported little added benefit from the rinsing programs at school.[16]

Because caries experience in North American children has generally reached lower levels than those shown in Tables 25–5 and 25–6, the cost-effectiveness of F mouthrinsing in fluoridated areas, especially where frequent use of F toothpaste is common, is hard to justify. This conclusion was confirmed at the 1989 workshop on cost-effectiveness of preventive programs.[148]

Cost-effectiveness is less of an issue for the private patient than it is in public health, but selection of a preventive regimen for an individual patient should still consider the likely extent of multiple benefits. To illustrate, professional F applications are of dubious additional value to the individual patient in a fluoridated area who brushes daily with an F toothpaste and who has little caries problem. More caries-susceptible patients, however, even in a fluoridated area may get reasonable additional benefit from professional F gel applications or prescribed daily use of F mouthrinse. The clinical judgment in these decisions should always be guided by experimental data.

As stated previously, broad exposure to multiple sources of F is the North American norm today. When introducing a new F program in a community, therefore, a public health administrator must assess whether the program will produce additional benefits to those already being received from other F sources. The evidence just cited shows that additional benefits will probably accrue, but the bigger and more difficult public health question is whether the extra benefits are worth the additional cost of the program.

REFERENCES

1. Aasenden R, DePaola PF, Brudevold F. Effects of daily rinsing and ingestion of fluoride solutions

upon dental caries and enamel fluoride. Arch Oral Biol 1972;17:1705-14.

2. Aasenden R, Peebles TC. Effects of fluoride supplementation from birth on deciduous and permanent teeth. Arch Oral Biol 1974;19:321-6.

3. Acute fluoride poisoning—North Carolina. MMWR 1974;23:199.

4. Adriaens ML, Dermaut LR, Verbeeck RM. The use of 'Fluor Protector,' a fluoride varnish, as a caries prevention method under orthodontic molar bands. Eur J Orthod 1990;12:316-9.

5. Allmark C, Green HP, Linney AD, et al. A community study of fluoride tablets for school children in Portsmouth. Results after six years. Br Dent J 1982;153:426-30.

6. American Academy of Pediatrics, Committee on Nutrition. Fluoride as a nutrient. Pediatrics 1972; 49:456-9.

7. American Academy of Pediatrics, Committee on Nutrition. Fluoride supplementation: Revised dosage schedule. Pediatrics 1979;63:150-2.

8. American Academy of Pediatrics, Committee on Nutrition. Fluoride supplementation. Pediatrics 1986;77:758-61.

9. American Academy of Pediatrics, Committee on Nutrition. Fluoride supplementation for children: Interim policy recommendations. Pediatrics 1995; 95:777.

10. American Dental Association, Council on Dental Therapeutics. Guidelines for the acceptance of fluoride-containing dentifrices. J Am Dent Assoc 1985;110:545-7.

11. American Dental Association, Council on Dental Therapeutics. Prescribing supplements of dietary fluorides. J Am Dent Assoc 1958;56:589-91.

12. American Dental Association, Council on Dental Therapeutics. Report of workshop aimed at defining guidelines for caries clinical trials: Superiority and equivalency claims for anticaries dentifrices. J Am Dent Assoc 1988;117:663-5.

13. American Dental Association, Council on Dental Therapeutics. New fluoride schedule adopted: Therapeutics council affirms workshop outcome. ADA News 1994 May 16;25:12, 14.

14. Ashley FP, Mainwaring PJ, Emslie RD, Naylor MN. Clinical testing of a mouthrinse and a dentifrice containing fluoride. Br Dent J 1977;143:333-8.

15. Awad MA, Hargreaves JA, Thompson GW. Dental caries and fluorosis in 7–9 and 11–14 year old children who received fluoride supplements from birth. J Can Dent Assoc 1994;60:318-22.

16. Axelsson P, Paulander J, Nordkvist K, Karlsson R. Effect of fluoride containing dentifrice, mouthrinsing, and varnish on approximal dental caries in a 3-year clinical trial. Community Dent Oral Epidemiol 1987;15:177-80.

17. Bagramian RA, Narendran S, Ward M. Relationship of dental caries and fluorosis to fluoride supplement history in a non-fluoridated sample of schoolchildren. Adv Dent Res 1989;3:161-7.

18. Bednarsh H, Connolly GN. A report on fluoride mouthrinsing programs among states. Presented at the 112th annual meeting of the American Public Health Association, Anaheim CA, 1984.

19. Bell RM, Klein SP, Bohannan HM, et al. Treatment effects in the National Preventive Dentistry Demonstration Program. Rand Corp report no R-3072-RWJ. Santa Monica CA: Rand, 1984.

20. Beltran ED, Szpunar SM. Fluoride in toothpastes for children: Suggestions for change. Pediatr Dent 1988;10:185-8.

21. Bibby BG, Zander HA, McKellegaet M, Labunsky B. Preliminary reports on the effect on dental caries of the use of sodium fluoride in a prophylactic cleaning mixture and in a mouthwash. J Dent Res 1946;25:207-11.

22. Binder K, Driscoll WS, Schutzmannsky G. Caries-preventive fluoride tablet programs. Caries Res 1978;12(Suppl 1):22-30.

23. Birkeland JM, Broch L, Jorkjend L. Benefits and prognoses following 10 years of a fluoride mouthrinsing program. Scand J Dent Res 1977;85:31-7.

24. Birkeland JM, Torell P. Caries-preventive fluoride mouthrinses. Caries Res 1978;12(Suppl 1):38-51.

25. Blinkhorn AS, Holloway PJ, Davies TG. Combined effects of a fluoride dentifrice and mouthrinse on the incidence of dental caries. Community Dent Oral Epidemiol 1983;11:7-11.

26. Bohannan HM, Graves RC, Disney JA, et al. Effect of secular decline in caries on the evaluation of preventive dentistry demonstrations. J Public Health Dent 1985;45:83-9.

27. Bohannan HM, Stamm JW, Graves RC, et al. Fluoride mouthrinse programs in fluoridated communities. J Am Dent Assoc 1985;111:783-9.

28. Bratthall D, Hänsel Petersson G, Sundberg H. Reasons for the caries decline: What do the experts believe? Eur J Oral Sci 1996;104:416-22.

29. Brudevold F, Naujoks R. Caries-preventive fluoride treatment for the individual. Caries Res 1978; 12(Suppl 1):52-64.

30. Brudevold F, Savory A, Gardner DE, et al. A study of acidulated fluoride solutions. I. *In vitro* effects on enamel. Arch Oral Biol 1963;8:179-82.

31. Bruun C, Givskov H. Calcium fluoride formation in enamel from semi- or low-concentrated F agents in vitro. Caries Res 1993;27:96-9.

32. Burt BA. The changing patterns of systemic fluoride intake. J Dent Res 1992;71:1228-37.

33. Caldera R, Chavinie J, Fermanian J, et al. Maternal-fetal transfer of fluoride in pregnant women. Biol Neonate 1988;54:263-9.

34. Clark DC. A review on fluoride varnishes: An alternative topical fluoride treatment. Community Dent Oral Epidemiol 1982;10:117-23.

35. Clark DC, Hann HJ, Williamson MF, Berkowitz J. Effects of lifelong consumption of fluoridated water or use of fluoride supplements on dental caries prevalence. Community Dent Oral Epidemiol 1995;23:20-4.

36. Clark DC, Stamm JW, Tessier C, Robert G. The final results of the Sherbrooke-Lac Megantic fluoride varnish study. J Canad Dent Assoc 1987;53:919-22.

37. Clarkson J. A European view of fluoride supplementation. Br Dent J 1992;172:357-8.

38. Clarkson JE, Ellwood RP, Chandler RE. A comprehensive summary of fluoride dentifrice caries clinical trials. Am J Dent 1993;6(Special Issue):S59-S106.

39. Conti AJ, Lotzkar S, Daley R, et al. A 3-year clinical trial to compare efficacy of dentifrices containing 1.14% and 0.76% sodium monofluorophosphate. Community Dent Oral Epidemiol 1988;16:135-8.

40. de Bruyn H, Arends J. Fluoride varnishes—a review. J Bio Buccale 1987;15:71-82.

41. de Bruyn H, Buskes JA, Jongbloed W, Arends J. Fluoride uptake and inhibition of intra-oral demineralization following the application of varnishes

with different concentrations of fluoride. J Biol Buc-cale 1988;16:81-7.

42. De Crousaz P, Marthaler TM, Weisner V, et al. Caries prevalence of children after 12 years of salt fluoridation in a canton of Switzerland. Helv Odont Acta 1985;29:21-31.

43. de Liefde B, Herbison GP. Prevalence of developmental defects of enamel and dental caries in New Zealand children receiving different fluoride supplementation. Community Dent Oral Epidemiol 1985;13:164-7.

44. de Liefde B, Herbison GP. The prevalence of developmental defects of enamel and dental caries in New Zealand children receiving differing fluoride supplementation, in 1982 and 1985. N Z Dent J 1989;85:2-8.

45. D'Hoore W, Van Nieuwenhuysen JP. Benefits and risks of fluoride supplementation: Caries prevention versus dental fluorosis. Eur J Pediatr 1992;151:613-6.

46. DenBesten PK, Thariani H. Biological mechanisms of fluorosis and level and timing of systemic exposure to fluoride with respect to fluorosis. J Dent Res 1992;71:1238-43.

47. DePaola PF, Lax M. The caries-inhibiting effect of acidulated phosphate-fluoride chewable tablets: A two-year double-blind study. J Am Dent Assoc 1968;76:554-7.

48. DePaola PF, Soparkar P, Foley S, et al. Effect of high-concentration ammonium and sodium fluoride rinses in dental caries in schoolchildren. Community Dent Oral Epidemiol 1977;5:7-14.

49. DePaola PF, Soparkar PM, Triol C, et al. The relative anticaries effectiveness of sodium monofluorophosphate and sodium fluoride as contained in currently available dentifrice formulations. Am J Dent 1993;6(Special Issue):S7-S12.

50. Dijkman TG, Arends J. The role of 'CaF$_2$-like' material in topical fluoridation of enamel in situ. Acta Odont Scand 1988;46:391-7.

51. Disney JA, Bohannan HM, Klein SP, Bell RM. A case study in contesting the conventional wisdom: School-based fluoride mouthrinse programs in the USA. Community Dent Oral Epidemiol 1990;18:46-54.

52. Disney JA, Graves RC, Stamm JW, et al. Comparative effects of a 4-year fluoride mouthrinse program on high and low caries forming grade 1 children. Community Dent Oral Epidemiol 1989;17:139-43.

53. Doherty NJ, Brunelle JA, Miller AJ, Li SH. Costs of school based mouthrinsing in 14 demonstration programs in USA. Community Dent Oral Epidemiol 1984;12:35-8.

54. Dreizen S, Brown LR, Daly TE, Drane JB. Prevention of xerostomia-related dental caries in irradiated dental patients. J Dent Res 1977;56:99-104.

55. Driscoll WS, Heifetz SB, Korts DC. Effect of chewable fluoride tablets on dental caries in schoolchildren: Results after six years of use. J Am Dent Assoc 1978;97:820-4.

56. Driscoll WS, Nowjack-Raymer R, Selwitz RH, Li SH. A comparison of the caries-preventive effects of fluoride mouthrinsing, fluoride tablets, and both procedures combined: Final results after eight years. J Public Health Dent 1992;52:111-6.

57. Driscoll WS, Swango PA, Horowitz AM, Kingman A. Caries-preventive effects of daily and weekly fluoride mouthrinsing in a fluoridated community: Final results after 30 months. J Am Dent Assoc 1982;105:1010-3.

58. Duckworth RM, Jones Y, Nicholson J, et al. Studies on plaque fluoride after use of F-containing dentifrices. Adv Dent Res 1994;8:202-7.

59. Duckworth RM, Knoop DT, Stephen KW. Effect of mouthrinsing after toothbrushing with a fluoride dentifrice on human salivary fluoride levels. Caries Res 1991;25:287-91.

60. Duckworth RM, Morgan SN. Oral fluoride retention after use of fluoride dentifrices. Caries Res 1991;25:123-9.

61. Duckworth RM, Morgan SN, Burchell CK. Fluoride in plaque following use of dentifrices containing sodium monofluorophosphate. J Dent Res 1989; 68:130-3.

62. Englander HR, Keyes PH, Gestwicki M. Clinical anticaries effect of repeated topical fluoride applications by mouthpieces. J Am Dent Assoc 1967;75:639-44.

63. Englander HR, Sherrill LT, Miller BG, et al. Incremental rates of dental caries after repeated topical sodium fluoride applications in children with lifelong consumption of fluoridated water. J Am Dent Assoc 1971;82:354-8.

64. Ericsson Y. State of fluorine in milk and its absorption and retention when administered in milk. Investigations with radio-active fluorine. Acta Odont Scand 1958;16:51-72.

65. Evans RW, Stamm JW. An epidemiologic estimate of the critical period during which human maxillary central incisors are most susceptible to fluorosis. J Public Health Dent 1991;51:251-9.

66. Fanning EA, Cellier KM, Somerville CM. South Australian kindergarten children: Effects of fluoride tablets and fluoridated water on dental caries in primary teeth. Aust Dent J 1980;25:259-63.

67. Fitzgerald RJ. The potential of antibiotics as caries-control agents. J Am Dent Assoc 1973;87:1006-9.

68. Fleiss JL. A dissenting opinion on the National Preventive Dentistry Demonstration Program. Am J Public Health 1986;76:445-7.

69. Fogels HR, Meade JJ, Griffith J, et al. A clinical investigation of a high-level fluoride dentifrice. J Dent Child 1988;55:210-5.

70. Forsman B. The caries preventing effect of mouthrinsing with 0.025 percent sodium fluoride solution in Swedish children. Community Dent Oral Epidemiol 1974;2:58-65.

71. Friis-Haché E, Bergmann J, Wenzel A, et al. Dental health status and attitudes to dental care in families participating in a Danish fluoride tablet program. Community Dent Oral Epidemiol 1984;12:303-7.

72. Garcia AI. Caries incidence and costs of prevention programs. J Public Health Dent 1989;49(Special Issue):259-71.

73. Gillespie GM, Roviralta G, eds. Salt fluoridation. Scientific Publication no. 501. Washington DC: Pan American Health Organization (WHO-AMRO), 1985.

74. Glenn FB, Glenn WD 3rd, Duncan RC. Prenatal fluoride tablet supplementation and improved molar occlusal morphology: Part V. J Dent Child 1984;51:19-23.

75. Glenn FB, Glenn WD 3rd. Optimum dosage for prenatal fluoride supplementation (PNF): Part IX. J Dent Child 1987;54:445-50.

76. Hanachowicz L. Caries prevention using a 1.2% sodium monofluorophosphate dentifrice in an aluminium oxide trihydrate base. Community Dent Oral Epidemiol 1984;12:10-6.

77. Haugejorden O, Lervik T, Riordan PJ. Comparison of caries prevalence 7 years after discontinuation of school-based fluoride rinsing or toothbrushing in Norway. Community Dent Oral Epidemiol 1985;13:2-6.

78. Haugejorden O, Nord A. Caries incidence after topical application of varnishes containing different concentrations of sodium fluoride: 3-year results. Scand J Dent Res 1991;99:295-300.

79. Hawes RR, Bibby BG. Evaluation of a dentifrice containing carbamide and urease. J Am Dent Assoc 1953;46:280-6.

80. Heifetz SB, Franchi GJ, Mosley GW, et al. Combined anticariogenic effect of fluoride gel-trays and fluoride mouthrinsing in an optimally fluoridated community. Clin Prevent Dent 1979;6:21-8.

81. Heifetz SB, Horowitz HS. Amounts of fluoride in self-administered dental products: Safety considerations for children. Pediatrics 1986;77:876-82.

82. Heifetz SB, Meyers R, Kingman A. A comparison of the anticaries effectiveness of daily and weekly rinsing with sodium fluoride solutions: Findings after two years. Pediatr Dent 1980;3:17-20.

83. Helfenstein U, Steiner M. Fluoride varnishes (Duraphat): A meta-analysis. Community Dent Oral Epidemiol 1994;22:1-5.

84. Hoffman R, Mann J, Calderone J, et al. Acute fluoride poisoning in a New Mexico elementary school. Pediatrics 1980;65:897-900.

85. Holland TJ, Whelton H, O'Mullane DM, Creedon P. Evaluation of a fortnightly school-based sodium fluoride mouthrinse 4 years following its cessation. Caries Res 1995;29:431-4.

86. Holloway PJ, Worthington HV. Sodium fluoride or sodium monofluorophosphate? A critical view of a meta-analysis on their relative effectiveness in dentifrices. Am J Dent 1993;6(Special Issue):S55-S58.

87. Holm AK. Effect of fluoride varnish (Duraphat) in preschool children. Community Dent Oral Epidemiol 1979;7:241-5.

88. Holm AK, Andersson R. Enamel mineralization disturbances in 12-year-old children with known early exposure to fluorides. Community Dent Oral Epidemiol 1982;10:335-9.

89. Horowitz HS. School fluoridation for the prevention of dental caries. Int Dent J 1973;23:346-53.

90. Horowitz HS. The need for toothpastes with lower than conventional fluoride concentrations for preschool-aged children. J Public Health Dent 1992;52:216-21.

91. Horowitz HS, Heifetz SB. Evaluation of topical applications of stannous fluoride to teeth of children born and reared in a fluoridated community; final report. J Dent Child 1969;36:65-71.

92. Horowitz HS, Law FE, Thompson MB, Chamberlin SR. Evaluation of a stannous fluoride dentifrice for use in dental public health programs. I. Basic findings. J Am Dent Assoc 1966;72:408-22.

93. Horowitz HS, Meyers RJ, Heifetz SB, et al. Combined fluoride, school-based program in a fluoride-deficient area: Results of an 11-year study. J Am Dent Assoc 1986;112:621-5.

94. Houpt M, Koeningsberg S, Shey Z. The effect of prior toothcleaning on the efficacy of topical fluoride treatment: Two-year results. Clin Prevent Dent 1983;5(4):8-10.

95. Intersalt Cooperative Research Group. Intersalt: An international study of electrolyte excretion and blood pressure. Results for 24 hour urinary sodium and potassium excretion. Br Med J 1988;297:319-28.

96. Ismail AI. Fluoride supplements: Current effectiveness, side effects, and recommendations. Community Dent Oral Epidemiol 1994;22:164-72.

97. James PMC, Anderson RJ. Clinical testing of a stannous fluoride-calcium pyrophosphate dentifrice in Buckinghamshire school children. Br Dent J 1967;123:33-9.

98. Jensen ME, Kohout F. The effect of a fluoridated dentifrice on root and coronal caries in an older adult population. J Am Dent Assoc 1988;117:829-32.

99. Johnson MF. Comparative efficacy of NaF and SMFP dentifrices in caries prevention: A meta-analytic overview. Caries Res 1993;27:328-36.

100. Jordan WA, Peterson JK. Caries inhibiting value of a dentifrice containing stannous fluoride: Final report of a two-year study. J Am Dent Assoc 1959;58:42-4.

101. Kalsbeek H, Verrips E, Backer Dirks O. Use of fluoride tablets and effect on prevalence of dental caries and dental fluorosis. Community Dent Oral Epidemiol 1992;20:241-5.

102. Kawall K, Lewis DW, Hargreaves JA. The effect of a fluoride mouthrinse in an optimally fluoridated community: Final two year results [abstract]. J Dent Res 1981;60:471.

103. Kesel RG. The effectiveness of dentifrices, mouthwashes, and ammonia-urea compounds in the control of dental caries. In: Easlick KA, ed: Dental caries. St. Louis: Mosby, 1948:88-102.

104. Klein SP, Bohannan HM, Bell RM, et al. The cost and effectiveness of school-based preventive dental care. Am J Public Health 1985;75:382-91.

105. Knutson JW. Sodium fluoride solutions: Technique for application to the teeth. J Am Dent Assoc 1948;36:37-9.

106. Knutson JW, Armstrong WD. Effect of topically applied sodium fluoride on dental caries experience. Public Health Rep 1943;58:1701-15.

107. Koch G, Petersson LG, Kling E, Kling L. Effect of 250 and 1000 ppm fluoride dentifrice on caries. A three-year clinical study. Swed Dent J 1982;6:233-8.

108. Koch G, Petersson LG, Ryden H. Effect of fluoride varnish (Duraphat) treatment every six months compared with weekly mouthrinses with 0.2 percent NaF solution on dental caries. Swed Dent J 1979;3:39-44.

109. Larsen MJ, Kirkegaard E, Poulsen S, Fejerskov O. Dental fluorosis among participants in a non-supervised fluoride tablet program. Community Dent Oral Epidemiol 1989;17:204-6.

110. Larsen MJ, Richards A, Fejerskov O. Development of dental fluorosis according to age at start of fluoride supplementation. Caries Res 1985;19:519-27.

111. Lalumandier JA, Rozier RG. The prevalence and risk factors of fluorosis among patients in a pediatric dental practice. Pediatr Dent 1995;17:19-25.

112. LeGeros RZ. Chemical and crystallographic events in the caries process. J Dent Res 1990;69(Special Issue):567-74.

113. LeGeros RZ, Glenn FB, Lee DD, Glenn WD. Some physico-chemical properties of deciduous enamel of children with and without pre-natal fluoride supplementation (PNF). J Dent Res 1985;64:465-9.

114. Lennon MA, Jones S, Woodward SM. Some operational aspects of school-milk fluoridation in St. Helens, Merseyside, UK. Adv Dent Res 1995;9:118-9.

115. Leske GS, Ripa LW, Green E. Posttreatment benefits in a school-based fluoride mouthrinsing program. Final results after 7 years of rinsing by all participants. Clin Prevent Dent 1986;8(5):19-23.

116. Leverett DH. Effectiveness of mouthrinsing with fluoride solutions in preventing coronal and root caries. J Public Health Dent 1989;49(Special Issue):310-6.

117. Leverett DH, Adair SM, Vaughn BW, et al. Randomized clinical trial of the effect of prenatal fluoride supplements in preventing dental caries. Caries Res 1997;31:174-9.

118. Leverett DH, Sveen OB, Jensen OE. Weekly rinsing with a fluoride mouthrinse in an unfluoridated community: Results after seven years. J Public Health Dent 1985;45:95-100.

119. Lind OP, Von der Fehr FR, Joost Larsen M, Moller IJ. Anticaries effect of a 2% Na_2PO_3F- dentifrice in a Danish fluoride area. Community Dent Oral Epidemiol 1976;4:7-14.

120. Lu KH, Ruhlman CD, Chung KL, et al. A three-year clinical comparison of a sodium monofluorophosphate dentifrice with sodium fluoride dentifrices on dental caries in children. J Dent Child 1987;54:241-4.

121. Mandel ID. Fluoride varnishes—a welcome addition [editorial]. J Public Health Dent 1994;54:67.

122. Margolis FJ, Burt BA, Schork MA, et al. Fluoride supplements for children: A survey of physicians' prescription practices. Am J Dis Child 1980; 134:865-8.

123. Margolis FJ, Reames HR, Freshman E, et al. Fluoride: Ten-year prospective study of deciduous and permanent dentition. Am J Dis Child 1975;130:794-800.

124. Marks RG, Conti AJ, Moorhead JE, et al. Results from a three-year caries clinical trial comparing NaF and SMFP fluoride formulations. Int Dent J 1994;44(3 Suppl 1):275-85.

125. Marthaler TM. Caries inhibiting effect of fluoride tablets. Helv Odont Acta 1969;13:1-13.

126. Marthaler TM. Caries inhibition by an amine fluoride dentifrice: Results after 6 years in children with low caries activity. Helv Odont Acta 1974;18:35-44.

127. Marthaler TM, Steiner M, Menghini G, de Crousaz P. DMF teeth in schoolchildren after 18 years of collective salt fluoridation. Caries Res 1989;23:48.

128. McConchie JM, Richardson AS, Hole LW, et al. Caries-preventive effect of two concentrations of stannous fluoride mouthrinse. Community Dent Oral Epidemiol 1977;5:278-83.

129. Miller AJ, Brunelle JA. A summary of the NIDR community caries prevention demonstration program. J Am Dent Assoc 1983;107:265-9.

130. Mitropoulos CM, Holloway PJ, Davies TG, Worthington HV. Relative efficacy of dentifrices containing 250 or 1000 ppm F- in preventing dental caries—report of a 32-month clinical trial. Community Dent Health 1984;1:193-200.

131. Muhler JC. Effect of a stannous fluoride dentifrice on caries reduction in children during a three-year study period. J Am Dent Assoc 1962;64:216-24.

132. Muhler JC, Radike AW, Nebergall WH, Day HG. Comparison between the anticariogenic effects of dentifrices containing stannous fluoride and sodium fluoride. J Am Dent Assoc 1955;51:556-9.

133. Murray JJ, Winter GB, Hurst CP. Duraphat fluoride varnish: a 2-year clinical trial in 5-year-old children. Br Dent J 1977;143:11-7.

134. Nourjah P, Horowitz AM, Wagener DK. Factors associated with the use of fluoride supplements and fluoride dentifrice by infants and toddlers. J Public Health Dent 1994;54:47-54.

135. O'Mullane DM, Kavanagh D, Ellwood RP, et al. A three-year clinical trial of a combination of trimetaphosphate and sodium fluoride in silica toothpastes. J Dent Res 1997;76:1776-81.

136. Pakhomov GN, Ivanova K, Møller IJ, Vrabcheva M. Dental caries-reducing effects of a milk fluoridation project in Bulgaria. J Public Health Dent 1995;55:234-7.

137. Parker PR, Bawden JW. Prenatal fluoride exposure: Measurement of plasma levels and enamel uptake in the guinea pig. J Dent Res 1986;65:1341-5.

138. Pendrys DG, Katz RV. Risk of enamel fluorosis associated with fluoride supplementation, infant formula, and fluoride dentifrice use. Am J Epidemiol 1989;130:1199-208.

139. Pendrys DG, Katz RV, Morse DE. Risk factors for enamel fluorosis in a fluoridated population. Am J Epidemiol 1994;140:461-71.

140. Pendrys DG, Katz RV, Morse DE. Risk factors for enamel fluorosis in a nonfluoridated population. Am J Epidemiol 1996;143:808-15.

141. Pendrys DG, Morse DE. Fluoride supplement use by children in fluoridated communities. J Public Health Dent 1995;55:160-4.

142. Petersson LG, Arthursson L, Ostberg C, et al. Caries-inhibiting effects of different modes of Duraphat varnish reapplication: A 3-year radiographic study. Caries Res 1991;25:70-3.

143. Petersson LG, Westerberg I. Intensive fluoride varnish program in Swedish adolescents: Economic assessment of a 7-year follow-up study on proximal caries incidence. Caries Res 1994;28:59-63.

144. Peyron M, Matsson L, Birkhed D. Progression of approximal caries in primary molars and the effect of Duraphat treatment. Scand J Dent Res 1992;100:314-8.

145. Radike AW, Gish CW, Peterson JK, et al. Clinical evaluation of stannous fluoride as an anticaries mouthrinse. J Am Dent Assoc 1973; 86:404-8.

146. Reintsema H, Schuthof J, Arends J. An in vivo investigation of the fluoride uptake in partially demineralized human enamel from several different dentifrices. J Dent Res 1985;64:19-23.

147. Report of the Canadian workshop on the evaluation of current recommendations concerning fluorides. Introduction to the workshop. Community Dent Oral Epidemiol 1994; 22:140-3.

148. Results of the workshop. J Public Health Dent 1989;49(Special Issue):331-7.

149. Richards A, Kragstrup J, Josephsen K, Fejerskov O. Dental fluorosis developed in post-secretory enamel. J Dent Res 1986;65:1406-9.

150. Ringelberg ML, Webster DB, Dixon DO, LeZotte DC. The caries-preventive effect of amine fluorides and inorganic fluorides in a mouthrinse or dentifrice after 30 months of use. J Am Dent Assoc 1979; 98:202-8.

151. Riordan PJ. Fluoride supplements in caries prevention: A literature review and proposal for a new dosage schedule. J Public Health Dent 1993;53:174-89.

152. Riordan PJ, Banks JA. Dental fluorosis and fluoride exposure in Western Australia. J Dent Res 1991; 70:1022-8.

153. Ripa LW. Fluoride rinsing: What dentists should know. J Am Dent Assoc 1981;102:477-81.

154. Ripa LW. Clinical studies of high-potency fluoride dentifrices: A review. J Am Dent Assoc 1989; 118:85-91.

155. Ripa LW. An evaluation of the use of professional

(operator-applied) topical fluorides. J Dent Res 1990;69(Special Issue):786-96.

156. Ripa LW, Leske GS. Two years' effect on the primary dentition of mouthrinsing with a 0.2% neutral NaF solution. Community Dent Oral Epidemiol 1979;7:151-3.

157. Ripa LW, Leske GS, Forte F, Varma A. Caries inhibition of mixed NaF - Na$_2$PO$_3$F dentifrices containing 1,000 and 2,500 ppm F: 3-year results. J Am Dent Assoc 1988;116:69-73.

158. Ripa LW, Leske GS, Sposato AL, Rebich T Jr. Supervised weekly rinsing with a 0.2% neutral NaF solution: Results after 5 years. Community Dent Oral Epidemiol 1983;11:1-6.

159. Ripa LW, Leske GS, Sposato A, Varma A. Effect of prior toothcleaning on bi-annual professional acidulated phosphate fluoride topical fluoride gel-tray treatments. Caries Res 1985;18:457-64.

160. Rise J, Haugejorden O. Monitoring and evaluation of results of community fluoride programs in Norway during the 1960s and 1970s. Community Dent Oral Epidemiol 1980;8:79-83.

161. Rölla G, Ekstrand J. Fluoride in oral fluids and dental plaque. In: Fejerskov O, Ekstrand J, Burt BA eds: Fluoride in dentistry. 2nd ed. Copenhagen: Munksgaard, 1996:215-20.

162. Rugg-Gunn AJ, Holloway PJ, Davies TGH. Caries prevention by daily fluoride mouthrinsing. Br Dent J 1973;135:353-60.

163. Seppä L. Studies of fluoride varnishes in Finland. Proc Finnish Dent Soc 1991;87:541-7.

164. Seppä L, Leppanen T, Hausen H. Fluoride varnish versus acidulated phosphate fluoride gel: A 3-year clinical trial. Caries Res 1995;29:327-30.

165. Seppä L, Pollanen L, Hausen H. Caries-preventive effect of fluoride varnish with different fluoride concentrations. Caries Res 1994;28:64-7.

166. Seppä L, Tolonen T. Caries preventive effect of fluoride varnish applications performed two or four times a year. Scand J Dent Res 1990;98:102-5.

167. Sidi AD. Effect of brushing with fluoride toothpastes on the fluoride, calcium, and inorganic phosphorus concentrations in approximal plaque of young adults. Caries Res 1989;23:268-71.

168. Sjögren K, Birkhed D. Effect of various post-brushing activities on salivary fluoride concentration after toothbrushing with a sodium fluoride dentifrice. Caries Res 1994;28:127-31.

169. Skold L, Sundquist B, Eriksson B, Edeland C. Four-year study of caries inhibition of intensive Duraphat application in 11–15-year-old children. Community Dent Oral Epidemiol 1994;22:8-12.

170. Slack GL, Berman DS, Martin WJ, Hardie JM. Clinical testing of a stannous fluoride-calcium pyrophosphate dentifrice in Essex school girls. Br Dent J 1967;123:26-32.

171. Speirs RL. The value of prenatally administered fluoride. Dent Update 1983;10:43-6, 49-51.

172. Stamm JW, Bohannan HM, Graves RC, Disney JA. The efficiency of caries prevention with weekly fluoride mouthrinses. J Dent Educ 1984;48:617-26.

173. Steiner M, Menghini G, Marthaler TM. The caries incidence in schoolchildren in Canton of Glarus 13 years after the introduction of highly fluoridated salt. Schweiz Monatsschr Zahnmedchr 1989;99:897-901.

174. Stephen KW, Boyle IT, Campbell D, et al. Five-year double-blind fluoridated mik study in Scotland. Community Dent Oral Epidemiol 1984;12:223-9.

175. Stephen KW, Campbell D. Caries reduction and cost benefit after 3 years of sucking fluoride tablets daily at school. A double-blind trial. Br Dent J 1978;144:202-6.

176. Stephen KW, Chestnutt IG, Jacobson AP, et al. The effect of NaF and SMFP toothpastes on three-year caries increments in adolescents. Int Dent J 1994;44(3 Suppl 1):287-95.

177. Stephen KW, Creanor SL, Russell JI, et al. A 3-year oral health dose-response study of sodium monofluorophosphate dentifrices with and without zinc citrate: Anti-caries results. Community Dent Oral Epidemiol 1988;16:321-5.

178. Stephen KW, McCall DR, Gilmour WH. Incisor enamel mottling in child cohorts which had or had not taken fluoride supplements from 0–12 years of age. Proc Finn Dent Soc 1991;87:595-605.

179. Stookey GK, DePaola PF, Featherstone JD, et al. A critical review of the relative anticaries efficacy of sodium fluoride and sodium monofluorophosphate dentifrices. Caries Res 1993;27:337-60.

180. Stookey GK, Schemehorn BR, Cheetham BL, et al. In situ fluoride uptake from fluoride dentifrices by carious enamel. J Dent Res 1985;64:900-3.

181. Suckling GW, Pearce EI. Developmental defects of enamel in a group of New Zealand children: Their prevalence and some associated etiological factors. Community Dent Oral Epidemiol 1984;12:177-84.

182. Svanberg M, Rölla G. Streptococcus mutans in plaque and saliva after mouthrinsing with SnF$_2$. Scand J Dent Res 1982;90:292-8.

183. Szpunar SM, Burt BA. Evaluation of appropriate use of dietary fluoride supplements in the US. Community Dent Oral Epidemiol 1992;20:148-54.

184. Thylstrup A. Is there a biological rationale for prenatal fluoride administration? J Dent Child 1981;48:103-8.

185. Thylstrup A, Fejerskov O, Bruun C, Kann J. Enamel changes and dental caries in 7-year-old children given fluoride tablets from shortly after birth. Caries Res 1979;13:265-76.

186. Tinanoff N, Klock B, Camosci DA, Manwell MA. Microbiologic effects of SnF$_2$ and NaF mouthrinses in subjects with high caries activity: Results after one year. J Dent Res 1983;62:907-11.

187. Torell P, Ericsson Y. Two-year clinical tests with different methods of local caries-preventive fluorine application in Swedish school-children. Acta Odont Scand 1965;23:287-322.

188. Toth K. A study of 8 years' domestic salt fluoridation for prevention of caries. Community Dent Oral Epidemiol 1976;4:106-10.

189. Toth K. Caries prevention by domestic salt fluoridation. Budapest: Akademiai Kiado, 1984.

190. Triol CW, Kranz SM, Volpe AR, et al. Anticaries effect of a sodium fluoride rinse and an MFP dentifrice in a nonfluoridated water area: A thirty-month study. Clin Preven Dent 1980;9(2):13-5.

191. Triol CW, Mandanas BY, Juliano GF, et al. A clinical study of children comparing anticaries effect of two fluoride dentifrices. A 31-month study. Clin Preven Dent 1987;9(2):22-4.

192. US Department of Health, Education, and Welfare; Food and Drug Administration. Oral prenatal drugs containing fluorides for human use. Fed Register 1966 Oct 20;31:13537.

193. Vogt RL, Witherell L, LaRue D, Klaucke DN. Acute fluoride poisoning associated with an on-site fluoridator in a Vermont elementary school. Am J Public Health 1982;72:1168-9.

194. Volpe AR, Petrone ME, Davies RM. A critical review of the 10 pivotal caries clinical studies used in a recent meta-analysis comparing the anticaries efficacy of sodium fluoride and sodium monofluorophosphate dentifrices. Am J Dent 1993;6(Special Issue):S13-S42.

195. Von der Fehr FR, Möller IJ. Caries-preventive fluoride dentifrices. Caries Res 1978;12(Suppl 1):31-7.

196. Weinstein P, Domoto P, Koday M, Leroux B. Results of a promising open trial to prevent baby bottle tooth decay. A fluoride varnish study. J Dent Child 1994;61:338-41.

197. Weisz WS. The reduction of dental caries through use of a sodium fluoride mouthwash. J Am Dent Assoc 1960;60:438-56.

198. Widenheim J, Birkhed D. Caries-preventive effect on primary and permanent teeth and cost-effectiveness of an NaF tablet preschool program. Community Dent Oral Epidemiol 1991;19:88-92.

199. Widenheim J, Birkhed D, Granath L, Lindgren G. Preeruptive effect of NaF tablets on caries in children from 12 to 17 years of age. Community Dent Oral Epidemiol 1986;14:1-4.

200. Winter GB, Holt RD, Williams BF. Clinical trial of a low-fluoride toothpaste for young children. Int Dent J 1989;39:227-35.

201. Woltgens JH, Etty EJ, Nieuwland WM. Prevalence of mottled enamel in permanent dentition of children participating in a fluoride programme at the Amsterdam dental school. J Biol Buccale 1989;17:15-20.

202. Woolfolk MW, Faja BW, Bagramian RA. Relation of sources of systemic fluoride to prevalence of dental fluorosis. J Public Health Dent 1989;49:78-82.

26

Fissure Sealants

Historical Development ◆ Rationale for Sealants ◆
Sealant Products and Procedures ◆ Clinical Trials ◆
Sealant Efficacy ◆ Cost-Effectiveness ◆ Public and
Professional Attitudes

A fissure sealant is a plastic, profession-ally-applied material used to occlude the pits and fissures of teeth. The purpose is to provide a physical barrier to the impaction of substrate for cariogenic bacteria in those crevices, and hence to prevent caries from developing. Sealants also can halt the carious process after it has begun, and can be used as a form of treatment for early lesions. All sealants are applied to the tooth in liquid form and polymerize (or "cure") in place a short time later.

The correct name for this group of materials is pit-and-fissure sealants, but they are more commonly referred to as fissure sealants, or just *sealants* (the term we will use). This chapter discusses the use of sealants in caries prevention, examines the issue of their cost-effectiveness, and makes recommendations for their use.

HISTORICAL DEVELOPMENT

The idea of physically occluding the pits and fissures is hardly new, for as long ago as 1923 Hyatt suggested a technique he called "prophylactic odontotomy."[48] In an age of severe and seemingly universal caries, Hyatt's technique involved minimal operative preparation of sound fissures and restoration with amalgam. The idea was not fully accepted even before the days of modern preventive dentistry,[54] but it led to widespread use of the "preventive restoration," meaning a full Black's-cavity restoration with "extension for prevention" in sound teeth, placed on the

grounds that such teeth would soon decay anyway. For many years, this type of restoration was considered good preventive practice, and perhaps it was when other preventive options were few. While we have no way of knowing just how much caries they "prevented," the extensive use of the "preventive restoration" served to artificially inflate DMF (Chapter 14) scores.[51]

In the prefluoride era, various chemicals were painted onto the tooth surface in efforts to prevent caries, but none proved successful.[10, 53] Even after fluoride entered dental practice, interest in a specific preventive agent for pit-and-fissure caries persisted, but it proved difficult to find a material that adhered successfully to enamel in the oral environment. The breakthrough came in 1955 with Buonocore's development of the acid-etch technique.[20] By the mid-1960s, cyano-acrylates had been used as sealant materials with some success,[29] but their production was not continued.[84] In the late 1960s the "bis-GMA" formulation (the sealant being the reaction product of bisphenol A and glycidyl methacrylate with a methyl methacrylate monomer) was developed and proved successful in a feasibility trial.[21] The bis-GMA formulation became the basis of a number of other products that soon came onto the market. The American Dental Association (ADA) issued provisional acceptance of the first bis-GMA material, Nuva-Seal, in 1972,[3] and full acceptance in 1976.[4] The number and type of accepted materials have grown and evolved steadily since then, and will likely continue to grow in the future. Currently, the most widely used sealant materials are either bis-GMA resin or urethane based.[98] There is also considerable interest in the potential use of glass ionomer-based materials and fluoride-containing varnishes as sealant materials, but the research literature to date shows their retention to be inferior to the conventional sealant materials.[8, 15, 17, 52, 89, 90, 105]

THE RATIONALE FOR SEALANTS

It has been recognized for years that fissured occlusal surfaces are the most vulnerable to caries.[48] With the continuing caries decline among children, caries is becoming a disease of the fissured surfaces as the rate of approximal caries development continues to decline faster than that of overall caries experience.[12, 92] Occlusal surfaces are also those least protected by fluorides,[11] so the case for sealant as a complementary procedure to fluoride is even stronger. As of the early 1990s, at least 83% of all decayed or filled surfaces in the permanent teeth of 5–17-year-olds were in pit-and-fissure surfaces.[18] In fact, the appropriate delivery of fluorides and sealants together, in theory at least, presents the dizzying prospect of virtually eliminating caries altogether.

SEALANT PRODUCTS AND PROCEDURES

The original bis-GMA materials, now referred to as first-generation sealants, polymerized under ultraviolet (UV) light, a procedure that demanded a bulky UV light source in the oral cavity. Second-generation sealants are chemically polymerized, meaning that when mixed, the operator has a fixed time to apply the sealant before it hardens. A number of these sealants are currently available. Third-generation sealants are those cured by visible light, which gives the operator the advantage of curing the sealant only when satisfied that it is all correctly in place. That advantage also applied to first-generation UV-cured sealants, but the visible light sources are far more compact and less expensive than the original UV lights. Some second- and third-generation sealants are colored to make them more visible at clinical examination.

As of late 1997, the ADA listed 12 sealant products as having been awarded the ADA Seal of Acceptance. Readers should always check with the ADA for the latest list of ac-cepted products, for in this fast-moving field many changes can occur in a short time. The ADA maintains lists of certified equipment and materials, including sealants, on its website.

It should also be noted that in 1996, a research report was published that demonstrated that shortly after placement of sealants, bisphenol-A and bisphenol-A dimethacrylate monomers were detected in saliva, and that these monomers showed estrogen-like activity when tested in in vitro cultures of human breast cell tumors.[64] This effect is of concern, because it theoretically could result in increased tumor cell growth. To date there is no evidence that the transient amounts of these chemicals in saliva represent an important exposure in humans. The finding, however, does point out that any material used in dentistry needs to be thoroughly evaluated for potential risk. As research on this matter will undoubtedly continue, practitioners must take care to use any procedure and material only when it is likely that the patient will benefit from it. The ADA provides continual updates on these and related matters on their website.

Sealant application is a simple but meticulous procedure that requires attention to all details of technique, especially moisture control. Even slight moisture contamination during sealant application and curing will result in failure. When applying a sealant, the operator begins by washing and drying the tooth surface, then etching with acid to demineralize the surface layers of enamel in and around the fissures. The etchant is supplied as either a liquid or a gel, and 37% orthophosphoric acid is the most commonly used concentration.[98] Acid etching dissolves out some of the inorganic fraction of the enamel, which subsequently allows "tags" of sealant to penetrate, thus enhancing retention. Some of these tags can extend up to 100 μm into enamel, although tags of 15 to 20 μm are more common.[85] After etching, the tooth surface is again washed and dried thoroughly, after which the liquid sealant is applied and worked into the fissures and pits. The sealant is then polymerized (by visible light or by self-curing) and trimmed if necessary. Detailed descriptions of the application process are available.[98]

During the 1990s, the development of sealants as a purely caries-preventive procedure was merging into the popularity of conservative restorations, many of which used the acid-etch technique. The trend was stimulated by the caries decline, which left practitioners increasingly having to manage small, slowly developing lesions rather than large cavities, and by the rapid developments in composite materials. Dentistry began moving away from amalgams in traditionally-prepared Black's cavities with "extension for prevention" and toward minimum-preparation restorations, which were far less invasive, lasted longer, and were more aesthetic.[33] The preventive resin and sealed composite restoration,[45, 62, 99] sealed glass ionomer restorations,[42] the "tunnel" restoration for small proximal restorations,[27] and even sealed amalgams[59, 62] are changing the face of restorative dentistry. The distinction between a purely preventive sealant placed on a sound tooth, the sealant placed on an incipient lesion, and a minimum-preparation sealed restoration is becoming increasingly blurred. The challenge is to understand the indications for each and to use them appropriately.

CLINICAL TRIALS

Clinical trials for testing the efficacy of sealants differ from the classical model (Chapter 12) in several respects:

- The study design is usually "half-mouth," in which the analytical unit is a contralateral pair of teeth, usually first or second molars. Because test and control teeth are in the same mouth, this allows the numbers of study subjects required to be reduced.

- There is no placebo sealant; the control tooth of each pair in earlier trials was simply left untreated (a passive control). Recent trials testing new products now more commonly apply an accepted sealant as a positive control on the control tooth.
- Examiners cannot be "blind" in a trial with a passive control, for they can clearly see the sealant on the test tooth. With the positive controls used in comparative studies, the examiners should be blind as to which sealant is test and which the positive control.
- The analytic procedures are necessarily different because not all surfaces of the teeth are involved, and because the analytical unit is a pair of teeth. Table 26-1 shows some hypothetical data typical of a half-mouth sealant trial, and the formulas used to compute the effectiveness of the sealant.

SEALANT EFFICACY

A large number of well-conducted sealant studies have been carried out, which allows conclusions on their efficacy to be stated with some confidence. The panel at the National Institutes of Health Consensus Conference on dental sealants in 1983, one of the relatively few such conferences held for dental procedures,[63] concluded that sealants were highly efficacious. The panel also noted, however, that practitioners were slow to adopt them, and that insurance carriers were also hesitant about adding sealants to their list of benefits. Progress in these areas since 1983 has been frustratingly slow.

Table 26–1. HYPOTHETICAL DATA FROM A HALF-MOUTH SEALANT CLINICAL TRIAL IN 561 CONTRALATERAL TOOTH PAIRS IN 561 CHILDREN TO DEMONSTRATE ANALYTIC METHOD IN SEALANT TRIALS

CONTRALATERAL TOOTH PAIRS: OUTCOMES		
SEALED TOOTH	CONTROL TOOTH	NUMBER
Sound	Sound	355
Sound	D, M, or F	109
D, M, or F	Sound	33
D, M, or F	D, M, or F	64
	Total Tooth Pairs	561

$$\% \text{ Effectiveness} = \frac{\text{No. pairs DMF control} - \text{No. pairs DMF sealed}}{\text{No. pairs DMF control}}$$

$$= \frac{(109 + 64) - (33 + 64)}{(109 + 64)}$$

$$= 43.9\%$$

The first clinical sealant studies in the 1960s yielded spectacular results, with caries reductions of 99% reported.[21] These initial studies, however, carefully selected both the patients and the teeth to be sealed. By the end of the 1970s, there was clear evidence from numerous clinical trials in different populations that sealants were highly efficacious when applied correctly.[69] Studies since then with second- and third-generation sealants have almost all been highly favorable; reviews of what is now an extensive literature have all reached highly favorable conclusions.[70, 72, 93, 102] Well-controlled clinical trials have yielded good results after 5 years,[44] 7 years,[60] and 10 years[72]; and 10-year and 15-year retrospective reports also showed encouraging results.[87, 88] The favorable evidence has led the ADA to strongly support the appropriate use of sealants in general practice.[1, 2]

Evidence of the efficacy of sealants in private practice, although scanty, also appears favorable. In an observational study in Canada, sealed first permanent molars had a 75% lower incidence of new restorations compared with sound but unsealed molars.[50] The authors acknowledged that sealants were more common in caries-free children, and in children whose parents had higher levels of education, which could account for some of the lower caries increment, but the differences in caries was so large that sealants unquestionably played a substantial role. It is nevertheless important to be cautious in interpreting outcomes from observational studies in which patients are not randomly assigned to receive or not receive sealants. As has been pointed out in a study of the use of sealants in a Medicaid program, the children who actually received sealants tended to be at lower risk; that is, they were more likely to have initially been caries-free and were more likely to have been classified by the study examiners as not needing sealants.[73] The authors pointed out that this pattern of nonrandom use of sealants, in the least caries-prone children, could lead to overestimates of sealant effectiveness. Nevertheless, there is ample reason to think that with appropriate patient selection sealants are highly effective in private practice.

Findings from the earlier clinical studies of sealants that have been supported by later research include the following:

• Sealant is generally retained better on mandibular than on maxillary molars. This is generally attributed to better accessibility and more favorable tooth morphology.
• Sealants are better retained when placed in older children. This is thought to be due to the ability to achieve better isolation in more completely erupted teeth, and the ability of the older child to cooperate in maintaining a dry field.
• Retention seems better on bicuspids than on molars. This too is likely to come from better accessibility, plus the fact that in studies where children have had bicuspids sealed they are obviously older than children who have had only their first molars sealed.
• Retention of sealant is synonymous with freedom from caries. An early concern was how the caries status of a tooth could be judged beneath intact sealant, but subsequent clinical research has shown that caries does not progress beneath intact sealant.
• Loss of sealant is greatest in the first 6 months after application. The sealant is probably lost a lot quicker than that, for these data suggest that the quickly-lost sealants are those that never "took" in the first place. The most likely reason for this kind of failure is moisture contamination. A properly-placed sealant will gradually wear down after a period of years, but protection from caries seems to remain, perhaps because of the sealant tags. The quickly-lost sealant almost certainly has no tags, so the tooth concerned is vulnerable again.

These results demonstrated unequivocally the considerable efficacy of sealants; they also gave hints of the more recent realization that sealants are more difficult to successfully apply and maintain on the very teeth that are most vulnerable, that is, the early-erupting molars in caries-prone children. On the other hand, sealants seem to be retained best on teeth that are least caries prone (e.g., bicuspids) and in children with low caries risk.[16] This realization is part of what has lead to efforts to target sealant use to the most susceptible groups, individuals, and teeth, an issue discussed later in this chapter.

Later studies of sealant efficacy have provided additional conclusions, described as follows.

All ADA-Approved Sealant Types Have Similar Efficacy

With the evolution of sealant systems and the large number of brand names now available, it is logical for dentists to ask which type is best. The response, from clinical studies, is that all accepted sealants are effective when applied properly. Results of numerous trials have demonstrated that the retention of the light-cured sealants is equivalent to that of the chemically polymerized products.[46, 74, 95, 106]

No UV-cured sealants have been among the list of ADA-approved sealants for a number of years, because they have been superseded by the chemically-polymerized and light-cured sealants. The dental practitioner's choice thus comes down to personal taste: an autopolymerized sealant hardens a specified time after preparation, just like many other products used in dentistry. The light-cured resins require the handling of an extra piece of equipment, the light source, but setting time is controlled by the operator.

Sealants Can Be Safely Placed Over Incipient Caries

A conclusion of the NIH consensus panel in 1983 was that evidence supported the use of sealants to arrest the progress of incipient lesions.[63] Nothing since then has occurred to alter that conclusion.

Modern sealants were developed as a primary preventive procedure, that is, to be placed on sound surfaces, but shades of Hyatt's philosophy soon emerged. Given that sealants occluded the fissures, the question about whether caries could progress or not beneath a sealant soon arose. The answer, after a number of studies, is now clear. When sealant is placed over an incipient carious lesion, meaning a stained fissure in which softness at the base could be detected but where cavitation had not yet occurred, caries does not progress provided the sealant remains intact. Sealant is retained on the carious teeth just as well as on sound teeth,[39] and neither lesion depth nor microbiologic counts progress under intact sealant.[38, 61] Reviews of these and other studies have concluded that the evidence is strong that caries-active lesions become caries-inactive beneath intact sealant.[36, 96] As restorative philosophy continues to evolve toward increasingly conservative cavity preparations, more recent reports confirm that even carious dentin, when isolated under a minimal restoration and sealant, does not progress.[62] These results provide further assurance that the clinician need not fear the placement of sealant over incipient

caries. Indeed, as discussed later in this chapter, consensus is developing that the placement of sealants over incipient lesions is one of their most effective uses.

Sealants Are of Uncertain Value on Primary Teeth

Some early research showed poorer retention of sealant on primary tooth enamel, although this improved in some later studies.[68, 86] The different enamel structure in primary teeth was thought to be a possible reason, although moisture contamination may also have been greater with younger children. Subsequent laboratory studies have shown that a short etch-time is effective in primary enamel,[97] and sealant retention for primary molars in a large Head Start program in Tennessee was equivalent to that for permanent molars.[40] What is not clear, however, is whether the usual caries pattern in primary molars is compatible with sealant effectiveness, despite retentive success. In many children, the occlusal surfaces of primary molars are not highly fissured and thus not especially caries prone. Further, when caries is a problem in primary molars, the first lesion is often interproximal. Sealants are not effective in these circumstances. Although sealant use in permanent teeth is growing (to be discussed later), as of 1991 only 1.4% of US children between 2 and 11 years had sealants on one or more primary teeth.[79]

Sealants Are an Important Part of Public Health Programs

With the decline of dental caries among children, especially in approximal caries, sealant programs are becoming more appropriate choices when deciding on a public caries-preventive program for children. Although many dental public health initiatives are directed toward encouraging the use of sealants in private practice, there is also considerable activity in the development of programs to actually place sealants in public programs. By the mid-1990s, 120 public health sealant programs were reported in 25 states.[9] These programs operate either in schools, usually with portable equipment, or in community clinics. The philosophy behind these public sealant programs is almost always aimed at bringing this preventive procedure to children who otherwise would be unlikely to receive comprehensive dental care. The programs surveyed report targeting their programs to schools with a high proportion of children from low-income families, schools with a high number of children with untreated dental needs, or in areas where there was a shortage of dentists.[9]

Research has shown that trained auxiliaries can apply sealant just as successfully as dentists.[24, 56] This is an important finding in public health, for the cost-effectiveness of sealant programs virtually depends on deployment of auxiliaries.[22] It is unfortunate that regulations in some states do not permit auxiliaries to apply sealant, a provision that is hard to defend as being in the public interest. The on-site presence of a dentist will obviously add to the cost of a public program without necessarily improving its outcome.

Several public health sealant programs have managed to deal with these problems and have subsequently flourished. One is in New Mexico, which required revision of its Dental Practice Act to permit auxiliaries to apply sealant in the state-administered program.[80] The New Mexico program, which uses mobile teams with portable equipment, found 67% retention of one-time sealant applications (i.e., each molar is sealed just once, and children are not subsequently checked to see if replacements are needed) after 6 years. Sixth-graders who received sealants on their first molars in grades 1, 2, or 3 had only 5.6% of those surfaces subsequently become carious, compared with 26.9% of the same surfaces among children not in the sealant program.[23] Even allowing for some self-selection bias, those figures are impressive. In the Canadian province of Saskatchewan, 79% of sealants applied by dental therapists (Chapter 10) were retained 3 years later, and sealed teeth developed 46% less caries than their unsealed counterparts after 4 years.[49] In Canada's Prince Edward Island program, there is annual resealing when needed. In that province, 85% of sealants were successful after 8 to 10 years,[76] similar to results reported from a 10-year study in Sweden.[104]

In addition to the usual targeting of sealant programs to communities and schools where there are large numbers of children in need, and with few private resources to get care, most public sealant programs also target sealants to specific children within these selected schools. In the United States, where children begin school at age 6, grades 1 to 2 are the best times for sealing first molars, and grades 6 to 7 for second molars.[13, 55] Sealing bicuspids and primary teeth is not usually a part of public programs because far fewer bicuspids decay than do molars,[5, 30] and a sound primary molar by grade 1 will probably stay that way. A good body of experience in operating programs with "sealant teams" has now been built up,[23, 49] and excellent guides to the development and operation of public sealant programs are available.[25, 65]

We referred earlier in this chapter to the prospect of sealants and fluoride together having the potential to virtually end caries altogether. Sealants are an obvious adjunct to fluoridated water; a comprehensive 1989 review found that sealants were more effective in fluoridated areas, compared with nonfluoridated areas, although the difference was slight.[102] Sealants have also been tested in combination with fluoride mouthrinsing. After 2 years in a New York study, the 84 children in grades 2 to 3 with sealants had an increment of only 0.03 DMFS, compared with the control group's 0.47 DMFS. The 84 children in the sealant/rinse group had only 3 new DF surfaces over the 2 years, 2 of them occlusal, whereas the 51 controls had 24 new DF surfaces, 15 of them occlusal.[71] In another study that used a sequential cross-sectional comparison group, a 23% decline in occlusal caries over a 4-year period in 14–17-year-olds was attributed to the addition of sealants to an ongoing school-based fluoride program.[78] These data suggest that complete prevention of caries is indeed theoretically possible, but its achievement might be costly. This is the biggest question a public health administrator has to deal with when considering sealant programs: can we afford it, and is the benefit from sealants worth the cost?

COST-EFFECTIVENESS OF SEALANTS

There were questions about the cost-effectiveness of sealants in public programs almost from their first use. A public health community that held water fluoridation as the "gold standard" in terms of the cost-effectiveness of public programs naturally looked askance at this one-on-one procedure, and an early economic assessment was not encouraging.[34] In this review, however, dentists applied the sealant, rather than auxiliaries, and retention of the first-generation sealant was not high.

Cost-effectiveness is defined as the least expensive way, from among competing alternatives, of meeting a defined objective.[101] It differs from *cost-benefit*, which is the ratio of an activity's cost to the monetary benefit it produces, although it is conceptually similar to *efficiency*, which is the return on effort expended.[100] The term *a cost-effective program* is virtually synonymous with *an efficient program*.

The cost-effectiveness issue arises in public dental programs when a dental director, with an objective of reducing caries experience in a child population by a specified amount over a specified time, might consider water fluoridation, sealants, fluoride mouthrinses, or dental health education to meet that objective. The director would weigh the costs of each program against the anticipated benefit. (In a fluoridated community where people routinely use fluoride toothpastes and have high utilization of dental services, introducing no new program could also be a viable alternative.) Thinking in terms of cost-effectiveness has moved dentistry away from "the more prevention the better" to careful selection of which programs are likely to be the most efficient. Cost-effectiveness is also at the base of discussions on "targeting" preventive programs to the most susceptible groups and individuals rather than applying them across the board (Chapter 19).

Are sealants expensive? That depends on what they are compared with. For example, when compared with water fluoridation and other self-applied fluoride uses, sealants are a relatively expensive, professionally-applied procedure. In terms of fees charged by dentists in private practice, the average fee for a sealant has remained approximately 50% of the fee for a one-surface amalgam restoration. The ADA's 1995 survey of fees charged by private practitioners found that the mean fee for sealant application was $24.42 per tooth, whereas the mean fee for a one-surface amalgam in a permanent tooth was $53.60.[6] In public programs, it has been shown that sealants can be even less expensive. The average cost of providing a sealant in public programs in the mid-1990s was $8.17 per tooth, well under the average of $24.42 charged in private offices.[9] The ability to provide sealants at these low costs in public programs is attributable in part to the economies that are possible through treating large numbers of children in a "captive" setting in schools, and through the extensive use of auxiliary personnel to place the sealants.

The other side of expense is effectiveness.

The evidence cited earlier shows that sealants are highly effective; their widespread use can have an immediate and substantial impact on the caries experience of a group. In the absence of specific studies on the relative cost-effectiveness of sealants and other preventive procedures, a 1989 workshop gave sealants a favorable cost-effectiveness review, slightly higher in nonfluoridated areas because of the higher probability of caries attack.[66] This means that sealants are not only a logical public health program to choose in light of caries distribution in the 1990s, they may well be one of the more efficient ones as well. It must be stated, however, that the cost-effectiveness issue is far from settled, and is really wide open for additional research. To illustrate, readers may have noted the vexing conundrum that whereas sealants may be more effective in fluoridated areas,[102] the 1989 workshop concluded that they are likely to be more cost-effective in nonfluoridated areas.[66] This is the case because although in a fluoridated area a higher *percentage* of carious lesions will be on occlusal surfaces, and thus preventable with sealants, in a nonfluoridated area, there will actually be a higher *total number* of occlusal lesions to prevent.

In the context of the targeting issue, it follows that sealants would be more cost-effective if they could be applied to teeth with the greatest probability of decaying, so that they do not have to be "wasted" on teeth that would not decay anyway. Although prediction methods are not yet precise enough to do that with sound teeth, an obvious approach with sealants is to take advantage of their demonstrated efficacy when applied to early lesions. A cost advantage of this approach has already been demonstrated,[58] with a benefit-cost ratio of only 0.3:1 in caries-inactive subjects, but 1.02:1 in caries-active subjects. In another study, the most favorable cost-effectiveness ratios were found when sealants were limited to children who already had restorations in one or more first permanent molars.[103] In yet another school-based study, although sealants were effective overall, their effect was especially striking on surfaces that were initially diagnosed as having incipient lesions.[41] Table 26–2 summarizes some of the data from that report. These data indicate that over a 5-year period, in surfaces that were initially diagnosed as sound, 8.1% of those that were sealed and 12.5% of those that were not sealed became carious. On the other hand, of those teeth initially diagnosed

Table 26–2. PERCENTAGE OF SURFACES (WITH ABSOLUTE NUMBERS IN PARENTHESES) BECOMING CARIOUS AFTER 5 YEARS, IN SEALED AND UNSEALED FIRST PERMANENT MOLARS, BY INITIAL DIAGNOSIS

	INITIAL DIAGNOSIS	
	SOUND	*INCIPIENT*
Sealed	8.1%	10.8%
	(24/297)	(41/380)
Nonsealed	12.5%	51.8%
	(8/64)	(29/56)

From Heller KE, Reed SG, Bruner FW, et al. Longitudinal evaluation of sealing molars with and without incipient dental caries in a public health program. J Public Health Dent 1995;55:148–53.

as having incipient caries, which meant that they had dark staining, a chalky appearance, or a slight explorer "stick" but no visible enamel surface defect, 10.8% of those that were sealed became carious, compared with 51.8% that were not sealed.

These results suggest strongly that applying sealants only to those teeth with early lesions or to teeth of children with a history of caries is likely to be much more efficient than a blanket sealing of all potentially "at risk" teeth. It is worth remembering, too, that as caries experience continues to decline, the need for selective use of sealant this way becomes even greater if the material is to be used efficiently. Use of sealant only on incipient lesions is, in effect, using it as an early restoration rather than as primary prevention, an approach that may require a different mind set in prevention-oriented dentists. It also further blurs the distinction between the use of sealants as primary preventive agents and their various uses in minimal-preparation restorations, as discussed earlier.

There are cost-effectiveness issues in private practice too, although they differ from those in public programs.[1, 5] After all, the value of preventive care eventually depends on what the individual thinks it is worth. A dentist is probably justified in sealing a number of teeth for a patient who wants prevention at any price, even if the dentist believes that the bicuspids he seals are unlikely to decay. The more pertinent issue facing a prac-

titioner is whether to seal or restore a deeply fissured molar, which at least until recent years was a decision between sealant or amalgam. Is it valid to compare these two options on a cost-effectiveness basis? Some commentators have said no, because one is a preventive procedure and the other is restorative.[43, 70, 91] Many would agree, but if a sealant can be viewed as a noninvasive restoration, then it becomes a valid comparison. One study directly compared the costs of sealing a caries-free molar with restoring the carious contralateral molar with amalgam. Taking all maintenance care into consideration, including necessary replacements of both sealant and amalgam, the average cumulative time to place and maintain a sealant over 7 years was 10 minutes 45 seconds; for the amalgams it was 14 minutes 26 seconds.[94] Another small-scale follow-up of 12 pairs of children concluded that treatment costs in children who did not receive sealant was 1.64 times greater than the costs in a group who had sealant maintained over the period.[87] Although these data are not conclusive, collectively they suggest that appropriate use of sealants on early lesions is effective, conserves tooth structure, and is likely to be cost-effective. As caries experience continues to decline, the future of sealants is likely to be even more focused on the early lesion rather than the totally sound tooth.

PUBLIC AND PROFESSIONAL ATTITUDES TO SEALANTS

The slow adoption of sealants by practitioners, despite the excellent results of many studies, has been frustrating. Even the main pediatric dental organizations in the United States did not adopt policies to encourage the use of sealants until 1983.[7] During a series of conferences and symposia in the early 1980s, which addressed the slow adoption of sealants, the reasons given for dentists' hesitancy included skepticism about efficacy, fear of "sealing-in decay," and failure of third-party carriers to reimburse for sealants. Virtually identical reasons were still given by dentists who were not using sealants as recently as 1992.[82] Many dentists also expressed a sublime faith in the longevity of amalgams, a faith that research shows is seriously misplaced.[5]

Even though the trend to more widespread use of sealants has developed slowly, it is consistent. Some growth in the numbers of dentists using sealants was evident through the 1980s,[28, 47, 75] and by the early 1990s it was reported in several states that more than 90% of general dentists were using sealants.[14, 37, 82] Growing acceptance of the use of sealants over incipient lesions was also evident. In a 1985 survey in Washington state, only 18% of dentists who used sealant reported doing so over incipient lesions,[26] but in 1992, more than 77% of Ohio dentists reported a willingness to seal over incipient caries, at least under some circumstances.[82] This trend toward more widespread use of sealants is likely to continue because the dentists most likely to use them are the younger, more recent dental school graduates,[82] and the acceptance of sealants by patients appears to be heavily influenced by the recommendations from the dentist.[57, 77, 82]

Data on the prevalence of sealants in national surveys also show that their use is increasing. Data from the 1986–1987 national survey of US schoolchildren aged 5 to 17 years indicated that 7.6% had one or more dental sealants on permanent teeth.[19] By 1991, however, the results from the first part of the third National Health and Nutrition Examination Survey (NHANES III) showed that this proportion had risen to 18.5%.[79] Although this increase is encouraging and is likely to continue, there is some note of caution that this increased use of sealants will be most useful if the sealants are being placed in children who are most likely to develop carious lesions.[83] For maximum benefit, it is important that dentists in private practice, as well as those in charge of public programs, make sure to target sealants toward patients most likely to profit from them.

The evidence is also consistent regarding the characteristics of patients who receive sealants. Higher levels of parental education and income, and dental insurance repeatedly have been shown to be associated with sealant use.[57, 77] These characteristics are associated with greater use of virtually all forms of dental care.

Lack of dental insurance coverage has been cited as a major factor in the slow acceptance of sealants.[35, 63, 82] This situation too appears to be improving. By 1994, all 50 states had included sealants as a benefit in their Medicaid programs,[81] and although exact numbers are unavailable, it is evident that an increasing number of privately insured groups are including sealants as a benefit.

The economic picture for insurers is not clear, however, because adding sealants to a benefit package usually requires premiums to increase, especially as caries experience and thus need for restorations continue to drop.[31, 32]

From the beginning, one of the primary concerns of insurers was how to ensure that sealants were used appropriately and not placed on teeth that did not need them, resulting in increased cost but little increased benefit. At a symposium in the early 1980s, several insurers stated that there was ample evidence already for inappropriate or even fraudulent claims.[5] In an effort to bridge this gap between the caution of the insurers and the growing body of evidence for the efficacy of sealants, the ADA developed standards for the use of sealants in insurance programs that were intended to reduce their inappropriate use while maximizing their preventive benefits. These standards are shown in Table 26–3. Although each insurer, in consultation with the purchasing group, is free to set whatever limitations are thought to be most appropriate, these recommendations, first published in 1985, are generally followed. There is usually an age limit to the benefit, as suggested by standard 1; and premolars, primary

Table 26–3. STANDARDS SUGGESTED BY THE AMERICAN DENTAL ASSOCIATION FOR USE OF SEALANTS IN DENTAL INSURANCE PROGRAMS

1. Sealant should be applied only to the occlusal fissures of permanent molars within 4 years of eruption (by age 10 years old for first molars, by 15 for second molars, by 22 for third molars). If a second molar is the prime tooth to be sealed, a nonrestored first molar could also be sealed at the same sitting. In this instance, the fee for the first molar sealing would be half the usual sealant fee.
2. The sealing of premolars and primary molars will not be reimbursed.
3. Teeth to be sealed must be free of proximal caries, and there can be no previous restorations on the surface to be sealed.
4. One replacement per sealed tooth can be accepted for reimbursement within the first 6 months, and one more replacement could be reimbursed each subsequent 3-year interval.
5. Within the time constraints given, any one dentist's replacement rate limit is 25% of total sealant applications.

From American Dental Association, Council on Dental Research. Cost-effectiveness of sealants in private practice and standards for use in prepaid dental care. J Am Dent Assoc 1985;110:103–7.

teeth, and previously restored teeth are usually excluded, as suggested in standards 2 and 3. Insurers usually deal with the intent of standards 4 and 5 by requiring dentists to be responsible for replacement, just as they would be with any other procedure, and that the fee for the initial service should include the costs of any anticipated maintenance.

Although it is evident that dentists and patients are becoming increasingly comfortable with the use of sealants, it is also true that the picture for their most appropriate use continues to evolve. In their earliest days, sealants were almost exclusively thought of as a material to be used on sound pit-and-fissure surfaces to prevent the development of a carious lesion. As the technology has developed and the overall caries pattern has changed, there has been an evolution in thinking. It is now widely accepted that not all children nor all teeth need sealants. Caries-free children, in the absence of other indications of risk, are not good candidates for sealants. A key criterion is that the fissured surface must be at significant risk for disease. This also gives rise to recommendations that sealants are appropriate for older children and adults in selected cases.[1, 67, 83] In this regard, sealants are increasingly seen as part of a trend toward much more conservative restorations.[62] A timely sealant on a tooth with an incipient lesion, with a conservative restoration if necessary, is increasingly seen as the most appropriate care, regardless of the age of the patient.

As with any other tool in the dental armamentarium, sealants must be used appropriately, in a way that is (a) compatible with the properties of the material, (b) consistent with the nature of the condition that it is meant to prevent or treat, and (c) at a cost that is acceptable to the provider and patient. Sealants and their associated composite products are among the most exciting technologic developments in dentistry. The technology and the standards for sealant use will undoubtedly continue to progress. At the same time, optimal use for sealants is also likely to remain somewhat different in public health programs than in private practice. In public programs, sealants should continue to be highly effective in reducing the burden of caries in children. This is because the children are selected on the basis of untreated disease and limited access to routine dental care, and large numbers of children can be provided with the traditional approach of sealing large numbers of teeth, including many that are sound. On the other hand, with patients who are available for regular care in private practice, the trend is toward a more selective, individual approach to sealants. Here the decision to treat is made on the basis of the expected risk for the individual child and tooth surface, and on the knowledge that sealants are part of a conservative approach to restorative care. The role for sealants and the related restorative materials to improve the oral health of the public is substantial. The challenge for the practitioner is to be alert for the inevitable evolution of the recommendations for the most appropriate use of these materials.

REFERENCES

1. American Dental Association, Council on Access, Prevention and Interprofessional Relations; Council on Scientific Affairs. Dental sealants. J Am Dent Assoc 1997;128:485-8.
2. American Dental Association, Council on Dental Health and Health Planning, Council on Dental Materials, Instruments, and Equipment. Pit and fissure sealants. J Am Dent Assoc 1987;114:671-2.
3. American Dental Association, Council on Dental Materials and Devices. Nuva-Seal pit and fissure sealant classified as provisionally accepted. J Am Dent Assoc 1972;84:1109.
4. American Dental Association, Council on Dental Materials and Devices. Pit and fissure sealants. J Am Dent Assoc 1976;93:134.
5. American Dental Association, Council on Dental Research. Cost-effectiveness of sealants in private practice and standards for use in prepaid dental care. J Am Dent Assoc 1985;110:103-7.
6. American Dental Association, Survey Center. Survey of dental fees 1995. Chicago, ADA, 1996.
7. American Society of Dentistry for Children, American Academy of Pedodontics. Rationale and guidelines for pit and fissure sealants. J Dent Child 1983;50:156.
8. Aranda M, Garcia-Godoy F. Clinical evaluation of the retention and wear of a light-cured pit and fissure glass ionomer sealant. J Clin Pediatr Dent 1995;19:273-7.
9. Association of State and Territorial Dental Directors. School-based and school-linked public health dental sealant programs in the United States, 1992-93. Columbus OH: ASTDD, 1997.
10. Ast DB, Bushel A, Chase HC. A clinical study of caries prophylaxis with zinc chloride and potassium ferrocyanide. J Am Dent Assoc 1950;41:437-42.
11. Backer Dirks O. The benefits of water fluoridation. Caries Res 1974;8(Suppl 1):2-15.
12. Bohannan HM. Caries distribution and the case for sealants. J Public Health Dent 1983;43:200-4.
13. Bohannan HM, Disney JA, Graves RC, et al. Indications for sealant use in a community-based preventive dentistry program. J Dent Educ 1984;48(Suppl 2):45-55.

14. Bowman PA, Fitzgerald CM. Utah dentists' sealant usage survey. J Dent Child 1990;57:134-8.

15. Bravo M, Llodra JC, Baca P, Oserio E. Effectiveness of visible light fissure sealant (Delton) versus fluoride varnish (Duraphat): 24-month clinical trial. Community Dent Oral Epidemiol 1996;24:42-6.

16. Bravo M, Oserio E, Garcia-Anillo I, et al. The influence of dft index on sealant success: a 48-month survival analysis. J Dent Res 1996;75:768-74.

17. Bravo M, Garcia-Anilo I, Baca P, Llodra JC. A 48-month survival analysis comparing sealant (Delton) with fluoride varnish (Duraphat) in 6- to 8-year-old children. Community Dent Oral Epidemiol 1997;25:247-50.

18. Brown LJ, Kaste LM, Selwitz RH, Furman LJ. Dental caries and sealant usage in U. S. children, 1988-1991. J Am Dent Assoc 1996;127:335-43.

19. Brunelle JA. Prevalence of dental sealants in US schoolchildren [abstract]. J Dent Res 1989;68(Special Issue):183.

20. Buonocore MG. A simple method of increasing the adhesion of acrylic filling materials to enamel surfaces. J Dent Res 1955;34:849-53.

21. Buonocore MG. Caries prevention in pits and fissures sealed with an adhesive resin polymerized by ultraviolet light: A two-year study of a single adhesive application. J Am Dent Assoc 1971;82:1090-3.

22. Burt BA. Fissure sealants: Clinical and economic factors. J Dent Educ 1984;48:96-102.

23. Calderone JJ, Davis JM. The New Mexico sealant program: A progress report. J Public Health Dent 1987;47:145-9.

24. Calderone JJ, Mueller LA. The cost of sealant application in a state dental disease prevention program. J Public Health Dent 1983;43:249-54.

25. Carter NL. Seal America: The prevention intervention. Cincinnati OH: American Association of Community Dental Programs, Cincinnati Health Department. 1995, ca 100 pp, 1 videotape (4:30 minutes, VHS).

26. Chapko MK. A study of the intentional use of pit and fissure sealants over carious lesions. J Public Health Dent 1987;47:139-42.

27. Christiansen GJ. Preventive restorative dentistry. Int Dent J 1990;40:259-66.

28. Cohen L, LaBelle A, Romberg E. The use of pit and fissure sealants in private practice: A national survey. J Public Health Dent 1988;48:26-35.

29. Cueto EL, Buonocore MG. Sealing of pits and fissures with an adhesive resin: Its use in caries prevention. J Am Dent Assoc 1967;75:121-8.

30. Eklund SA, Ismail AI. The development of occlusal and proximal lesions: Implications for fissure sealants. J Public Health Dent 1986;46:114-21.

31. Eklund SA. Factors affecting the cost of fissure sealants: A dental insurer's perspective. J Public Health Dent 1986;46:133-40.

32. Eklund SA, Pittman JL, Smith RC. Trends in dental care among insured Americans: 1980 to 1995. J Am Dent Assoc 1997;128:171-8.

33. Elderton RJ. Restorations without conventional cavity preparations. Int Dent J 1988;38:112-8.

34. Foch CB. The costs, effects, and benefits of preventive dental care: A literature review. Rand report no N-1732-RWJF. Santa Monica CA: Rand, 1981.

35. Glasrud PH, Frazier PJ, Horowitz AM. Insurance reimbursement for sealants in 1986: Report of a survey. J Dent Child 1987;54:81-8.

36. Going RE. Sealant effect on incipient caries, enamel maturation, and future caries susceptibility. J Dent Educ 1984;48:35-41.

37. Gonzales CD, Frazier PJ, Messer LB. Sealant use by general practitioners: A Minnesota survey. J Dent Child 1991;58:38-45.

38. Handelman SL, Leverett DH, Espeland MA, Curzon JA. Clinical radiographic evaluation of sealed carious and sound tooth surfaces. J Am Dent Assoc 1986;113:751-4.

39. Handelman SL, Leverett DH, Espeland M, Curzon J. Retention of sealants over carious and sound tooth surfaces. Community Dent Oral Epidemiol 1987;15:1-5.

40. Hardison JR, Collier DR, Sprouse LW, et al. Retention of pit and fissure sealant on the primary molars of 3- and 4-year-old children after 1 year. J Am Dent Assoc 1987;114:613-5.

41. Heller KE, Reed SG, Bruner FW, et al. Longitudinal evaluation of sealing molars with and without incipient dental caries in a public health program. J Public Health Dent 1995;55:148-53.

42. Henry RJ, Jerrell RG. The glass ionomer rest-a-seal. J Dent Child 1989;56:283-7.

43. Horowitz HS. Pit and fissure sealants in private practice and public health programmes: Analysis of cost-effectiveness. Int Dent J 1980;30:117-26.

44. Horowitz HS, Heifetz SB, Poulsen S. Retention and effectiveness of a single application of an adhesive sealant in preventing occlusal caries, final report after five years of study in Kalispell, Montana. J Am Dent Assoc 1977;95:1133-9.

45. Houpt M, Eidelman E, Shey Z, et al. Occlusal composite restorations: 4-year results. J Am Dent Assoc 1985;110:351-3.

46. Houpt M, Fuks A, Shapira J, et al. Autopolymerized versus light-polymerized fissure sealant. J Am Dent Assoc 1987;115:55-6.

47. Hunt RJ, Kohout FJ, Beck JD. The use of pit and fissure sealants in private dental practices. J Dent Child 1984;51:29-33.

48. Hyatt TP. Prophylactic odontotomy. Dent Cosmos 1923;65:234-41.

49. Ismail AI, King W, Clark DC. An evaluation of the Saskatchewan pit and fissure sealant program: A longitudinal followup. J Public Health Dent 1989;49:206-11.

50. Ismail AI, Gagnon P. A longitudinal evaluation of fissure sealants applied in dental practices. J Dent Res 1995;74:1583-90.

51. Jackson D. Caries experience in English children and young adults during the years 1947-1972. Br Dent J 1974;137:91-8.

52. Karlzen-Reuterving G, van Dijken JWV. A three-year follow-up of glass ionomer cement and resin fissure sealants. J Dent Child 1995;62:108-10.

53. Klein H, Knutson JW. Studies on dental caries. Effect of ammoniacal silver nitrate on caries in the first permanent molars. J Am Dent Assoc 1942;29:1420-6.

54. Klein H, Palmer CE. "Therapeutic odontotomy" and "preventive dentistry." J Am Dent Assoc 1940;27:1054-5.

55. Kuthy RA, Ashton JJ. Eruption pattern of permanent molars: Implications for school-based dental sealant programs. J Public Health Dent 1989;49:7-14.

56. Leske GS, Pollard S, Cons N. The effectiveness of dental hygienist teams in applying a pit and fissure sealant. J Preven Dent 1976;3:33-6.

57. Lang WP, Weintraub JA, Choi C, Bagramian RA. Fissure sealant knowledge and characteristics of

parents as a function of their child's sealant status. J Public Health Dent 1988;48:132-7.

58. Leverett DH, Handelman SL, Brenner CM, Iker HP. Use of sealants in the prevention and early treatment of carious lesions: Cost analysis. J Am Dent Assoc 1983;106:39-42.

59. Mertz-Fairhurst EJ, Call-Smith KM, Shuster GS, et al. Clinical performance of sealed composite restorations placed over caries compared with sealed and unsealed amalgam restorations. J Am Dent Assoc 1987;115:689-94.

60. Mertz-Fairhurst EJ, Fairhurst CW, Williams JE, et al. A comparative clinical study of two pit and fissure sealants: 7-year results in Augusta, GA. J Am Dent Assoc 1984;109:252-5.

61. Mertz-Fairhurst EJ, Schuster GS, Fairhurst CW. Arresting caries by sealants: Results of a clinical study. J Am Dent Assoc 1986;112:194-7.

62. Mertz-Fairhurst EJ, Adair SM, Sams DR, et al. Cariostatic and ultraconservative sealed restorations: Nine-year results among children and adults. J Dent Child 1995;62:97-107.

63. National Institute of Health Consensus Development Conference Statement. Dental sealants in the prevention of tooth decay. J Dent Educ 1984;48:126-31.

64. Olea N, Pulgar R, Perez P, et al. Estrogenicity of resin-based composites and sealants used in dentistry. Environ Health Perspect 1996;104:298-305.

65. Proceedings of the workshop on guidelines for sealant use. J Public Health Dent 1995;5:257-313.

66. Results of the workshop. J Public Health Dent 1989;49 (Special Issue):331-7.

67. Richardson PS, McIntyre IG. Susceptibility of tooth surfaces to carious attack in young adults. Community Dent Health 1996;13:163-8.

68. Ripa LW. Sealant retention on primary teeth: A critique of clinical and laboratory studies. J Pedod 1979;3:275-90.

69. Ripa LW. Occlusal sealants: Rationale and review of clinical trials. Int Dent J 1980;30:127-39.

70. Ripa LW. Occlusal sealants: An overview of clinical studies. J Public Health Dent 1983;43:216-25.

71. Ripa LW, Leske GS, Forte F. The combined use of pit and fissure sealants and fluoride mouthrinsing in second and third grade children: Final clinical results after two years. Pediatr Dent 1987;9:118-20.

72. Ripa LW. Sealants revisited: An update of the effectiveness of pit and fissure sealants. Caries Res 1993;27(Suppl 1):77-82.

73. Robison VA, Rozier RG, Weintraub JA, Koch GG. The relationship between clinical tooth status and receipt of sealants among child Medicaid recipients. J Dent Res 1997;76:1862-8.

74. Rock WP, Weatherill S, Anderson RJ. Retention of three fissure sealant resins. The effects of etching agent and curing method. Results over 3 years. Br Dent J 1990;168:323-5.

75. Romberg E, Cohen LA, LaBelle AD. A national survey of sealant use by pediatric dentists. J Dent Child 1988;55:257-64.

76. Romcke RG, Lewis DW, Maze BD, Vickerson RA. Retention and maintenance of fissure sealants over 10 years. J Canad Dent Assoc 1990;56:235-7.

77. Selwitz RH, Colley BJ, Rozier RG. Factors associated with parental acceptance of dental sealants. J Public Health Dent 1992;52:137-45.

78. Selwitz RH, Nowjack-Raymer R, Driscoll WS, Li S-H. Evaluation after 4 years of the combined use of fluoride and dental sealants. Community Dent Oral Epidemiol 1995;23:30-5.

79. Selwitz RH, Winn DM, Kingman A, Zion GR. The prevalence of dental sealants in the US population: Findings from NHANES III, 1988-91. J Dent Res 1996;75:652-60.

80. Siegal MD, Calderone JJ. Controversy over the supervision of dental hygienists: Impact on a community-based sealant program. J Public Health Dent 1986;46:156-60.

81. Siegal MD. Promotion and use of pit and fissure sealants: An introduction to the special issue. J Public Health Dent 1995;55:259-60.

82. Siegal MD, Garcia AI, Kandray DP, Giljahn LK. The use of dental sealants by Ohio dentists. J Public Health Dent 1996;56:12-21.

83. Siegal MD, Farquhar CL, Bouchard JM. Dental sealants: who needs them? Public Health Rep 1997;112:98-106.

84. Silverstone LM. Operative measures for caries prevention. Caries Res 1978;12(Suppl 1):103-12.

85. Silverstone LM. State of the art on sealant research and priorities for further research. J Dent Educ 1984;48:107-18.

86. Simonsen RJ. Fissure sealants in primary molars: Retention of colored sealants with variable etch times, at twelve months. J Dent Child 1979;46:382-4.

87. Simonsen RJ. Retention and effectiveness of a single application of white sealant after 10 years. J Am Dent Assoc 1987;115:31-6.

88. Simonsen RJ. Retention and effectiveness of dental sealant after 15 years. J Am Dent Assoc 1991; 122(11):34-42.

89. Simonsen RJ. Glass ionomer as fissure sealant—a critical review. J Public Health Dent 1996;56:146-9.

90. Songpaisan Y, Bratthal D, Phantumvanit P, Somridhivej Y. Effects of glass ionomer cement, resin-based pit and fissure sealant and HF applications on occlusal caries in a developing country field trial. Community Dent Oral Epidemiol 1995;23:25-9.

91. Stamm JW. The use of fissure sealants in public health programs: A reactor's comments. J Public Health Dent 1983;43:243-6.

92. Stamm JW. Is there a need for dental sealants? Epidemiological indications in the 1980s. J Dent Educ 1984;48:9-17.

93. Stephen KW, Strang R. Fissure sealants: A review. Community Dent Health 1985;2:149-56.

94. Straffon LH, Dennison JB. Clinical evaluation comparing sealant and amalgam after 7 years: Final report. J Am Dent Assoc 1988;117:751-5.

95. Sveen OB, Jensen OE. Two-year clinical evaluation of Delton and Prisma-Shield. Clin Preven Dent 1986;8(5):9-11.

96. Swift EJ Jr. The effect of sealants on dental caries: A review. J Am Dent Assoc 1988;116:700-4.

97. Tandon S, Kumari R, Udupa S. The effect of etch-time on the bond strength of a sealant and on the etch-pattern in primary and permanent enamel: An evaluation. J Dent Child 1989;56:186-90.

98. Waggoner WF, Siegal M. Pit and fissure sealant application: Updating the technique. J Am Dent Assoc 1996;127:351-61.

99. Walker JD, Jensen ME, Pinkham JR. A clinical review of preventive resin restorations. J Dent Child 1990;57:257-9.

100. Warner KE. Issues in cost effectiveness in health care. J Public Health Dent 1989;49(Special Issue):272-8.

101. Warner KE, Luce BR. Cost-benefit and cost-effectiveness analysis in health care. Ann Arbor MI: Health Administration Press, 1982:46-50.

102. Weintraub JA. The effectiveness of pit and fissure sealants. J Public Health Dent 1989;49:317-30.

103. Weintraub JA, Stearns SC, Burt BA, et al. A retrospective analysis of the cost-effectiveness of dental sealants in a children's health center. Soc Sci Med 1993;36:1483-93.

104. Wendt LK, Koch G. Fissure sealant in permanent first molars after 10 years. Swed Dent J 1988; 12:181-5.

105. Winkler TM, Deschepper EJ, Dean JA, et al. Using a resin-modified glass ionomer as an occlusal sealant: A one-year clinical study. J Am Dent Assoc 1996;127:1508-14.

106. Wright GZ, Friedman CS, Plotzke O, Feasby WH. A comparison between autopolymerizing and visible-light-activated sealants. Clin Prevent Dent 1988;10(1):14-7.

27

Diet and Plaque Control

Nutrition and Caries ◆ What Is a Cariogenic Food? ◆
Consumption of Sugars ◆ Cariogenicity of
Different Sugars ◆ Noncariogenic Sugar Substitutes ◆
"Cleansing" and "Protective" Foods ◆ Control of
Caries by Dietary Restriction ◆ Plaque Control

Probably more effort has been expended down the years in trying to prevent caries by dietary control and consistent toothbrushing than by any other methods. Traditionally these efforts have been in dental health education, which aimed at changing personal behavior by exhorting people to voluntarily restrict their consumption of sugars and to brush religiously. Americans' response is to eat more sugar than ever, although oral hygiene is also probably better than ever. Although mass education to restrict sugar consumption has clearly not worked, restriction of sugar consumption still is an appropriate part of the strategy for controlling caries in a caries-susceptible patient. Developments in low- and noncariogenic sugar substitutes also provide a few more options for these patients.

This chapter takes a critical look at the role of dietary approaches to preventing oral disease, the potential for caries control through the use of sugar substitutes, and the most appropriate place for oral hygiene in caries control.

NUTRITION AND CARIES

Diet refers to the food and drink that passes through the mouth, whereas nutrition is concerned with the absorption and metabolism of nutrients from dietary sources. We stated in Chapter 19 that there is little firm evidence to show that nutritional deficiencies, either during tooth development or subsequently, cause dental caries. Malnourishment

is unusual in the well-fed societies of North America, although it is seen among some who live in deprived circumstances and among some patients with eating disorders.

Despite the infrequency of nutritional disturbances among North Americans, some well-meaning dentists have extolled the virtues of controlling dental caries and periodontal diseases through nutritional counseling. In cases of rare metabolic diseases that can disrupt the immune system, there may be improvement in oral conditions when the patient's nutritional status is improved, but in healthy, well-nourished patients there is no basis for treating existing disease through nutritional (as distinct from dietary) counseling.

The nutritional status of a patient is the concern of the attending dental professional, and all dentists and hygienists should be sensitive to the signs of nutritional disturbances. Where a nutritional disturbance or eating disorder is suspected, referral to a physician or nutritionist is the right course of action. Even when such a patient is treated successfully for the nutritional problem, improvement in oral status is likely to follow as a consequence only in the most severe cases.

WHAT IS A CARIOGENIC FOOD?

Any food that contains sugars or other readily fermentable carbohydrates can be metabolized by cariogenic bacteria in plaque. This property of a food is termed *acidogenesis*, and it is a necessary, although not sufficient, condition for the development of caries. This means that a wide range of foods and drinks are acidogenic. Whether or not an acidogenic food is cariogenic depends on a number of factors specific to the individual who eats it, namely, predominant bacterial flora, flow rate and buffering capacity of saliva, fluoride availability, individual immune factors, and perhaps some other factors. The outcome also depends on the quantity and frequency of the food eaten, whether it is eaten in isolation or with other foods, and the nature of any accompanying foods. We cannot be certain, therefore, whether a particular acidogenic food is cariogenic for a particular patient. However, we can be confident about the converse: because acidogenesis is a necessary condition for caries, a nonacidogenic food must also be a noncariogenic food.

The concept of a cariogenic food is too broad to be of practical use in caries control, so attempts were made to define the *cariogenic potential* of a food, defined as the food's ability to foster caries in humans under conditions conducive to caries formation.[45] The underlying idea with cariogenic potential was to draw up a rank order of cariogenic foods, but a 1986 workshop on food cariogenicity at the University of Texas at San Antonio concluded that this approach was unproductive. Although efforts to identify cariogenic foods were not followed up because that category was so broad, the workshop agreed that there was value in identifying nonacidogenic foods, which by definition have no cariogenic potential.[26] Such foods can then be confidently recommended to patients who need a sugar-restricted diet.

Cariogenic potential of a single food cannot be satisfactorily tested in human studies because of the "background noise" from other, uncontrolled consumption of sugars in a normal mixed diet. Studies to determine whether the consumption of presweetened breakfast cereals, for example, increased caries incidence were unable to control for other crucial variables.[22] The 1986 Texas conference suggested guidelines for testing the cariogenic potential of foods using a combination of several testing regimens, including animal models and in vitro procedures.[26] These protocols are intended to identify foods with no cariogenic potential, especially snack foods, but they have not received much attention.

Research attention in food cariogenicity has concentrated heavily on sugars, but it is likely that some other foods have an etiologic role that has not yet been well defined.[20] Starches and other simple carbohydrates found in processed foods, however, are considered potentially cariogenic. Starch, defined as a branched or unbranched polysaccharide chain of glucose molecules, usually means large-molecular carbohydrates such as those found in potatoes, rice, and whole grains—all carbohydrates that have long been considered virtually noncariogenic because little breakdown occurs in the oral cavity.[56, 74] However, cooked or milled starches in the refined flours used in cookies, biscuits, croissants, and other processed foods can be broken down to simple carbohydrates by the salivary enzyme amylase. Some evidence suggests that starch-sugar mixtures are more cariogenic than sugars alone.[15, 16, 30, 68] The nonspecific term *fermentable carbohydrates* is used widely in the literature, a generic term to cover sugars and refined starches.

The Swiss government has been testing the cariogenic potential of snack foods since 1982, and permitting snack foods there to be labeled *Zahnschonend* ("tooth-friendly" or "happy tooth") if they do not lower the pH of interdental plaque below 5.7 for up to 30 minutes after consumption.[44] Under this program, tests of food products are carried out telemetrically with a plaque electrode. Accepted products are usually confectionery sweetened with the sugar alcohols xylitol, sorbitol, mannitol, and maltitol, or with Lycasin, a hydrogenated starch derivative. Fructose does not pass the test.

The impact of this program on the dental health of the Swiss people, the country where it has been in place the longest, is difficult to document. However, it is likely to be positive because a high proportion of Swiss children and adults have learned to recognize the "happy tooth" logo and to understand its oral health benefits.[73] This program is likely to grow further as more nonacidogenic sugar substitutes are developed. The concept has spread to a number of other countries, including the United States, where the Food and Drug Administration (FDA) in 1996 permitted the claim "does not promote tooth decay" to be used for sugar-free foods that met the test conditions.[42]

CONSUMPTION OF SUGARS

The material known in lay terms as sugar is sucrose, a disaccharide that is the most common form of sugar consumed by humans. Sucrose and other sugars, both monosaccharides and disaccharides, are added to a wide variety of processed foods; labels on supermarket staples such as canned soups, salad dressings, and processed meats frequently put sugars high on the list of ingredients. The ingredients on a label are listed in order of relative proportions, so the higher up on the list an ingredient appears, the more of it there is in the product.

Consumption of sugars in all forms has continued to rise in the United States for many years. It exceeded 120 pounds (54.5 kg) per head per year in the 1920s,[5] and has risen steadily since then. Figure 27–1 uses data from the US Department of Agriculture (USDA) from 1972 to 1996 to show that whereas average consumption of all sugars rose steadily over that period, sucrose consumption dropped until 1984 and has leveled out since then. Consumption of monosaccharides continues to increase. According to the USDA, average per capita consumption of all sugars in the United States reached 154.5 pounds (70.2 kg) in 1997, one of the highest levels of national consumption in the world. Some international contrasts for sucrose (not

necessarily total sugars) consumption are shown in Figure 27–2. These data do not include the monosaccharides that are more than half of the US consumption, although monosaccharides are a much smaller fraction of the total sugars consumed elsewhere.

Most monosaccharide now consumed in the United States is high fructose corn syrup (HFCS), widely used in place of sucrose in processed foods and soft drinks. HFCS consists mostly of fructose, glucose, and other oligosaccharides and is used by food manufacturers instead of sucrose because it is cheaper. Because it is produced domestically, it is available from a stable market. Corn is a cheap and abundant crop in the United States; no other country uses HFCS in the same amounts. Sucrose has such a variety of desirable characteristics from the food manufacturer's point of view that it is difficult to replace. As well as the sweet taste, sucrose can be baked and boiled without losing its desirable properties of adding body, luster, and texture to a food product; promoting the emulsification of fats; and acting as a preservative.[70] When HFCS is used instead of sucrose in processed foods, the other desirable qualities of sucrose have to come from addi-

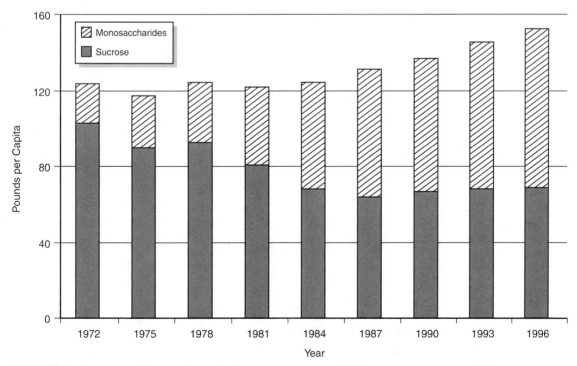

Figure 27-1. Mean annual consumption of total sugars, sucrose, and high-fructose corn syrup and other monosaccharides. United States, 1972–1996. (From US Department of Agriculture, Economic Research Service. Sugar and Sweetener: Situation and outlook report. SSS-220, June 1997.)

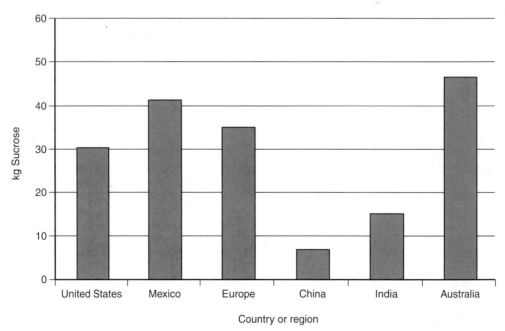

Figure 27-2. Mean annual consumption of sucrose in the United States, Europe, and four other countries in 1996. (Data are for sucrose only, and do not include consumption of high-fructose corn syrup and other monosaccharides.) (From US Department of Agriculture, Economic Research Service. Sugar and Sweetener: Situation and outlook report. SSS-220, June 1997.)

tives. In an age of sensitivity about food additives, the replacement of sucrose, which presents few health hazards apart from caries,[35] may be a mixed blessing in terms of the public health. However, economics have driven the trend for sucrose replacement in processed foods.

A caveat with regard to these data is that they are all "disappearance" data, meaning sugar that is produced and then is distributed from storage warehouses. Disappearance data do not account for industrial use, wastage, and other losses. Just how much of the "disappeared" sugars actually are consumed by humans is a matter of speculation, but disappearance figures by themselves are almost certainly overestimates of human consumption. Still, these data are collected in the same way from year to year, so the trends represented are probably accurate even if the absolute amounts cannot be taken literally.

In addition to the considerable shift from sucrose to HFCS and other syrups in processed food, two other major changes have taken place in sugar consumption patterns since the early 20th century:

- The proportion of energy intake from carbohydrate foods has shifted from a preponderance obtained from starches (bread, pota-

toes, whole grain cereals) to one obtained from sugars.
- The main use of sugars has changed from discretionary (i.e., from the sugar bowl on the table) to consumption by way of processed foods, the "hidden sugars." By the mid-1970s, three-fourths of all sugars consumed came from processed foods.[24]

CARIOGENICITY OF DIFFERENT SUGARS

Sucrose for years was billed as the "arch-criminal" of dental caries because it was considered to be so much more cariogenic than other sugars.[69] Research since then, however, suggests that the differences between sucrose and the various monosaccharides in terms of cariogenic potential is less pronounced than originally believed.[44, 55] This is a difficult issue to study in humans because of the variability of the human diet, so views are based principally on extrapolations from animal studies and laboratory research. One study in Sweden with a small number of preschool children found that those consuming invert sugar (a mix of glucose and fructose) in place of sucrose had a lower caries increment over 2 years,[31] although the differences did not reach statistical significance. One could speculate, however, that reduced consumption of sucrose in the United States (Fig. 27–1) has been a factor in the sharp reduction in approximal and smooth-surface caries relative to the overall caries decline (Chapter 19). This is based on the knowledge that the production of extracellular polysaccharides depends on sucrose,[71] and that smooth-surface caries can only develop with plaque that adheres by means of extracellular polysaccharides.

There is no important difference in cariogenicity between refined sugars and brown sugar, or between refined sugars and other "natural" sugars such as those found in fruits and honey (honey contains a mix of sugars, mostly glucose and fructose). Fruits can contain a lot of sugar, and consumption of a high-fruit diet does not necessarily protect from caries.[38] However, fruits have considerably more nutritional value than the average candy bar, and fruit sugars are also thought to be rapidly cleared from the oral cavity.

NONCARIOGENIC SUGAR SUBSTITUTES

The development of noncaloric sugar substitutes is big business in the United States. Commercial development of these products, from the laboratory to marketing, is time-consuming and expensive. This is mainly because of the stringent requirement of the FDA that all such products be shown to present no potential hazard to human health, a requirement that demands extensive animal testing. Despite the sometimes formidable costs involved, sugar substitutes continue to be developed. Some, like the noncaloric saccharin, have been in common use in the United States and elsewhere for years. Aspartame, a dipeptide composed of 2 naturally occurring amino acids, became available in the United States in 1982.

Research into the dental applications of sugar substitutes goes back several decades.[32] The rationale is that *Streptococcus mutans* and *S. sobrinus* emerge in plaque flora when sugar substrate is plentiful, but can be suppressed when the diet is low in sugars. A widely used sugar substitute is the group of caloric sweeteners known as the sugar alcohols. The most commonly-used sugar alcohol in the United States has been sorbitol, which is the standard sweetener in several "sugarless" chewing gums and over-the-counter medicines. Sorbitol's advantage over sugars, in terms of cariogenesis, is that in small amounts

it does not lower the pH of plaque to a point at which enamel demineralization occurs.[17] However, sorbitol is considered low-cariogenic rather than noncariogenic, because when larger amounts are consumed, both the acid production in plaque and the number of sorbitol-fermenting microorganisms can be increased.[18] Cariogenic microorganisms "learn" to metabolize sorbitol when their sugar supply is restricted, a form of adaptation to sorbitol that has also been demonstrated in animals.[29] Several clinical trials with sorbitol chewing gum, however, have shown that these problems cannot be demonstrated when consumption levels are low, around two sticks of gum per day. Use of sorbitol gum at this level at least does not promote caries,[34] and may help to reverse early demineralized lesions.[27, 53, 59]

The sugar alcohol that has received most research attention, however, is xylitol. Xylitol, like other sugar alcohols, is caloric, but has been shown to be noncariogenic and to possess the properties of a marketable sweetener. In the late 1960s and early 1970s, xylitol was the subject of interesting experiments in the Finnish city of Turkü, collectively known as the Turkü Sugar Studies.[85] In the first of the Turkü studies, a small group of volunteer adults made virtually complete substitution of sucrose in their diet by xylitol, a change made possible by having food manufacturers prepare special nonsucrose, xylitol-sweetened foods for the 2 years of the study. A second test group consumed fructose-sweetened foods through the same protocol, and a third group acted as controls by consuming a conventional sucrose-containing diet. By necessity, this study deviated from the requirements of an ideal clinical trial in that the participants were self-selected and were aware of their group assignment. Still, the magnitude of the differences in new caries experience between the groups was impressive. Over the 2 years of the study, there were practically no new carious lesions in the xylitol group, whereas there were more than 7 new lesions per person in the group eating the usual sucrose diet and 4 in the fructose group. Lesions in the adult test subjects, whose average age was 27.5 years, were almost all of the "white spot" variety (i.e., reversible early demineralization) on smooth surfaces.[83] The quantity of plaque formed in the xylitol group was also significantly lower.[85]

In a separate 1-year clinical trial in Turkü, young adult subjects consumed an average of 4 sticks a day of xylitol-sweetened chewing gum, with no other changes in conventional diet. Control group subjects consumed the same amount of sucrose-sweetened gum. After a year, the test group subjects had 0.3 new DMF carious surfaces compared with nearly 4 surfaces in the sucrose group.[84] The lesions were again mostly of white spots, which explains why the caries incidence appears high.

Subsequent field trials of xylitol-sweetened gum and confectionery have continued to yield impressive results.[47, 51, 64, 65] Other field studies, in one instance with fluoride added to xylitol gum, have yielded acceptable positive results despite questionable study design and data analysis.[11, 50, 82]

Xylitol cannot be metabolized by cariogenic microorganisms[12, 37] and thus does not reduce the pH of plaque.[58] The counts of salivary S. mutans drop as a consequence of consistent use of xylitol gum, probably because replacement of sucrose by xylitol in plaque "starves" the cariogenic microorganisms. Further analysis of data from the Turkü studies,[76, 77] in addition to laboratory studies[86] suggests that xylitol may promote remineralization, and there are also reports that xylitol can arrest established dentin caries.[66] This evidence has led to the possibility that xylitol goes beyond being noncariogenic and is actually therapeutic, or anticariogenic. Although these claims require further confirmation before they can be fully accepted, research supports the conclusion that even partial substitution of xylitol for sucrose, such as in confectionery, is an effective means of caries prevention at the public health level.[81]

Xylitol has been approved for special dietary use in the United States since 1963,[72] although it has not been used much. It did appear for a short time as an ingredient in a Wrigley chewing gum, but the product was withdrawn by the company after an animal study suggested that xylitol might be tumorigenic. Xylitol is much more expensive than sucrose, however, and because it is destroyed by heat, it cannot be used in cooked food products. Its use may thus be restricted to products such as chewing gum, which require only small amounts of sweetener,[72] but with the FDA's acceptance of the "tooth-friendly" logo[42] it is likely that more xylitol-sweetened products will be seen in the United States.

"CLEANSING" AND "PROTECTIVE" FOODS

As discussed in Chapter 19, long-held and strenuously-asserted beliefs in the anti-cariogenic properties of "cleansing foods" have little substance. The thinking here was that chewing a fibrous food (apple, carrot, celery) will "clean" plaque from tooth surfaces and thus prevent caries, although research has long since shown that chewing fibrous foods does not remove plaque (Chapter 28). There is obvious nutritional merit in snacking on fresh fruit and vegetables rather than on candy bars: more fiber, more vitamins and minerals, less fat. However, unless the sugar intake of persons eating fibrous snacks was drastically reduced in addition, which as mentioned before is difficult to do without a radical move away from processed foods, the impact on caries will be minimal. Even that very symbol of oral health, the apple, has been shown to lower plaque pH soon after ingestion,[33] and to induce caries in rats when eaten ad libitum.[88]

One food with reported protective factors is cheese; there is evidence in humans to show that finishing a meal with cheese reduces the acidity of plaque[78] and therefore presumably its cariogenicity. Animal studies support this finding.[57] Apart from fluoride, other dietary trace elements have been associated with caries experience: molybdenum with low disease levels[80] and selenium with high levels.[40] Evidence for an important etiologic role is weak, however, and these reports have no practical implications for caries control.

Among the various food additives intended to reduce the carious attack, the addition of phosphates has probably received most attention. In numerous animal studies, phosphates have been shown to reduce caries when added to the diet, but studies among humans have been disappointing.[49, 60] The reductions in caries have been too small to be of any significance, and the phosphate materials tend to give the food an unpleasant taste.

The conclusions on cleansing and protective foods is that nutritious and fibrous foods are naturally to be recommended for good general health. Although the impact on oral health of a balanced diet high in unprocessed foods could only be good, it cannot be demonstrated under modern conditions of fluoride exposure that such a diet, by itself, will improve oral health status. Nor is there any evidence to support chewing of carrots, celery, or apples as a means of cleaning plaque from teeth. This form of dietary counseling should not become a centerpiece of dental health education, although dental personnel should always encourage healthy food choices by their patients.

CONTROL OF CARIES BY DIETARY RESTRICTION

Dietary regimens that involved strict control of carbohydrate intake were developed for caries control in the immediate pre-fluoride years.[48] Success was based on reducing counts of *Lactobacillus acidophilus*, and Jay's regimen[48] demanded almost total abstinence from all forms of carbohydrate for a short period, with a gradual return to limited carbohydrate intake. However, this draconian regimen of dietary control was too much for most patients, and it had little broad-scale success.[13] Of more concern in today's world, drastic reduction of all forms of carbohydrate, which included fruits and vegetables, is clearly unwise because it could lead to either excessive intake of fat and protein or to energy deprivation. Dietary guidelines now urge the consumption of more unrefined carbohydrate (e.g., fruit, potatoes, and whole grains) while retaining the recommendation for reduced consumption of refined carbohydrate (sugars and other fermentable carbohydrates).

In Chapter 19, we discussed the impact of Vipeholm[39] on dental health education, and how applying the results of that landmark study may have become misdirected. In normal-living populations, there is no epidemiologic evidence that consumption of sticky foods is more strongly associated with caries experience than are sugared drinks,[46] although this conclusion was dependent on quantities consumed (i.e., food cariogenicity rather than cariogenic potential). Sugared rinses served very well to demonstrate the *Stephan curve*, the first laboratory demonstration that ingestion of sugars caused an immediate sharp drop in plaque pH, followed by a gradual return to normal pH from salivary buffer action.[87] The Stephan curve is shown in Figure 27–3. Sugared rinses were also the basis of experimental caries studies in humans,[90] so advice to "take your sugars in drinks rather than sticky foods" can hardly be recommended from this evidence. An additional factor on this subject is that consumer perceptions of "sticky" foods is poorly related to objective measures of retentive foods.[52]

We also discussed in Chapter 19 how prospective studies in the 1980s could not

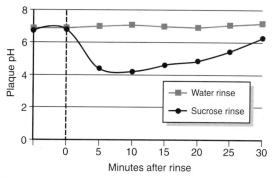

Figure 27–3. Data from Stephan's experiments to show the "Stephan Curve." The group with the sucrose rinse showed a sharp and immediate drop in plaque pH; the control group with a water rinse showed no change. (From Stephan RM. Changes in hydrogen-ion concentration on tooth surfaces and in carious lesions. J Am Dent Assoc 1940;27:718-23.)

demonstrate a relationship between caries experience and frequency of eating among children, and that the conclusion in the Vipeholm study on the importance of frequency may have been based on a distorted eating pattern that is rarely seen in the general population. Health educators today are advised to concentrate on reducing total sugars intake for caries-susceptible people rather than fuss with "sticky" foods or details of snacking frequency.

Research studies in humans have identified many people who get little caries even though they consume a lot of sugars[21, 79]; extensive dietary counseling for such individuals is clearly time not well spent. The philosophy behind extensive effort to get major reductions in their consumption of sugars to prevent a small amount of disease has to be seriously questioned. Patients who are more susceptible to caries, however, can benefit considerably. Extensive dietary counseling in the dental office therefore should concentrate on patients who show an obvious susceptibility to caries.

On a community basis, dietary advice in dental health education should be linked with general efforts to educate the public on wise food choices for healthy living. Dietary guidelines now emphasize choosing unrefined carbohydrates from a variety of foods, moderate amounts of protein, and low fat. High-sugar foods are often high-fat foods, so dentally-oriented advice is completely in harmony with broad advice to enhance the public health. Drastic reductions in sugar consumption, even if these could be engineered on a mass scale in the United States, would probably have only minor effects on caries levels and lead to replacement of that lost energy by fat consumption.[23] This would clearly not be a move to enhance the public health.

PLAQUE CONTROL

Dietary restriction has historically been mixed with plaque removal as a means of caries prevention. From the time of Miller in the 1880s, caries was seen as theoretically preventable by regular and careful oral hygiene procedures to remove plaque. Countless hours of dental health education have been devoted to that end, based on the adage that "a clean tooth never decays." The approach to caries control by focusing on oral hygiene is based on the "nonspecific plaque hypothesis," which incorrectly implied that all bacteria in plaque are of equal cariogenicity and should therefore be removed.[63] It also stems from the pioneering work of Stephan in the 1940s (Fig. 27–2), which quickly became the basis of dental health education aimed at brushing immediately after eating to neutralize the impact of "acid attacks."

Even with all the knowledge gained from modern research, however, the relation between levels of oral hygiene and caries development is confusing. Plaque harbors cariogenic bacteria and other bacteria associated with periodontal conditions, but it also is the main intraoral repository of fluoride and other remineralizing minerals. Presumably plaque evolved in the human race for some beneficial purpose, although one would doubt it from the message given out by most dental health education materials.

Individual oral hygiene status is traditionally seen as poorly related to caries experience,[4, 14] despite intuitive feelings to the contrary. Despite poor research evidence, interest in the oral hygiene-caries link was revived by a series of 1970s reports concluding that caries incidence in children could be virtually eliminated by meticulous plaque removal carried out by trained dental auxiliaries at frequent intervals.[7-9, 61] These reports are known collectively as the Karlstad studies after the Swedish town in which they were conducted. Intervals between professional cleanings were 2 weeks in younger children; in older children spectacular results were maintained when the time between cleanings was extended to 8 weeks after an initial 2 years at 2-week inter-

vals.[62] The procedures involved in the professional cleaning of children's teeth are detailed in Chapter 28.

Benefits from this protocol probably came from a combination of (a) plaque control, (b) intensive use of topical fluoride paste, and (c) dental health education and oral hygiene practices at home, although the researchers concluded that most benefit came from the oral hygiene procedures.[8] Caries reductions of 98% were reported over 2 years,[7] although attempts to replicate the Karlstad regimen were not able to achieve the same reported level of success.[1, 6, 10, 41] More recently, studies on the Danish island of Bornholm have reported great success with rigorous control of plaque deposits on erupting first molars.[25] Like the Karlstad regimen, the Bornholm approach is resource-intensive enough to make it of questionable utility for mass application outside Scandinavia.

Studies carried out by Scandinavian researchers with small groups of children continue to relate good oral hygiene to low caries experience.[3, 19, 54, 67] On the other hand, despite extensive improvements in the oral health of Quebec children between 1977 and 1990, no improvement in oral hygiene could be found,[75] and a European report has defended plaque deposits as necessary to remineralization.[28] Even if a poor level of oral hygiene promotes caries, extensive professional care to clean up a dirty mouth may not be time well spent if there are underlying reasons for the inattention to oral hygiene. Mass education for good oral hygiene, although obviously in the public interest, has often failed. School-based instructional programs to promote oral hygiene in American children have not been successful,[43] and promotion of the self-use of dental floss in children has repeatedly failed.[2, 36, 43]

Oral hygiene is so clearly a desirable goal for social and periodontal reasons (Chapter 28) that education or treatment to achieve it cannot be rejected out of hand. However, it is a question of cost-effectiveness, of how a professional's time might best be used. The intensity of the Karlstad protocol, in education and home care as well as in the professional treatments themselves, demands a high investment in equipment and personnel and absorbs 3 hours of chair time per child each year.[6] The cost of the Karlstad approach therefore is unrealistic for most public services; caries prevention is far better focused into appropriate uses of fluoride. The main purpose of regular toothbrushing, in terms of caries prevention, is to introduce fluoride into the mouth regularly via the toothpaste. The plaque-removal effect appears secondary in caries prevention, although it can have primary benefits in controlling gingivitis (Chapter 28). Regular toothbrushing with a fluoride toothpaste should be encouraged as a regular daily routine for all people, whether or not they are susceptible to caries.

REFERENCES

1. Agerbaek N, Poulsen S, Melsen B, Glavind L. Effect of professional toothcleaning every third week on gingivitis and dental caries in children. Community Dent Oral Epidemiol 1978;6:40-1.
2. Ainamo J, Parviainen K. Occurrence of plaque, gingivitis and caries as related to self-reported frequency of toothbrushing in fluoride areas in Finland. Community Dent Oral Epidemiol 1979;7:142-6.
3. Aleksejuniene J, Arneberg P, Eriksen HM. Caries prevalence and oral hygiene in Lithuanian children and adolescents. Acta Odont Scand 1996;54:75-80.
4. Andlaw RJ. Oral hygiene and dental caries: A review. Int Dent J 1978;28:1-6.
5. Antar MA, Ohlson MA, Hodges RE. Changes in retail market food supplies in the United States in the last seventy years in relation to the incidence of coronary heart disease, with special reference to dietary carbohydrates and essential fatty acids. Am J Clin Nutr 1964;14:169-78.
6. Ashley FP, Sainsbury RH. The effect of a school-based plaque control programme on caries and gingivitis. Br Dent J 1981;150:41-5.
7. Axelsson P, Lindhe J. The effect of a preventive programme on dental plaque, gingivitis and caries in school children. Results after one and two years. J Clin Periodontol 1974;1:126-38.
8. Axelsson P, Lindhe J. Effect of fluoride on gingivitis and dental caries in a preventive program based on plaque control. Community Dent Oral Epidemiol 1975;3:156-60.
9. Axelsson P, Lindhe J, Waseby J. The effect of various plaque control measures on gingivitis and caries in schoolchildren. Community Dent Oral Epidemiol 1976;4:232-9.
10. Badersten A, Egelberg J, Koch G. Effect of monthly prophylaxis on caries and gingivitis in schoolchildren. Community Dent Oral Epidemiol 1975; 3:1-4.
11. Barmes D, Barnaud J, Khambonanda S, Infirri JS. Field trials of preventive regimens in Thailand and French Polynesia. Int Dent J 1985;35:66-72.
12. Beckers HJ. Influence of xylitol on growth, establishment, and cariogenicity of Streptococcus mutans in dental plaque of rats. Caries Res 1988;22:166-73.
13. Becks H. The physical consistency of food and refined carbohydrate restrictions: Their effect on caries. J Dent Res 1948;27:405-12.
14. Bellini HT, Arneberg P, von der Fehr FR. Oral hygiene and caries: A review. Acta Odont Scand 1981;39:257-65.
15. Bibby BG. The cariogenicity of snack foods and confections. J Am Dent Assoc 1975;90:121-32.
16. Bibby BG. Diet, nutrition, and oral health: A rational approach for the dental practice. J Am Dent Assoc 1984;109:20-32.
17. Birkhed D, Edwardsson S, Kalfas S, Svensater G. Cariogenicity of sorbitol. Swed Dent J 1984;8:147-54.
18. Birkhed D, Svensater G, Edwardsson S. Cariological studies of individuals with long-term sorbitol consumption. Caries Res 1990;24:220-3.
19. Bjertness E. The importance of oral hygiene on variation in dental caries in adults. Acta Odont Scand 1991;49:97-102.
20. Bowen WH. Food components and caries. Adv Dent Res 1994;8:215-20.
21. Burt BA, Eklund SA, Morgan KJ, et al. The effects of sugars intake and frequency of ingestion on dental caries increment in a three-year longitudinal study. J Dent Res 1988;67:1422-9.
22. Burt BA, Ismail AI. Diet, nutrition, and food cariogenicity. J Dent Res 1986;65(Special Issue):1475-84.
23. Burt BA, Szpunar SM. The Michigan Study: The relationship between sugars intake and dental caries over three years. Int Dent J 1994;44:230-40.
24. Cantor SM. Patterns of use. In: National Academy of Sciences. Sweeteners: Issues and uncertainties. Academy forum, fourth of a series. Washington DC: National Academy of Sciences, 1975:19-29.
25. Carvalho JC, Thylstrup A, Ekstrand KR. Results after 3 years of non-operative caries treatment of erupting permanent first molars. Community Dent Oral Epidemiol 1992;20:187-92.
26. DePaola DP. Executive summary. J Dent Res 1986;65(Special Issue):1540-3.
27. Edgar WM, Geddes DA. Chewing gum and dental health—a review. Br Dent J 1990;168:173-7.
28. Etty EJ, Henneberke M, Gruythuysen RJ, Woltgens JH. Influence of oral hygiene on early enamel caries. Caries Res 1994;28:132-6.
29. Firestone AR, Navia JM. In vivo measurements of sulcal plaque pH after topical applications of sorbitol and sucrose in rats fed sorbitol or sucrose. J Dent Res 1986;65:1020-3.
30. Firestone AR, Schmid R, Muhlemann HR. Effect on the length and number of intervals between meals on caries in rats. Caries Res 1984;18:128-33.
31. Frostell G, Birkhed D, Edwardsson S, et al. Effect of partial substitution of invert sugar for sucrose in combination with Duraphat treatment on caries development in preschool children: The Malmö study. Caries Res 1991;25:304-10.
32. Frostell G, Keyes PH, Larson RH. Effect of various sugars and sugar substitutes on dental caries in hamsters and rats. J Nutr 1967;93:65-76.
33. Geddes DA, Edgar WM, Jenkins GN, Rugg-Gunn AJ. Apples, salted peanuts and plaque pH. Br Dent J 1977;142:317-9.
34. Glass RL. A two-year clinical trial of sorbitol chewing gum. Caries Res 1983; 17:365-8.
35. Glinsmann WH, Irausquin H, Park YK. Evaluation of health aspects of sugars contained in carbohydrate sweeteners. J Nutr 1986;116:S1-216.
36. Granath LE, Martinsson T, Matsson L, et al. Intraindividual effect of daily supervised flossing on caries in schoolchildren. Community Dent Oral Epidemiol 1979;7:147-50.
37. Grenby TH, Phillips A, Mistry M. Studies of the dental properties of lactitol compared with five other bulk sweeteners in vitro. Caries Res 1989;23:315-9.
38. Grobler SR. The effect of a high consumption of citrus fruit and a mixture of other fruits on dental caries in man. Clin Preven Dent 1991;13:13-7.

39. Gustaffson BE, Quensel CE, Lanke LS, et al. The Vipehölm dental caries study. The effect of different levels of carbohydrate intake on caries activity in 436 individuals observed for five years. Acta Odont Scand 1954;11:232-364.

40. Hadjimarkos DM. Selenium: A caries-enhancing trace element. Caries Res 1969;3:14-22.

41. Hamp SE, Johansson LA, Karlsson R. Clinical effects of preventive regimens for young people in their early and middle teens in relation to previous experience with dental prevention. Acta Odont Scand 1984;42:99-108.

42. Health claims: Dietary sugar alcohols and dental caries. Fed Register 1996;61(165):43446-7.

43. Horowitz AM, Suomi JD, Peterson JK, et al. Effects of supervised daily dental plaque removal by children after 3 years. Community Dent Oral Epidemiol 1980;8:171-6.

44. Imfeld T, Mühlemann HR. Evaluation of sugar substitutes in preventive cariology. J Preven Dent 1977;4:8-14.

45. Integration of methods—working group consensus report. J Dent Res 1986;65(Special Issue):1537-9.

46. Ismail AI, Burt BA, Eklund SA. The cariogenicity of soft drinks in the United States. J Am Dent Assoc 1984;109:241-5.

47. Isokangas P, Tiekso J, Alanen P, Makinen KK. Long-term effect of xylitol chewing gum on dental caries. Community Dent Oral Epidemiol 1989;17:200-3.

48. Jay P. The reduction of oral Lactobacillus acidophilus counts by the periodic restriction of carbohydrate. Am J Orthodont Oral Surg 1947;33:162-84.

49. Jenkins GN. Current concepts concerning the development of dental caries. Int Dent J 1972;22:350-62.

50. Kandelman D, Bar A, Hefti A. Collaborative WHO xylitol field study in French Polynesia. I. Baseline prevalence and 32-month caries increment. Caries Res 1988;22:55-62.

51. Kandelman D, Gagnon G. A 24-month clinical study of the incidence and progression of dental caries in relation to consumption of chewing gum containing xylitol in school preventive programs. J Dent Res 1990;69:1771-5.

52. Kashket S, Van Houte J, Lopez LR, Stocks S. Lack of correlation between food retention on the human dentition and consumer perception of food stickiness. J Dent Res 1991;70:1314-9.

53. Kashket S, Yaskell T, Lopez LR. Prevention of sucrose-induced demineralization of tooth enamel by chewing sorbitol gum. J Dent Res 1989;68:460-2.

54. Kleemola-Kujala E, Rasanen L. Relationship of oral hygiene and sugar consumption to risk of caries in children. Community Dent Oral Epidemiol 1982; 10:224-33.

55. Koulourides T, Bodden S, Keller S, et al. Cariogenicity of nine sugars tested with an intraoral device in man. Caries Res 1976;10:427-41.

56. Krasse B. Oral effect of other carbohydrates. Int Dent J 1982;32:24-32.

57. Krobicka A, Bowen WH, Pearson S, Young DA. The effects of cheese snacks on caries in desalivated rats. J Dent Res 1987;66:1116-9.

58. Larmas M, Makinen KK, Scheinin A. Turkü sugar studies. VIII. Principal microbiological findings. Acta Odont Scand 1976;34:285-328.

59. Leach SA, Lee GT, Edgar WM. Remineralization of artificial caries-like lesions in human enamel in situ by chewing sorbitol gum. J Dent Res 1989;68:1064-8.

60. Lilienthal B. Phosphates and dental caries. Monogr Oral Sci 1977;6:1-107.

61. Lindhe J, Axelsson P. The effect of proper oral hygiene and topical fluoride application on caries and gingivitis in Swedish schoolchildren. Community Dent Oral Epidemiol 1973;1:9-16.

62. Lindhe J, Axelsson P, Tollskog G. The effect of proper oral hygiene on gingivitis and dental caries in schoolchildren. Community Dent Oral Epidemiol 1975; 3:150-5.

63. Loesche WJ. Chemotherapy of dental plaque infections. Oral Sci Rev 1976;9:63-107.

64. Loesche WJ, Grossman NS, Earnest R, Corpron R. The effect of chewing xylitol gum on the plaque and saliva levels of Streptococcus mutans. J Am Dent Assoc 1984;108:587-92.

65. Mäkinen KK, Söderling E, Isokangas P, et al. Oral biochemical status and depression of Streptococcus mutans in children during 24- to 36-month use of xylitol chewing gum. Caries Res 1989;23:261-7.

66. Mäkinen KK, Mäkinen P-L, Pape H Jr, et al. Stabilisation of rampant caries: Polyol gums and arrest of dentine caries in two long-term cohort studies in young subjects. Int Dent J 1995;45:93-107.

67. Mathiesen AT, Ogaard B, Rölla G. Oral hygiene as a variable in dental caries experience in 14-year-olds exposed to fluoride. Caries Res 1996;30:29-33.

68. Mundorff SA, Featherstone JDB, Bibby BG, et al. Cariogenic potential of foods. I. Caries in the rat model. Caries Res 1990;24:344-55.

69. Newbrun E. Sucrose, the arch criminal of dental caries. Odont Revy 1967;18:373-86.

70. Newbrun E. The role of food manufacturers in the dietary control of caries. J Prevent Dent 1974;4:33-44.

71. Newbrun E. Sucrose in the dynamics of the carious process. Int Dent J 1982;32:13-23.

72. Newbrun E. Cariology. 3rd ed. Chicago: Quintessence, 1989:148-50.

73. Newbrun E. The potential role of alternative sweeteners in caries prevention. Isr J Dent Sci 1990;2:200-13.

74. Newbrun E, Hoover C, Mettraux C, Graf H. Comparison of dietary habits and dental health of subjects with hereditary fructose intolerance and control subjects. J Am Dent Assoc 1980;101:619-26.

75. Payette M, Brodeur JM. Comparison of dental caries and oral hygiene indices for 13- to 14-year-old Quebec children between 1977 and 1989-1990. J Can Dent Assoc 1992;58:921-2, 926-9, 932-3.

76. Rekola M. Changes in buccal white spots during 2-year consumption of dietary sucrose or xylitol. Acta Odont Scand 1986;44:285-90.

77. Rekola M. Correlation between caries incidence and frequency of chewing gum sweetened with sucrose or xylitol. Proc Finn Dent Soc 1989;85:21-4.

78. Rugg-Gunn AJ, Edgar WM, Geddes DA, Jenkins GN. The effect of different meal patterns upon plaque pH in human subjects. Br Dent J 1975;139:351-6.

79. Rugg-Gunn AJ, Hackett AF, Appleton DR, et al. Relationship between dietary habits and caries increment assessed over two years in 405 English school children. Arch Oral Biol 1984;29:983-92.

80. Schamschula RG, Adkins BL, Barmes DE, et al. WHO study of dental caries etiology in Papua New Guinea. WHO Offset Publ No. 40. Geneva:WHO, 1978.

81. Scheinin A. Field studies on sugar substitutes. Int Dent J 1985;35:195-200.

82. Scheinin A, Banoczy J, Szoke J, et al. Collaborative WHO xylitol field studies in Hungary. I. Three-year caries activity in institutionalized children. Acta Odont Scand 1985;43:327-47.

83. Scheinin A, Mäkinen KK. Turkü sugar studies: An overview. Acta Odont Scand 1976;34:405-8.

84. Scheinin A, Mäkinen KK, Tammisalo E, Rekola M. Turkü sugar studies. XVIII. Incidence of dental caries in relation to 1-year consumption of xylitol chewing gum. Acta Odont Scand 1975;33:269-78.

85. Scheinen A, Mäkinen KK, Ylitalo K. Turkü sugar studies. V. Final report on the effect of sucrose, fructose, and xylitol diets on the caries incidence in man. Acta Odont Scand 1976;34:179-216.

86. Smits MT, Arends J. Influence of extraoral xylitol and sucrose dippings on enamel demineralization in vivo. Caries Res 1988;22:160-5.

87. Stephan RM. Changes in hydrogen-ion concentration on tooth surfaces and in carious lesions. J Am Dent Assoc 1940;27:718-23.

88. Stephan RM. Effect of different types of human foods on dental health in experimental animals. J Dent Res 1966;45:1551-61.

89. US Department of Agriculture, Economic Research Service. Sugar and sweetener: Situation and outlook report. SSS-220, June 1997.

90. Von der Fehr FR, Loe H, Theilade E. Experimental caries in man. Caries Res 1970;4:131-48.

28

Prevention of Periodontal Diseases

Rationale for Plaque Control ◆ The Nature of Dental Plaque ◆ Approaches to Plaque Control ◆ Mechanical Plaque Removal by the Individual and the Dental Professional ◆ The Karlstad Studies ◆ Prophylactic Treatment of Adults ◆ Professional plus Personal Care ◆ Chemotherapeutic Plaque Control: Chlorhexidine and Other Compounds ◆ Anticalculus (``Tartar-Control'') Toothpastes ◆ Community Control of Periodontal Diseases

Although our understanding of periodontal conditions is growing rapidly (Chapter 20), prevention and control of periodontal conditions still have to be based on the periodic removal of plaque and calculus, either by each individual or by a dental professional. There is no parallel, in periodontal prevention, to a public health measure such as water fluoridation.

The reassessment of the nature of periodontal diseases that has resulted from recent research (Chapter 20) has affected our thinking on the prevention of these conditions. The realization that only 7% to 15% of a population suffers from serious periodontitis, for example, has led some to downplay the importance of prevention; this is the view that "periodontal disease doesn't matter any more." This view is clearly faulty, because this level of prevalence means that 25 million Americans and 2 to 3 million Canadians suffer from serious periodontitis. From the data given in Chapter 20, 8 times that number have moderate adult periodontitis, much of which requires treatment and could probably be prevented. Prevention of periodontitis still is clearly a worthwhile public health endeavor; the problems and the frustrations come with the limitations in our current approach to doing it. Even though our understanding of periodontitis has expanded greatly over recent years, the only practical approach to prevention of periodontitis (rather than its control through clinical treatment), is to prevent and control gingivitis.[100]

RATIONALE FOR PLAQUE CONTROL

The rationale for controlling periodontal conditions by regular plaque removal is based on the premise that supragingival plaque, if undisturbed, will become subgingival plaque,[100] and subgingival plaque has the potential to be colonized by periodontally pathogenic bacteria. Although relatively few gingivitis sites progress to periodontitis (Chapter 20), we still do not have the technology to identify those sites that will do so. Accordingly, the principles for prevention have not changed for years: the regular and consistent control of plaque buildup, supragingival and subgingival, soft and mineralized (calculus), on the teeth and in the gingival crevices. This approach is bacteriologically nonspecific, meaning that it is not aimed at specific pathogens, but rather it seeks to control the buildup of all plaque. It also depends strongly on individual motivation for success. Plaque control is therefore unlikely ever to be completely effective in preventing periodontal diseases in a population, although individual success is common. Until research produces methods of (a) controlling periodontal infection, (b) enhancing host response, and (c) identifying susceptible individuals, however, mass plaque control by personal, professional, or chemical means is the best we can do.

This chapter deals with the available methods for controlling the deposition of dental plaque, an approach that can effectively prevent gingivitis. As was detailed in Chapter 20, however, plaque's role in periodontitis is not so straightforward. Plaque deposits may be a necessary condition for periodontitis, although clearly they are not sufficient. In other words, susceptible people may have to be stringent with oral hygiene, but millions of people with poor oral hygiene do not have serious periodontitis. There is an analogy here with consumption of sugars in caries etiology. Caries-susceptible persons have to restrict their intake of sugars, but there are many people who consume a lot of sugars but have little or no caries as a consequence.

THE NATURE OF DENTAL PLAQUE

Although dental plaque is commonly depicted as the root cause of both caries and periodontitis, it is well to remember that it must have evolved in humans for some purpose. Commercial advertising would have us believe that oral health depends on the complete removal of all plaque at all times, but clearly that is not only not possible but also not desirable. Dental plaque forms naturally on the teeth and benefits the host by helping to prevent intraoral colonization by exogenous species.[95] Plaque's role in promoting remineralization of demineralized lesions was described in Chapter 19.

Dental plaque is a natural biofilm that forms on the tooth surface and consists of a diverse microbial community embedded in a polymer matrix of bacterial and salivary origin.[96] After a tooth surface is cleaned, the pellicle, a conditioning film of proteins and glycoproteins, is adsorbed rapidly onto the tooth surface. The interactions between this biofilm and early bacterial colonizers are the first steps in plaque formation. Secondary bacterial colonizers adhere to these early colonizers through specific molecular interactions, a process that contributes toward the pattern of bacterial succession. The biofilm character

of plaque allows for the survival of a diverse bacterial flora.[94] Although plaque formation begins with microbial adhesion, microbial multiplication is thought to be the dominant factor in the buildup of dental plaque, and the nature of this microbial proliferation is highly dependent on the local environment. Because environmental conditions vary from place to place within the oral cavity, each site with plaque represents its own distinct ecosystem, and the dominant microbial composition at the site depends on the outcome of numerous host-microbe and microbe-microbe interactions.[114]

The clinical picture of all this activity has been well described. After plaque has been completely removed, it reforms slowly on the tooth surface for about 3 days and, if left undisturbed, it increases rapidly to reach a maximum bulk after 7 days.[124] The various microbial interactions actually keep the bacterial composition of plaque relatively stable, but when this homeostasis breaks down the shifts in microbial balance can set up conditions for caries or gingivitis to begin. Plaque accumulation around the gingival margin leads to an inflammatory host response and an increased flow of gingival crevicular fluid.[95] Few bacteria can be isolated from around healthy gingival tissue, although with gingivitis there is a considerable increase in the numbers and complexity of bacteria as the lesion develops.[100] Subgingival plaque microflora shift from being predominantly gram-positive to increased levels of anerobic gram-negative organisms; the character of subgingival plaque is thus quite different from that found in supragingival plaque.[95] Specifically, *Porphyromonas gingivalis* and *Bacteroides forsythus* in subgingival plaque have been associated with both loss of periodontal attachment and bone loss.[49, 50] It is accepted that supragingival plaque influences the formation of new subgingival plaque after existing subgingival plaque has been disrupted or removed, although the control of new supragingival plaque has no effect on the existing subgingival flora in periodontitis patients.[23] There has been little study of the way in which controlling supragingival plaque affects the progression of periodontitis,[33] although one study with young Brazilians found that it did not affect the progression of disease at all.[4] Subgingival plaque is also characterized by oral spirochetes, whose role in periodontitis is still not clear although their presence in the subgingival plaque is seen as a marker for disease.[126]

Calculus was formerly seen only as an "irritating factor" in the etiology of periodontitis,[66] and with the development of research interest in plaque during the 1960s and 1970s it did not receive much attention. Today, however, calculus is recognized as a calcified matrix that can harbor periodontopathic bacteria, and subgingival calculus is closely associated with gingivitis and periodontitis.[31] The initial formation and the continued presence of subgingival calculus, therefore, are something to be prevented. The only known method is to control the initial formation of supragingival plaque and calculus.

APPROACHES TO PLAQUE CONTROL

Because plaque occurs naturally in all mouths, it cannot be prevented entirely. Because it has some indentifiable health functions, and because disease comes more from an upset in the homeostatic balance than from infection with exogenous organisms, disease prevention should be geared more toward plaque control than plaque eradication. This concept is referred to as the *ecological plaque hypothesis*.[95] The goal in preventing periodontitis is to prevent fresh plaque becoming "established plaque," which permits the establishment of specific bacteria that are viewed as periodontopathic,[111, 131] and to prevent supragingival plaque from becoming established subgingivally.

Several approaches to plaque control can be quickly ruled out as having no scientific basis: rinsing with water, for example, removes loose food debris but not plaque.[72, 74] Chewing fibrous foods can also help remove loose food debris, but it does not remove plaque.[76, 89] There is no evidence to alter the long-held view[78, 118] that preventive benefits cannot be achieved by changes in diet or nutrition, although given the importance of the host response in peridontitis and the fact that nutrition is a vital part of the immune reaction, this issue should continue to be researched. Natural self-cleansing mechanisms do not remove plaque well enough to prevent disease.[84] Nor does the customary use of the "chewing stick," used in much of Africa and Asia for oral hygiene, although with supervision it can be efficient in populations accustomed to its use.[99]

Primary prevention of gingivitis requires consistent, thorough control of plaque accumulation on a lifetime basis. The rationale is to prevent plaque reaching the stage of maturity at which gingivitis begins. Some people are capable of maintaining adequate oral hygiene status largely by their own efforts, but many are not. The dental professional will consistently see some level of gingivitis in these patients and may become frustrated in the effort to eliminate gingivitis entirely. With these patients, the dental professional's goal should be to maintain the gingivitis at as low a level as possible. As long as the lowest possible level of gingivitis can be maintained over time, subsequent loss of periodontal support is likely to be minimized. This is true for the majority of patients who are at low risk of severe periodontitis. It is much less the case for those patients with early-onset periodontitis who fit the compromised host model described in Chapter 20. Prevention of disease in these patients is extremely difficult because we do not yet have the means of influencing the deficient host response to a periodontal challenge.

So long as plaque accumulation remains supragingival, it can be controlled by mechanical or chemotherapeutic means.[109] Once plaque becomes established subgingivally, however, the individual patient cannot remove it by self-care and professional intervention is necessary. Because the mechanism by which supragingival plaque becomes established subgingivally is not known,[100] the goal of individual prevention of periodontal conditions through plaque control is to not permit supragingival plaque to accumulate.

There are essentially 3 approaches to preventing the buildup of dental plaque, each of which we will assess in turn:

- Mechanical plaque removal by the individual
- Mechanical plaque removal by the dental professional
- Chemotherapeutic methods of plaque control.

MECHANICAL PLAQUE REMOVAL BY THE INDIVIDUAL

Self-care is a fundamental part of periodontal health. Unless the individual is able to maintain at least a reasonable level of oral cleanliness by regular and consistent home care, the benefits of treatment by dental professionals will be limited. Individual effort means mechanical plaque removal with the toothbrush and aids such as dental floss, the interproximal brush, and wood points.

Given that individual oral hygiene practices are so fundamental to the promotion of oral health, it is surprising how little is really known about such basic things as the most efficient type of toothbrush and how often to brush. Research studies in these areas have often been run only for short periods and with atypical populations, such as dental or dental hygiene students. Long-term effects and the projection of results to the general population are thus difficult to assess.

Frequency of Toothbrushing

The best available information indicates that a thorough oral cleansing should be carried out at 24- to 48-hour intervals.[63, 68] Considering the time needed for plaque to mature bacteriologically, the old adage of brushing after every meal, which was usually impractical anyway, is unnecessary to prevent gingivitis. However, because toothbrushing with a fluoride toothpaste is also a major source of fluoride exposure for caries prevention, it is best carried out at least twice per day. Brushing in the morning and evening fits with most peoples' daily routines, and should be the basis for education of the public and dental patients. Patients who have received treatment for periodontitis of course are likely to be at high risk for further disease, and more stringent home care regimens may be required for them.[128]

Type of Toothbrush

Little research has been carried out on the best type of toothbrush; what evidence there is suggests that it really does not matter much.[56, 118] Children clearly should use a smaller brush, and the dentist or hygienist may want to recommend different sizes and degrees of softness depending on each patient's manual dexterity, enthusiasm, and oral health. Manufacturers are constantly coming out with new designs, so anyone can find a comfortable and efficient toothbrush. These recommendations, however, are based on common sense rather than on firm evidence.

Electric toothbrushes with a rotary action were found to be more effective plaque removers in closely supervised clinical trials,[125] although it is uncertain how these findings are reflected in everyday effectiveness. Both manual and power-driven toothbrushes are effective if used properly; differences between individuals' brushing efficiency are likely to be much greater than inherent differences between the brushes. New versions of power-driven brushes are constantly being marketed, some with much advertising, and few have been subjected to rigorous testing. Power brushes may be particularly useful for handicapped persons or others with low manual dexterity.

Toothbrushing Methods

A variety of toothbrushing methods, some requiring a lot of manual gymnastics, have been described in the dental literature. Proponents of one method or another have traditionally been vehement in the defense of their method's efficacy, a good example of the rule that the level of passion that people have about an issue is inversely proportional to its basis in science. Research indicates that there is little inherent difference between the various methods in their ability to remove dental plaque.[43, 52, 108, 110, 112, 116] From these limited studies, the scrub method emerges as the simplest method available and one that is no less effective than any other. It requires minimal manual dexterity and patient concentration. Because dental professionals must aim for the best possible results within practical limits in educating their patients, the scrub method seems best for most persons. For some individuals receiving treatment for advanced disease, a special method may be needed, assuming they are able to manage it.

Interdental Cleaning

The rationale for supplementing toothbrushing with use of dental floss, interdental brushes, or wood points to clean below the contact areas is that even assiduous use of the toothbrush usually cannot penetrate these areas efficiently. There is some evidence that interdental cleaning, by floss or interdental brushes, does reduce interdental gingivitis and plaque more than would be achieved by toothbrushing alone.[27, 82]

A lot of dental health education materials extol the efficacy of dental floss: "brush and floss" long ago replaced the exhortation to just "brush." There is still little evidence, however, to show that flossing, as practiced by the individual with normal interdental spaces, adds much to the efficiency of brushing,[55, 108, 116] nor are the limited research studies able to find a difference between waxed and unwaxed floss in cleaning efficiency.[23, 39, 62, 82] Where papillae have diminished to leave open interdental spaces, interdental brushes have been demonstrated as superior to floss.[24] Many people prefer wood points to floss because floss can break and get stuck in awkward contact areas, and wood points probably are effective interdental cleaners.[93]

Individual Motivation

The individual practice of regular, thorough, and consistent oral hygiene procedures depends largely on the interest of the individual in his oral health. Dentally conscious people have this interest already, but many others do not. Oral hygiene practices must fit into the lifestyle of each individual, and lifestyles are rarely changed by exhortation alone.[54] To illustrate the lifestyle issue, a British study found that schoolchildren who reported more frequent toothbrushing also reported more frequent bathing, use of deodorant, and handwashing after visiting the toilet.[91] This information should come as no surprise.

Knowledge is usually thought to precede action, but a study of periodontal patients in North Carolina found that there was a poor correlation between knowledge of the disease process and periodontal health.[17] Carefully thought-out and well-organized "motivational programs" in schoolchildren have produced poor results in the United States.[53, 57] Supervised daily toothbrushing with schoolchildren in Sweden did produce a reduction in gingivitis for the duration of the program, but the improvement disappeared when the supervision ended.[73] Although compliance with periodontitis treatment instructions is related to health beliefs,[67] the effects of individual chairside instruction have been demonstrated to be weak.[123, 130] Doubts are thus raised about what "motivational programs" really do; they may succeed only in reinforcing existing favorable attitudes and not in altering negative ones.[97] A Danish longitudinal study found that oral hygiene behavior in youth was found to predict periodontal health in adulthood,[77] a finding confirming that attitudes and oral health behavior are principally determined by factors outside the dental office. (These issues in health promotion are discussed more fully in Chapter 5.)

For dental professionals who try to induce individual patients to improve their daily oral hygiene performance, success may best come from a personal and common sense approach by the dentist or hygienist. Some patients will respond better than others. Objective monitoring by measuring gingival bleeding, pocket depth, periodontal attachment levels, calculus deposits, and plaque is important because subjective impressions of progress can be misleading. Reinforcement of simple messages and constant encouragement of the individual's efforts seem to be important factors. Oral health professionals must work within the limitations of the individual patient, and within their own limitations too.

Oral hygiene in the United States is thought by most experts to be constantly improving, a trend thought to result from heightened awareness, heavy advertising, and constantly improving oral hygiene products. Public health education programs intended to produce mass improvement in oral hygiene have had little measurable impact on this trend.[44, 53, 83] Time given to this form of education in public health programs, especially to populations bombarded by television commercials about oral hygiene, could probably be much better spent on primary prevention or on providing dental care to needy people. This may not be the case, however, in a developing country, where basic knowledge of oral hygiene may be lacking. "Toothbrush drills" are quite properly a common part of dental public health education in such countries, whereas they may be redundant in most developed nations.

MECHANICAL PLAQUE REMOVAL BY THE DENTAL PROFESSIONAL

Professional care is necessary to remove subgingival plaque and calculus; the patient cannot remove plaque from deep pockets. Frequent professional care seems to control the progress of periodontitis in many patients. For successful outcomes in susceptible people, a concomitant high level of personal oral hygiene needs to be achieved by the patient. The benefits of professional plaque removal have been shown in studies of children and adults who were in reasonable periodontal health to begin with, as well as in studies of adults receiving treatment for advanced disease.

The Karlstad Studies

The discussion on the Karlstad studies in Chapter 27 was related principally to caries; this section relates to periodontal disease. Among children, spectacular success at preventing gingivitis was reported by the Axelsson-Lindhe group in their studies at Karlstad, Sweden.[11, 12, 14, 71] Conducted with children aged 7 to 14 years, this research group set out to show that a regimen of intensive prophylactic procedures that went considerably beyond the routine prophylaxis would be effective in preventing both caries and gingivitis. The protocol for the Karlstad regimen was as follows:

- Detailed initial explanations of oral disease etiology and purpose of treatment by the dentist or auxiliary carrying out the treatment. Involvement of the family was considered integral to the program's success.
- Identification of plaque in the patient's mouth by disclosing tablet, then demonstration of correct toothbrushing technique for removing the stain. The patient then used dental floss under supervision. These oral hygiene instructions were repeated throughout the course of treatment as necessary.
- Rubber cup cleaning of accessible surfaces and engine-mounted pointed bristle was used for cleaning fissures in occlusal surfaces. A fluoride-containing prophylactic paste was used for these procedures.
- Interdental cleaning, again by the dentist or auxiliary providing the treatment, with dental floss and reciprocating interproximal tips. Again, the fluoridated prophylactic paste was forced interdentally and kept in close contact with the proximal surfaces by the floss and the tips.

These procedures were applied by professionals every 2 weeks over a 2-year period. In the third year, the time between these "professional cleanings," as the Karlstad researchers call them, was extended to 4 weeks for the 7–11-year-olds and to 8 weeks for the 13–14-year-olds. The continuing good results with this reduced frequency of cleaning was attributed to the background effects of the first 2 years.[71] These researchers were firm in their contention that professional cleanings 5 to 8 times per year are still not enough by themselves to control gingivitis.

Results from the Karlstad group during the 1970s were impressive. Other European groups who carried out similar studies also achieved good results, although none of them quite reached the Karlstad heights.[2, 8, 18, 64] A British study followed up its participants a year after the study ended, and found that the 3-year reduction in plaque mass of 54% had since relapsed to 26%.[9]

No studies of the Karlstad regimen have been carried out in the United States or Canada because the expense of this personnel-intensive regimen is beyond the capacity of public health agencies. In addition, the implied paternalism of the regimen probably goes against the North American cultural grain of individualism. One study in the United States, however, did find that prophylaxes twice per year in children aged 10 to 11 produced neither beneficial reductions in gingivitis nor improvements in oral hygiene levels.[107] Another study of a Karlstad-type regimen in young Brazilians found that the intensive preventive care did not slow down the progression of periodontitis when compared with either routine oral hygiene instruction or to no instruction.[4] The authors speculated that they may have been dealing with a "compromised host" type of periodontitis (Chapter 20). This condition would not be expected to respond much to even intensive oral hygiene if the cause is in a deficient host response, whereas the "local factor" type of periodontitis would respond.

Prophylactic Treatment of Adults

Prophylactic treatment of adults relates to routine prophylactic care of nondiseased adults, rather than the different issue of treatment for periodontitis patients. Patients, by definition, are susceptible to periodontitis, so all clinical studies showing the value of maintenance prophylactic care in treated patients are carried out with susceptible people.[104, 105]

Studies that examined the value of routine prophylaxis in adult populations in the community (i.e., adults who were not patients) are now rather old. Qualified success from routine prophylaxes (with a less intensive cleaning procedure than that used in the Karlstad regimen) in adults was reported from Norway.[90] For 5 years, factory workers received a prophylaxis plus oral hygiene instruction at 6-month intervals, or at 3-month intervals for "more severely affected" individuals. The greatest benefits were gained by persons whose oral hygiene status was best to begin with, and least success was achieved among those with initially poor oral hygiene. This difference in results might emphasize the importance of self-care and the limitations of professional cleaning without it.

In the study among adults in Karlstad,[15] the professional cleanings were carried out every 2 to 3 months for the first 6 years, and once or twice a year for the subsequent 9 years for most participants. A small subgroup of persons who had developed caries or further loss of attachment during the study were retained on more intensive professional cleaning regimen for the entire 15 years. All subjects exhibited almost no further loss of periodontal attachment during this period. In line with the philosophy of these researchers, intensive oral hygiene instruction for self-care accompanied the professional cleanings. The authors concluded that intensive self-performed oral hygiene (with a fluoride toothpaste) together with a stringent regimen of professional treatment maintained oral health. The more "high-risk" patients received the more stringent regimen.

In the United States, a study of office workers in California showed that a professional prophylaxis plus intensive oral hygiene instruction every 2 to 4 months reduced levels of plaque and gingivitis relative to a control group, and greatly slowed the rate of loss of attachment.[119] A separate study of young men found a tendency toward improved gingival health accompanying greater frequency of prophylaxes, although differences resulting from prophylaxes at 12-, 6-, and 4-month intervals were not pronounced.[121] An Air Force study[70] found that beneficial results were proportional to the frequency of the prophylactic treatment received; best results were achieved in the group that received 4 prophylaxes per year plus oral hygiene instruction at each appointment. None of these American studies achieved Karlstad-type results, but they did not test nearly so intensive a regimen. Collectively, they demonstrated modest across-the-board results. In light of our current views, it would have been helpful if the authors had reported their results in terms of distributional patterns; it is likely that best results were achieved in the best-motivated patients.

PROFESSIONAL PLUS PERSONAL CARE

The studies just described have some limitations, but collectively they indicate that professional prophylaxis can help with plaque control in many people. It must be re-emphasized, however, that the best results were obtained when excellent personal oral hygiene status was maintained by the individual, which raises questions about the value of regular professional prophylaxis for periodontally healthy adults with good oral hygiene.

The conclusions from these studies suggest that a thorough professional prophylaxis at 2- to 4-month intervals (longer in some patients), combined with a high level of individual oral hygiene, is enough to prevent the destructive periodontal disease that leads to tooth loss. Whether the same results could be achieved in periodontally healthy adults without the professional intervention is an open question. This evidence also is questionable because of epidemiologic studies from untreated populations (Chapter 20), that show that some people with virtually no oral hygiene practices, and hence extensive gingivitis, develop little serious periodontitis. It could be concluded that persons susceptible to periodontitis may need frequent professional maintenance care, but that is by no means so clear for nonsusceptible persons.

CHEMOTHERAPEUTIC METHODS OF PLAQUE CONTROL

The inability of many persons to remove their own dental plaque consistently results from insufficient knowledge, poor mechanical dexterity, or lack of motivation. The idea of a chemical method of plaque removal, a mouthrinse or toothpaste that does it all, is therefore highly attractive.[1, 109] Research over many years has led to the development of some products that have some plaque-control success in specific circumstances. Commercial competition in the marketing of plaque-preventive products is keen, so much so that the American Dental Association (ADA) has established guidelines under which products claiming to control plaque can be accepted by the council.[5] These criteria are listed in Table 28–1, and they conform well with the requirements of acceptable clinical trials given in Chapter 12. If consistently applied, they will serve both professionals and public in their choice of both prescription and over-the-counter oral hygiene products. They do not, however, apply to those toothpastes marketed as "anticalculus" products, because the ADA considers the action of these toothpastes in

Table 28-1. CRITERIA FOR CLINICAL STUDIES UNDER WHICH PRODUCTS CLAIMING TO CONTROL PLAQUE FORMATION CAN BE ACCEPTED BY THE AMERICAN DENTAL ASSOCIATION

- Characteristics of the study population should represent typical product users.
- Active products should be used in normal regimen and compared with placebo control, or, where applicable, an active control.
- Crossover or parallel design studies are acceptable.
- Studies should be a minimum of 6 months in duration.
- Two studies conducted by independent investigators will be required.
- Microbiologic sampling should estimate plaque qualitatively to complement indexes that measure plaque quantitatively.
- Plaque and gingivitis scoring and microbiologic sampling should be conducted at baseline, 6 months, and at an intermediate period.
- Microbiologic profile should demonstrate that pathogenic or opportunistic microorganisms do not develop over the course of the study.
- The toxicologic profile of products should include carcinogenicity and mutagenicity assays in addition to generally recognized tests for drug safety.

From American Dental Association, Council on Dental Therapeutics. Guidelines for acceptance of chemotherapeutic products for the control of supragingival dental plaque and gingivitis. J Am Dent Assoc 1986;112:529–32.

inhibiting the reformation of supragingival calculus after a prophylaxis to be cosmetic rather than therapeutic.

Day-to-day plaque control in the healthy individual must be separated from the use of antibiotics or other medications in the treatment of established disease. Antibiotics have no place in prophylactic control.

Chlorhexidine

Chlorhexidine gluconate (CHX) has been effectively used as a mouthwash (10 ml, 0.2% once or twice daily), topical gel application by dental professionals (1.0% to 2.0% daily), in toothpaste (0.4% to 1.0%), and in direct injection into periodontal pockets. When introduced into the oral cavity, CHX adheres to anionic substrates and is released over 8 to 12 hours. Mucosal and gingival penetration is minimal, and it is poorly absorbed from the gastrointestinal tract.[47] It does not appear to have any local or systemic toxic reactions.[42] CHX has a wide range of bactericidal action, and its selective effect against *Streptococcus mutans* can be useful for caries control in patients with special problems.[28, 132, 133]

Early short-term studies found that CHX rinses inhibited the formation of plaque almost completely.[34, 86, 87] However, because these initial studies were conducted with periodontally healthy dental students who ceased routine oral hygiene procedures for their duration, the generalizability of these findings was doubtful. Results of short-term studies by other researchers using CHX in gel and dentifrice form were less clear-cut, and

revealed some undesirable side effects.[20, 37, 41] Staining of teeth and restorations, for example, was a persistent problem.

Results of longer-term studies, conducted over 2 years, showed that the routine use of CHX was not appropriate. One study found no changes in plaque and gingivitis levels among the dental students who were the test subjects, although again their initial excellent oral hygiene status could have masked any beneficial effects of the CHX.[60] Another found reduced levels of plaque and gingivitis in a 2-year study (also with dental and medical students), although one perplexing finding was that supragingival calculus deposition increased in the test group.[88] Other 6-month studies have also reported increased deposition of thin supragingival calculus,[51, 69] although in both studies it was considered of no clinical consequence.

By the end of the 1970s, the limitations of the routine use of CHX were widely accepted, although it was clear that CHX could play a useful role in plaque control. The side effect of staining and the chance that resistant organisms could develop were enough to produce warnings from leading periodontists against the indiscriminate use of CHX.[85] In addition, CHX does not affect subgingival plaque, which means that its preventive effect in periodontal diseases is limited to preventing the deposition of supragingival plaque after a professional cleansing. Subsequent research has confirmed these earlier findings. European and American studies of 6 months' duration confirmed that CHX use, whether a twice daily 0.12% CHX rinse or applied in other forms and concentrations, reduced gingivitis, gingival bleeding, and plaque deposits.[3, 13, 51, 69]

CHX has been used for years in much of Europe as an antiseptic rinse before oral surgery, to improve plaque control up to 3 to 4 weeks after periodontal surgery, and as an oral hygiene aid for patients with immobilized jaws recovering from fractures. This limited and selective application of CHX, because of its well-documented undesirable side effects, is also its recommended role in the United States and Canada.

CHX is marketed in the United States under the brand name of Peridex. It has been accepted by the ADA[7] as a safe and effective antiplaque agent under the 1986 ADA guidelines (Table 28–1). Its use should be restricted to periodontitis patients, and it has no public health applications.

Other Antibacterial Compounds

In short-term studies, alexidine dihydrochloride mouthwash (10 to 15 ml, 0.035% to 0.05%) has yielded results similar to those found with CHX. Reductions in plaque and gingivitis were recorded,[29, 35, 81, 117, 127] although some were of little clinical importance.[29, 117] Mild staining was also reported in all of these studies. Mouthwashes using octenidine[102] and cetylpyridinium chloride[10] have been tested with mixed results; sanguinaria has been tested with some reported success.[48, 65] The over-the-counter mouthwash Listerine has been accepted by the ADA as a safe and effective antiplaque rinse[6] under its 1986 guidelines.

Stannous fluoride has also been found to have antiplaque properties, probably because it affects the growth and adherence of bacteria rather than exerting a direct bactericidal action. Stabilization of the stannous fluoride in an anhydrous formulation, rather than in aqueous preparations, has increased its efficacy.[98] Stabilized stannous fluoride at 0.454% in a toothpaste reduces gingivitis, although this product was found no better than a control (with sodium fluoride only) toothpaste in restricting the buildup of supragingival plaque.[21, 103]

Baking soda and peroxide (together) toothpastes are marketed as plaque inhibitors, but clinical trials and in vivo testing have provided no evidence for efficacy at reducing plaque buildup and gingivitis following a prophylaxis.[16, 21, 122] The performance of a baking soda and peroxide toothpaste was notably inferior to that of a stabilized stannous fluoride product in the same test.[22]

Anticalculus ("Tartar-Control") Toothpastes

Efforts to find a toothpaste ingredient that prevents the formation of calculus on teeth are longstanding,[58, 120] but until recently they were not successful. Research during the 1960s, however, found that pyrophosphate prevented calcification by interfering with the conversion of amorphous calcium phosphate to hydroxyapatite.[40] When added to the finding that the concentration of pyrophosphate in the plaque of low calculus formers was higher than in the plaque of high calculus formers,[36] the stage was set for testing the anticalculus effect of pyrophosphate in toothpaste.[92] Commercially marketed anticalculus toothpastes mostly contain a mix of soluble pyrophosphates at 3.3% concentration, with or without additional ingredients. These compounds are not part of the abrasive system of the toothpaste, and they are independent of the fluoride added for caries control.

A number of studies have demonstrated that pyrophosphates can effectively inhibit the formation of supragingival calculus after it has been removed by a prophylaxis.[26, 30, 79, 80, 83, 129] These studies were all of fairly similar design. They lasted 2 to 6 months with groups of adult subjects, mostly selected for their propensity to form calculus quickly. All subjects received a thorough prophylaxis to remove all calculus and were then randomly allocated to test and control groups. In all of the studies, test subjects exposed to the pyrophosphates had considerably less supragingival calculus formation than the control subjects.

Triclosan is an antibacterial that inhibits plaque buildup by adsorbing to the tooth surface and may also have direct anti-inflammatory effects on mediators of gingival inflammation.[46] It has been shown to be highly effective at preventing plaque deposition after a professional prophylaxis and reducing gingival bleeding, especially when it is combined with a co-polymer of methoxyethylene and maleic acid.[45] Studies have shown triclosan's efficacy (compared with a toothpaste with only sodium fluoride as an active ingredient) when used as a mouthrinse at 0.1% or 0.2%,[59] or at 0.3% concentration in a toothpaste with 2% co-polymer.[25, 61, 101, 106] Efficacy of the triclosan-co-polymer formulation is independent of the type of fluoride used in the toothpaste,[115] and it is more effective than a fluoride-only dentrifice at removing existing plaque and controlling gingivitis.[75] Studies of triclosan-co-polymer and other ingredients such as pyrophosphates and zinc citrate have given generally positive results,[19, 32, 38, 113] and further work on these formulations is continuing.

It must be noted what these anticalculus toothpastes do and don't do. They inhibit the deposition of new supragingival calculus after a professional cleaning without adverse tissue reaction. Triclosan-co-polymer has been shown to reduce existing plaque and gingivitis.[75] They do not remove existing supragingival calculus, and they have no effect on existing subgingival calculus. The ADA's website lists a number of toothpastes that have been accepted as being tartar-control as well as anticavity products, and the number is likely to continue growing.

The marketing of constantly more effective plaque-control toothpastes, which otherwise do not affect the oral ecology, can only lead to further improvements in oral hygiene and reductions in gingivitis. It is reasonable to assume that adult periodontitis should also be reduced in time, although there is no evidence yet to show that this happens. The effects of these products on early-onset periodontitis are also unknown, and because of the compromised-host etiology of that condition, they are likely to be less evident.

COMMUNITY CONTROL OF PERIODONTAL DISEASES

Until some means can be found to enhance the host response of susceptible persons, there will always be a minority of individuals who are at special risk of losing teeth from periodontitis. Oral hygiene in such individuals is especially important, even though oral plaque deposits may represent only part of the disease problem.

Public programs of dental health education, aimed at improving general standards of oral hygiene, have long been a mainstay of dental public health. Their effectiveness is hard to demonstrate, even though it is likely that public standards of oral hygiene are continuing to improve. Because oral hygiene is of high cultural value, extensive and sophisticated commercial advertising has almost certainly made a strong impact on public oral

hygiene behavior. As a result, the potential additional impact of organized programs of oral hygiene education need to be carefully thought through before they are launched. They are likely to be of most value when directed at populations with little exposure to commercial advertising, or who do not espouse the middle-class values of oral hygiene that such advertising assumes. Public education for oral hygiene is useful in many developing countries, although the programs should always be monitored periodically for effectiveness.

REFERENCES

1. Addy M, Koltai R. Control of supragingival calculus. Scaling and polishing and anticalculus toothpastes: An opinion. J Clin Periodontol 1994;21:342-6.
2. Agerbaek N, Poulsen S, Melsen B, Glavind L. Effect of professional toothcleansing every third week on gingivitis and dental caries in children. Community Dent Oral Epidemiol 1978;6:40-1.
3. Ainamo J, Asikainen S, Paloheimo L. Gingival bleeding after chlorhexidine mouthrinses. J Clin Periodontol 1982;9:337-45.
4. Albandar JM, Buischi YA, Oliveira LB, Axelsson P. Lack of effect of oral hygiene training on periodontal disease progression over 3 years in adolescents. J Periodontol 1995;66:255-60.
5. American Dental Association, Council on Dental Therapeutics. Guidelines for acceptance of chemotherapeutic products for the control of supragingival dental plaque and gingivitis. J Am Dent Assoc 1986;112:529-32.
6. American Dental Association, Council on Dental Therapeutics. Council on Dental Therapeutics accepts Listerine. J Am Dent Assoc 1988;117:515-6.
7. American Dental Association, Council on Dental Therapeutics. Council on Dental Therapeutics accepts Peridex. J Am Dent Assoc 1988;117:516-7.
8. Ashley FP, Sainsbury RH. The effect of a school-based plaque control programme on caries and gingivitis. Br Dent J 1981;150:41-5.
9. Ashley FP, Sainsbury RH. Post-study effects of a school-based plaque control programme. Br Dent J 1982;153:337-8.
10. Ashley FP, Skinner A, Jackson PY, Wilson RF. Effect of a 0.1% cetylpyridinium chloride mouthrinse on the accumulation and biochemical composition of dental plaque in young adults. Caries Res 1984; 18:465-71.
11. Axelsson P, Lindhe J. The effect of a preventive programme on dental plaque, gingivitis and caries in school children. Results after one and two years. J Clin Periodontol 1974;1:126-38.
12. Axelsson P, Lindhe J. Effect of fluoride on gingivitis and dental caries in a preventive program based on plaque control. Community Dent Oral Epidemiol 1975;3:159-60.
13. Axelsson P, Lindhe J. Efficacy of mouthrinses in inhibiting dental plaque and gingivitis in man. J Clin Periodontol 1987;14:205-12.
14. Axelsson P, Lindhe J, Waseby J. The effect of various plaque control measures on gingivitis and caries in

schoolchildren. Community Dent Oral Epidemiol 1976;4:232-9.

15. Axelsson P, Lindhe J, Wystrom B. On the prevention of caries and periodontal disease. Results of a 15-year longitudinal study in adults. J Clin Periodontol 1991;18:182-9.

16. Bacca LA, Leusch M, Lanzalaco AC, et al. A comparison of intraoral antimicrobial effects of stabilized stannous fluoride dentifrice, baking soda/peroxide dentifrice, conventional NaF dentifrice and essential oil mouthrinse. J Clin Dent 1997;8(Special Issue):54-61.

17. Bader JD, Rozier RG, McFall WT Jr, Ramsey DL. Association of dental health knowledge with periodontal conditions among regular patients. Community Dent Oral Epidemiol 1990;18:32-6.

18. Badersten A, Egelberg J, Koch G. Effect of monthly prophylaxis on caries and gingivitis in schoolchildren. Community Dent Oral Epidemiol 1975;3:1-4.

19. Banoczy J, Sari K, Schiff T, et al. Anticalculus efficacy of three dentifrices. Am J Dentistry 1995; 8:205-8.

20. Bassiouny MA, Grant AA. The toothbrush application of chlorhexidine. Br Dent J 1975;139:323-7.

21. Beiswanger BB, Doyle PM, Jackson RD, et al. The clinical effect of dentifrices containing stabilized stannous fluoride on plaque formation and gingivitis—a six-month study with ad libitum brushing. J Clin Dent 1995;6(Special Issue):46-53.

22. Beiswanger BB, McClanahan SF, Bartizek RD, et al. The comparative efficacy of stabilized stannous fluoride dentifrice, peroxide/baking soda dentifrice and essential oil mouthrinse for the prevention of gingivitis. J Clin Dent 1997;8(Special Issue):46-53.

23. Bergenholtz A, Brithon J. Plaque removal by dental floss or toothpicks. An intraindividual comparative study. J Clin Periodontol 1980;7:516-24.

24. Bergenholtz A, Olsson A. Efficacy of plaque-removal using interdental brushes and waxed dental floss. Scand J Dent Res 1984;92:198-203.

25. Bolden TE, Zambon JJ, Sowinski J, et al. The clinical effect of a dentifrice containing triclosan and a co-polymer in a sodium fluoride/silica base on plaque formation and gingivitis: A six-month clinical study. J Clin Dent 1992;3:125-31.

26. Bollmer BW, Sturzenberger OP, Vick V, Grossman E. Reduction of calculus and Peridex stain with Tartar-Control Crest. J Clin Dent 1995;6:185-7.

27. Bouwsma O, Caton J, Polson A, Espeland M. Effect of personal oral hygiene on bleeding interdental gingiva. Histologic changes. J Periodontol 1988;59:80-6.

28. Bowden GH. Mutans streptococci, caries, and chlorhexidine. J Can Dent Assoc 1996;62:700, 703-7.

29. Carlson HC, Porter K, Alms TH. The effect of an alexidine mouthwash on dental plaque and gingivitis. J Periodontol 1977;48:216-8.

30. Chitke UM, Rudolph MJ, Reinach SG. Anti-calculus effects of dentifrice containing pyrophosphate compared with control. Clin Prevent Dent 1992;14:29-33.

31. Christersson LA, Grossi SG, Dunford RG, et al. Dental plaque and calculus: Risk indicators for their formation. J Dent Res 1992;71:1425-30.

32. Cohen S, Schiff T, McCool J, et al. Anticalculus efficacy of a dentifrice containing potassium nitrate, soluble pyrophosphatae, PVM/MA copolymer, and sodium fluoride in a silica base: A twelve-week clinical study. J Clin Dent 1994;5(Special Issue):93-6.

33. Corbet EF, Davies WIR. The role of supragingival plaque in the control of progressive periodontal disease: A review. J Clin Periodontol 1993;20:307-13.

34. Davies RM, Jensen SB, Rindom Schiott C, Löe H. The effect of topical application of chlorhexidine on the bacterial colonization of the teeth and gingiva. J Periodontol Res 1970;5:96-101.

35. Deasy MJ, Formicola AJ, Johnson DH, Howe EG. Inhibitory effects of an alexidine mouthrinse on dental plaque formation. Clin Prevent Dent 1979; 1:(2)6-9.

36. Edgar WM, Jenkins GN. Inorganic pyrophosphate in human parotid saliva and dental plaque. Arch Oral Biol 1972;17:219-23.

37. Emilson CG, Fornell J. Effect of toothbrushing with chlorhexidine gel on salivary microflora, oral hygiene, and caries. Scand J Dent Res 1976;84:308-19.

38. Fairbrother KJ, Kowolik MJ, Curzon ME, et al. The comparative clinical efficacy of pyrophosphate/triclosan, copolymer/triclosan and zinc citrate/triclosan dentifrices for the reduction of supragingival calculus formation. J Clin Dent 1997;8(Special Issue):62-6.

39. Finkelstein P, Grossman E. The effectiveness of dental floss in reducing gingival inflammation. J Dent Res 1979;58:1034-9.

40. Fleisch H, Russell GG, Bisaz S, et al. Influence of pyrophosphate on the transformation of amorphous to crystalline calcium phosphate. Calcif Tissue Res 1968;2:49-59.

41. Flotra L, Gjermo P, Rolla G, Waerhaug J. Side effects of chlorhexidine mouthwashes. Scand J Dent Res 1971;79:119-25.

42. Foulkes DM. Some toxicological observations on chlorhexidine. J Periodont Res 1973;8(Suppl 12):55-7.

43. Frandsen AM, Barbano JP, Suomi JD, et al. A comparison of the effectiveness of the Charters' scrub and roll methods of toothbrushing in removing plaque. Scand J Dent Res 1972;80:267-71.

44. Frazier PJ. A new look at dental health education in community programs. Dent Hyg 1978;52:176-86.

45. Gaffar A, Afflitto J, Nabi N, et al. Recent advances in plaque, gingivitis, tartar and caries prevention technology. Int Dent J 1994;44(Suppl 1):63-70.

46. Gaffar A, Scherl D, Afflito J, Coleman EJ. The effect of tricolosan on mediators of gingival inflammation. J Clin Periodontol 1995;22:480-4.

47. Greenstein G, Berman C, Jaffin R. Chlorhexidine: An adjunct to periodontal therapy. J Periodontol 1986;57:370-7.

48. Grenby TH. The use of sanguinarine in mouthwashes and toothpaste compared with some other antimicrobial agents. Br Dent J 1995;178:254-8.

49. Grossi SG, Genco RJ, Machtei EE, et al. Assessment of risk for periodontal disease. II. Risk indicators for alveolar bone loss. J Periodontol 1995;66:23-9.

50. Grossi SG, Zambon JJ, Ho AW, et al. Assessment of risk for periodontal disease. I. Risk indicators for attachment loss. J Periodontol 1994;65:260-7.

51. Grossman E. Chlorhexidine efficacy on gingivitis tested. J Periodont Res 1986;21:33-43.

52. Hansen F, Gjermo P. The plaque-removing effect of four toothbrushing methods. Scand J Dent Res 1971;79:502-6.

53. Heifetz SB, Bagramian RA, Suomi JD, Segreto VA. Programs for the mass control of plaque: An appraisal. J Public Health Dent 1973;33:91-5.

54. Heifetz SB, Suomi JD. The control of dental caries and periodontal disease: A fundamental approach. J Public Health Dent 1973;33:2-6.

55. Hill HC, Levi PA, Glickman I. The effects of waxed and unwaxed dental floss on interdental plaque accumulation and interdental gingival health. J Periodontol 1973;44:411-3.

56. Horowitz AM. Oral hygiene measures. J Can Dent Assoc 1980;46:43-6.

57. Horowitz AM, Suomi JD, Peterson JK, et al. Effects of supervised daily dental plaque removal by children after 3 years. Community Dent Oral Epidemiol 1980;8:171-6.

58. Jackson D. The efficacy of 2 per cent sodium ricinoleate in toothpaste to reduce gingival inflammation. Br Dent J 1962;112:487-93.

59. Jenkins S, Addy M, Newcombe RJ. A dose-response study of triclosan mouthrinses on plaque regrowth. J Clin Periodontol 1993;20:609-12.

60. Johansen JR, Gjermo P, Eriksen HM. Effect of 2 years use of chlorhexidine-containing dentifrices on plaque, gingivitis, and caries. Scand J Dent Res 1975;83:288-92.

61. Kanchanakamol U, Umpriwan R, Jotikasthira N, et al. Reduction of plaque formation and gingivitis by a dentifrice containing triclosan and copolymer. J Periodontol 1995;66:109-12.

62. Keller SE, Manson-Hing LR. Clearance studies of proximal tooth surfaces. Part II. In vivo removal of interproximal plaque. Ala J Med Sci 1969;6:266-74.

63. Kelner RM, Wohl BR, Deasy MJ, Formicola AJ. Gingival inflammation as related to frequency of plaque removal. J Periodontol 1974;45:303-7.

64. Kjaerheim V, von der Fehr FR, Poulsen S. Two-year study on the effect of professional toothcleaning on schoolchildren in Oppergord, Norway. Community Dent Oral Epidemiol 1980;8:401-6.

65. Kopczyk RA, Abrams H, Brown AT, et al. Clinical and microbiological effects of a sanguinaria-containing mouthrinse and dentifrice with and without fluoride during 6 months of use. J Periodontol 1991;62:617-22.

66. Kreshover SJ, Russell AL. Periodontal disease. J Am Dent Assoc 1958;56:625-9.

67. Kuhner MK, Raetzke PB. The effect of health beliefs on the compliance of periodontal patients with oral hygiene instructions. J Periodontol 1989;60:51-6.

68. Lang NP, Cumming BR, Loe H. Toothbrushing frequency as it relates to plaque development and gingival health. J Periodontol 1973;44:396-405.

69. Lang NP, Hotz P, Graf H, et al. Effects of supervised chlorhexidine mouthrinses in children: A longitudinal clinical trial. J Periodont Res 1982;17:101-11.

70. Lightner LM, O'Leary TJ, Drake RB, et al. Preventive periodontic treatment procedures: Results over 46 months. J Periodontol 1971;42:555-61.

71. Lindhe J, Axelsson P, Tollskog, G. The effect of proper oral hygiene on gingivitis and dental caries in schoolchildren. Community Dent Oral Epidemiol 1975;3:150-5.

72. Lindhe J, Koch G. The effect of supervised oral hygiene on the gingiva of children. Progression and inhibition of gingivitis. J Periodont Res 1966;1:260-7.

73. Lindhe J, Koch G. The effect of supervised oral hygiene on the gingiva of children. Lack of prolonged effect of supervision. J Periodont Res 1967;2:215-20.

74. Lindhe J, Koch G, Mansson U. The effect of supervised oral hygiene on the gingiva of children. Effect of mouth rinsings. J Periodont Res 1966;1:268-75.

75. Lindhe J, Rosling B, Socransky SS, Volpe AR. The effect of a triclosan-containing dentifrice on established plaque and gingivitis. J Clin Periodontol 1993;20:327-34.

76. Lindhe J, Wicen PO. The effects on the gingivae of chewing fibrous foods. J Periodont Res 1969;4:193-201.

77. Lissau I, Holst D, Friis-Haasche E. Dental health behaviors and periodontal disease indicators in Danish youths. A 10-year epidemiological follow-up. J Clin Periodontol 1990;17:42-7.

78. Listgarten MA. Prevention of periodontal disease in the future. J Clin Periodontol 1979;6:32-6.

79. Lobene RR. A clinical study of the anticalculus effect of a dentifrice containing soluble pyrophosphate and sodium fluoride. Clin Prevent Dent 1986;8:5-7.

80. Lobene RR. A clinical comparison of the anticalculus effect of two commercially-available dentifrices. Clin Prevent Dent 1987;9:3-8.

81. Lobene RR, Soparkar PM. The effect of an alexidine mouthwash on plaque and gingivitis. J Am Dent Assoc 1973;87:848-51.

82. Lobene RR, Soparkar PM, Newman MB. Use of dental floss; effect on plaque and gingivitis. Clin Prevent Dent 1982;4:5-8.

83. Lobene RR, Soparkar PM, Newman MB, Kohut BE. Reduced formation of supragingival calculus with use of fluoride-zinc chloride dentifrice. J Am Dent Assoc 1987;114:350-2.

84. Löe H. A review of the prevention and control of plaque. In: McHugh WD, ed: Dental plaque. Edinburgh: Churchill Livingstone, 1970:259-70.

85. Löe H. Principles and progress in the prevention of periodontal diseases. In: Lehner T, Cimasoni G, eds: The borderland between caries and periodontal disease. II. New York: Grune and Stratton, 1980:255-68.

86. Löe H, Rindom Schiott C. The effect of suppression of the oral microflora upon the development of dental plaque and gingivitis. In: McHugh WD, ed: Dental plaque. Edinburgh: Churchill Livingstone, 1970:247-55.

87. Löe H, Rindom Schiott C. The effects of mouthrinses and topical application of chlorhexidine on the development of dental plaque and gingivitis in man. J Periodontol Res 1970;5:79-83.

88. Löe H, Rindom Schiott C, Glavind L, Karring T. Two years oral use of chlorhexidine in man. I. General design and clinical effects. J Periodontol Res 1976;11:135-44.

89. Longhurst P, Berman DS. Apples and gingival health; report of a feasibility study. Br Dent J 1973;134:475-9.

90. Lovdal A, Arno A, Schei O, Waerhaug J. Combined effect of subgingival scaling and controlled oral hygiene on the incidence of gingivitis. Acta Odont Scand 1961;19:537-55.

91. Macgregor IDM, Balding JW. Toothbrushing frequency and personal hygiene in 14-year-old schoolchildren. Br Dent J 1987;162:141-4.

92. Mallatt ME, Beiswanger BB, Stookey GK, et al. Influence of soluble pyrophosphate on calculus formation in adults. J Dent Res 1985;64:1159-62.

93. Mandel ID. Why pick on teeth? J Am Dent Assoc 1990;121:129-32.

94. Marquis RE. Oxygen metabolism, oxidative stress and acid-base physiology of dental plaque biofilms. J Indust Microbiol 1995;15:198-207.

95. Marsh PD. Microbial ecology of dental plaque and its significance in health and disease. Adv Dent Res 1994;8:263-71.

96. Marsh PD, Bradshaw DJ. Dental plaque as biofilm. J Indust Microbiol 1995;15:169-75.

97. Melsen B, Agerbaek N. Effect of an instructional motivation program on oral health in Danish adolescents after 1 and 2 years. Community Dent Oral Epidemiol 1980;8:72-8.

98. Miller S, Truong T, Heu R, et al. Recent advances in stannous fluoride technology: Antibacterial efficacy and mechanism of action towards hypersensitivity. Int Dent J 1994;44(Suppl 1):83-98.

99. Olsson, B. Efficiency of traditional chewing sticks in oral hygiene programs among Ethiopian schoolchildren. Community Dent Oral Epidemiol 1978;6:105-9.

100. Page RC. Gingivitis. J Clin Periodontol 1986;13:345-9.

101. Palomo F, Wantland L, Sanchez A, et al. The effect of three commercially available dentifrices containing triclosan on supragingival plaque formation and gingivitis: A six month clinical study. Int Dent J 1994;44(Suppl 1):75-81.

102. Patters MR, Anerud K, Trummel CL, et al. Inhibition of plaque formation in humans by octenidine mouthrinse. J Periodont Res 1983; 18:212-9.

103. Perlich MA, Bacca LA, Bollmer BW, et al. The clinical effect of a stabilized stannous fluoride dentifrice on plaque formation, gingivitis and gingival bleeding: A six-month study. J Clin Dent 1995;6(Special Issue):54-8.

104. Pihlstrom BL, Ortiz-Campos C, McHugh RB. A randomized four-year study of periodontal therapy. J Periodontol 1981;52:227-42.

105. Ramfjord SP, Knowles JW, Nissle RR, et al. Longitudinal study of periodontal therapy. J Periodontol 1973;44:66-77.

106. Renvert S, Birkhed D. Comparison between 3 triclosan dentifrices on plaque, gingivitis and salivary microflora. J Clin Periodontol 1995;22:63-70.

107. Ripa LW, Berenie JT, Leske GS. The effect of professionally administered bi-annual prophylaxes on the oral hygiene, gingival health and caries scores of school children. Two-year study. J Prevent Dent 1976;3:22-6.

108. Robinson E. A comparative evaluation of the scrub and Bass methods of toothbrushing with flossing as an adjunct. Am J Public Health 1976;66:1078-81.

109. Robinson PJ. Gingivitis: A prelude to periodontitis? J Clin Dent 1995;6(Special Issue):41-5.

110. Rodda JC. A comparison of four methods of toothbrushing. N Z Dent J 1968;64:162-7.

111. Russell RR. Control of specific plaque bacteria. Adv Dent Res 1994;8:285-90.

112. Sangnes G, Zachrisson B, Gjermo P. Effectiveness of vertical and horizontal brushing techniques in plaque removal. J Dent Child 1972;39:94-7.

113. Saxton CA, Huntington E, Cummins D. The effect of dentifrices containing triclosan on the development of gingivitis in a 21-day experimental gingivitis study. Int Dent J 1993;43(Suppl 1):423-9.

114. Scheie AA. Mechanisms of dental plaque formation. Adv Dent Res 1994;8:246-53.

115. Schiff T, Cohen S, Volpe AR, Petrone ME. Effects of two fluoride dentifrices containing triclosan and a copolymer on calculus formation. Am J Dent 1990;3(Special Issue):S43-5.

116. Schmid MO, Balmelli OP, Saxer UP. Plaque removing effect of toothbrush, dental floss, and a toothpick. J Clin Periodontol 1976;3:157-65.

117. Spolsky VW, Bhatia HL, Forsythe A, Levin BS. The effect of an antimicrobial mouthwash on dental plaque and gingivitis in young adults. J Periodontol 1975;46:685-90.

118. Suomi JD. Prevention and control of periodontal disease. J Am Dent Assoc 1971;83:1271-87.

119. Suomi JD, Greene JC, Vermillion JC, et al. The effect of controlled oral hygiene procedures on the progression of periodontal disease in adults. Results after third and final year. J Periodontol 1971; 42:152-60.

120. Suomi JD, Horowitz HS, Barbano JP, et al. A clinical trial of a calculus-inhibitory dentifrice. J Periodontol 1974;45:139-45.

121. Suomi JD, Smith LW, Chang JJ, Barbano JP. Study of the effect of different prophylaxis frequencies on the periodontium of young adult males. J Periodontol 1973;44:406-10.

122. Taller SH. The effect of baking soda/hydrogen peroxide dentifrice (Mentadent) and 0.12 percent chlorhexidine gluconate mouthrinse (Peridex) in reducing gingival bleeding. J NJ Dent Assoc 1993; 64:23-5,27.

123. Tan HH, Saxton CA. Effect of a single dental health care instruction and prophylaxis on gingivitis. Community Dent Oral Epidemiol 1978;6:172-5.

124. Theilade E, Wright WH, Jensen SB, Löe H. Experimental gingivitis in man. II. A longitudinal clinical and bacteriological investigation. J Periodontol Res 1966;1:1-13.

125. Walmsley AD. The electric toothbrush: A review. Br Dent J 1997;182:209-18.

126. Wardle HM. The challenge of growing oral spirochaetes. J Med Microbiol 1997;46:104-16.

127. Weatherford TW, Finn SB, Jamison HC. Effects of an alexidine mouthwash on dental plaque and gingivitis in humans over a six-month period. J Am Dent Assoc 1977;94:528-36.

128. Westfelt E. Rationale of mechanical plaque control. J Clin Periodontol 1996;23(3 Part 2):263-7.

129. Zacherl WA, Pfeiffer HJ, Swancar JR. The effect of soluble pyrophosphates on dental calculus in adults. J Am Dent Assoc 1985;110:737-8.

130. Zaki HA, Bandt CL. The effective use of a self-teaching oral hygiene manual. J Periodontol 1974;45:491-5.

131. Zambon JJ. Principles of evaluation of the diagnostic value of subgingival bacteria. Ann Periodontol 1997;2:138-48.

132. Zickert I, Emilson CG, Krasse B. Effect of caries preventive measures in children highly infected with the bacterium Streptococcus mutans. Arch Oral Biol 1982;27:861-8.

133. Zickert I, Emilson CG, Krasse B. Microbial conditions and caries increment 2 years after discontinuation of controlled antimicrobial measures in Swedish teenagers. Community Dent Oral Epidemiol 1987;15:241-4.

29

Smokeless Tobacco, Oral Cancer, and Antitobacco Initiatives

Pathologic Effects of Smokeless Tobacco ◆ Prevalence of Smokeless Tobacco Use ◆ Preventing Smokeless Tobacco Use ◆ What Dental Professionals Can Do to Curb Tobacco Use in their Patients

Tobacco was described as a principal risk factor for oral cancer in Chapter 22, with the degree of risk proportional to the extent of use. We also described in Chapter 20 that tobacco has been clearly identified as a risk factor for periodontitis. It follows that when dental professionals find these habits in their patient, they have a responsibility to do what they can to change them. This rarely is easy, because the addictions are powerful and there are usually strong social or psychological reasons why these habits were adopted in the first place. However, as will be described, there are programs in place that can help.

A particularly worrisome form of tobacco use, because of its appeal to young people, is smokeless tobacco, heavily marketed over recent years in North America and elsewhere. This product, also referred to as "spit tobacco" in an effort to make it sound less appealing, presents some special challenges to the dental professions because its current use among young people has the potential of increasing the prevalence of oral cancer in the future.[35] There are well-documented hazards that follow regular use of smokeless tobacco, and it certainly is not an acceptable substitute for those trying to quit smoking, as has been asserted.[36]

This chapter describes the programs that dental professionals can use in their practices to help patients cut any form of tobacco use, though it focuses on the specific public health issue of how to reduce the consumption of smokeless tobacco among young people. We will use the abbreviation ST for these products; readers can take it as standing for either "smokeless tobacco" or "spit tobacco," according to taste.

PATHOLOGIC EFFECTS OF SMOKELESS TOBACCO

ST is sold in several forms. The main concern comes with snuff, a powdered tobacco product, which is used by placing a "dip" between the cheek and gum. Dry snuff contains high concentrations of N-nitrosamines,[2, 24] a group of compounds strongly implicated as carcinogens, especially for oral cancers.[24, 34] The N-nitroso compounds found in snuff are DNA-damaging agents in cancers of the aerodigestive tract.[30] A Consensus Panel from the National Institutes of Health found strong evidence that use of snuff causes oral cancers,[32] a conclusion for which there was ample support at the time[43, 46] and subsequently.[24, 26, 50] Nicotine is absorbed from ST in amounts similar to those seen in cigarette smokers,[6] thus making ST a potential risk factor for the many illnesses that result from smoking. That could be the reason for the finding that ST users face a relative risk of 2.1 for cardiovascular disease compared with nonusers. The relative risk for smokers, compared with nonsmokers in the same study, was 3.2.[7]

The continued use of snuff leads to localized tissue changes, most commonly the development of leukoplakia, which is characterized by the appearance of white, wrinkled mucosa at the site where the snuff is placed. Leukoplakia can become cancerous in 3% to 5% of cases,[41] although there is also evidence that these lesions can be reversed if the ST habit is ended.[20] In terms of oral conditions other than precancerous soft tissue changes, there is no good evidence that it can cause caries and periodontal diseases. Gingival recession at the site where the quid or the dip is placed, however, is common.[45] It has also been found that poor oral hygiene among ST users contributes to the formation of nitrosamines in the oral cavity.[30]

Further evidence for the carcinogenic potential of chewing tobacco comes from studies among women smokers and dippers in the South.[47] The relative risk of developing cancer of the gums and buccal mucosa was 4.6 for smokers (i.e., smokers had 4.6 times the chance of developing oral cancer than did nonsmokers). For users of ST, however, the relative risk was 13 to 48, the higher risk being found in those with greater length of ST use.

PREVALENCE OF SMOKELESS TOBACCO USE

Heavy marketing of smokeless tobacco products, principally targeted to adolescent and young adult males, has coincided with the national decline in cigarette smoking. This marketing seems to have been successful; consumption of ST products in the United States almost tripled between 1972 and 1991.[44] It was estimated from a national survey that in 1991, 5.3 million American adults (2.9% of the population) were using ST, 4.8 million men and 533,000 women.[44] The concerns about ST's appeal to youth seems well founded: 1995 national survey data found that 11.4% of high school students had used ST within the last 30 days, 19.7% of males and 2.4% of females. ST use among white students was 14.5%, among African-American students 2.2%, and among Hispanic students 4.4%.[25] Among adults aged 45 or older, however, ST use was more common among African-Americans than among whites.[19]

Usage of ST is highest in the South, in rural areas, and declines with increasing education.[44] Women users of ST are predominantly in the South.[47] Prevalence in Canada appears much lower; estimates from the 1986

Labor Force Survey smoking supplement were that 0.7% of males over age 15 used chewing tobacco and 0.4% used snuff.[29]

Surveys suggest that 7% of adolescent white males use ST daily, that a majority have tried it, and 10% to 40% have reported using it within the last week.[3, 8, 9, 28, 33] The 1991 national survey found that 8.2% of males aged 18 to 24 years were regular ST users, the highest proportion in any one age group. Even if there is some overreporting,[15] presumably for "macho" reasons, these figures are high. Its use is extensive in the military[5, 23] and is particularly heavy among Native Americans, where a study in 7 western states found that 56% of ninth and tenth graders reported that they were regular users,[10] as were 28.1% of sixth graders.[4] ST use among Native American women is substantially above the national rate for women.[39, 40] As mentioned, although ST usage is related to lower education, a survey among college students found that 8% of students in the Northeast, and 15% in the south central region, reported using ST.[21] Prevalence is also widespread among highly visible professional baseball players; surveys carried out with major- and minor-league teams in 1987 and 1988 found that 39% to 46% of players were regular users.[18, 48] Another study with baseballers found that ST users in 1988 had 60 times the risk of developing leukoplakia when compared with nonusers.[22]

Virtually all of the surveys in the United States show that principal use is among adolescent and young adult white males. Reported usage is much lower among white females, African-Americans, and Asian-Americans, although ST use among Hispanics is comparable to that among other whites.[8] Native Americans emerge as the ethnic group with the heaviest relative use of ST, and the only one in which there is almost equivalent use among males and females.[10, 49] In one study with Navajo adolescents, more than 25% of ST users had leukoplakia, compared with only 4% of the nonusers. The duration and frequency of use were highly significant risk factors for leukoplakia.[49]

The remarkably high occurrence of oral cancers in India (Chapter 22) is thought to follow from the high prevalence of tobacco chewing in several forms. It is noteworthy that the rate of conversion of leukoplakia and other precancerous lesions to oral cancers is no higher in India than that reported elsewhere.[41] This suggests that it is the very high exposure to tobacco, rather than any inherent qualities of the Indian people, that produces the high prevalence of leukoplakia, and subsequently oral cancer, in that country.

PREVENTING SMOKELESS TOBACCO USE

Prevention against the diseases that come with ST is based principally on public and individual education to drop the habit, or preferably not to begin in the first place. The public health efforts of the various professions involved received a boost with the passage of PL 99-252, the Comprehensive Smokeless Tobacco Health Education Act, in February 1986. Major provisions of this legislation include the following:

- Development and implementation of health education programs and materials to inform the public of health risks resulting from the use of smokeless tobacco products.
- Inclusion of health warning labels on all smokeless tobacco products and advertisements, except those on outdoor billboards.
- Prohibition of radio and television advertising, beginning in August 1986.
- Disclosure to the Secretary of Health and Human Services of the ingredients used in the production of smokeless tobacco, as well as the quantity of nicotine in such products.
- Technical assistance in public health education for the states.
- Authorization of research on the effects of smokeless tobacco.[27]

Ironically, this national legislation was supported by the tobacco industry, which was spurred to do so because of the likelihood that a majority of states would pass much more severe laws of their own.[12] The growth of public concern about the marketing of ST was spurred by the publicity generated by the 1985 case of *Marsee vs US Tobacco Company*. Sean Marsee, a top high school athlete, had died at age 19 from oral cancer, which was considered to have resulted from his use of ST. The suit was brought by Marsee's mother, who charged misleading advertising by the tobacco company and failure to place warnings on its products.[13] Although Ms. Marsee's case was not successful, the case engendered a great deal of sympathy and concern.

Voluntarily breaking the ST habit, given that nicotine addiction is involved, seems to be no easier than breaking the cigarette habit. An intensive program of ST cessation with 25 adolescent habitual ST users found that only 4 had remained successful in quitting 3 months after the program.[17] Strategy therefore should be aimed at having young people not start using ST, although it is obvious that health education programs need to go well beyond the "just say no" level to be successful. In the 1991 national survey, 22.9% of current ST users reported that they currently smoked, and another 33.3% formerly smoked.[44] Many ST users report using it concurrently with alcohol, cigarettes, and marijuana; and peer pressure is a strong influence in getting started.[3] The relationship between cigarette smoking and ST use, as well as other correlates of the habit, is complex and needs further study if education to discourage commencement of either habit is to be successful.[38] Ignorance of the health consequences is also common; one study in Pennsylvania reported that nearly half the males in grades 7 to 12 did not believe that ST was harmful.[15] Like any health education with adolescents, the immediate negative effects of ST use (stained teeth, bad breath) can make a greater impression than the long-term health hazards.[16]

Multifaceted strategies were needed to use the provisions of PL 99-252, with state and local public health agencies playing a leading role.[11] Some states established programs of media advertising and school health education programs aimed specifically at discouraging the start of ST use. Monitoring the impact of these educational efforts requires considerable survey effort. Following the passage of PL 99-252, the Centers for Disease Control and Prevention (CDC) identified 6 indicators for evaluating the impact of that legislation:

- Prevalence of ST current use, meaning surveys to show the numbers who reportedly used ST within the last 7 days.
- Perceptions of the safety of use, whether users and nonusers alike are aware that ST is not a safe alternative to cigarettes.
- The amounts of ST sold.
- Prevalence of ST ever used, meaning surveys to show the numbers who reportedly ever used ST.
- Incidence of ST-induced leukoplakia (also referred to as *snuff-dippers keratosis*), meaning the number of newly-diagnosed cases in the population.

- Curricula on ST, meaning the numbers of schools, at all levels from elementary to medical schools, with curricula covering the health hazards of ST use.[13]

The monitoring process is proceeding well through a series of institutionalized surveys,[19, 25] but progress toward reducing ST use is slow. Trends in ST use in Indiana, Iowa, Montana, and West Virginia between 1988 and 1993 showed little change, a finding attributed to increased advertising and promotion by the tobacco industry[31] (despite PL 99-252). Minors still have relatively little trouble getting ST even in states where such sales are illegal.[1]

WHAT DENTAL PROFESSIONALS CAN DO TO CURB TOBACCO USE IN THEIR PATIENTS

Dental professionals obviously have a potentially major role to play in educating patients about the hazards of ST and in helping already addicted patients to quit.[37] It may sound daunting, but it can be done. In one intervention study, the number of young male ST users who quit was 50% above the normal rate when they viewed a 9-minute videotape and were given a self-help manual and an explanation of the risks and "unequivocal advice" to quit.[42]

The National Cancer Institute (NCI), one of the National Institutes of Health (NIH), has produced some excellent materials designed to be used in the dental office to help patients quit. *Tobacco Effects in the Mouth* (NIH publication No. 94-3330) is a graphically illustrated guide to the pathology that can follow ST use and includes patient-assessment forms for charting progress. *How to Help Your Patients Stop Using Tobacco* (NIH publication No. 93-3191) is a manual for the dental team produced by dental and behavioral experts for NCI's Smoking and Tobacco Control progam. It presents the steps involved in getting the dental staff prepared, helping patients, and following through, as well as progress assessment materials. The NCI also funds the National Dental Tobacco-Free Steering Committee, a broad-based group whose mission is to promote tobacco-cessation activities through the dental office. Oral Health America sponsors the National Spit Tobacco Education Program (NSTEP), largely funded by the Robert Wood Johnson Foundation, a group that achieved national prominence in the late 1990s largely through its charismatic, highly-visible national honorary chairman, baseball legend Joe Garagiola. Mr. Garagiola hammered the message that ST is not a traditional part of the great American pastime, no matter how the tobacco companies tried to make it appear so. There is now a cluster of programs that dental professionals can tap into to assist them in helping patients kick the tobacco habit. These activities should be part of the routines of every dental office, for after all it is a matter of life and death.

REFERENCES

1. Accessibility to minors of smokeless tobacco products—Broward County, Florida, March-June 1996. MMWR 1996;45:1079-82.
2. Adams JD, Owens-Tucciarone P, Hoffmann D. Tobacco-specific N-nitrosamines in dry snuff. Food Chem Toxicol 1987;25:245-6.
3. Ary DV, Lichtenstein E, Severson HH. Smokeless tobacco use among male adolescents: Patterns, correlates, predictors, and the use of other drugs. Prevent Med 1987;16:385-401.
4. Backinger CL, Bruerd B, Kinney MB, Szpunar SM. Knowledge, intent to use, and use of smokeless tobacco among sixth grade schoolchildren in six selected U.S. sites. Public Health Rep 1993;108:637-42.
5. Ballweg JA, Bray RM. Smoking and tobacco use by U.S. military personnel. Mil Med 1989;154:165-8.
6. Benowitz NL, Jacob P 3rd, Yu L. Daily use of smokeless tobacco: Systemic effects. Ann Intern Med 1989;111:112-6.
7. Bolinder G, Alfredsson L, Englund A, de Faire U. Smokeless tobacco use and increased cardiovascular mortality among Swedish construction workers. Am J Public Health 1994;84:399-404.
8. Boyd G. Use of smokeless tobacco among children and adolescents in the United States. Prevent Med 1987;16:402-21.
9. Brownson RC, DiLorenzo TM, Van Tuinen M, Finger WW. Patterns of cigarette and smokeless tobacco use among children and adolescents. Prevent Med 1990;19:170-80.
10. Bruerd B. Smokeless tobacco use among Native American school children. Public Health Rep 1990;105:196-201.
11. Capwell EM. P.L. 99-252 and the roles of state and local governments in decreasing smokeless tobacco use. J Public Health Dent 1990;50:70-6.
12. Chen MS Jr. Evaluating the impact of P.L. 99-252 on decreasing smokeless tobacco use. J Public Health Dent 1990;50:65-69.
13. Chen MS Jr, Schroeder KL. An epilogue to evaluating the impact of P.L. 99-252 on decreasing smokeless tobacco use. J Public Health Dent 1990;50:101-4.
14. Cohen RY, Sattler J, Felix MR, Brownell KD. Experimentation with smokeless tobacco and cigarettes by children and adolescents: Relationship to beliefs, peer use, and parental use. Am J Public Health 1987;77:1454-56.
15. Cohen SJ, Katz BP, Drook CA, et al. Overreporting

of smokeless tobacco use by adolescent males. J Behav Med 1988;11:383-93.

16. Colborn JW, Cummings KM, Michalek AM. Correlates of adolescents' use of smokeless tobacco. Health Educ Q 1989;16:91-100.

17. Eakin E, Severson H, Glasgow RE. Development and evaluation of a smokeless tobacco cessation program: A pilot study. NCI Monographs 1989;95-100.

18. Ernster VL, Grady DG, Greene JC, et al. Smokeless tobacco use and health effects among baseball players. JAMA 1990;264:218-24.

19. Giovino GA, Schooley MW, Zhu BP, et al. Surveillance for selected tobacco-use behaviors—United States 1900–1994. MMWR CDC Surveill Summ 1994 Nov 18;43:1-43.

20. Giunta JL, Connolly G. The reversibility of leukoplakia caused by smokeless tobacco. J Am Dent Assoc 1986;113:50-2.

21. Glover ED, Laflin M, Flannery D, Albritton DL. Smokeless tobacco use among American college students. J Am College Health 1989;38:81-5.

22. Grady D, Greene J, Daniels TE, et al. Oral mucosal lesions found in smokeless tobacco users. J Am Dent Assoc 1990;121:117-23.

23. Grasser JA, Childers E. Prevalence of smokeless tobacco use and clinical oral leukoplakia in a military population. Mil Med 1997;162:401-4.

24. Gupta PC, Murti PR, Bhonsle RB. Epidemiology of cancer by tobacco products and the significance of TSNA. Crit Rev Toxicol 1996;26:183-98.

25. Kann L, Warren CW, Harris WA, et al. Youth Risk Behavior Surveillance—United States, 1995. MMWR 1996;45(SS-4):1-84.

26. Kaugars GE, Riley WT, Brandt RB, et al. The prevalence of oral lesions in smokeless tobacco users and an evaluation of risk factors. Cancer 1992;70:2579-85.

27. Malvitz DM. Introduction. J Public Health Dent 1990;50:64.

28. Marty PJ, McDermott RJ, Williams T. Patterns of smokeless tobacco use in a population of high school students. Am J Public Health 1986;76:190-2.

29. Millar WJ. The use of chewing tobacco and snuff in Canada, 1986. Can J Public Health 1989;80:131-5.

30. Nair J, Ohshima H, Nair UJ, Bartsch H. Endogenous formation of nitrosamines and oxidative DNA-damaging agents in tobacco users. Crit Rev Toxicol 1996;26:149-61.

31. Nelson DE, Tomar SL, Mowery P, Siegel PZ. Trends in smokeless tobacco use among men in four states, 1988 through 1993. Am J Public Health 1996; 86:1300-3.

32. NIH Consensus Development Panel. National Institutes of Health consensus statement. Health implications of smokeless tobacco use. Biomed Pharmacother 1988;42:93-8.

33. Poulson TC, Lindenmuth JE, Greer RO, Jr. A comparison of the use of smokeless tobacco in rural and urban teenagers. CA 1984;34:248-61.

34. Preston-Martin S, Correa P. Epidemiological evidence for the role of nitroso compounds in human cancer. Cancer Surv 1989;8:459-73.

35. Projected smoking-related deaths among youth—United States. MMWR 1996;45:971-4.

36. Rodu B. An alternative approach to smoking control [editorial]. Am J Med Sci 1994;308:32-4.

37. Schroeder KL. P.L. 99-252—implications for dentists and their clinical practice. J Public Health Dent 1990;50:84-9.

38. Severson HH. Psychosocial factors in the use of smokeless tobacco and their implications for Public Law 99-252. J Public Health Dent 1990;50:90-7.

39. Smokeless tobacco use among American Indian women—southeastern North Carolina, 1991. MMWR 1995;44:113-7.

40. Spangler JG, Dignan MB, Michielutte R. Correlates of tobacco use among Native American women in western North Carolina. Am J Public Health 1997;87:108-11.

41. Squier CA. Smokeless tobacco and oral cancer: A cause for concern? CA 1984;34:242-7.

42. Stevens VJ, Severson H, Lichtenstein E, et al. Making the most of a teachable moment: A smokeless-tobacco cessation intervention in the dental office. Am J Public Health 1995;85:231-5.

43. Stockwell HG, Lyman GH. Impact of smoking and smokeless tobacco on the risk of cancer of the head and neck. Head Neck Surg 1986;9:104-10.

44. Use of smokeless tobacco among adults—United States 1991. MMWR 1993 Apr 16;42:263-6.

45. Weintraub JA, Burt BA. Periodontal effects and dental caries associated with smokeless tobacco use. Public Health Rep 1987;102:30-5.

46. Winn DM. Smokeless tobacco and cancer: The epidemiologic evidence. CA 1988;38:236-43.

47. Winn DM, Blot WJ, Shy CM. Snuff dipping and oral cancer among women in the southern United States. N Engl J Med 1981;304:745-9.

48. Wisniewski JF, Bartolucci AA. Comparative patterns of smokeless tobacco usage among major league baseball personnel. J Oral Pathol Med 1989;18:322-6.

49. Wolfe MD, Carlos JP. Oral health effects of smokeless tobacco use in Navajo Indian adolescents. Community Dent Oral Epidemiol 1987;15:230-5.

50. Wray A, McGuirt WF. Smokeless tobacco usage associated with oral carcinoma. Incidence, treatment, outcome. Arch Otolaryngol Head Neck Surg 1993;119:929-33.

Index

Note: Page numbers in *italics* refer to illustrations; page numbers followed by t refer to tables.

Academic institution(s), dental practice in, 11–12
Acid etching, before application of fissure sealant, 335
Acidogenesis, 347–348
Acidulated phosphate fluoride (APF), 319–320
Acquired immunodeficiency syndrome (AIDS). See also *Human immunodeficiency virus (HIV) infection.*
  epidemiology of, 60, 60t
  ethics and, 30–31
ADA. See *American Dental Association (ADA).*
ADHA (American Dental Hygienists' Association), 9
Administrative services only (ASO), 103
  in Canada, 141
Adverse selection, insurance and, 90
Age, and caries, 217, *218, 219*
  and periodontitis, 243–245, *245, 247*
  and tooth loss, partial, 206, *207–209*
    total, *204,* 204–205, 205t
  and utilization of dental services, 20–21, *20–22*
  distribution of, 13, 15, *15*
Aging, and health care expenditures, 91
AIDS. See *Acquired immunodeficiency syndrome (AIDS); Human immunodeficiency virus (HIV) infection.*
Alberta, dental public health in, 146–147
Alcohol, and oral cancer, 271
Alexidine dihydrochloride, for plaque control, 366
α level, 166
Amalgam restoration(s), mercury in, 66–68
American Dental Association (ADA), 7–8
  code of ethics of, 30–31
  Dental Practice Parameters of, 30
  fissure sealants accepted by, 335
  fluoride supplement dosage recommendations of, 317–318, 318t
  health promotion by, 44
  interaction with OSHA, 59
  policies of, on expanded-function dental auxiliaries, 127–128
    on plaque removal products, 365t
    on supervision of auxiliary personnel, 116, 116t

American Dental Association (ADA) *(Continued)*
  standards of third-party reimbursement, for fissure sealants, 342t
American Dental Hygienists' Association (ADHA), 9
Animal(s), research using, 152–153
Anticalculus toothpaste, 366–367
ASO (administrative services only), 103
  in Canada, 141
Assessment, in dental public health, 38t
  in public health, 34
Autonomy, 27
Auxiliary personnel, 115–117, 116t
Auxiliary program(s), public, 80

Baby bottle tooth decay, 227–228
Backflow prevention, 65–66
Bacterial infection, and caries, 223–224
Beneficence, 27
Betel, and oral cancer, 271
Bias, in research design, 164
Biofilm, plaque and, 359
Biologic variation, and epidemiology, 168–169
bis-GMA sealant(s), 334
Black, G.V., 4
Bloodborne pathogen(s), OSHA standard on, 58–59
Blue Cross and Blue Shield, 101
Body burden, of fluoride, 284
Bone density, fluoride and, 287–288
Bottle tooth decay, 227–228
British Columbia, dental public health in, 147
Burst theory, of periodontitis, 239

Calculus. See also *Plaque.*
  and periodontitis, 245, 248, *249,* 250
  measurement of, 188–189
Canada, dental care in, 134–148
  cost of, 140–141
    national structure of, 134–135
    utilization of, 140, 141t
  dental personnel in, assistants, 140
    denturists, 139–140
    hygienists, 139
    therapists, 139
  dental public health in, 142–144
    future of, 148
    provincial, 144–147, 145t
  health care system in, 135–137, 136t

Canada *(Continued)*
  financing of, 137
  oral health status in, 141–142
  population of, 135
  supply of dentists in, 137–138, 137t
  water fluoridation in, 144
Canadian Hospital Insurance and Diagnostic Act, 135
Cancer, fluoride and, 286–287
  oral. See *Oral cancer.*
Candidiasis, oral, 63
Capitated network(s), 77–78
Capitation, reimbursement by, 98, 102–103
Carbohydrate(s), and caries, 224–225
Cardiovascular disease, and periodontitis, 252–253
  risk factors for, Stanford Five-Cities Study of, 45–46
Caries, age and, 217, *218,* 219
  and tooth loss, 208
  and water fluoridation, early studies of, 279–282, *282–283*
  bacterial infection and, 223–224
  before water fluoridation, 279
  control of, diet in, *353,* 353–354
    fluoride supplements and, 317–319, 318t
    water fluoridation and, 290–292, 290t, 302–305, 303t, *304, 306.* See also *Water fluoridation.*
  diagnosis of, 179–181, 180t
    D1-D3 scale in, 180, 180t
    dichotomous scale in, 180, 180t
    use of explorer in, 181
  diet and, 224–225
    epidemiologic studies on, 225–226, 226t
  distribution of, global, 212–214, 213t
    in children, 214–216, *216*
    in United States, 214, *215*
  ethnicity and, 219, *220,* 221
  familial patterns in, 223
  fluorosis and, 261–262, *262–263*
  from bottle feeding, 227–228
  gender and, 219
  genetic patterns in, 223
  hidden, 181
  history of, 212
  in early childhood, 227–228
  incipient, fissure sealants for, 338
  industrialization and, 212–213, 213t
  longitudinal studies of, diagnostic reversals in, *174*
  measurement of, 178–183
    DMF index, 178–179

Caries (Continued)
nutrition and, 347
race and, 215
risk of, prediction of, 176
root. See Root caries.
severity of, distribution of, 216–217, 217–218
socioeconomic status and, 221, 222, 223
sugar and, 224–227
susceptibility of different teeth to, 214
treatment needs in, 182–183
Cariogenic food(s), 347–348
Cariogenicity, of sugars, 350–351
Case-control study(ies), 162
Causality, and research design, 159–161, 160t
CD4+ lymphocyte count, in human immunodeficiency virus infection, 59
Certification, of dental assistants, 117
of dentists, in Canada, 138
Child(ren), caries in, control of, water fluoridation and, 302–303, 303t
screening of, by dental hygienists, 142
Child development, fluoride and, 288
Children's Health Insurance Program (CHIP), 111
Chlorhexidine, for plaque removal, 365–366
Cholera, epidemiologic study of, 169, 170
"Cleansing" food(s), 352–353
Cleft lip/palate, 272–273
Climate, and water fluoride levels, 298t
Clinical trial(s), 162–163
Closed panels, 74
Code of ethics, of American Dental Association, 30–31
of International Association for Dental Research, 31–32
Cohort(s), 161–162
"Colorado brown stain," 279
Commentary(ies), 153
Commercial insurance, 101–102
Community, health promotion in, 45
Community and Migrant Health Program, 79–80
Community Periodontal Index of Treatment Needs (CPITN), 187–188, 188t
Comprehensive Health Manpower Act, 130
Comprehensive Smokeless Tobacco Health Education Act, 373
Compromised host model, in periodontal disease, 238
Computer(s), for literature searches, 155–156
Consent, informed, in research, 166–167
Consumer satisfaction, and quality assurance, 85
Continuing education, as ethical responsibility, 31

Control group(s), 163–164
Copayment(s), 90
Corn syrup, high-fructose, 349
Coronal caries. See Caries.
Cost containment, quality assurance and, 83–86
CPITN (Community Periodontal Index of Treatment Needs), 187–188, 188t
Cross-connection, prevention of, 65–66
Crossover research design, 164
Cross-sectional study(ies), 161

D1-D3 scale, in diagnosis of caries, 180, 180t
Data collection, in dental public health, 39–40, 40
Dean, H.T., work on fluorosis, 280–282, 282–283
Dean's Fluorosis Index, 191, 192–193, 192t
def index, 178–179
Delivery system(s), components of, 71
Delta Dental Plan(s), 98–101, 100
Dental assistant(s), certification of, 117
demographic characteristics of, 126
in Canada, 140
Dental care, access to, 32–33, 72–73
human immunodeficiency virus and, 64
and tooth loss, 209
cost of, 93–95, 93–98
fee-for-service, 93, 95, 95
for third-party payors, 95, 95–97
Gross National Product and, 93, 95
in Canada, 140–141
water fluoridation and, 307–308
demand for, 18
financing of, by government, 75–76, 105–106, 106
Children's Health Insurance Program and, 111
for veterans, 112
Medicaid program and, 107–111, 107–111. See also Medicaid.
in Canada, 134–148. See also Canada.
in hospital, 78
models of, 3
Dental caries. See Caries.
Dental clinic(s), in department stores, 78–79
Dental fluorosis, measurement of, 191–196. See also Fluorosis, measurement of.
Dental health maintenance organization(s) (DHMOs), 78
Dental hygiene, history of, 6
independent practice of, 125–126
Dental hygienist(s), as gatekeepers, in screening of children, 142
demographic characteristics of, 124–125, 125t

Dental hygienist(s) (Continued)
in Canada, 139
in dental public health, 38
Dental insurance. See Insurance.
Dental laboratory technician(s), 117, 128
Dental literature. See Literature.
Dental nurse(s), 117
Dental personnel, attitudes of, toward infectious disease, 64
auxiliary, 115–117, 116t, 124–129, 125t, 127t
dental assistants as, 126
denturists as, 128–129
expanded function, 126–127, 127t
hygienists as, 124–125, 125t
laboratory technicians as, 128
in health maintenance organizations, 76–77
types of, 115–117, 116t
Dental practice, franchised, 78–79
in public programs, 79–81
managed care and, 74–76. See also Health maintenance organization(s) (HMOs); Managed care.
OSHA and, 58–59
private, 71–74, 72–73. See also Private practice.
water fluoridation and, 308–309
Dental Practice Act, 6–7
Dental Practice Parameters, of American Dental Association, 30
Dental profession(s), careers in, 9–12
image of, 8
organization of, in United States, 6–9
Dental public health, and private practice, differences between, 41–42
similarities between, 40–41
and private practitioner, 39
components of, 37, 38t
data collection in, 39–40, 40
definition of, 37
dental hygienists in, 38
epidemiology in, 38
fissure sealants in, 338–339
funding of, 41
in Canada, 142–144
provincial, 144–147, 145t
misconceptions about, 39
need for, 33
planning cycle in, 40, 40
program evaluation in, 41
treatment planning in, 41
Dental school(s), employment in, 11–12
enrollment in, and supply of dentists, 120–121, 121
recent, 6, 118
history of, 4
quality assurance in, 83
subsidies to, 130
Dental service(s), utilization of, 18–19, 19
age and, 20–21, 20–22
by dentate and edentulous persons, 21, 22

Dental service(s) *(Continued)*
dental insurance and, 23–24, *25*
ethnicity and, 23
gender and, 20
general health and, 23
geographic location and, 23, *24*
in future, 24–25
socioeconomic status and, 21, 22, 23
Dental service corporation(s), 98–101, *100*
Dental specialist(s), organizations for, 8
supply of, 118–119
Dental student(s), with human immunodeficiency virus infection, 65
Dental therapist(s), 117
in Canada, 139
Dentist(s), licensure of, in Canada, 138
supply of, 117–123, 117t, *118*, 119t, *121*
controversy about, 122–123
dental school enrollment and, 120–121, *121*
geographic area and, 119–120, 119t
in Canada, 137–138, 137t
legislation and, 129–130
requirements for, 123–124
specialists, 118–119
state practice acts and, 121–122
Dentist/population ratio, income and, *72*, 117t
trends in, 123–124
Dentistry, history of, 4–5
in twentieth century, 5–6
Dentition, primary, caries in, water fluoridation and, 304
fissure sealants for, efficacy of, 338
Denturist(s), 128–129
in Canada, 139–140
Department of Veterans Affairs, 11
Department store(s), dental clinics in, 78–79
Developmental Defects of Dental Enamel (DDE) Index, 194, 195t, 196
DHMO(s) (dental health maintenance organizations), 78
Diabetes, and periodontitis, 251
Diagnosis, reliability of, in research design, 165
Diagnostic reversal(s), in longitudinal studies, *174*, 174–175
Dialysis patient(s), fluoride levels in, 285
Dichotomous scale, in diagnosis of caries, 180, 180t
Diet, and caries, 224–225
epidemiologic studies on, 225–226, 226t
for caries control, *353*, 353–354
Disease, measurement of, 170–171
risk of, assessment of, *175*, 175–176
DMF Index, 178–179

DMF Index *(Continued)*
age and, 217, *218*, 219
and caries severity, 216, *216–217*
ethnicity and, 219, *220*, 221
gender and, 219
in children, 216, *218*
water fluoridation and, 303t
socioeconomic status and, 221, *222*, 223
Down syndrome, fluoride and, 287

Ecological plaque hypothesis, 360
Economic issue(s), in water fluoridation, 307–309
Edentulism. See *Tooth loss.*
Education, and utilization of dental services, 22
EFDA(s). See *Expanded-function dental auxiliary (EFDA).*
Efficacy study(ies), 164–165
"Empty vessel" approach, to patient education, 49
Enamel, fluoride and, 285, 291
English Poor Law(s), 36
Epidemiology, and measurement of oral disease, 172–173, 173t
and variability in measurement, 170–171
assessment of disease risk in, *175*, 175–176
biologic variation and, 168–169
clinical applications of, 169–170, 171t
definition of, 159, 168
examiner reliability and, 173–175, *174*
history of, 169, *170*, 171t
in dental public health, 38
populations sampled and, 171–172
predictive value in, *175*, 175–176
research design in, 159–167. See also *Research design.*
EPSDT program, 109
Erythroplakia, 272
Ethical standards, of organizations, 27–28
Ethics, and access to care, 32–33
and AIDS patient, 30–31
and continuing education, 31
and research, 31–32, 32t
and research design, 166–167
code of, of American Dental Association, 30–31
of International Association for Dental Research, 31–32
definition of, 27
principles in, 27–28
Ethnicity, and caries, 219, *220*, 221
and oral cancer, 268, *270–271*
and periodontitis, 243, *247*
and root caries, 229, 230
and utilization of dental services, 23
population distribution by, 16–17, *18*
Expanded-function dental auxiliary (EFDA), 116, 126–127, 127t

Expanded-function dental auxiliary (EFDA) *(Continued)*
ADA policy on, 127–128
Experimental research design, 162–167. See also *Research design, experimental.*
Extended Health Benefits Plan, in Alberta, 146–147
Extent and Severity Index, of periodontal disease, 186

Fauchard, P., 4
FDI (World Dental Federation), 9
Fee(s), percentile, *100*, 100–101
Fee schedule(s), 98
Fee-for-service dental care, cost of, 93, 95, *95*
Fiber, dietary, and caries, 225
Fissure sealant(s), 334–343
attitudes toward, 341–343, 342t
clinical trials of, 336, 336t
cost-effectiveness of, 339–341, 341t
development of, 334–335
efficacy of, 336–339
in dental public health programs, 338–339
on primary dentition, 338
type of product and, 337–338
with incipient caries, 338
procedure for, 335–336
products for, 335–336
rationale for, 335
third-party reimbursement for, ADA standards on, 342t
Fluoridation, of water. See *Water fluoridation.*
Fluoride, acidulated phosphate, 319–320
and cancer, 286–287
and caries control, mechanism of, 290–292, 290t
and child development, 288
and Down syndrome, 287
and enamel, 291
and mortality, 286
and osteoporosis, 287–288
and plaque, 290–291
balance of, 284
body burden of, 284
concentration of, optimal, 297–298, 298t
effect of, on different tooth surfaces, 291–292
environmental, 282
exposure to, in infants, 283
multiple, 326–327, 326t–327t
in enamel, 285
in milk, 317–317
in saliva, 291
in salt, 315–316
in toothpaste, 323–325
global impact of, 325
optimal intake of, 285–286
physiology of, 284–285
self-applied, 322
sources of, 282–284, 284t
toxicity of, 288–290, 289t, 321
use of, 292
Fluoride gel(s), professionally applied, 319–321, 320t–321t

Fluoride mouthrinse(s), 322–323
  with fluoride toothpaste, 327t
  with water fluoridation, 326t
Fluoride supplement(s), 317–319,
  318t
  and fluorosis, 261, 318
  dosage of, 317–318, 318t
  prenatal, 319
Fluoride varnishes, 321–322
Fluorosis, and caries, 261–262,
  262–263
  as public health problem, 262, 264
  definition of, 259–260
  discovery of, 279–282, 282–283
  fluoride supplements and, 318
  measurement of, 191–196
    Dean's Fluorosis Index in, 191,
      192–193, 192t
    Developmental Defects of Den-
      tal Enamel Index in, 194,
      195t, 196
    Thylstrup-Fejerskov Index in,
      193–194, 194t, 195
    Tooth Surface Index of Fluoro-
      sis in, 191, 193, 193t
  prevalence of, in United States,
    260, 260–261
  risk factors for, 261
  toothpaste and, 325
Fluorosis Risk Index (FRI), 194
Food(s), cariogenic, 347–348
  "protective," 352–353
Franchised dental practice(s), 78–79
FRI (Fluorosis Risk Index), 194
Fructose intolerance, hereditary, 226

Gatekeepers, dental hygienists as, in
    screening of children, 142
GDP (Gross Domestic Product), and
    expenditures for dental care, 94
Gel(s), fluoride, professionally
    applied, 319–321, 320t–321t
Gender, and caries, 219
  and oral cancer, 267, 268t, 269,
    269
  and periodontitis, 243, 247, 249
  and tooth loss, 205
  and utilization of dental services,
    20
Geographic location, and utilization
    of dental services, 23, 24
Gies report, 83
Gingival Index, 185
Gingivitis, definition of, 237
  distribution of, 240
  measurement of, 185–186, 185t
  plaque and, 245, 248, 249, 250
Government, reimbursement for
    dental care by, 75–76
  role of in water fluoridation, 300–
    301
Government agency(ies), dental
    practice in, 10–11
Grainger's hierarchy, for caries
    measurement, 178
Great Depression, 29
Gross Domestic Product (GDP), and
    expenditure for dental care, 94
Group model, in health
    maintenance organizations, 77

Group practice, 73, 73–74
Guild model, of dental care, 3

Hairy leukoplakia, oral, 63
"Halo effect," in water fluoridation,
    306
HDA (Hispanic Dental Association),
    8
Health, definition of, 34
  holistic view of, 43
  responsibility for, individual vs.
    social, 28
Health Canada, Medical Services
    Branch of, 147
Health care, as right, 29
  cost of, and quality assurance,
    83–86
    managed care and, 75
  expenditures for, 90–93, 91–92
  in Canada, 135–137, 136t. See also
    Canada.
  financing of, 137
  primary, World Health Organiza-
    tion and, 81
  public financing of, 104–112
    by Medicaid, 107–111, 107–111.
      See also Medicaid.
    by Medicare, 106–107
    history of, 104–105
    type of care and, 106
Health care delivery system(s),
    components of, 71
Health education, definition of, 44
Health maintenance organization(s)
    (HMOs), 76–78
    dental, 78
Health Professions Education Act,
    130
Health Professions Educational
    Assistance Act, 5
Health promotion, 43–45
  community-based, 45
  history of, 44
  of oral health, 46–49, 47t–48t. See
    also Oral health, promotion of.
Healthy People 2000, oral health
    goals of, 47–48, 48t
Hepatitis B, 61–63, 62
  epidemiology of, 61, 62
  immunization against, 62
  morbidity in, 61
  transmission of, 62
Hepatitis C, 61, 62
Hereditary fructose intolerance, 226
High-fructose corn syrup, 349
Hispanic Dental Association (HDA),
    8
Hispanic population, growth of, 16
HIV. See Human immunodeficiency
    virus (HIV) infection.
HLD Index, 197
HMO(s). See Health maintenance
    organization(s) (HMOs).
Hopewood House, caries study at,
    225–226
Hospital(s), dental care in, 78
Human immunodeficiency virus
    (HIV) infection, 59–61, 60t
    and opportunistic infections, 59

Human immunodeficiency virus
    (HIV) infection (Continued)
    and periodontitis, 251–252
    CD4+ lymphocyte count in, 59
    dental students with, 65
    epidemiology of, 60, 60t
    ethics and, 30–31
    legal issues in, 64–65, 65t
    oral manifestations of, 63
    pediatric, 63
    professionals' attitudes toward,
      63–64
    transmission of, 60
Human subject(s), in research,
    ethical treatment of, 31–32, 32t

Immunization, against hepatitis B,
    62
Income, and population/dentist
    ratio, 72, 117t
Index(es), in measurement of oral
    disease, 172, 173t
Index Medicus, 155
Index of Orthodontic Treatment
    Need (IOTN), 197
Index to Dental Literature, 155
Indian Health Service, 111
Indigent, medically, 105
Individual responsibility, vs. social
    responsibility, 28
Individualism, in United States,
    28–29
Industrialization, and incidence of
    caries, 212–213, 213t
Infant(s), fluoride exposure in, 283
Infection(s), bacterial, and caries,
    223–224
  opportunistic, 59
  professionals' attitudes toward,
    63–64
Infection control, 57–65
  advances in, 57
  guidelines for, 58
  history of, 57–58
  OSHA and, 58–59
  policies on, adherence to, 64
Informed consent, in research,
    166–167
Insurance, and quality assurance, 83
  and utilization of dental services,
    23–24, 25
  Blue Cross and Blue Shield, 101
  capitated plans for, 102–103
  Children's Health Insurance Pro-
    gram, 111
  commercial, 101–102
  copayments for, 90
  cost of, control of, 104
  Delta Dental Plans, 98–101, 100
  direct reimbursement in, 103
  growth of, 96–97
  national, 112
  preauthorization by, 101
  prepaid group, 102–103
  principles of, 89–90
  tax cap on, 96
Interactive model, of dental care, 3
Interdental cleansing, for plaque
  removal, 361–362

Interexaminer reliability, in epidemiology, 173–175, *174*
Interim Primary Drinking Water Regulations, 301
International Association for Dental Research (IADR), code of ethics of, 31–32
IOTN (Index of Orthodontic Treatment Need), 197
IPA(s) (independent practice associations), 77
Irreversible index(es), 173

Journal(s), information in, hierarchy of, 152–153, 153t
peer-reviewed, 150–152
quality of, 151–152
Justice, as ethical principle, 27

Kaposi's sarcoma, 63
Karlstad studies, 354, 363
Kerr-Mills Bill, 105

Laboratory technician(s), 117, 128
Learned societies, journals of, 151
Legal issue(s), in human immunodeficiency virus infection, 64–65, 65t
Legislation, and supply of dentists, 129–130
Leukoplakia, 272
hairy, 63
smokeless tobacco and, 372
Licensure, of dentists, in Canada, 138
Literature, 150–156
commentaries in, 153
journals as, 150–152. See also *Journal(s)*.
on World Wide Web, 156
quality of, judging, 153
research findings in, interpretation of, 153–154
searches of, 155–156
textbooks as, 150–152
Litigation, malpractice, and quality assurance, 84
Longitudinal study(ies), 161
negative reversal in, *174*, 174–175
Loss of periodontal attachment (LPA), 186, *187*
as predictor of periodontitis, 253
in classification of periodontitis, 241–242, *241–242*
LPA. See *Loss of periodontal attachment (LPA)*.
Lymphocyte(s), CD4+, in human immunodeficiency virus infection, 59

Malocclusion, epidemiology of, 273
measurement of, 197–198
Malpractice litigation, and quality assurance, 84
Managed care, 74–76
history of, 29
Manitoba, dental public health in, 146

Mass media, oral health promotion programs using, 46–47
McKay, F., discovery of naturally fluoridated water by, 279–280
Measurement, variability in, 170–171
Media, oral health promotion programs using, 46–47
Medicaid, *107–110*, 107–111
eligibility for, 110
EPSDT program of, 109
expenditures by, 107, *107–108*
for dental care, 107, *107–108*, *110*
future of, 110–111
states' responsibilities for, 109
Medical savings account(s) (MSAs), 103–104
Medical Services Branch, of Health Canada, 147
Medically indigent, 105
Medicare, 106–107
in Canada, 136, 136t
MEDLINE, 155
Mercury safety, 66–68
Military service, dental practice in, 11
Milk, fluoridation of, 316–317
Mouthrinse(s), fluoride, 322–323
with fluoride toothpaste, 327t
with water fluoridation, 326t
Mouthwash, for plaque control, 365–366
MSA(s) (medical savings accounts), 103–104
Mutans streptococci, and caries, 223–224

NaF rinses, 322–323
National Cancer Institute, educational materials from, on smokeless tobacco, 374
SEER program of, 198
National Dental Association (NDA), 8
National Dental Caries Prevalence Survey, 214
National Dental Examination Board, 138
National Health and Nutrition Examination Survey (NHANES), 204
National health insurance, in Canada, 135–137, 136t
in United States, 112
National Health Service Corps, 80, 129
National Preventive Dentistry Demonstration Program, and caries severity, 216–217, *217–218*
National Sample of Oral Health in US Employed Adults and Seniors, 171–172, 189
NDA (National Dental Association), 8
Negative reversal, in longitudinal studies, *174*, 174–175
New Brunswick, dental public health in, 146

New Zealand, school dental nurse program in, 80–81
Newfoundland, dental public health in, 146
NHANES (National Health and Nutrition Examination Survey), 204
Nominal scale(s), 173
Nonexperimental research design, 161–162
North York Public Health Department, 142–143
Nova Scotia Children's Oral Health Program, 143–144
Nuremberg Code, 31
Nursing caries, 227–228
Nutrition. See also *Diet.*
and caries, 224–225, 347
and periodontitis, 250

Occlusal Index, 197
Occupational Safety and Health Administration (OSHA), infection control standards of, 58–59
OHI-S (Oral Health Index-Simplified), 188
Ontario, dental public health in, 144–145
Open panels, 74
Opportunistic infection(s), 59
Oral cancer, 267–272, *268–271*, 268t–269t
alcohol and, 271
ethnicity and, 268, *270–271*
gender and, 267, 268t, 269, *269*
measurement of, 198
mortality from, 267, *268*
premalignant conditions and, 272
smokeless tobacco and, 371–374. See also *Smokeless tobacco.*
tobacco and, 270–271
Oral candidiasis, 63
Oral disease, measurement of, 172–173, 173t
Oral hairy leukoplakia, 63
Oral health, and quality of life, measurement of, 198–199
attitudes about, 48–49
in Canada, 141–142
knowledge about, 48–49
measurement of, quality assurance and, 84–85
promotion of, 46–49, 47t–48t
patient education about, 49–51
school-based, 50
water fluoridation and, 51–52
Oral Health Impact Profile, 199
Oral Health Index (Simplified) (OHI-S), 188
Oral hygiene, and periodontitis, 245, 248, *249*, 250
and plaque control, 354
public education about, 367
Ordinal scale(s), 173
OSHA (Occupational Safety and Health Administration), infection control standards of, 58–59

Osteoporosis, fluoride and, 287–288

PAC(s) (political action committees), for water fluoridation, 51–52
Participating dentist(s), in Delta Dental Plans, 99–100
Pathfinder Survey, of World Health Organization, 183
Patient education, about plaque prevention, 50
  about water fluoridation, 51–52
  "empty vessel" approach to, 49
  evolution of, 49
Peer review, of journals, 150–152
Percentile fee(s), 100, 100–101
Periodontal disease, distribution of, 240–243, 241–242
  host response to, 237–239, 238t
  measurement of, 185–189
    Extent and Severity Index in, 186
    in calculus, 188–189, 189t
    in gingivitis, 185–186, 185t
    in plaque, 188–189, 189t
    loss of periodontal attachment in, 186, 187
    partial-mouth, 189
    Periodontal Index in, 186
  models of, 239–240, 239t
  plaque control and, 358–367
  treatment needs in, 187–188, 188t
Periodontal Index, 186, 187
Periodontitis, age and, 243–245, 245, 247
  burst theory of, 239
  cardiovascular disease and, 252–253
  classification of, 238–239, 238t
  definition of, 237
  diabetes and, 251
  ethnicity and, 243, 247
  gender and, 243, 247, 249
  human immunodeficiency virus infection and, 251–252
  incidence of, 242–243
  longitudinal studies of, diagnostic reversals in, 175
  nutrition and, 250
  oral hygiene and, 245, 248, 249, 250
  prediction of, 253
  prevalence of, 240–242, 241–242
  risk of, prediction of, 176
  socioeconomic status and, 245, 246–248
  tobacco use and, 250–251
Permanent dentition, caries in, DMF index of, 178–179
Piedmont Project, 242
Pit and fissure sealant(s). See Fissure sealant(s).
Placebo(s), in research design, 164
Planning cycle, in dental public health, 40, 40
Plaque, and periodontitis, 245, 248, 249, 250
  control of, 354–355
    alexidine dihydrochloride in, 366

Plaque (Continued)
    chemotherapy in, 364–367, 365t
    chlorhexidine in, 365–366
    in adults, 363–364
    professional and personal, 364
    rationale for, 358–359
  ecological hypothesis of, 360
  fluoride and, 290–291
  nature of, 359–360
  prevention of, patient education about, 50
  "protective" foods and, 352–353
  removal of, by patient, 360–362
    interdental cleansing in, 361–362
    mechanical, by professional, 362–364
    toothbrushing in, 361
  subgingival, 359
Plaque Index, 188–189, 189t
Plasma, fluoride in, 284–285
Policy development, in dental public health, 38t
  in public health, 34
Political action committees (PACs), for water fluoridation, 51–52
Polypharmacy, and root caries, 230
Population, distribution of, by age, 13, 15, 15
  by economic status, 17
  by ethnicity, 16–17, 18
  geographic, 15–16, 16–17
  growth of, 13, 14
  in research design, choice of, 163
  sample of, in epidemiology, 171–172
Population/dentist ratio. See Dentist/population ratio.
Positive reversal, in longitudinal studies, 174, 174–175
PPO(s). See Preferred provider organization(s) (PPOs).
Practice act(s), of states, and supply of dentists, 121–122
Preauthorization, 101
Precancerous lesion(s), oral, 272
Predictive value, in epidemiology, 175, 175–176
Preferred provider organization(s) (PPOs), 102–103
Pregnancy, and water fluoridation, 304
Prenatal fluoride supplement(s), 319
Prepaid group insurance, 102–103
Primary dentition, caries in, def
  index of, 178–179
  water fluoridation and, 304
  fissure sealants for, efficacy of, 338
Primary health care, World Health Organization and, 81
Prince Edward Island Dental Program, 145–146, 145t
Private practice, 9–10, 71–74, 72–73
  advantages of, 72
  and dental public health, 39
    differences between, 41–42
    similarities between, 40–41
  group, 73, 73–74
  open and closed panels in, 74

Private practice (Continued)
  solo, 73, 73
Profession(s), characteristics of, 3–4
  definition of, 3
  models of, 3
Professional organization(s), journals of, 151
Professional standards review organization(s) (PSROs), and quality assurance, 84
Program evaluation, in dental public health, 41
Prophylaxis, in adults, 363–364
Proportion(s), in measurement of oral disease, 172
Prospective study(ies), 161–162
"Protective" food(s), 352–353
Provider(s), profiles of, as quality assurance activity, 85
PSRO(s) (professional standards review organizations), and quality assurance, 84
Psychological profile, in temporomandibular joint disorders, 274
Public health. See also Dental public health.
  components of, 34–37, 35t
  definition of, 34
  history of, 36–37
  issues in, identification of, 35–36
  surveillance in, 39–40
Public health dentistry, oral hygiene programs in, 367
Public program(s), for dental care, 79–81
Puritan ethic, 29
Pyrophosphate, in toothpaste, 366

Quality assurance, 81–86, 82t–83t
  and cost control, 83–86
  and measurement of oral health, 84–85
  and monitoring of technical quality, 84–85
  definition of, 81–82
  evaluation of, 83
  in dental education, 83
  in dental public health, 38t
  in public health, 34
  on-site evaluation in, 84
  structure, process, and outcome approach in, 82, 82t
  terms used in, 82, 83t
  trends in, 83–84
Quality of life, oral health and, measurement of, 198–199
Quebec, dental public health in, 146

Race. See also Ethnicity.
  and caries, 215, 219, 220, 221
  and tooth loss, 205, 206
  and utilization of dental services, 23
  population distribution by, 16–17, 18
Random allocation, in research design, 163
Rate(s), in measurement of oral disease, 172

RCI (Root Caries Index), 182
Recommended maximum
    contaminant level (RMCL),
    301–302
Reliability, of diagnosis, in research,
    165
    of examiner, and epidemiology,
    173–175, *174*
Renal failure, and fluoride
    absorption, 285
Research, ethics and, 31–32, 32t
    interpretation of, 153–154
    using animals, 152–153
Research design, bias in, 164
    case-control, 162
    causality and, 159–161, 160t
    crossover, 164
    duration of trial in, 165
    ethical issues in, 166–167
    experimental, 162–167
        choice of population for, 163
        clinical trials in, 162–163
        components of study in, 163–
        164
        control groups in, 163–164
        number of subjects in, 163
    longitudinal, 161
    nonexperimental, 161–162
    operational procedure in, 164–165
    placebos in, 164
    prospective, 161–162
    protocol for, 159, 159t
    randomized *vs.* nonrandomized
        selection in, 163
    reliability in diagnosis and, 165
    retrospective, 162
    risk factors and, 159–161
    statistical analysis in, 165–166
    surveys in, 161
Responsibility, individual *vs.* social,
    28
Retrospective study(ies), 162
Risk, assumption of, in health
    maintenance organizations,
    77–78
Risk factor(s), and research design,
    159–161
Risk indicator(s), 160
Risk marker(s), 161
RMCL (recommended maximum
    contaminant level), 301–302
Root caries, diagnosis of, 181–182,
    181t
    polypharmacy and, 230
    prevalence of, 228, *229*, 230
    water fluoridation and, 303–304
Root Caries Index (RCI), 182

Safe Drinking Water Act, 301
Salaried practice, 10–11
Saliva, fluoride in, 291
Salt, fluoride in, 315–316
Sample, in epidemiology, 171–172
Sarcoma, Kaposi's, 63
Saskatchewan, dental public health
    in, 146
Scale(s), in measurement of oral
    disease, 172–173
School(s), drinking water in,
    fluoridation of, 316

School dental nurse program(s),
    80–81
School-based program(s), on oral
    health promotion, 50
Sealant(s), fissure. See *Fissure
    sealant(s).*
SEER (Surveillance, Epidemiology,
    and End Results) program, of
    National Cancer Institute, 198
Self-care, for plaque removal,
    360–362
SES. See *Socioeconomic status (SES).*
Significance, statistical, 166
Smokeless tobacco, pathologic
    effects of, 371–372
    use of, prevalence of, 372–373
    prevention of, 373–374
Smoking, and oral cancer, 270
    and periodontitis, 250–251
    as public health issue, 36
Snack food(s), cariogenic potential
    of, 348
Snow, J., epidemiologic studies on
    cholera, 169, *170*
Snuff, pathologic effects of, 371–372
Social policy, in United States,
    history of, 28–29
Social responsibility, *vs.* individual
    responsibility, 28
Social Security Act, 104–105
Socioeconomic status (SES), and
    access to dental care, 72–73
    and caries, 221, *222*, 223
    and periodontitis, 245, *246–248*
    and root caries, 230
    and tooth loss, 205–206, *207*
    and utilization of dental services,
    21, *22*, 23
Sodium fluoride rinses, 322–323
Sorbitol, cariogenicity of, 351
Staff model, in health maintenance
    organizations, 76–77
Standard precautions, 58
Stanford Five-Cities Study, 45–46
State practice act(s), and supply of
    dentists, 121–122
Statistical analysis, in research
    design, 165–166
Stephan curve, 353, *353*
Structure, process, and outcome
    approach, in quality assurance,
    82, 82t
Subgingival plaque, 359
Sucrose, cariogenicity of, 350–351
    properties of, 349–350
Sugar(s), and caries, 224–227
    cariogenicity of, 350–351
    consumption of, 348–350, *350*
Sugar substitute(s), noncariogenic,
    351–352
"Sunbelt migration," 15
Surveillance, in public health, 39–40
Surveillance, Epidemiology, and
    End Results (SEER) program,
    of National Cancer Institute,
    198
Survey(s), in research design, 161

Table of allowances, 97

"Tartar-control" toothpaste, 366–367
Tax cap, on insurance, 96
Technology, advances in, and health
    care expenditures, 91–92
Temporomandibular joint
    disorder(s), 273–274
Textbook(s), 150–152
Third-party payor(s), and cost of
    dental care, *95*, 95–97
    reimbursement by, 97–98
Thylstrup-Fejerskov Index, 193–194,
    194t, *195*
Tobacco, and oral cancer, 270–271
    and periodontitis, 250–251
    smokeless. See *Smokeless tobacco.*
Tooth loss, dental care and, 209
    etiology of, 208–209
    historical perspective on, 203
    partial, 206, *207–209*, 208
        age and, 206, *207–209*
    total, 203–206, *204*, 205t, *206–207*
        age and, *204*, 204–205, 205t
        gender and, 205
        race and, 205, *206*
        socioeconomic status and, 205–
        206, *207*
Tooth Surface Index of Fluorosis
    (TSIF), 191, 193, 193t
Toothbrushing, frequency of, and
    plaque removal, 361
Toothpaste, fluoride-containing,
    323–325
    and fluorosis, 261
    with fluoride mouthrinses, 327t
    tartar-control, 366–367
Treatment planning, in dental
    public health, 41
Triclosan, in toothpaste, 366–367
Tristan da Cunha, caries study in,
    225
TSIF (Tooth Surface Index of
    Fluorosis), 191, 193, 193t
Turkü Sugar Studies, 351
Twenty-one Cities Study, 281

UCR (usual, customary, and
    reasonable) fees, 97
Universal precautions, 58
US Preventive Services Task Force,
    152
US Public Health Service, dental
    practice in, 10–11
Usual, customary, and reasonable
    (UCR) fees, 97

Varnishes, fluoride, 321–322
Veracity, 27
Veterans, dental care for, 112
Veterans Administration, dental
    practice in, 11
Vipehölm Caries Study, 226, 226t
Volpe-Manhold Index, 189

Water fluoridation, and caries
    control, 302–305, 303t, *304,
    306*
    in adults, 303–304, *304*
    in children, 302–303, 303t

Water fluoridation *(Continued)*
  in primary dentition, 304
  prenatal effects of, 304
caries before, 279
court decisions on, 310
dental practice and, 308–309
early studies of, 298–299
economic issues in, 307–309
exposure to, multiple, 303t, 305–307
  partial, 305, *306*
funding of, 300–301
future of, 310–311
global distribution of, 299–300, 299t
"halo effect" in, 306
in Canada, 144

Water fluoridation *(Continued)*
  in school drinking water, 316
  in United States, 300–302, 301t
  natural, 282
    history of, 279–280
  opposition to, 310
  optimal concentration in, 297–298, 298t
  political issues in, 309–310
  promotion of, 51–52
  public opinion about, 309–310
  standards for, 301–302
  with fluoride mouthrinses, 326t
Water supply, backflow prevention in, 65–66
WHO. See *World Health Organization (WHO)*.

World Dental Federation (FDI), 9
World Health Organization (WHO), and primary health care, 81
  data collection by, 40
  oral health promotion goals of, 47t
  Pathfinder Survey of, 183
World War II, caries studies during, 225
  dentistry during, 5
World Wide Web, 156

Xylitol, cariogenicity of, 351–352

Property of
High-Tech Institute of Sacramento, CA
Library/Resource Center